the
COMPLETE GUIDE TO
A HIGH-FAT DIET

THE KETO DIET

WITH MORE THAN **125**
DELECTABLE RECIPES AND
5 MEAL PLANS TO SHED WEIGHT,
HEAL YOUR BODY
& REGAIN CONFIDENCE

LEANNE VOGEL

Victory Belt Publishing Inc.
Las Vegas

First Published in 2017 by Victory Belt Publishing Inc.

ISBN-13: 978-1-628600-16-2

The author is not a licensed practitioner, physician, or medical professional and offers no medical diagnoses, treatments, suggestions, or counseling. The information presented herein has not been evaluated by the U.S. Food and Drug Administration, and it is not intended to diagnose, treat, cure, or prevent any disease. Full medical clearance from a licensed physician should be obtained before beginning or modifying any diet, exercise, or lifestyle program, and physicians should be informed of all nutritional changes.

The author/owner claims no responsibility to any person or entity for any liability, loss, or damage caused or alleged to be caused directly or indirectly as a result of the use, application, or interpretation of the information presented herein.

Front and Back Cover Photography by Leanne Vogel and Nathan Elson

Interior Design by Yordan Terziev and Boryana Yordanova

Printed in Canada

TC 1218

CONTENTS

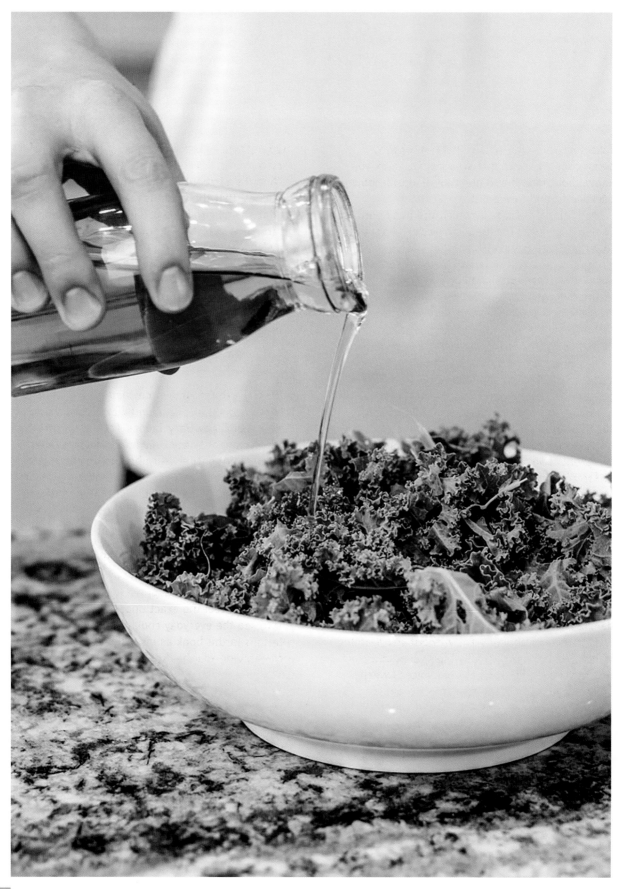

INTRODUCTION

Take charge of your health in a new way by being open to the idea that what you think you know about health and nutrition is upside-down, backwards, and inside out.

Nutritional ketosis, in which the body burns fat rather than sugar for fuel, is a powerful approach to radically improving health that's achieved by eating a high-fat, low-carbohydrate, moderate-protein diet. This can seem counterintuitive: Most of us have been taught that what's best for health is restricting dietary fat and consuming lots of carbohydrates, especially "healthy whole grains." But the truth, as proved by many cutting-edge medical studies, is that eating more fat and less carbs is beneficial for a wide range of health concerns. It can help you lose weight, improve mental focus, increase energy, stabilize blood sugar, balance hormones, and much more.

The book you're holding in your hands is a comprehensive guide to high-fat living that's different from the rest. Unlike traditional guides to the ketogenic diet, it doesn't focus on calories, manipulating macros, or rigidly following certain rules. Instead, it allows you the freedom and flexibility to do what feels right for you, your body, and your health.

With the strategies and recipes you'll find here, you can end food obsession, cravings, and restrictions through sound nutrition practices and delicious whole-food meals so that you can get the weight and health you want without self-loathing or guilt. This is how I finally lost weight and kept it off, healed my hormonal imbalances (which had resulted in eight years without a period!), eliminated symptoms of ADHD, and was able to replace negativity with optimism and joy.

My goal with this epic resource is to show you how the same strategies can help you wherever you are right now, whether you're struggling with weight, hormonal problems, autoimmune conditions, or other chronic health problems, or even if you just don't feel good—all without guilt or self-loathing. I hope it shows you how changing the way you eat—and think about eating—can help you fully love, appreciate, and honor the beautiful person you are.

And it's all about eating fat! I feel, deep in my bones, that the world is ready to get off of the fat-shaming roller coaster and start seeing fat for what it truly is: a tool that we can use to transform our waistlines, disease rates, taste buds, relationship with food, and more. We were all born with an inherent drive to seek out nutrient-rich high-fat foods. But somewhere along the way, our t's were dotted, our i's were crossed, and our bodies got a little lost. *The Keto Diet* will help you get back into the groove—your body's natural drive toward consuming ultra-nourishing, delectable fats.

Perhaps you're already on the high-fat train thanks to books like *Keto Clarity* by Jimmy Moore, *Why We Get Fat* by Gary Taubes, *Eat Fat, Get Thin* by Mark Hyman, or *Wheat Belly* by Dr. William Davis, but you're not entirely sure how to go about it. Oh man, do I understand. There's nothing quite as frustrating as feeling like you know *what* to do to make things better but not *how*. In *The Keto Diet*, you'll find all of the tools you need to understand how to eat more fat, as easily as breathing. Really.

You may feel like eating a bunch of fats and reducing carbs will tear your favorite things from your life, but I'm here to prove that, once you let fat in, you'll feel the exact opposite. I encourage you to see the everyday cooking and meal prep solutions in this book as insanely powerful tools for improving your health without radically upsetting your schedule, priorities, or love of pies, cakes, chips, and other carby things.

(Don't worry, if you're really torn up about ditching the pies, cakes, chips, and other carby things, I've got you covered—see page 38.)

I hope that *The Keto Diet* will be the launch pad that gets you feeling on top of your game and at home in your body, confident, loving life, and ready to bust out on the scene with your amazingness.

I know, radical concept. But I have a really, really good feeling about this.

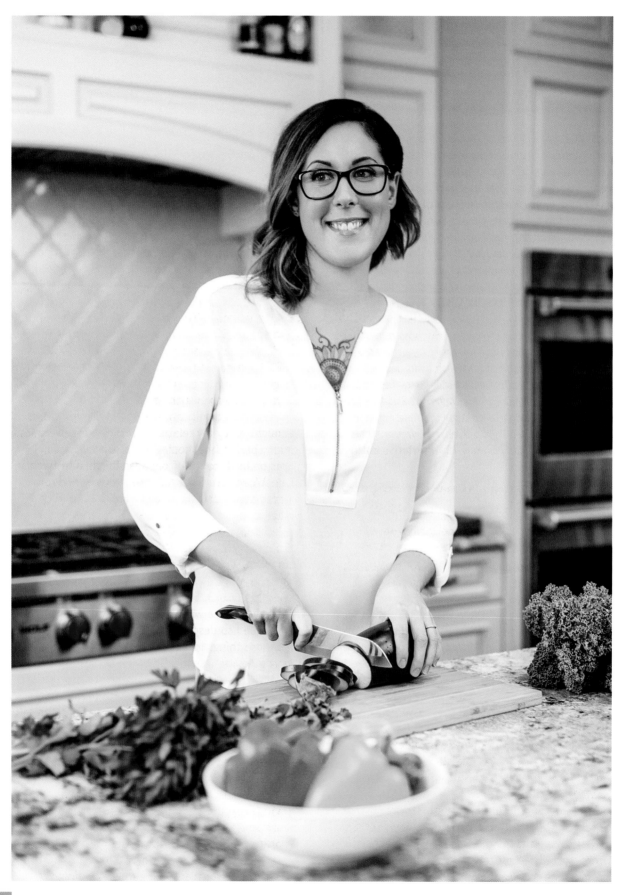

HEY, I'M LEANNE

I am a nutrition educator, wellness activist, and creator of *Healthful Pursuit,* where in the last three years I've provided guidance and support to more than five million people looking to thrive on a high-fat, low-carb ketogenic eating style.

After graduating with honors from the Canadian School of Natural Nutrition in 2007, I began a private nutrition consulting practice and started *Healthful Pursuit.* I now have a top-ranked YouTube channel called Healthful Pursuit and a podcast where I provide ketogenic support (find it at healthfulpursuit.com/podcast). My most recent publication, *Fat Fueled,* is a thirty-day program that uses dietary fats to heal, nourish, and balance the body (find it at healthfulpursuit.com/fatfueled).

But my keto story really began in 2014, when I transitioned to a high-fat, low-carb eating style. It transformed my life. By eating this way instead of trying to control my body with restrictive eating patterns, I

- **Lost twenty stubborn, hormone-related pounds**
- **Freed myself from fifteen years of ADHD**
- **Got my period back after being diagnosed with early-onset menopause at age twenty-four**
- **Balanced my mood—I'm now living without the mild depression that used to plague me**
- **Got rid of brain fog**
- **Boosted my energy**
- **Improved my skin, hair, and nails**
- **Stopped experiencing food cravings**
- **Released my obsession with food**
- **Experienced a boost in self-confidence**

Before you decide that my liberating experience is outside of your reach and slam this book back on the shelf, let me give you the full picture by sharing where I've been.

I'm not going to bore you with stories of where I grew up, what my parents are like, my first steps, or how awesome my little sister is (although she is pretty rad). Let's get to the meaty bits right away—no foreplay on this one.

How Keto Helped Me Shed Pounds and Other Cool Things

The story of my relationship with food and fitness began the moment I switched from finding balanced pleasure in food to using food to control my surroundings. I struggled with an eating disorder from ages thirteen to twenty-eight. It started with bulimia, where I would binge on restricted foods and then purge them from my body, then shifted to years of starvation with anorexia and intense drug abuse, then back to bulimia as I continued to severely restrict my diet, and finally to orthorexia (obsession with eating the "right" foods), where I'd experience panic attacks if I wasn't able to prepare my own meals.

The most significant of the physical problems brought on by my relationship to food was the loss of my period (the medical term is *amenorrhea*). I was on birth control from ages thirteen to twenty-one. When I went off birth control, my period never came back. As in, eight years with no cycle at all.

I spent a good portion of my twenties not caring about the fact that my period had gone missing. After all, life was a lot simpler without it. I continued to push my body with marathon running, cycling, swimming, and dieting because I believed there was no other way to achieve the physique I so desperately wanted. But while I did all these things in the name of health, none of my behavior was truly healthy.

It was a turbulent time filled with insecurities that I masked with job promotions, backpacking trips, and a facade of happiness. Body love and self-care were foreign to me. I obsessed about working out, following the "rules" of good nutrition—including avoiding dietary fat—and being the best at everything. While the classic eating-disorder tendencies were dissipating, I was no closer to loving or respecting my body. Instead, the energy I had spent on food restriction and bingeing was transferred to exercise abuse and nutrient control.

Five years after I went off birth control, in the midst of a never-ending loop of training and training-related injuries, I went on hormone replacement therapy (HRT). Eight months later, my hormones hadn't budged, but the scale had. I'd reached 32 percent body fat and was carrying around an extra twenty pounds that, I swear, was made up entirely of cellulite.

I was doing all the "right" things—eating vegan, later going Paleo, working out once or twice a day, not eating after 5 p.m., consuming six small meals a day—but the weight just kept piling on with each passing week. When my hips wouldn't fit into a pair of shorts I'd purchased the previous summer, I felt that I had to do something.

So, like everyone who wants to lose weight, I reduced my calorie intake and increased the intensity of my workouts. And I quickly became starving and moody. Every two to three days I binged and felt like I was back to square negative one. Frustrated, I went to a naturopath, who suggested I go on a low-carb diet. My immediate reaction was a big hell no. I associated low-carb diets with the processed dressings, sweeteners, sodas, treats, and weight-loss supplements I'd seen on infomercials. That, coupled with what my nutrition professors had to say about low-carb diets being unhealthy, unnatural, and absolutely ludicrous, had me convinced to stay away.

But I was desperate, so eventually I decided that if I could do low-carb in a way that felt good to me, I was in. That very same day, a friend mentioned keto on one of her Instagram posts. The word intrigued me, so I looked it up, and bam, there was my solution, sitting right there on the screen.

Although I was initially overwhelmed to see how many ketogenic resources used dairy as a primary fat source and relied heavily on processed foods to reduce carb intake, I was interested enough—and desperate enough—to give keto a try. But I was determined to do it my way: grain-free, dairy-free, and whole food–based. I spent weeks researching ketogenic eating and delving deep into the diet.

For the first time in my life, I gave myself permission to be okay with eating fat, and it was liberating! I slathered coconut oil on flax muffins, cooked vegetables with scoops of local beef fat, and ate my fair share of bacon, even the extra-fatty marbled stuff I'd always avoided. It was a summer of firsts—first rack of ribs, first spoonful of nut butter. I let my fat flag fly, and it felt good. The more fat I ate, the more balanced my emotions were, the steadier my mood and more confident my decisions became, and the more sure of myself I was. Plus, I wasn't endlessly hungry anymore. I ate until I was satisfied—and I started to lose weight. I was eating 200 grams of fat per day, and in just two months I lost twenty pounds and reduced my body fat from 32 percent to 20 percent.

But here's where the happy story takes a turn for the worse. I'm prone to restriction. When I find something new that sparks weight loss and makes me feel like I'm on my way to becoming my "better self," I take it to the extreme. What's a ten-pound weight loss if I can lose twenty? What's twenty pounds if thirty is on the table? I was off to the races, counting each pound lost as a step toward a happier, healthier me.

The obsessive high-fat, low-carb, low-calorie suffering ran its course for six months, to the point that I wasn't sleeping, my hair was falling out, and I was secretly bingeing on carbs. The stricter I became with my eating, the more I binged. I looked fantastic and enjoyed how clear and focused my thinking was, but deep down I knew I was losing myself with each passing day.

The fact that I had the emotional balance needed to recognize that there was a problem and to begin making changes was due to my consumption of dietary fat. You see, when you start eating enough fat after a period (in my case, a decade plus) of eating next to no fat, something pretty spectacular happens: your brain comes back online, your emotions settle down, and you become able to make thoughtful decisions in a snap.

I knew there was power behind eating the keto way, but I needed to change my version of it. So, while remaining dedicated to using fats to nourish and heal, I developed the Fat Fueled program, which is what *The Keto Diet* is based on. The program became my, and so many others', saving grace by promoting healing, weight stabilization, and happiness within a ketogenic diet.

On top of eating all the fats, I gave myself full permission to listen to my body, do what felt right, and heal myself from the inside out. It started with ditching the standard ketogenic approach of massive restriction, shame, and guilt that I had come to practice so, so well. Instead of believing that it was me against my body, I attempted to feel gratitude toward the wondrous things my body did for me on a daily basis, from the basics, like breathing, to the more complex, like feeling emotion in response to a situation. I also got rid of my ketone and glucose blood monitors, took steps to end calorie counting and macro manipulation, and unfollowed low-carb gurus who told me that if I ate more than 20 grams of carbs in a day, I wasn't "legit keto." My hair stopped falling out and my sleep improved, yet I maintained my favorite benefits of eating high-fat and low-carb: steady emotions, balanced blood sugar, a clear mind, and newfound weight loss.

After nine months of following the Fat Fueled approach, I got my period back, binged on self-care, and became addicted to loving myself. Now, three years into this lifestyle, I'm the Leanne I always knew I was but couldn't quite get to. Some say self-actualization starts when we invite love in, but for me, it was all about fat.

I took an exceedingly roundabout way of getting to good health. The great thing is that *you* don't have to! By applying everything I've learned about this style of eating through trial and error, you can begin to feel better tomorrow.

And it all starts with redefining the word *diet*.

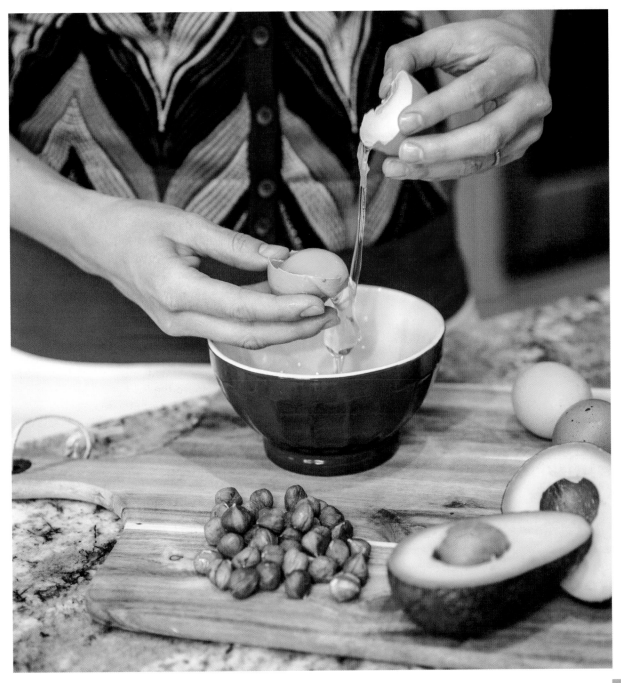

A NEW KIND OF "DIET"

There's something you should know about me: I hate the word *diet*. Those four little letters hold so much power over people, it makes me want to punch walls, stomp my feet, and then write a book with *diet* in the title to prove that *diet* can mean so much more than what we've been led to believe.

You bet this program will help you lose weight and provide you with the tools you need to feel your best. But it won't lead you to say things like, "I don't trust myself around chocolate when I'm dieting," or, "I start the new diet on Monday." Instead, you'll be saying things like, "No, thanks, cake doesn't make me feel good," and, "Whoa, did I just go a whole afternoon without thinking about food?" It's not about eating fewer calories and less fat, which leads you to feel like a binge-fest could erupt at any moment and contributes to more cravings, food restrictions, brain fog, and so on.

The standard approach to dieting is limiting, restrictive, and shaming, and I don't want any part of it. Let's redefine *diet* and take our lives back, yes? Instead of the same old binge/restrict/self-loathe/repeat cycle of dieting, I'd like to create a diet that's focused on self-love, respect, and health-promoting goals.

You've probably read a lot of spiels that go something like this: "I followed the diet for four weeks, lost fifty pounds, and now I'm the happiest woman in the world. My life has completely changed: my husband is obsessed with me, my kids enjoy being around me, and my friends want to *be* me."

I have news for you: People want to be around you because you're kind. Your significant other loves your confidence, your wild side, and the way you are with your children. Your kids love you because you're their idol and in their eyes you can do no wrong. When people say, "Losing weight changed my life," often what they really mean is that losing weight changed their *perception* of themselves, which influences how they interact with the world. Of course, there's a chance that losing weight will enable you to go for a hike for the first time ever, and that's pretty cool. I want to help you do the things you want to do.

But I bet you're reading this book because you want to lose weight and believe that when you do, your life will be better in every way. It took me years to learn that I am not my weight. That I can do anything I set my mind to, regardless of my weight. And that, in so many cases, it's our own perception of our bodies and our limitations that takes us away from the life we dream of. The weight isn't holding us back—*we're* holding ourselves back.

On the flip side, I totally understand where you're coming from. Maybe you just read that last paragraph and thought, "This woman is crazy. Of course my weight is a problem." And I get it. When I gained twenty pounds during that horrible hormone replacement therapy experience, I too felt like that weight did not belong on my body. And I would have done just about anything to get it off.

But what if I told you that losing weight and getting healthy doesn't have to be a battle? What if I told you that you could be confident right now, in the body you have, loving your life and the people in it, doing the things you want to do, and lose weight in the process?

If you delve into keto and give dietary fat a chance, not only will you lose weight, but your brain will feel better, too. And when your brain feels better, things work a little differently. Your mood and ability to make quality decisions improve, the brain fog lifts, and for the first time, you can see clearly. I'm not kidding; this is a real thing. Your brain loves fat. And right now, it's probably not getting enough of it to work properly, which is affecting the way you see your life. I know, it sounds a little hocus pocus, but it wouldn't if you were eating high-fat, I promise.

If emotional eating and the "relationship with food" conversation isn't your jam, I respect that. If all you want to do is improve your health, maybe shed some weight and start to feel better, no problem—everything I share in this book will help you to do that.

But if you want to stop the endless cycle of diet after diet, cheats followed by guilt, I'd like to help. *The Keto Diet* is about eating in a way that feels good in your body and personalizing your food choices so that you can achieve health and hotness without going crazy in the process. And for me, this is what a "diet" really is, or at least should be.

Your body wants to be healthy. If it were up to your body, you would not gain three hundred pounds in a matter of months. It's not your body making the imbalanced choices that you can't control; it's your alter ego—you along with a bunch of media-instilled expectations of what your body should look like, mixed with a dose of dieting rules, a splash of emotion deflection, and—bam!—the perfect recipe for not trusting yourself, binge eating at night, and feeling like you can't control yourself around food.

In the following pages, you'll be encouraged to listen to your body and figure out what it wants. This may sound pretty ludicrous at first; I know that when I started working through this stuff, I thought all my body wanted was licorice and potato chips. Turns out, though, that my body wants to be healthy, and it knows exactly what weight I'm best at. Now I eat, I get full, and I don't think too much about it. You can do the same and get down to your realistic weight by connecting to what your body wants and needs.

I want to help you have that hot-damn awesome life you've always dreamed of. And if that life includes dipping your bacon in mayo on the daily, then you've come to the right place.

FREEDOM FROM THE DIET!

It's estimated that two in five women are dieting all the time. I don't want to be one of those people. I don't want to use an app to count calories in a restaurant in the South of France while my husband waits for me to figure out what to order. I don't want to skip my little sister's wedding cake because it's over my carb allotment for the day. I don't want to pass on an evening around the fire making s'mores in fear that I'll lose control and eat all the chocolate. I don't want to miss out on life because I'm on a diet.

Initially, when I went ketogenic, it was from a place of restriction. I thought of all the things I couldn't have anymore, counted calories, and weighed myself two, sometimes three, times a day. I didn't go out, I didn't visit with friends, and I was nervous about food all the time. Living like this, if you could even call it living, wasn't fun. As soon as I left the restrictive mindset out on the porch, I was overcome by the amazing freedom of high-fat living.

But the restrictive mindset has been drilled into our brains since we were young, and it's not always easy to get past. TV teaches us from an early age that our bodies cannot be trusted and that we need to have power over them if we are

to lose weight, feel great, and be worthy of love. Remember the Special K commercial from the 1980s that said, "Thanks to the K, you can't pinch an inch"? Or the Diet Pepsi commercial that said in reference to body fat, "Now you see it, now you don't"?

If you're a die-hard tracker like I was, think back to a time when you had 150 calories left in your daily allotment. You weren't hungry, but you ate anyway in fear that if you didn't, you'd be hungry tomorrow, and then you wouldn't have an extra 150 calories because "calories don't carry over like that." Plus, of course, the activities you did that day required the allotted calories; you'd planned to eat a chocolate mug cake and it'd be a shame to miss out; and if you didn't eat said mug cake, you wouldn't "hit your macros."

Okay, now recall a time when you hit your calorie goal at 4 p.m. after indulging in a handful of nuts at your desk. You drove home wishing you hadn't eaten those nuts because bedtime was still five hours away. Hunger. So much hunger. For the rest of the drive home, you were thinking about activities to keep you occupied until bedtime so that you wouldn't gorge and go over your calories or macros.

I don't know about you, but when I was living in this obsessive space of constant tracking, I wasn't happy. In fact, I was miserable. But I didn't know the way out. Heck, I didn't even know there *was* a way out.

There are some classic signs that a dieting mentality is ruling your life:

- **You track every little morsel that enters your body and make sure that it will support you in getting to your goals.**

- **You have lots of gas and can't pinpoint which food is causing it.**

- **You get stressed in eating situations. Going out for dinner with friends means checking the menu beforehand and figuring out what questions you'll ask the server. Conversations around an event put you in defensive mode, make you anxious, or have you canceling at the last minute.**

- **Your cycle is off—missing periods, crazy PMS, you name it.**

- **You find yourself constantly talking about food choices, weight, and dieting.**

- **You get anxious at the possibility of missing a workout.**

If all this sounds way too familiar, I urge you to do two things: First, develop an open mind and a willingness to listen to your body. Second, take time for yourself so that you can listen to your body.

This is where self-care comes in. Self-care is the practice of—yep, you guessed it—taking care of yourself. But it goes beyond showering and doing your hair. It's about truly caring for yourself with intentional actions that meet your physical, mental, and emotional needs. I like to think of it as "me time." For example, some of my physical self-care practices are taking an evening bath, going on a walk, taking time to make dinner, stretching before bed, and getting a massage. Some of my mental self-care practices are journaling, meditating, and working on challenging Sudoku puzzles. For emotional health, my practices include removing toxic people from my life, having in-depth conversations with my husband, dancing with my friends, and working with a business coach.

Your turn! What are a couple of things—even *one* thing—that you can begin doing on a daily basis to make yourself feel good? It doesn't have to take up a lot of time; even five minutes of self-care is a great start!

Between developing a self-care practice and following a keto diet, which will light up your brain and give you more focus and awareness, you'll be able to connect to what your body actually wants. Imagine knowing what to eat and how much in order to achieve the body and health you've always dreamed of, without having to restrict your foods, count calories, or spend oodles of money!

If you're way down the rabbit hole, as I was—not trusting yourself around food, having a strong hatred or disgust toward your body, or feeling sick of being ruled by a diet—here are some things that may help, in conjunction with going keto:

DITCH THE MATH

more on page 56

How many times have you gotten halfway through a meal and thought, "I'm not that hungry, but I have to eat this or [*insert reason:* I won't stay in ketosis, I won't make it until my next meal, my muscles won't grow]"?

That little voice telling you that you're not hungry is your body's way of trying to reach its happy place, where it gets the right amount of food for its needs. By pushing and prodding yourself to finish your meal, you are going against your body in the worst possible way.

That means measuring and weighing your food is a complete waste of time. Your body knows when it's had enough. Trust your body.

TRUST YOURSELF

more on page 65

After you've been eating keto for a while, ditch the "rules" and make up your own. After becoming fat-adapted, you'll know what being in ketosis feels like. Now it's time to play. You know how good you feel eating this way, but can you feel even better by tweaking some things?

INCORPORATE POSITIVE MOVEMENT

more on page 75

Do you hate your workouts? Think about what type of movement brings you joy and do more of that. If you are hating every moment, why are you doing it? Because you think you should? Is that a good enough reason?

START PRACTICING SELF-CARE

Write a list of things that make you feel good and rank them in order of the amount of time required, from items that take a long time to those that take less than fifteen minutes. Begin with one shorter activity a week and slowly increase to at least one per day. My own self-care practice includes making tea before the workday begins, going for a walk in the afternoon, and winding down with a bath before bed. In all, self-care takes me about two hours a day, but it didn't start off that way. At first, I was lucky to get five minutes alone to do the things that made me feel good. Now I can see that when I take time for myself, I reap the rewards in self-respect, self-knowledge, and (my favorite) self-confidence.

DEFINE YOUR PURPOSE

It can happen to anyone: despite our best intentions, we find ourselves back on the dieting train, counting calories and cursing ourselves for eating that extra piece of chicken. When this happens to me, I define my purpose.

My purpose in getting off the dieting train was to live a freer, more spontaneous life and be consumed by the present moment rather than be ruled by fears or regrets. When I count calories or jump back on the restrictive dieting train, I'm not able to live the life I want to live. So when I slide into those old negative behaviors, I remind myself that they don't allow me to have the life I desire.

As you start changing your eating style, you may need to reconnect to your purpose every day to remind yourself what's important to you (why you're saying no to sugar and yes to that afternoon walk). The longer you practice, the easier it becomes to live out your purpose without having to constantly remind yourself of it.

Here are some questions you could ask yourself to help identify your purpose:

- What drew you to purchase this book?
- What about eating more fat entices you?
- What does a healthy, happy life look like to you?
- How do your thoughts and actions change when you feel happy and healthy?
- What small activities can you commit to doing on a daily basis that will help you connect to and stay focused on your purpose?

In all, I hope that you see just how wonderful this way of eating can be on so much more than your body. Heck yes, it's awesome for weight loss and feeling great physically and all that jazz, but it also puts you in a fine position to actually enjoy the journey and feel more balanced in your life.

THE STATE OF YOUR BODY IS IN YOUR CONTROL

Widespread chronic health problems are not being resolved by common medical practices. In the United States alone, 5 million women have polycystic ovary syndrome, 26 million people have diabetes, 3 million are plagued with neurological disorders, and 1.6 million are diagnosed with cancer every year. Health seekers of all backgrounds are beginning to wake up to the realization that what we're doing, and eating, isn't working.

So many of us have either experienced or witnessed someone we love go through the pain, suffering, and frustration of receiving a life-altering diagnosis of Alzheimer's, Crohn's, diabetes, cancer, multiple sclerosis, or the like. Of course, the diagnosis itself is a scary thing. But what scares me more is that health-care organizations and media outlets are unwilling to change the conversation and revisit their approach to preventing and healing disease. In many cases, they apply outdated treatments instead of adopting a cutting-edge approach that incorporates the current knowledge about nutrition and disease.

I discovered this for myself when my dad underwent chemotherapy in 2010. After the daily treatment, patients were offered tea with packets of sugar and store-bought cookies. The point of this sugar-laced snack was to boost energy. But the hospital didn't take into account another effect of sugar: cancer thrives on sugar!

Or consider my grandpa's experience with Alzheimer's. In just a matter of months, he went from minor dementia to catastrophic stage-three Alzheimer's to death. I'm positive that the shockingly fast progression of his Alzheimer's was exacerbated by the countless bowls of candies and other sweet treats that were stationed around his room at the nursing home. Alzheimer's has been coined "type 3 diabetes" for good reason, but the benefits of high-fat foods, especially MCT oil (see page 140), were unheard of back then.

Both my father's and my grandfather's experiences could have been improved with education on the benefits of dietary fat. Perhaps you've witnessed, heard of, or experienced something similar?

We have to learn how to take care of ourselves, and it begins and ends with education. You don't have to go out and become a nutritionist, but you can explore different approaches to ultimately develop an eating style that works well for you, your body, your health, and your life. And if issues arise, you'll be in a fabulous place to understand what adjustments to make to smooth them out and where to go to get the help you need.

I'm sharing this not to scare you into change but to spark a conversation about being open to new ideas about supporting your body, both to improve any health concerns you have now and to avoid health problems in the future. I have a feeling that, since you've purchased this book, you are interested in taking responsibility for your body. Our bodies are the most precious things we have, and when we educate ourselves with information from a wide variety of sources, we're better equipped to handle whatever comes our way.

The idea of healing through nutrition is spreading quickly. In just the last year, new books focused on high-fat and ketogenic eating have been bestsellers on Amazon, and three titles related to grain-free and sugar-free living have consistently been on the *New York Times* list of bestselling food and diet books since late 2013.

Our world is hungry for change, and I'm hoping that this book assists in answering that call.

WHAT FATS DO IN YOUR BODY

Think of the fat landscape as the Enchanted Forest. We want to stick with the princes, princesses, and devoted sidekicks—the heroes who will improve our health—and avoid the evil queens, nasty sea creatures, and wicked witches—the villains who will make our health even worse. I'll talk about which fats are good and which are bad later on, but for now, let's review what fats can do in the body.

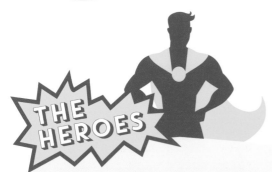

THE HEROES

* ★ Improve cardiovascular risk factors
* ★ Strengthen bones
* ★ Improve the health of the liver, lungs, and brain
* ★ Increase balanced nerve signaling to improve training, learning, muscle memory, and more
* ★ Strengthen the immune system
* ★ Create cell integrity
* ★ Lower LDL (bad) cholesterol, specifically Lp(a)
* ★ Increase HDL (good) cholesterol
* ★ Assist with the assimilation of nutrients
* ★ Encourage better body composition, with a good balance of lean muscle mass and body fat
* ★ Improve insulin sensitivity
* ★ Reduce inflammation
* ★ Support a healthy metabolism
* ★ Assist with thyroid function
* ★ Aid in the balance of LDL and HDL cholesterol, which helps fight inflammation
* ★ Provide a satiated or "full" feeling, leading to fewer cravings
* ★ Support balanced hormones
* ★ Aid in building muscle
* ★ Assist with weight loss
* ★ Reduce the risk of depression, cancer, and heart attack
* ★ Improve the health of skin and eyes

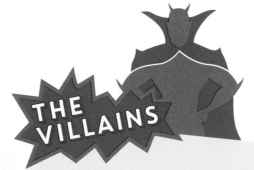

THE VILLAINS

* ☠ Create free radicals, which damage and age cells
* ☠ Remove vitamins and minerals from the body
* ☠ Cause systemic inflammation
* ☠ Increase LDL (bad) cholesterol, specifically Lp(b)
* ☠ Deteriorate cell walls, causing decay
* ☠ Damage DNA
* ☠ Make it difficult to fight infection
* ☠ Lower a person's ability to deal with stress
* ☠ Place stress on the body
* ☠ Increase the effects of aging
* ☠ Reduce the body's ability to produce energy
* ☠ Negatively affect gut microflora
* ☠ Increase the risk of cancer, heart disease, and Alzheimer's
* ☠ Clog arteries
* ☠ Cause headaches
* ☠ Negatively affect memory

WEIGHT LOSS ISN'T JUST ABOUT CALORIES

There was a time where I was consuming 1,200 calories a day, tracking every morsel that went into my mouth, and obsessing about food preparation, dieting, and weight loss. Now, there are days when I consume around 3,000 calories and don't track my foods, yet I'm smaller than I was back then, and I effortlessly maintain a steady weight and feel great. If my previous messed-up self can get out of the funk, you can, too.

Your body is not a machine. Your thoughts, emotions, activities, hormonal profile, circadian rhythm, food choices—they all have an impact on your energy requirements and therefore how many calories your body needs. Heck, as I write this I'm legitimately hungry, like I haven't eaten in days, whereas yesterday, a similar day in terms of activities, I couldn't be bothered to eat. What's up with that?

The classic "eat less, exercise more" approach to weight loss is based on a calories-in-calories-out mentality: the idea that losing weight is simply a matter of consuming fewer calories than you burn. But our bodies are far more complicated than that.

First, your body has varied hormonal responses to food. Take protein, for example. It stimulates the release of glucagon, a hormone that, among other things, signals the body to burn stored fat. Or consider fructose: It fails to lower the hunger hormone ghrelin, so after eating a giant bowl of fruit salad, we're generally just as hungry, even though we've consumed all those calories. So the specific foods we eat can help or hurt our weight-loss efforts by affecting our hormones.

Second, the ratio of macronutrients (carbohydrates, proteins, and fats) that you consume has an impact on your appetite and your weight. Fat is more satisfying and makes you feel fuller longer than carbs or protein, so when you get a greater percentage of your total calories from fat, you can eat less without feeling hungry. At the same time, when you're eating high-fat and in a fat-burning state, your body can handle more calories than it can on a low-fat diet—in other words, you can eat more and still lose weight effortlessly.

Third, your metabolic rate—how much fuel your body needs for basic functions, like keeping your organs working and maintaining a stable temperature—drops during caloric restriction. In other words, when you consume fewer calories, your body reduces how many calories it needs. Weight loss occurs at first, but only until your body is able to function on that new calorie amount; then the weight starts to come back. The more you restrict calories, the lower your metabolic rate goes in response, until weight loss is practically impossible.

Fourth, your environment and emotions may affect how much you eat. For example, writing this book has been one of the most challenging things I've ever done. Not because I don't know the material—I can spew this stuff any day—but because I'm putting myself out there in the world in a way I never have before. That's scary! And, like a lot of people, I react to fear by overeating. Eating makes me feel good, so when I feel scared, the easiest thing for me to do is eat. But over time, I've learned better ways to cope than turning to food for comfort.

With these four facts in mind, it's clear that there's much more to weight loss than calories in, calories out. Supporting hormones, balancing macros, and boosting metabolism are also very, very important pieces of the weight-loss puzzle. A keto diet supports a positive weight-loss experience and lifelong maintenance because it so perfectly meets these requirements. (We'll explore how exactly keto does all this later in the book.)

A little note to my fellow dieting/body hating/weight-loss lifers: I'm crossing my fingers and toes that by this point, you've had a couple of light bulb moments when it comes to food, nourishment, and self-care. I've done a lot of not-so-awesome things to my body in the name of weight loss, and they damaged my relationships, sex drive, metabolism, sanity, ability to have more than one bowel movement a week...the list goes on. Learn from my mistakes and take a saner approach to weight loss, supporting your body through the transition in a healthful way.

ABOUT THIS BOOK

I so desperately wanted to create this book because I know that you, too, are probably struggling with something. And I feel very deeply that eating fat, being okay with fat, and celebrating the nourishing fats in your life could be your ticket to everything. Studies show that boosting fat intake and delving into nutritional ketosis can alleviate food cravings, blood sugar irregularities, brain fog, excess body weight, abnormal cell growth, psychological imbalances, infertility, and more.

In the following pages, I'm going to show you how to feel liberated with a gluten-free, grain-free, sugar-free, dairy-free, legume-free, Paleo-friendly eating style that uses nutritional ketosis to propel you to better health. And that eating style includes a lot of fat. Whether you're not so keen on how your body looks or you're sick of afternoon energy lulls, headaches, daily digestive upsets, hormonal imbalances, crazy moods, or anything else you have going on, I really, really think that fat will help.

That may sound counterintuitive to you—or even flat-out crazy. But if you find yourself resisting the ideas in this book, ask yourself if that resistance is coming from a place of fear or if you truly feel that your body wouldn't like what I'm suggesting. If it's the latter, know that you can adjust any and all of these strategies and concepts to make them work for you, your body, and your life. You'll find lots of options for personalizing the keto diet in Chapter 2, and you can adapt it even further as you figure out what works best for you.

My path to eating high-fat and low-carb—what I call the Fat Fueled approach—is a bit different from what you'll find in most other resources because I learned that it has to be. The standard ketogenic approach didn't work for me or many of my clients, so I changed it. Changing keto to your liking really takes the stress out of it. You can benefit from the high-fat, low-carb magic without worrying so much about total carb intake and tracking everything you eat.

The Fat Fueled approach shared in this book is less about restriction and obsession and more about nourishing the body to encourage healing—you know, so we can redefine what a diet is and

I can be proud that the word *diet* is plastered all over the cover of this book.

And just in case the word *healing* has you all, "Whoop-dee-doo, but when am I going to lose weight?": healing generally leads to weight loss that stays off forever.

With both the standard ketogenic approach and the Fat Fueled approach, you will likely lose weight, feel better, and eat a heck of a lot of fat. But the Fat Fueled approach will help you do away with the fear-based dieting mentality and will set you up with an eating style that is not limiting, restrictive, or shame-based.

The recipes in this book are designed to help you transition into and maintain a keto style of eating without craving unhealthy processed foods or feeling guilty about your ketogenic choices. They're full of variety, packed with whole foods, and free of gluten, grains, dairy, and legumes. And of course, they're high in fat and low in carbs—so you'll feel great and stay full and satiated. They're also designed to be quick and easy to prepare so that you can stick with keto no matter how busy or new to the kitchen you are.

The meal plans and shopping lists in Chapter 12 will guide you through a month of ketogenic eating, customized for the Fat Fueled Profile you decide on. Of course, you don't have to follow any of these meal plans, but if you're just starting out on keto, doing so can be helpful. And you won't have to think about the dreaded question, "What's for dinner?"

Whether you're reading this book or scouring the internet for more information, recipes, and general how-tos, please, if something doesn't feel right to you or doesn't make you feel good, don't do it. And if you're part of a community that doesn't make you feel good about your choices, pack up and find a group of people who will support you in making keto a positive lifelong practice. I don't know about you, but I'm planning to hang out on this earth for a whole lot longer, so let's make sure we're having fun doing life, yeah?

Imagine waking up every morning knowing that you can, and will, do the things you want to do, in the body you were always meant to have. Imagine not being at war with your body. Imagine preparing food with ease, feeling good about your food choices, and doing away with nighttime bingeing, guilt-based eating, and diet starts and stops.

The keto diet has the potential to change everything for you, and I'm excited to be part of your transformation.

And it all starts with fat! Let's get this party started, shall we?

APPROACHES to the KETO DIET

STANDARD KETOGENIC APPROACH	FAT FUELED APPROACH
Result: Weight loss, blood sugar control, and balanced cholesterol	Result: Weight loss, blood sugar control, and balanced cholesterol, lowered inflammation, improved nutrition, balanced hormones, and more
Obscene amount of dairy—cheese, yogurt, cheese, cheese, sour cream, cottage cheese, cheese...	Focus on whole foods and nourishing practices that heal the body
Processed sweeteners, diet soda, and fiber-rich bars that claim "low net carbs"	Paleo in principle, with conscious food sourcing and intuitive eating practices
Extremely limited focus on vegetables	Motto: I don't count my kale
Extremely low-carb forever	The Fat Fueled Profiles (pages 47 to 49) provide flexibility for carb intake based on what's going on in your body and your life
Strict adherence to ketogenic eating	Customize for your needs with the five Fat Fueled Profiles
Track calories and macros every day	Trust your body, not the calculator; counting and tracking are less important
Fear of carbs	Use carbs to your advantage with the Fat Fueled Profiles—especially important for women's health and training efforts
Fear of proteins that affect ketosis	Use protein to your advantage with the Fat Fueled Profiles—especially important for adrenal health
Lack of support for anaerobic training*	Mega support and strategies for anaerobic training*

*Anaerobic training consists of short high-intensity workouts, such as HIIT, sprints, jumping, and heavy weight training.

I was twenty-eight years old when my doctor suggested I start taking a statin for high cholesterol and metformin to control my blood sugar. She also told me that it would help if I lost some weight. I was five-foot-four and 130 pounds, not overweight by any means. I had previously been diagnosed with polycystic ovary syndrome and also suffered from mild depression and anxiety. I was eating a vegan diet and working out regularly. Instinctively I knew that something was out of balance in my body and that medication would not help to resolve the imbalance. That's when I did some research and discovered the ketogenic diet.

I've never had a poor relationship with food. Sure, I would binge here and there when I was stressed or bored, but fat was something I had never feared. I was vegan in my mid-twenties because I thought it was the "cool" thing to do. I felt lethargic and in a daze when I followed a vegan eating style, and I think that's what raised my cholesterol and sent me on a blood sugar roller coaster. One day I was craving fatty comfort food. I don't know what possessed me to do this, but I was working in a market at the time and decided to snack on half a stick of butter. Yes, I ate half a stick of pure, solid, delicious butter. And you know what? It made me feel amazing!

That was almost four years ago. Since then, I have been fueling my body with more fat and less carbs, and it has made all the difference. Transitioning to a keto eating style wasn't difficult. Nausea was my biggest side effect, but it subsided quickly. I did a lot of research on how to prevent what's called keto flu. Reading Leanne's blog and books and watching her YouTube videos helped a lot.

I lost the belly fat my doctor wanted me to lose within the first month after I started following Leanne's advice. But I really didn't have that much weight to lose. I also felt like I was burning fat while building muscle even though I wasn't working out nearly as much as I used to. My body just looked more toned. Even though my cholesterol is still high, my triglyceride and HDL: LDL ratios are within optimal range now and my blood sugar is right where it should be.

My PCOS, depression, and anxiety symptoms have all subsided too. Fueling my body with fat has no doubt helped with that. I also sleep better, have a ton more energy, have clearer skin, and generally feel much better overall when I eat this way. I teach kindergarten, which can be really stressful at times. Previously, during times of stress I craved sugar and carbs and gave in to those cravings. Now, because I am fueling my body properly, I don't usually get cravings for sugar and carbs. But if by chance I do, it's really easy not to give in to cravings. I just eat a fat bomb and move on. It's that simple.

I can't even imagine living a life without fat for fuel now. There's definitely something to be said about this ketogenic lifestyle, and I wish more people knew about it. Just imagine how much better they would feel inside and out!

Stephanie
Los Angeles, California

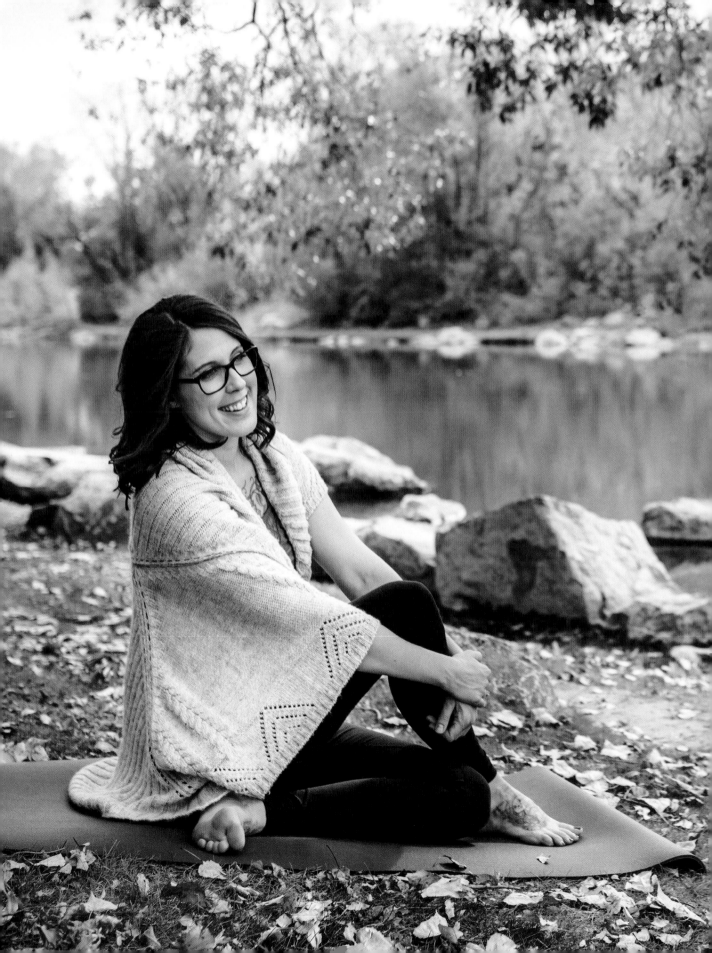

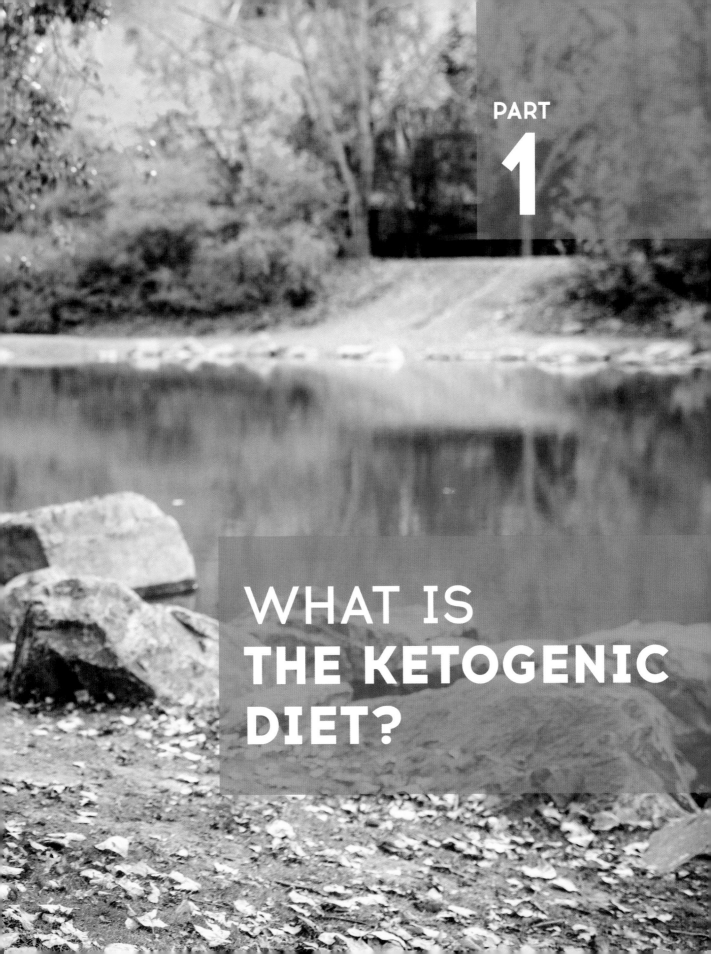

WHAT IS THE KETOGENIC DIET?

CHAPTER 1

WHAT KETO IS AND WHY YOU WANT IN ON THE PARTY

When we talk about eating keto, we're talking about eating fat. Like, a lot of fat. Probably more than you've ever dreamed of eating, and then about 10 percent more than that.

But before we get to how and why that works, let's run through the basics. Fat, protein, and carbohydrates are all macronutrients, or "macros," and they make up the bulk of our food. (The rest is micronutrients—vitamins and minerals that are essential for health.) Carbohydrates are most abundant in grains and sugars—bread, pasta, rice, corn, quinoa—but fruits and vegetables also contain carbohydrates, especially starchy vegetables like potatoes and sweet potatoes and high-sugar fruits like bananas. Proteins are found in animal foods like eggs, beef, fish, chicken, and turkey and in moderate quantities in some plant foods, such as beans, lentils, nuts, and seeds. Fats are abundant in coconut oil, avocados, olives, nuts, and seeds and animal foods such as ribs, steak, bacon, and dairy.

I used to be a low-fat, high-carb vegan. I remember exactly how little fat I ate and how scared I was of it. I'm guessing that many of you are right there with the old me. But if what you're doing isn't working, you're in a fine place to try something new. Something like the keto diet.

When I first saw the word *keto*, I was totally intrigued. It sounded foreign, somewhat rebellious. And as you'll read further on, I love being rebellious, so I was instantly hooked. *Keto* is short for *ketogenic*, an eating style that reduces carbohydrate intake, increases fat intake, and moderates protein intake in order to achieve a metabolic shift known as *ketosis*.

Right now you are burning glucose for energy (unless you're eating ketogenic already, in which case, total win!). Your body is primed to use energy from the limited glucose in your body, so when that starts to get used up, you become hungry and need to eat again. When I was a glucose burner, I ate every three hours, and the word *hangry* was at the top of my personal dictionary. I packed snacks to take with me, worried about where my next meal would come from, and would (lightly) budge people in line if it meant I'd get food sooner. Food ruled my life.

What the ketogenic diet does is switch the body from burning glucose to burning fat. This is the metabolic shift I was talking about. When the body burns fat, whether dietary fat or body fat, it produces molecules known as ketones, which are used for fuel. When ketones are the primary source of fuel for the body, it's known as being in ketosis. Now that I'm in ketosis, my daily energy requirements are primarily met by burning fat, so I don't need to get glucose from the bread, cookies, dried fruits, and treats I used to eat constantly.

My body doesn't need glucose to survive, and yours doesn't either! I've jumped off the roller coaster of blood sugar highs and lows, and I'm living the good life free from constant snacking, epic weight gain, and uncontrollable cravings. You can, too! There's tons of room at the keto table for you. Pull up a seat!

KETOSIS IS NOT KETOACIDOSIS

When we talk about being a fat burner, we're talking about nutritional ketosis, not ketoacidosis. Ketoacidosis is a dangerous condition experienced by diabetics when blood glucose and ketones rise to extremely high levels at the same time. A ketogenic diet won't get you even close to the levels of ketones that diabetics can experience in ketoacidosis. In fact, if you do not have diabetes, it's virtually impossible for you to go into ketoacidosis. Even a trace amount of insulin will keep ketone levels in the safe zone.

The level to which carbohydrate intake has to be reduced in order to get into ketosis varies greatly from person to person depending on enzymatic processes, stress level, heritage, and more. (We'll get into the nitty-gritty of macro ratios and how you know when you're in ketosis in the next couple of chapters.) But regardless of where you're coming from, even if you don't want to go balls to the wall, I'll outline how you can benefit from increasing your fat intake and dance on the edge of ketosis without macro and calorie tracking running the show.

There are many forms of ketogenic eating. I'm going to be introducing you to the whole food–based form that's rich in health-promoting foods and fats. Think of it as a Paleo eating style, jacked up on fats and with way fewer sweet potatoes and chocolate treats and way less maple syrup. You will radically lower your carbohydrate intake, massively increase fat, and moderate protein, a triple whammy that triggers your body to start burning fat for energy rather than glucose.

IS KETO BASICALLY A LOW-CARB DIET?

The fact that the keto diet is high-fat and moderate-protein is what makes it different from a traditional low-carb diet. Many low-carb diets are high-protein and low-fat, which puts up a roadblock to effectively using fat as the primary fuel source. Just like carbs, excess protein intake stimulates the release of insulin, which tells the body not to burn stored fat. So on a traditional low-carb diet, fat-burning takes place only in the wee hours of the night, when insulin levels drop. The keto diet, on the other hand, allows the body to burn fat at all hours so we can lose weight once and for all. And because it turns out that the body really *likes* being fueled by fat, it also helps us gain copious amounts of brain function we never knew we had, increases hormone efficiency, boosts energy, eliminates insomnia, balances blood sugar, and so much more.

WHAT HAPPENS IN YOUR BODY WHEN YOU EAT KETO

To explain why the keto diet is so great for health, I want to start by explaining how the body functions on carbohydrates—which is probably the way your body is functioning right now.

Carbohydrates from any source—fruits, vegetables, grains, sugars, anything starchy—are broken down into glucose, which is used for energy. When you have more glucose than you need immediately, your body stores the excess in the liver and then the muscles as glycogen. This is the body's first-line energy stockpile of fuel for short-burst physical efforts and for keeping certain systems (the brain, red blood cells, kidney cells) running efficiently all day. The glycogen stores in the liver can be utilized by the rest of the body, but the glycogen in muscles is reserved for action in that particular muscle. When space for glycogen in the liver and muscles is full, glucose is converted to fat.

Glucose is the first source the body goes to when it needs energy. But because we can store only a couple thousand calories of glucose (or glycogen when it's stored) at any given time, it's not a sustainable source of energy. That means we need to keep replenishing it by eating constantly throughout the day. And relying on glucose can prevent us from stabilizing our blood sugar, which spikes when we eat and then drops, resulting in endless cravings and overall weight gain. In addition, glucose can be converted to not just stored fat but also triglycerides in the blood, which can be a risk for heart disease.

You've also probably heard a lot about insulin, insulin resistance, and insulin sensitivity—all can be negatively impacted when relying on glucose for fuel. Insulin is the hormone that balances blood sugar; it triggers the absorption of glucose by the liver, fat, and muscle cells and thereby lowers the level of glucose in the bloodstream (blood sugar). Insulin also pauses any fat-burning that's going on so that we can burn or store the glucose that's coming in. Once glucose is handled, insulin levels drop and we go back to burning fat. Insulin also alerts the brain if we're in need of fuel, which triggers hunger signals. When we have good insulin sensitivity, all of these processes work perfectly, maintaining healthful blood sugar stability. But problems arise when glucose levels in the blood are constantly high. The correspondingly high levels of insulin cause the insulin receptors on cells to become deaf to insulin. Think of the boy who cried wolf: he cries and cries, so all the townspeople stop listening to his warnings. In the case of insulin resistance, cells no longer listen to insulin's instruction to absorb glucose, so glucose levels in the bloodstream can get and stay too high.

But when things are functioning as they should, when the concentration of glucose in the bloodstream falls too low, a hormone called glucagon is released. It stimulates the liver to convert stored glycogen into glucose, which is then released into the bloodstream. It also tells the body to start using the stored fuel source, fat. Burning fat for fuel is called lipolysis; technically, during lipolysis, fatty acids and glycerol molecules are moved from fat cells and metabolized to generate energy.

As it burns fat, the body creates ketone bodies. When we're in ketosis, these ketone bodies become what carbs are to you right now, your primary fuel. The brain can use ketones, as can skeletal muscles, the liver—the list goes on. In fact, the heart prefers ketones to glucose.

That's not to say that the body doesn't need glucose at all. Red blood cells, for instance, require glucose, and so does the brain (although a certain amount of its energy requirements can be met by ketones). But the body can actually create glucose on its own through a process called gluconeogenesis. In gluconeogenesis, the liver turns amino acids—the building blocks of protein—and fatty acids into glucose. There's no need to eat carbohydrates to get glucose!

It can be challenging to make the switch from preferring glucose as the primary fuel to preferring fat because the body isn't entirely accustomed to using fat. It has to ramp up the processes needed to metabolize fat until it finally is able to prefer fat to glucose as a fuel source—a process that's known as "fat adaptation" or "becoming fat-adapted."

Once you're in nutritional ketosis and burning fat as your primary fuel, blood sugar and insulin levels drop and levels of HDL (good) cholesterol increase. Your body starts to burn its stored fat along with dietary fat, which means that you start to lose weight—and, even better for your health, the visceral fat around your vital organs, which is linked to increased risk of heart disease and type 2 diabetes, shrinks. And remember how insulin alerts the brain if fuel is running low, resulting in hunger? Because insulin is stable on a ketogenic diet and the fuel we need (fat) is right on our bodies, appetite is reduced naturally. In addition, studies show that nutritional ketosis can be therapeutic for many of today's widespread chronic health problems, such type 2 diabetes, irritable bowel syndrome (IBS), polycystic ovary syndrome (PCOS), Alzheimer's disease, and dementia.

On a day-to-day basis, people in ketosis often report the following changes in their health:

- **Effortless weight loss**
- **Reduced appetite**
- **Improved mood**
- **Ability to eat more without gaining weight**
- **Lower and more stable blood sugar**
- **Fewer cravings**
- **Lower blood pressure**
- **Clearer thoughts**
- **Improved sleep**
- **Reduction in gas and bloating**

THE PROCESS OF NUTRITIONAL KETOSIS

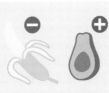

1

Carbohydrate intake is decreased.

2

After the body has used most of its stored glucose (glycogen), it shifts to using fat for energy.

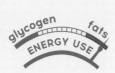

glycogen · ENERGY USE · fats

3

Dietary fat and stored body fat are broken down for energy, resulting in the production of ketones.

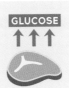

4

The body also creates glucose from noncarbohydrate sources* for the small set of bodily processes that require it.

GLUCOSE

5

Ketones become the body's primary fuel, replacing glucose.

KETONES

*VIA GLUCONEOGENESIS.

When the body makes glucose all on its own! More on page 26.

UNIFYING PALEO AND LOW-CARB

The transition from burning glucose to burning fat is best supported by eating copious amounts of fat. It's not completely necessary: You can slide into fat-burning mode through fasting, eating low-carb/low-fat, or countless other ways. But I feel, and have experienced firsthand, that ketosis is best supported by a high-fat, whole food–based eating style, like the one I've outlined in this book. Another way to put it is that I advocate for a high-fat, low-carb Paleo diet.

To many health advocates and nutrition professionals, Paleo trumps low-carb in many ways. Paleo prides itself on its abundance of fruits and vegetables, balanced intake of omega-6 fatty acids, and consumption of healthy fats. Low-carb, on the other hand, as many practice it, is strictly about hitting macronutrient goals, with limited concern about food quality or food sensitivities, which can play a huge role in overall health and success on the diet itself. These two communities have traditionally seen the world through very different sets of eyes.

Of course, because it eliminates grains and sugars, Paleo is lower in carbohydrates than the Standard American Diet, and the lost carbohydrates are often replaced by dietary fat. This naturally low-carb, high-fat scenario is what many believe to be one of the key drivers of the success of Paleo eating. And, coincidentally, it's on the borderline of the practice of nutritional ketosis.

Low-carbers have recognized that their weight-loss plateaus are easily overcome when, for a period of time, they increase their dietary fat and lower their protein intake. Again, this borders on the keto diet. But interestingly, when these same low-carbers go long periods with extremely limited carbs and hit a bumpy spot of plateaus and health concerns such as hair loss and sleepless nights, an increase in carbs usually helps the situation. (See the discussion of carb-ups on pages 39 to 43 for an explanation.)

The approach I've taken to keto brings the Paleo and low-carb worlds together in a whole new way. If you're a member of a Paleo tribe, you'll be empowered to safely transition into, and maintain, a state of nutritional ketosis that's based on your already balanced approach to primal fare. If you're a low-carber already or don't assign yourself to any eating style whatsoever, I'm going to present you with a couple of mind-altering shifts to how you think about carbohydrates, guidance for developing a carb-up practice that may help you balance your health, and information about how focusing on high-quality foods and mindful food preparation can make all the difference in a low-carb diet.

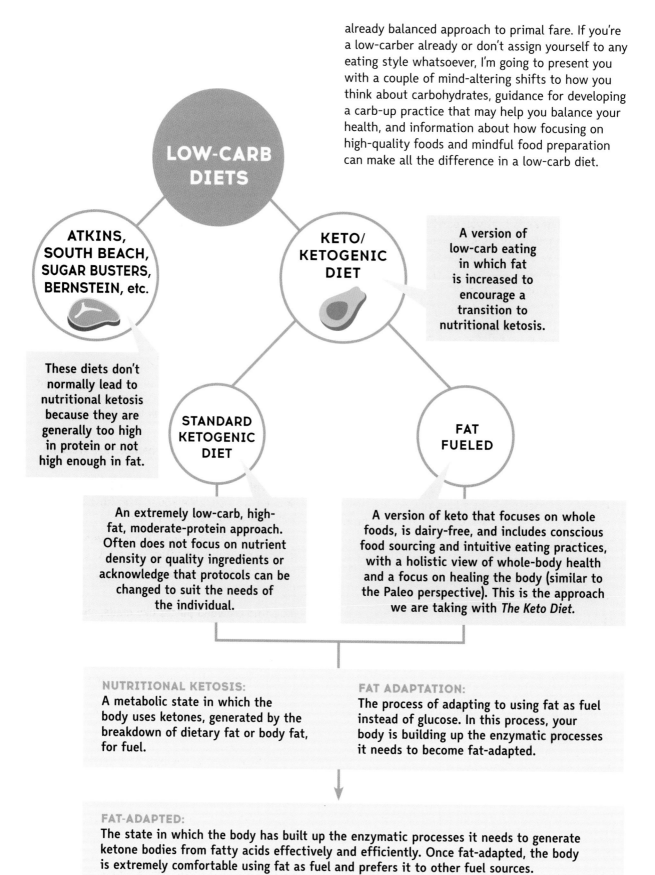

LOW-CARB DIETS

ATKINS, SOUTH BEACH, SUGAR BUSTERS, BERNSTEIN, etc.

These diets don't normally lead to nutritional ketosis because they are generally too high in protein or not high enough in fat.

KETO/ KETOGENIC DIET

A version of low-carb eating in which fat is increased to encourage a transition to nutritional ketosis.

STANDARD KETOGENIC DIET

An extremely low-carb, high-fat, moderate-protein approach. Often does not focus on nutrient density or quality ingredients or acknowledge that protocols can be changed to suit the needs of the individual.

FAT FUELED

A version of keto that focuses on whole foods, is dairy-free, and includes conscious food sourcing and intuitive eating practices, with a holistic view of whole-body health and a focus on healing the body (similar to the Paleo perspective). This is the approach we are taking with *The Keto Diet*.

NUTRITIONAL KETOSIS:
A metabolic state in which the body uses ketones, generated by the breakdown of dietary fat or body fat, for fuel.

FAT ADAPTATION:
The process of adapting to using fat as fuel instead of glucose. In this process, your body is building up the enzymatic processes it needs to become fat-adapted.

FAT-ADAPTED:
The state in which the body has built up the enzymatic processes it needs to generate ketone bodies from fatty acids effectively and efficiently. Once fat-adapted, the body is extremely comfortable using fat as fuel and prefers it to other fuel sources.

IS KETO RIGHT FOR YOU?

Your body sends you signals constantly, every moment of every day. But if you're not attuned to them, those signals may go completely unnoticed, so you keep doing things that are leading to the unhappiness or discontentment you feel toward your body, health, or your life in general.

The good news is that you don't need to sit on a meditation pillow for hours to know what your body needs. For many, increasing fat intake and lowering carbohydrate intake, coupled with a bit of self-care action (see page 14), is a great starting point for giving your body what it needs, without the kumbaya action. And once you've started giving your body what it needs, it's suddenly easier to hear what other things it's asking for.

Signs Your Body Needs More Fat

If you're wondering whether your body really wants or needs more fat, I've compiled some classic signs and symptoms. If you recognize yourself in two or more of the following, it could be a good indication that you're in need of some additional fat in your life. And that means you've come to the right place!

- You've tried every eating style, but none of them help you feel good and look great.
- You experience headaches, weight gain, sluggishness, constipation, and random symptoms that make your day-to-day challenging.
- You need afternoon pick-me-ups to get your brain working again.
- You know that your hormones are wonky—perhaps you're on hormone replacement therapy to treat it—and you're gaining weight like crazy.
- You could eat and eat and then eat some more. And sometimes you're hungry again just thirty to sixty minutes after eating.
- You seem to be allergic or sensitive to foods you never used to react to. Symptoms can include acne, bloating, constipation, itchy skin, or joint pain.
- Post-meal bloat is a real thing. "Move over, I've got a food baby!" is a constant line in your life.
- About thirty minutes after eating, you experience intense sleepiness, to the point where you'd like to just cuddle up and have a little snooze.
- No matter how hard you try to quit it, sugar just keeps coming back into your life.
- You have Candida and need to address it, but the restrictive diet that comes along with Candida removal is way too stressful for you right now.
- You often experience tiredness, breast tenderness, irritability, or cystic acne, or you've been told that your hormones are a bit wonky.
- Much of what you eat is steamed or low-fat, and it all tastes like cardboard.
- You have moments of extreme emotional highs and lows and have a hard time understanding what sparked the imbalance, or remembering that it occurred.
- Your feet, hands, or love handles are freezing most of the time.
- You feel like you could gain weight by just looking at a cupcake—no matter how little you eat, the weight doesn't budge.
- Your doctor has put you on a supplement to boost your levels of vitamin A, D, E, or K.
- It's been a couple of months since you had your period.
- You find crowded places like malls, shows, and events overwhelming. It's hard to focus, and you feel increasingly overstimulated the longer you stay.
- You have trouble recalling names and events. It takes you time to think of what you did yesterday or when you spoke to your best friend last.
- You've been told that your hair is just frizzy. But I can just about guarantee that's not the case!
- Summer, winter, fall, or spring, your skin flakes all the time.
- You get deep pains in your joints, generally early in the morning or a couple of hours after eating.
- You think about food constantly and have a "live to eat" instead of an "eat to live" outlook.

The Breakfast Test

Still not convinced that chowing down on fat could lead to good things for you? If you're a bit apprehensive of taking the plunge, a breakfast test is a simple way to dip your toe in the water. Don't worry, there's no studying involved in this test. In fact, it's focused solely on eating! That's a test we can all get behind, right?

NOTE: *Try to keep your calorie consumption between meals on testing days as similar as possible.*

Choose two mornings, preferably at least three days but no more than four days apart, where you carve out just ten to fifteen minutes for breakfast to perform the following test. (If the test days are more than four days apart, your hormonal cycle can affect the results of the test.)

The more similar the conditions on each test day, the more accurate the final results will be. For example, if the first test is on a workday, it's best to do the second test on a workday as well.

TEST DAY 1:	TEST DAY 2:
Eat a **high-carb, low-fat breakfast** no more than two hours after you wake.	Eat a **low-carb, high-fat breakfast** no more than two hours after you wake.

Keep the fat as low as possible, protein moderated, and carbs high! If you drink coffee or tea in the morning alongside your breakfast, keep it low-fat. Adding sugar is okay, but things like full-fat creamer are not.

Here are two possible breakfast options:

Keep the fat as high as possible, protein moderated, and carbs low! If you drink coffee or tea in the morning alongside your breakfast, combine it with a dollop of coconut oil in the blender and blend for thirty seconds before transferring back to the cup.

Here are two possible breakfast options:

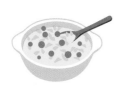 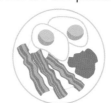 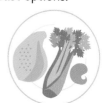

Oatmeal with water, fruit, and protein powder or egg whites cooked in.	Fruit smoothie with protein powder and a tablespoon or so of flax, chia, or hemp seeds (best if you're grain-sensitive)	Bacon and eggs with a small side of sautéed greens. Cook the eggs in leftover bacon grease for extra points!	Skin-on chicken thighs with raw celery and nut or seed butter

Go back to your normal way of eating for a couple of days before moving on to test day 2.

On both test days, note any changes in the way you feel and specifically track the following:

- Energy before and after the meal
- Energy throughout the day
- Mental clarity
- When you're hungry for your next meal
- What your food choices were like that day. Did you crave sweets in the afternoon? Did you binge on food when you got home from work?
- Were you bloated after the meal?
- Did you experience anxiety or a short temper?
- Did you experience a blood sugar crash, where you needed to eat right this hot moment or you'd punch someone in the mouth?

NOTE: *Many people report that on test day 2, they felt like they needed something sweet directly following breakfast. This is a signal that the body is searching for the carbs it thought it would get with breakfast but didn't. This is most often a simple sign that you're glucose-fueled, but it shouldn't influence the overall success of the test or your answers to these questions.*

Did you feel significantly better during and after test day 2? Told you! What a difference, right? Now imagine feeling like that every darn day.

Who the Keto Diet May Be Good For

If you have an awesome medical team or a history of health imbalances, it's always best to chat with your team about making the transition to keto. Getting direct support from a team of professionals who are familiar with your unique health history is invaluable, especially if you have diabetes, have kidney imbalances, or are pregnant.

I've seen keto help the following kinds of people. I am sure there are many, many more groups to add to this list, but it's a start!

1. **Men**
   Your body is a lot less complicated than women's, so it usually responds quickly and well to keto.

2. **Women**
   Be sure to review the Fat Fueled Profiles that include carb-up practices (see pages 48 and 49) and see if they will work for you—I've found carb-ups to be particularly helpful for women.

3. **People with severe allergies**

4. **Vegans and vegetarians**
   While it's a bit more challenging, you can maintain a state of ketosis while eating plant-based proteins. Aim for high-fat, lower-carb options (see page 116).

5. **People who have hit a weight-loss plateau**

6. **Restrictive dieters**

7. **Diabetics**
   Be sure to talk to your health-care team first.

8. **People with hypoglycemia**

9. **Candida sufferers**
   Keep an eye on your flare-ups, and if they worsen, go a bit lower in fat and replace it with protein.

10. **Acne sufferers**

11. **People with inflammatory conditions**

12. **People with digestive issues**

13. **People with thyroid imbalances**
    Be sure to review the Fat Fueled Profiles that include carb-up practices (see pages 48 and 49) and see if they will work for you.

14. **People without a gallbladder**
    Be sure to include ox bile with your meals.

15. **People with kidney disorders**
    Be sure to talk to your health-care team first.

16. **Pregnant women**
    Be sure to talk to your health-care team first.

17. **Women in menopause**

18. **People struggling with food obsession**

19. **People struggling with sugar cravings**

20. **Women on hormone replacement therapy**

21. **Athletes**

22. **Women who haven't had a period for more than three months (amenorrhea)**

23. **Children**
    Be sure to review the Fat Fueled Profiles that include carb-up practices (see pages 48 and 49) and see if they will work for you.

Of course, not everyone in the above groups will feel great on keto. This is okay! We're all different. But you don't know until you try, right?

WHAT ABOUT CHOLESTEROL? AND OTHER CONCERNS ABOUT EATING FAT

The picture I've painted of the high-fat keto eating style probably has your brain reeling with stories of high cholesterol, clogged arteries, heart attacks, and near-death experiences.

I want you to step back for a moment and look at the facts, facts that have not been muddled by an agenda. Because I have no vested interest in whether or not you eat keto. Really, I don't. While I think you may benefit from it, I don't know your body. Only you do. I'm simply presenting you with details I know about this eating style so that if what you're doing now isn't working, you have other options for improving your health.

Let's begin with what we know about cholesterol and how it works.

Simplifying the Cholesterol Conundrum

There are a lot of misconceptions about cholesterol and the role that it plays in the health of our hearts and beyond. Let's simplify.

First, cholesterol is not the enemy! This perfectly innocent sterol—a combination of a steroid and alcohol—is necessary for many essential bodily functions. It's needed to make sex hormones, such as estrogen, progesterone, testosterone, and DHEA; it repairs damaged cells and maintains the integrity of the cell to extend cell life; it transfers nutrients to the brain to protect from dementia; and it maintains the integrity of the intestinal tract. It also helps with serotonin receptor firing, which is essential for feeling happy, fabulous, and on top of our game, and it assists with vitamin D uptake, which is essential for healthy bones and nerves, muscle tone, insulin production, fertility, and a strong immune system.

Cholesterol also plays a huge role in combating systemic inflammation. Imagine your body is a house and inflammation is a fire. Cholesterol is the fire truck that comes racing in to put the fire out. Without the fire truck, the fire destroys the house. Without satisfactory levels of cholesterol, inflammation is left to do its thing with very little working against it. When allowed to run rampant, excess inflammation in the body makes it more susceptible to disease. Common conditions where inflammation is often at the root of the issue are overall body pain, asthma, gall bladder disease, allergies, ADD/ADHD, psoriasis, heart disease, diabetes, migraines, dental issues, cancer, Alzheimer's, eczema, thyroid issues, and more.

In summary: Cholesterol is important. Without it, we would die.

Cholesterol comes from two sources: the food we eat, and our own bodies, which produce it. Because much of the cholesterol that we consume cannot be absorbed, about 25 percent of the cholesterol in our body comes from the food we eat and 75 percent is synthesized by the body. The body tightly regulates the amount of cholesterol in the blood by controlling internal production. When we eat more cholesterol, we produce less, and vice versa. Eating more dietary cholesterol has little effect on cholesterol levels.

To be transported in the bloodstream, cholesterol enlists the help of lipoproteins: LDL (low-density lipoprotein) and HDL (high-density lipoprotein). Cholesterol is carried by these lipoproteins from the liver and gut to the rest of the body and back again.

HDL is associated with better cardiovascular health. The health implications of LDL depend on the size of the particles: There are large, puffy particles and small, dense particles. Higher amounts of large, puffy LDL particles are associated with normal cholesterol and triglyceride levels. Higher amounts of small, dense LDL particles are associated with low HDL, elevated triglycerides, and a tendency to develop high blood sugar and type 2 diabetes.

Imagine your bloodstream is a children's birthday party. LDL particles are the children who carry presents over to the present table, and cholesterol is the presents themselves. We used to believe that the more presents a child brought to the party (that is, the higher the concentration of cholesterol being carried by an LDL particle), the higher the risk of heart disease. However, more-recent studies show that it's the overall number of children (the number of LDL particles) that matters. Imagine a house filled with a hundred screaming children instead of the ten you had planned. No matter how many presents each child brings, a house filled with screaming children is a house filled with screaming children. Moreover, when the children are bubbly and happy—they're fluffy LDL particles—the better the party is; when the children are sour and sullen—small, dense LDL particles—the worse the party is. We want happy, bubbly children to make the party a hit!

> If you're curious about how many of the fluffy LDL and how many of the small, dense LDL you have, your count of HDL, and other cholesterol stats, an NMR lipid profile test is the blood test you're looking for.

For the vast majority of individuals, a ketogenic diet reduces the number of small LDL particles and increases HDL. And for some people—I experienced this when I went keto—the total cholesterol level will go up. This is not as big a deal as we've been led to believe. As long as small LDL stays low, the total cholesterol count is less important. In fact, the ratio between your triglyceride count and HDL count can be a stronger indicator of heart health than your total cholesterol number. To determine your ratio, divide your triglycerides by your HDL. If that number is under 1.0, you're in a good place.

What we want to pay attention to instead of total cholesterol is our blood sugar, triglycerides, HDL count, and hs-CRP (high-sensitivity C-reactive protein), which measures the amount of inflammation in the body. If inflammation increases on a ketogenic diet, it's usually because of nuts, seeds, a food sensitivity (dairy is a common trigger), or products that contain artificial sweeteners, flavors, and/or colors.

Other Myths About Dietary Fat

When I was first introduced to high-fat eating, I was scared, skeptical, and quick to dismiss it as irresponsible mumbo jumbo. It challenged every belief I had about my body and nutrition, and the food rules I had set for myself as a result.

But I'm a logical gal, so I decided to investigate, and I'm so happy I did. Here's what I found out about dietary fat consumption. (Hopefully it goes without saying, but all this applies to healthy, natural fats, not artificial fats like partially hydrogenated oils and trans fats.)

MYTH **"Fat makes you fat."**
Au contraire! First, body fat is created when excess carbohydrates need to be stored.

Second, increasing dietary fat consumption can help you lose weight in many ways. It keeps you satiated, reducing crazy hunger pains and preventing overeating and bingeing. Omega-3 fats help turn on genes that are involved with fat-burning while turning off the genes that store fat. And finally, eating a greater proportion of fat allows for balance of hormones such as testosterone and estrogen, and that makes losing fat and maintaining a lean physique much easier. (Note: These points assume that you decrease your consumption of carbohydrates as you increase your consumption of fats.)

MYTH **"Fat clogs your arteries and leads to heart disease."**
What causes arterial plaque is not fat but cholesterol—and although cholesterol is found in fat, dietary cholesterol has very little effect on blood cholesterol levels. (See page 31 for more.) As far as leading to heart disease: Increasing dietary fat consumption reduces your blood triglyceride level, the main risk factor in heart disease. Low-fat diets, on the other hand, can actually cause triglycerides to go up.

MYTH **"Fat has no nutrients."**
Fat is full of nutrients! It's loaded with vitamins A, E, and K2. In fact, fat-soluble vitamins need fat in order to be absorbed by the body.

Plus, there are all kinds of benefits that come with fat that aren't often advertised:

- **Adequate intake of healthy fats helps prevent depression (which can be a side effect of a low-fat diet). Depression can be caused by a deficiency of cholesterol and fat in the brain, resulting in lower levels of the neurotransmitter serotonin, which makes people feel good.**

- **Increasing dietary fats and reducing carbohydrates lowers blood sugar and insulin levels and helps keep blood sugar stable. As a result, you'll have fewer cravings and steadier energy.**

- **Fats help you maintain your ideal weight by keeping your metabolism balanced and healthy.**

If you're still on the fence, try this cravings challenge: For a week, anytime you crave a high-carb or high-sugar food, have a high-fat snack—an avocado, a spoonful of sunflower butter, a handful of macadamia nuts, or even a glob of coconut oil. Within ten minutes, the cravings should be gone.

I always thought I was healthy. I ate the recommended six to eight servings of grains, lots of fruit and dairy, and little to no fat. I ate my salads with fat-free dressing, carbed up before my hour-long runs (which I did five to six days a week), and took vitamins.

Now, looking back on this, I laugh a little because it's funny that I thought that was healthy, but mostly because I'm so glad I am not that person anymore.

In 2008, at 19 years old, I was diagnosed with type 1 diabetes. I was told to increase my carbs to 175–250 grams daily, avoid fat at all costs, and eat a starchy meal before bed to keep my body from going into ketosis (which they linked incorrectly to diabetic ketoacidosis). I was a machine of the system and did as I was told until my blood glucose meter started to look like a roller coaster. Seeing those sugar spikes and drops was the seed that started me thinking maybe the approach was all wrong. I was feeling like crap and put on about 20 pounds.

In 2012, I was diagnosed with Hashimoto's thyroiditis. Feeling betrayed by my own body and the health-care system, I switched to a functional medicine doctor. She discovered that I have celiac disease and recommended an Autoimmune Paleo diet for the next three to four months to heal my body and stop the inflammation. I finally started to feel better. This got me going down the path of nonconventional care.

Somehow I stumbled upon the keto diet, which coincidentally is also the diet they used to put diabetics on before big pharma came into the picture.

Now, a couple months into eating keto, I've already seen a huge improvement. My blood sugars are so incredibly stable, my A1C is now the lowest it's ever been, and I am not a slave to my snacks. I have been able to cut my insulin needs in half, and I haven't had a blood sugar low since I started eating keto.

My cholesterol numbers have improved. In 2010, at age 21, my total cholesterol was 197 and I was given a statin. I took it for three days, then stopped because it didn't feel right. I have since switched to an amazing endocrinologist who fully supports high-fat, low-carb and even told me that when I eat, to eat mindfully and peacefully. She is not concerned with my cholesterol numbers (most doctors would see 230 total and freak out). One of the many reasons why I love her so much.

I love Leanne's keto approach, which revolves around real food, because that helps significantly with my three autoimmune diseases. Maybe if I had adopted this diet from the start I might only have one autoimmune disease instead of three...or maybe none at all! At least I'm hopeful that I'll never have four.

Rachel
New Hampshire

I'm a former vegetarian who ate lots of carbs and experienced daily sugar/salt cravings for years. My thyroid and blood sugar numbers were constantly on the rise. I didn't get it: I was doing everything right, eating as healthy as could be.

Then came Leanne, a compassionate, knowledgeable, funny, awesome keto guardian angel! After seeing her website listed on one of my favorite blogs in April 2016, I started adding more healthy fats to my diet, cut way back on sugar and simple carbs, and amped up my intake of whole foods. My cravings were gone...I repeat, GONE...within 2 days! Since incorporating the advice Leanne shares on her blog, podcast, and YouTube channel, as well as purchasing The Keto Bundle, I've also lost weight, my blood work numbers are heading in a better direction, and I don't feel beholden to well-meaning but often outdated health advice.

I'm still in awe over how great I feel, physically and mentally. Thank you SO much for encouraging us to put on our Big Girl Pants, take responsibility for our well-being, and really listen to our bodies.

Karen
New York

CHAPTER 2

FIFTY SHADES OF THE KETO DIET: DO WHAT WORKS FOR YOU

This is where the Fat Fueled approach takes a major turn from other, stricter—and therefore almost impossible to follow long-term—"standard" ketogenic diets.

I'm a high-fat keto enthusiast who promotes the benefits of a low-carb diet, yet I eat 75 to 150 grams of carbs per day and encourage others to do the same to see how it feels. Ah, yes, and I recommend that most of those carbs be eaten at night. At night! What gives?

I've embraced the gray area of keto, and there are at least fifty shades of it, so hold on to your fat! I mean, hat.

There are multiple ways to achieve ketosis, none of them better than the others. Each lets you experience the amazing benefits of the keto diet. Which one you choose depends on your needs and how your body responds to keto. Heck, I bounce between different approaches depending on how my day is going. There is a lot of versatility here.

This chapter gets to the heart of personalizing keto so that it works for you. I'll cover three keto eating styles, each with a different ratio of fat, protein, and carbs, and then, in the Fat Fueled Profiles, I'll describe five different ways to enjoy keto, depending on your needs. (I first developed the profiles for my digital program, Fat Fueled, but in this book I've added two new profiles based on user experiences.)

Some of the profiles include a practice of eating carbohydrates at certain times; others don't. Some call for additional protein intake; others don't. There are multiple paths to the same destination, giving you the space to find the one that works best for you. All of them are designed to help you benefit from a high-fat eating style without obsessing about measuring ketones, tracking your meals, or ensuring that you're in ketosis 24/7.

But first, I want to explain why keto can work with different approaches. Most guides to the ketogenic diet emphasize strict tracking and control of macronutrients, especially when it comes to carbs and protein. But I've found that allowing for a little more carbs or protein can be the difference between feeling great and feeling miserable.

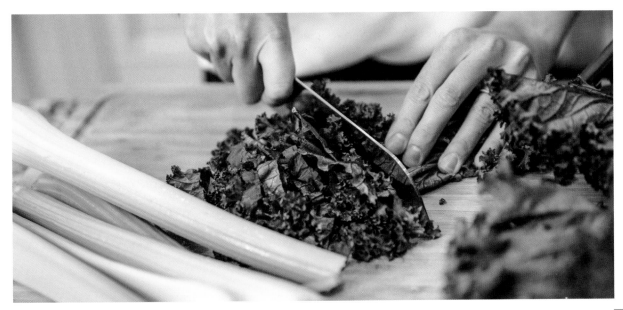

PROTEIN AND WHERE THE STANDARD KETOGENIC DIET FALLS SHORT

Protein is a hot topic in keto, or at least a confusing one. Why? Because the word on the street is that any protein in excess of what we need immediately, even a small amount, will be turned into glucose through spontaneous gluconeogenesis (GNG), kicking us out of ketosis.

There's a lot of fearmongering in the space of ketogenic diets and protein intake, but since there's a Fat Fueled Profile that calls for high protein, you can see that there's a bit of gray there, too. Sadly, as with most things in the ketogenic realm, more studies are needed on the role of GNG on a ketogenic diet, especially in the case of women, because I'm sure our hormone profile plays a role in the GNG pathway. I will, however, try to paint a picture of the ins and outs of protein on a ketogenic diet, so that you can make an informed choice for yourself.

If you remember from the previous chapter, gluconeogenesis is the process by which glucose is made out of noncarbohydrate sources. Once you're in ketosis, your body uses ketones as its primary fuel source and makes the glucose it needs from the protein and fat you consume. As long as you're consuming enough protein, your body won't use protein from your muscles for GNG.

So here's a potential problem with standard moderate-protein ketogenic diets: Because we know that GNG uses dietary protein to create glucose, a lot of individuals believe that the less protein consumed, the less glucose created. The problem with eating too little protein is that you run the risk of GNG using muscle to fuel the process.

Know that GNG isn't out to get you. GNG is a demand-driven, not supply-driven, process. When our body needs the additional glucose, GNG ramps up to create it, providing the body with a small amount of glucose for parts of the body that can run only on glucose, such as red blood cells and parts of the brain. If we don't need extra glucose, GNG will not just spontaneously convert protein into glucose, leading to ridiculously high glucose levels. GNG is used to maintain tight controls on glucose levels in the blood via a hormone called glucagon. If glucagon isn't saying, "Yo man, we need some more glucose up in here," GNG won't randomly start converting proteins into glucose.

15 REASONS WHY BALANCED PROTEIN IS GOOD

1. Aids in body weight regulation
2. Provides balanced vitamins, minerals, and fatty acids
3. Benefits bone health
4. Benefits workout recovery
5. Enhances muscle mass and performance
6. Ensures nitrogen balance
7. Increases satiety when paired with physical activity
8. Prevents lean muscle loss during weight-loss programs
9. Promotes muscle repair and growth
10. Lowers the hunger hormone, ghrelin
11. Reduces risk of osteoporosis and fractures
12. Reduces cravings
13. Increases fat-burning (the body requires more energy, or calories, to process dietary protein)
14. Slows age-related muscle loss
15. Lowers triglycerides

On the flip side, protein consumption stimulates glucagon, and it's entirely possible that excess consumption of protein will therefore stimulate GNG, making it more challenging to achieve ketosis—though perhaps not as much as we've been led to believe.

In cases like this, I'd like to think that it all comes down to balance. Consuming too much protein won't work for you if you want to slide into ketosis easily, but consuming too little won't work, either.

Regardless of how things are working on a molecular level, the important thing is to listen to your body. You may need more protein in certain situations—when recovering from surgery, for instance, or during times of high stress—or if you're experiencing certain symptoms, like achy joints or poor sleep. See page 37 for a list.

SIGNS YOU NEED MORE PROTEIN

You have metabolic problems.

Your sleep sucks.

You love running, cycling, and other cardio activities.

You train hard.

You want to build muscle.

You're over 50.

You're always hungry.

You're recovering from surgery.

You're stressed.

You're vegan.

You've cut your calorie intake to lose weight.

Your blood sugar is all over the place.

Your joints ache.

Balancing Your Protein Intake

Sadly, there's no magic formula for finding the balance between too much and too little protein. However, I think a good general rule is to get 20 to 35 percent of your calories from protein, at least to start.

In my private practice, almost every single woman I worked with was too low in protein. This was primarily due to a misinterpretation of the information out there on becoming fat-adapted. I like to call it the "less is more" mentality. It goes something like this: "Well, if I have to eat less protein to become fat-adapted, I'll eat even less of it so I adapt quicker!" Unfortunately, this logic is flawed to the core. I think many of us on the ketogenic path go through it; I know I had my moment in the lower-than-it-should-be protein sun. The truth is, we need protein, and the body will not become fat-adapted any faster if it's deprived of protein.

Here's my approach: eat as much as possible without it negatively affecting your numbers. When I say "numbers," I mean on the scale or in your blood work (that includes the level of ketones in your blood). This strategy goes for carbohydrates, proteins, supplements, you name it. If I can get away with eating 100 grams of protein in a day without spiking my blood sugar or affecting my ability to get into ketosis, you're damn right I'll do it!

Now, if you're having three meals a day, with a balanced focus on animal-based proteins and a sprinkle of plant-based proteins, you're probably fine just the way you are. However, if protein has taken a backseat in your life, I urge you to look at what you're eating, play around with boosting your protein intake, and see where you land with the whole thing. You might even find it helpful to try a protein shake, like the Keto Milkshake on page 423.

IF YOU WANT TO EAT ALL THE CARBS . . . DO IT!

In Chapter 1, I talked a lot about how and why the keto diet works. Now I'm about to tell you why it sometimes doesn't work and what you can do to adjust it. (I know, I'm like the man in Katy Perry's song "Hot N Cold.") If you've struggled with keto, know that you're not alone in the fight, and you may find the answer you need in the following pages. (Shout out to all of my chronic dieting buddies! You'll be feeling this message, too.)

Avoiding the Binge

Ever been on a thirty-day diet but were able to follow it for only two days? You know, the start-stop cycle of good intentions and fresh starts followed by binges and restarts?

Me, too.

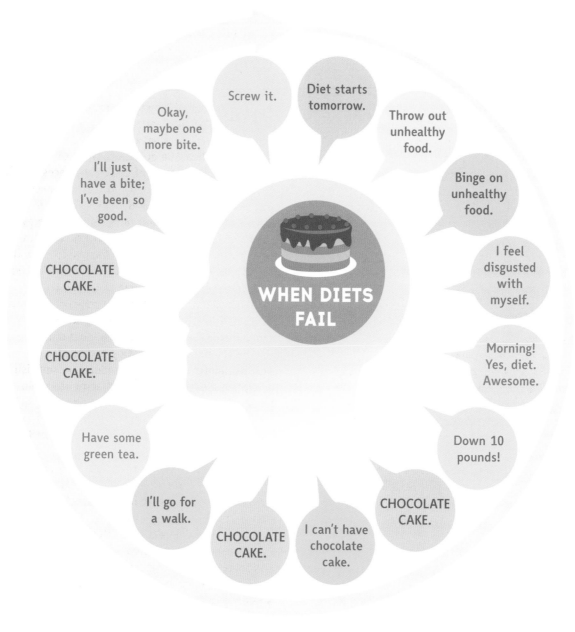

When I was following a strict ketogenic eating style, I binged. A lot. I'd start out restricting my food, running a 500- to 750-calorie deficit, and calculating the calories and macros of every morsel that entered my body. I'd maintain this routine for about ten days, and then it would all fall apart. I'd find myself deep in an eating frenzy that ended only when all the food was gone, regardless of how full I was.

The bizarre thing is that the biweekly binges actually improved my body composition. The day after a binge, I would wake up with more muscle tone and very little interest in eating; I was easily able to fast for a full twenty-four to forty-eight hours following a binge.

But while this process helped me achieve the body I'd always dreamed of having, I wasn't happy. I felt restricted, unsettled, out of control, and absolutely, totally crazy. And the guilt was unbearable at times.

So I decided to start back at square one and built myself a ketogenic diet that didn't lead to epic restriction and massive guilt. I opened up the rules and stopped counting my macros and tracking every little morsel. I kept my general diet about the same, but I transformed my binges into carb-ups, and that made all the difference. Creating a carb-up practice within a ketogenic diet was the best thing I ever did for my health. It helped me get my period back after eight years, healed my hypothyroidism, supported my adrenal dysfunction, assisted with energy output in training, and so much more.

For me and a lot of other people, including carbs every once in a while on your low-carb, high-fat ketogenic eating style is a great idea. And I've got the science to explain why.

If you're on a ketogenic diet because of a health imbalance, condition, or concern, it's best to chat with a medical professional to determine if the carb-up approach aligns with your health-care plan. However, as someone with a tendency for hypothyroidism, adrenal fatigue, anxiety, and paralyzing stress, I've found that a carb-up practice is the key to my success at ketogenic living.

What Is a Carb-Up?

A carb-up (also known as cyclical ketosis) is a period of time, generally in the evening, when you eat a touch of carbs with dinner or dessert simply by swapping the fat you would normally eat for carbohydrates. It's used to address certain side effects that some people experience on a ketogenic diet—but it can also be used by anyone who feels better being fat-fueled than glucose-fueled but also wants to eat cake on their birthday, for instance, or do other ordinary carb-related things.

> The key to successful carb-ups is to think of your fat intake as inversely related to your carb intake. If you're increasing your carb intake for the evening, then you are also reducing your fat intake. It is like a teeter-totter.

If you're a low-carb advocate, you're probably saying, "Did she just recommend that we eat carbs, get fat and sick, and have our blood sugar do crazy things?" But hear me out! Carbohydrates—or rather glucose, the basic form of carbs—are necessary for specific actions in the body, including converting thyroid hormone to its active form, which in turn is necessary for metabolism regulation, energy maintenance, and digestive regularity. Without the conversion, these things don't happen as smoothly, which can leave us feeling sick or fatigued. Glucose is also fuel for the brain and red blood cells. Although the body can create glucose on its own to meet these needs (see page 26), sometimes consuming a small amount can be beneficial.

The key here is that eating carbohydrates may be helpful for some individuals, in smallish *quantities*. Please read that last sentence again, because my message of carb-ups sometimes gets lost and twisted, like in the telephone game, and soon I'm touted as a high-carb enthusiast. Yikes—I don't think so.

Whether you decide to practice carb-ups or not, we know that carbohydrates in excess aren't fabulous for us and that fats are pretty darn nourishing. Wherever you're at with your diet right now, we'll be doing a little switcheroo of the food pyramid—more fats, less carbs—but not going as far as committing to all fats, zero carbs. If you choose not to practice carb-ups, your "more fat, less carbs" approach will include low-carb vegetables and omit starchy vegetables and most fruits. If you choose to practice carb-ups, your "more fat, less carbs" approach will still include low-carb vegetables but will also include a couple of starchy vegetables and fruits sprinkled in during your carb-up practice.

The key to a successful carb-up practice is doing it only after you're fat-adapted, when your body already chooses fat as its primary fuel over carbohydrates. The process of becoming fat-adapted drains the glycogen that's stored in your muscles and liver. The more that glycogen is drained and the longer your body is fully in fat-burning, ketone-generating mode, the better your body is able to switch back and forth between glucose-burning and fat-burning.

> See pages 48–49 for the three different approaches to carb-ups and how to implement them.

It takes about ten to fifteen days (or more, depending on your body) of following a low-carb, high-fat eating style to become fat-adapted. After that, your body has ramped up the processes needed to slide easily into fat-burning mode, even if you consume a couple of carbs here or there. Even though your body burns the glucose you've ingested, it still prefers fat—you're still fat-adapted.

> **Your body prefers fat as its fuel source once it's fat-adapted. Practicing carb-ups will *not* kick you out of ketosis. It just provides your body with a touch of glucose before it jumps back over to fat burning.**

While most people do well starting carb-ups only after they're fat-adapted, some people literally aren't able to wait. I've worked with clients whose quality of sleep plummeted after just two days of eating low-carb. So for them, it's out of the question to go thirty, fifteen, sometimes even just ten days with minimal carbs until they're fat-adapted.

This is why I created the Fat Fueled Profiles (see pages 47 to 49). If you'd like to wait until you're fat-adapted and then carb-up once a week or so, there's an outline for that. If you'd like to wait until you're fat-adapted and then switch over to having carbs every night, there's an outline for that. If you literally can't go more than a couple of days on low-carb and need the carbs daily, there's an outline for that.

Why You May Want to Carb Up

For me, carb-ups were especially helpful for overcoming weight plateaus, balancing hormones, improving sleep quality, freeing up my food choices, eliminating all-out carb binges, improving athletic performance and muscle strength, and more. If you are experiencing issues like these on your keto diet, it may be time for you to entertain the idea of carb-ups.

And if you've been eating low-carb for a while and never truly feel satisfied, listen up! Another benefit to carb-ups is increased leptin sensitivity. Leptin is the hormone that makes us feel full and satisfied after a meal, and it's released in response to increased carb consumption. After eating low-carb for a long time, our cells can become slightly leptin resistant. Adding a touch of carbohydrates here and there while following a keto diet boosts leptin intermittently, keeping your body sensitive to leptin, so you'll feel satisfied after meals. This is why, in my estimation, fasting is so much easier the morning following a carb-up, which has benefits of its own (see pages 68 to 71).

> If you've been on a low-carb eating style for quite some time, the carb-up concept will probably feel a bit foreign to you—and your body. It took me a few tries to feel okay mentally with the whole thing, and my digestion took about double that to be okay with the carbs again. Now, I can't go without this practice.

Of course, some people benefit from extremely limiting their carbs all the time—it varies greatly from person to person. For instance, someone with type 1 diabetes might believe that they would do better with extremely limited carbs—and they could be totally right. But what if you're a woman with type 1 diabetes who hasn't had her period in three years, or who has an extremely stressful job, or who just got diagnosed with hypothyroidism? Each of these things can change your body's landscape and your relationship with carbs.

What I'm trying to convey here is that the right amount of carbohydrates for you may be different from that of anyone else reading this book right now. It's okay to eat fats, limit your carbs, see how you feel, adjust your macros, and repeat. If you feel great on an extremely low amount of carbs, awesome! If you don't feel so great, slightly increase your carbs with carb-ups.

For signs that you're fat-adapted and information on how to test for ketones, head to page 63.

Timing Is Everything

I firmly believe that there's a time and a place for carbs. And the time I'm going to recommend will probably feel a little weird to you. I'm about to tell you to eat carbs at night.

When we first wake up in the morning, cortisol, which moves energy out of storage, is elevated, and therefore so is blood glucose. Because of this rise in blood glucose, we're more insulin sensitive first thing in the morning; as the day goes on we become less and less sensitive to the effects of insulin. This means that insulin is better able to push glucose into cells in the morning.

This is why we are told that if we're eating carbs, we should eat them in the morning. But just because we're insulin sensitive in the morning doesn't mean that's when we should be eating insulin-spiking carbs. I'm of the belief that the body is most insulin sensitive during that time because it's trying to get the naturally elevated blood glucose, which gives us energy to get going when we wake up, back down to normal levels. Eating carbs counteracts that, sending blood glucose and insulin up even higher—causing a midmorning blood sugar crash.

Consuming carbs in the morning can very easily turn the day into one of those all-day carb feasts—eating every two hours, experiencing brain fog and poor work performance, and making imbalanced nutrition choices. When we start the day with carbs, we tend to run with carbs all day long. Oatmeal at breakfast turns into an apple for a snack, a sandwich at lunch, dried fruit in the afternoon, and a heaping bowl of white rice with veggies and chicken for dinner. Once we climb on the carb train in the morning, it's hard to get off.

Eating carbs in the morning also disrupts our natural fat-burning. The hormone status of the body as we awaken is primed for fat-burning thanks to cortisol, ghrelin, and growth hormone. As you sleep, cortisol levels increase, reaching their all-time high first thing in the morning. Cortisol releases glucose into the bloodstream by breaking down glycogen stores. When glycogen stores are depleted, we're in a fine place to release fat from fat cells. Ghrelin also peaks as you awaken and stimulates the release of growth hormone, which encourages fat-burning and muscle-building.

Between cortisol helping make fat available to burn and growth hormone, which is stimulated by ghrelin, encouraging fat-burning, we're primed to burn fat first thing in the morning. But in order for all this to occur, cortisol must not be interrupted by insulin. Eating carbs first thing in the morning causes a spike in insulin, putting a wedge in fat-burning and stopping these processes from doing what is natural.

WHEN WE EAT CARBS IN THE MORNING

- Further increase of already elevated glucose and insulin levels
- Ongoing hunger throughout the day as we ride the blood sugar roller coaster from meal to meal
- Brain fog
- Instant stop to the natural morning fat-burning process
- More challenging to access fat stores for energy throughout the day
- Fatigue, energy crash as your body continues to hunger for a quick glucose fix
- Tendency to eat carbs all day

All these are reasons I vote not to eat carbs in the morning. How about the flip side—why is it good to eat carbs at night?

Replenishes Your Systems
When you're already fat-adapted and have a touch of carbohydrate in the evening, your body uses it to replenish the systems that may be in need of glucose, such as your endocrine system, muscular system, or nervous system, and slides back into fat-burning mode by morning. Although the body's metabolism does slow down overall during sleep, this only holds true for fat and protein oxidation. Carbohydrate oxidation continues at the same rate and begins to increase before awakening.

Provides Better Sleep and More Serotonin
Eating carbs at night helps us prepare for sleep by increasing the brain's uptake of tryptophan, the protein found in poultry that's so often credited with causing post–Thanksgiving dinner sleepiness. Tryptophan is also used to create the neurotransmitter serotonin, so eating carbs at night helps boost serotonin—which leads to improved

mood, better sleep, increased weight loss, increased fat loss, faster post-workout recovery, and better immune health. And the improved sleep we get from eating carbs at night benefits insulin sensitivity.

Supports Muscles

If you work out after work or in the evenings, nighttime is the perfect time for eating carbs. After a workout, your muscles are like sponges, ready to soak up that glucose goodness, which insulin shuttles straight to muscle tissues.

Lets You Sleep Through Side Effects

If you feel like you need a touch of carbs to balance out your low-carb approach, consuming them in the evening not only provides you with all these benefits, it also helps you sleep through the brain fog and blood sugar spike and subsequent crash that result from consuming carbs.

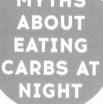

MYTHS ABOUT EATING CARBS AT NIGHT

★ ★

MYTH

Eat your carbs in the morning so that you have all day to burn them off.

1

TRUTH

Eating carbs in the morning sets you up for a blood sugar roller coaster and an endless feeding frenzy, along with difficulty concentrating. Try it for yourself: see the breakfast test on page 30.

MYTH

If you eat carbs at night, you'll gain weight.

2

TRUTH

Carbohydrates don't magically add to your waistline after the clock strikes 6 p.m. Excess carbs are stored as body fat at any time; conversely, if your body needs the glucose from carbs, it'll use it, no matter the time of day.

MYTH

Your metabolic rate declines when you sleep, so carbs aren't burned at the same rate.

3

TRUTH

Metabolism does slow down to about 35% below normal as you sleep, but only for fat and protein oxidation! Carbohydrate oxidation doesn't significantly change, and it actually begins to increase before you wake. Your body loves to burn carbohydrates while you sleep.

MYTH

You shouldn't eat after 5 p.m.

4

TRUTH

We are programmed to be night eaters. Think of our Paleolithic ancestors, hunting all day and eating all night. Or consider your ravenous hunger at the end of a long workday. This is not a coincidence. Eating at night increases leptin sensitivity, which leads to feeling satiated in the morning, encourages a longer fasting period, and sustains fat-burning.

- Avoidance of brain fog
- No energy crash!
- Accelerated fat loss
- No cravings, better nutrition choices
- Ability to mobilize and burn fat all day long
- Improved leptin sensitivity
- Promotion of fat loss and muscle retention
- Increased tryptophan uptake in the brain (for functional sleep and boosted serotonin)
- Boosted serotonin leads to increased weight loss, increased fat loss, faster post-workout recovery, and improved immune health
- Better sleep
- Increased insulin sensitivity

Newbies:
When to Start Carbing Up

You don't have to carb up, ever. Some people do better without carb-ups, while others need to carb up one, two, or sometimes even seven days a week. How your body responds to carb-ups is entirely unique to you. (As an observation, though, I find that women are more likely to need carb-ups than men, probably because of our more complex hormone landscape.)

My straightforward answer on when a newbie "should" carb up:

- When ketone tests show consistently high levels for five days (see pages 63 to 65 for information on ketone testing).

  OR

- When you exhibit three or more signs of being fat-adapted. Generally, this occurs around the ten- to fifteen-day mark of eating keto. At this time, most people have switched over to fat as the primary fuel source. However, stress can affect our ability to switch into fat-burning mode—see page 90.

Keto Veterans:
Signs It's Time for a Carb-Up

If you've been eating low-carb or ketogenic for some time—thirty days or more—and you are experiencing any of the following symptoms, it may be a good time to carb up. However, if you're rocking the keto life with the breeze in your hair and the sun on your face, don't change anything! Carb-ups are completely optional—a tool for those who need them.

It may be time to try a couple of carb-ups if, since you've started eating this way, you've experienced any of the following:

- Never-ending weight-loss plateau
- Imbalanced hormones
- Poor sleep quality
- Hair falling out
  Although many in the low-carb space say that this is a natural reaction to going low-carb and should end at some point, you need to listen to your body.
- Feeling restricted in your food choices
- Carb bingeing
- Issues with muscle growth; not getting the results you want from your workouts
- Stalled progress at the gym
- Low body temperature
- Difficulty maintaining even moderate intensity while training

CUSTOMIZING KETO

My Fat Fueled approach to keto is designed to help you customize your diet to fit you. It has three main paths to keto, each of which has a different ratio of fat, protein, and carbs. There are also five Fat Fueled Profiles to choose from, some of which include carb-ups and some of which do not.

Take a look at the three paths and see which seems to make the most sense for you. Then read through the Fat Fueled Profile(s) that fit the path you chose and select a profile to try. If, after two weeks, the path and profile you picked don't seem to be working, try something else! The goal is to find what works specifically for you.

Paths to Keto

Depending on your needs, you might do best with a low-carb/high-fat keto approach (Path 1), a moderate-fat/high-protein keto approach (Path 2), or a low-carb/high-fat keto approach that includes carb-ups (Path 3).

> Avoid the funky symptoms that can occur on Path 1 by eating enough protein! Listen to your body and eat more protein when you need to. For more, see page 37.

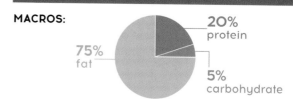

PATH 1: LOW CARB/HIGH FAT

MACROS:

75% fat

20% protein

5% carbohydrate

FAT FUELED PROFILE: Classic Keto (page 47)

This path doesn't include carb-ups, ever. It's the most straightforward way to get into ketosis, as well as the most traditional—which means that you'll find a lot of online and print resources for it. It also gets you into ketosis faster than the other paths.

However, it's heavily restrictive. And if you're sticking to this path after you've already become fat-adapted, there are a couple of possible side effects: It can affect your anaerobic training/workouts by limiting muscle growth and reducing energy output, and if you don't consume enough protein or fast for too long (see pages 68 to 72 for fasting on keto), it can lead to low blood sugar and cortisol irregularities. If this happens to you, eat more protein (see Path 2) or stop fasting until your symptoms improve.

THIS PATH IS GOOD FOR:

- Those who are in the process of becoming fat-adapted
- Those who became fat-adapted on this path and feel fabulous after being adapted for at least thirty days
- Sedentary or less-active individuals
- Those seeking weight loss
- Those without hormone imbalances
- Menopausal and post-menopausal women
- Aerobic athletes (more on page 74)
- Anyone whose health-care team has recommended a strict ketogenic approach

PATH 2: MODERATE FAT/HIGH PROTEIN

MACROS:

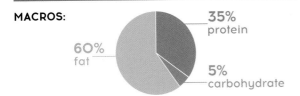

60% fat

35% protein

5% carbohydrate

FAT FUELED PROFILE: Pumped Keto (page 47)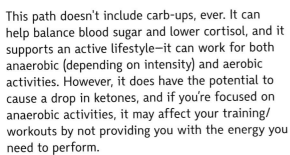

This path doesn't include carb-ups, ever. It can help balance blood sugar and lower cortisol, and it supports an active lifestyle—it can work for both anaerobic (depending on intensity) and aerobic activities. However, it does have the potential to cause a drop in ketones, and if you're focused on anaerobic activities, it may affect your training/ workouts by not providing you with the energy you need to perform.

If you're a vegan or vegetarian, this path is a no-go due to the high protein and extremely low carb requirements.

I like to think of this path as a transitional one. Rarely would I recommend that someone start with Path 2, but if you feel like Path 1 isn't working—especially if you're experiencing blood sugar irregularities (shakiness, anxiety, nervousness, irritability, confusion, dizziness, and/or nausea) or cortisol imbalances (sleeplessness, restlessness, and/or a tired-but-wired feeling)—this can be a great alternative. However, some react really well to starting on this path and stay here permanently!

THIS PATH IS GOOD FOR:

- Hypoglycemic individuals
- Those who experience symptoms of blood sugar irregularities or cortisol imbalances on Path 1 after becoming fat-adapted
- Those who don't feel quite right on Path 1 but are not interested in doing carb-ups
- Those who experience constant hunger on Path 1
- Those who are struggling to break through weight-loss plateaus

NOTE: *This path may not be right for insulin-dependent diabetics. Learn more on page 31.*

PATH 3: PATH 1 with CARB-UPS

MACROS:

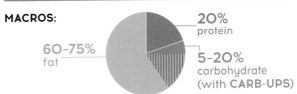

60–75% fat

20% protein

5–20% carbohydrate (with CARB-UPS)

FAT FUELED PROFILES: Full Keto (page 48)

Adapted Fat Burner (page 48)

Daily Fat Burner (page 49)

Think of Path 3 as Path 1 with carb-ups. On a daily, biweekly, or weekly basis, carbohydrates take the place of fats for a short time, preferably at night. (See pages 39 to 41 for my take on carb-ups.)

The benefits of this approach primarily mirror the benefits of carbing up: It reduces feelings of restriction that are often experienced on Paths 1 and 2; it supplies glucose for processes that require it, such as converting thyroid hormone to its active form; and it ameliorates potential symptoms of physiological insulin resistance (see page 96). It's also fabulous for muscle growth.

However, carb-ups can stimulate bingelike behavior if they're approached from a place of lack and restriction. And if you don't stick to healthy carbs (see page 117), they may lead to gas and bloating.

THIS PATH IS GOOD FOR:

- Fat-adapted individuals
- Anaerobic athletes who need carbs to perform (more on page 74)
- Individuals with hormone imbalances
- Women of reproductive age
- Individuals with adrenal dysfunction
- Those seeking weight loss that's focused on body healing
- Those who are struggling to break through weight-loss plateaus

NOTE: *This path may not be right for insulin-dependent diabetics. Learn more on page 31.*

PATH 1: Low Carb/High Fat

Fat Fueled Profile: CLASSIC KETO (page 47) **ck**

NO CARB-UPS

+ Fastest route to ketosis

! Heavily restrictive

! Without enough protein, may lead to low blood sugar, muscle wasting, and cortisol irregularities

 GOOD IF YOU'RE:

Diabetic, in the process of becoming fat-adapted, less active, an aerobic junkie, free of hormone imbalances, or seeking weight loss

PATH 2: Moderate Fat/High Protein

Fat Fueled Profile: PUMPED KETO (page 47) **pk**

NO CARB-UPS

+ Helps balance blood sugar and lower cortisol

! May cause a drop in ketones

 GOOD IF YOU'RE:

Fat-adapted and experiencing blood sugar irregularities or cortisol imbalances on Path 1, feeling off on Path 1 but don't want to do carb-ups, experiencing constant hunger on Path 1, or struggling with a weight-loss plateau

PATH 3: Low Carb/High Fat with CARB-UPS

Fat Fueled Profiles: FULL KETO (page 48), ADAPTED FAT BURNER (page 48), and DAILY FAT BURNER (page 49) **fk** **afb** **dfb**

Daily, biweekly, or weekly carb-ups, preferably at night

+ Reduces feelings of restriction

+ Supplies glucose for processes that require it, which can ease physical symptoms

+ Ameliorates potential symptoms of physiological insulin resistance (page 96)

+ Good for muscle growth in response to anaerobic activity

! Can stimulate bingelike behavior or lead to gas and bloating

 GOOD IF YOU'RE:

Fat-adapted, an anaerobic athlete, a woman of reproductive age, seeking weight loss focused on healing, or struggling with a weight-loss plateau; also good if you have a hormone imbalance or adrenal dysfunction

Fat Fueled Profiles

Think of these profiles as outlines for developing your own keto map. Where the paths point to general macro strategies, the profiles give a larger view of how those strategies work day to day. If you're interested in Path 3 (the one with carb-ups), there are three different profiles to choose from depending on how often you want to carb up.

Try a profile for at least two weeks and see how you feel; if the approach isn't working for you, switch it around as needed.

> The Full Keto, Adapted Fat Burner, and Daily Fat Burner profiles all pair very well with an intermittent fasting practice (see pages 68 to 72). Combining carb-ups with fasting helps you maintain high levels of ketones while eating foods that make you feel good.

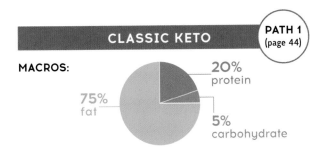

CLASSIC KETO — PATH 1 (page 44)

MACROS:
- 75% fat
- 20% protein
- 5% carbohydrate

The core of the keto diet and the foundation of all the Fat Fueled Profiles, this is a low-carbohydrate, moderate-protein, high-fat approach. It follows Path 1 (page 44); see that description for a list of those who would benefit most from Classic Keto.

HOW TO EAT ON CLASSIC KETO: All of the recipes in this book will work for you, but pay close attention to those marked with the Classic Keto symbol (see page 173). Consuming fat bombs (see page 114) is encouraged, and a daily Rocket Fuel Latte (page 428) is your friend. Intermittent fasting (see pages 68 to 72) may be fairly easy for you once you're fat-adapted.

If you begin to feel like you need more carbs (see page 43 for signs), switch to the Full Keto profile (page 48). If you begin to feel like you need more protein (see page 37 for signs), switch to the Pumped Keto profile.

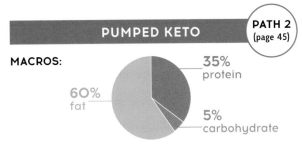

PUMPED KETO — PATH 2 (page 45)

MACROS:
- 60% fat
- 35% protein
- 5% carbohydrate

This profile includes more protein and less fat than Classic Keto. It follows Path 2 (page 45); see that description for a list of those who would benefit most from Pumped Keto. This is a fabulous option for people who are not interested in doing carb-ups but don't feel quite right on Path 1.

If you don't want to commit to this eating style full-time, you can use "protein-ups" instead of carb-ups and aim for these macros in just one meal or for one whole day.

HOW TO EAT ON PUMPED KETO: All of the recipes in this book will work for you, but pay close attention to those marked with the Pumped Keto symbol (see page 173). A daily Rocket Fuel Latte (page 428) is your friend. Intermittent fasting (see pages 68 to 72) may be fairly easy for you once you're fat-adapted. Because protein may cause insulin to spike, you might do better with small meals, which will reduce the impact.

If you begin to feel like you need more carbs (see page 43 for signs), switch to the Full Keto profile (page 48). If you find that you can't eat this much protein or it's standing in the way of your success, switch to the Classic Keto profile.

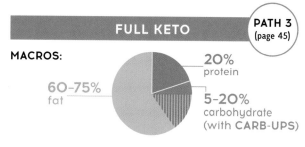

FULL KETO

PATH 3 (page 45)

MACROS:

60-75% fat
20% protein
5-20% carbohydrate (with **CARB-UPS**)

This profile is great once you're fat-adapted; if you are not yet fat-adapted, start with Classic Keto or Pumped Keto (page 47). (See page 63 for ways to know whether you're fat-adapted.)

With Full Keto, carb-ups happen weekly. You can time your carb-ups with anaerobic workouts if you like.

WHO IT'S GOOD FOR: Individuals with no health imbalances who engage in anaerobic activity one to three times per week or are sedentary. It's also good if you're interested in pairing weight loss with physical training, you're trying to break through a weight-loss plateau, or you have blood sugar irregularities or insulin resistance.

HOW TO EAT ON FULL KETO: All of the recipes in this book will work for you. For carb-ups, look for recipes with carb-up instructions (see page 173).

CARBING UP: Once you're fat-adapted, start carbing up once a week, preferably at night. A good place to start is with 1 gram of carbs for every pound (0.45 kg) that you weigh. If you feel like you need carb-ups two or three times a week, shift to the Adapted Fat Burner profile. If you feel like you need carb-ups more than three times a week, shift to the Daily Fat Burner profile (page 49).

If you want to align your carb-ups with your workouts, you can add half a banana to your post-workout shake. However, the ideal scenario is to work out in the afternoon and then have a carb-up dinner that swaps carbs for the usual fat.

NOTE: How you do your carb-ups depends on your body, activity level, health imbalances, and more. The type of carbs you choose is up to you. I enjoy sticking to Paleo-friendly carbs such as sweet potatoes, plantains, and potatoes, but I also like to have white rice on occasion. See page 117 for my favorite carb-up options.

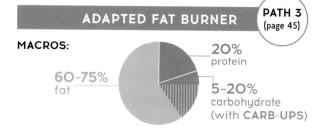

ADAPTED FAT BURNER

PATH 3 (page 45)

MACROS:

60-75% fat
20% protein
5-20% carbohydrate (with **CARB-UPS**)

This profile is great once you're fat-adapted; if you are not yet fat-adapted, start with Classic Keto or Pumped Keto (page 47). (See page 63 for ways to know whether you're fat-adapted.)

With Adapted Fat Burner, carb-ups happen two or three times a week. You can time your carb-ups with anaerobic workouts if you like.

WHO IT'S GOOD FOR: Individuals with minimal health imbalances who engage in anaerobic activity three to seven times per week. It's also good if you're interested in pairing weight loss with physical training. If you have a minor health imbalance that doesn't influence your hormone status, such as minor inflammation, energy inconsistencies, or digestive complications such as IBS, this profile is a good option for you. If you have minor health imbalances but are not active, Classic Keto (page 47) or Full Keto may be a better choice.

HOW TO EAT ON ADAPTED FAT BURNER: All of the recipes in this book will work for you. For carb-ups, look for recipes with "Make It a Carb-Up" instructions (see page 173).

CARBING UP: Once you're fat-adapted, start carbing up two or three times a week, always at night. A good place to start is with ½ gram of carbs for every pound (0.45 kg) that you weigh. If you feel like you need carb-ups more than three times a week, shift to the Daily Fat Burner profile (page 49).

If you want to align your carb-ups with your workouts, you can add half a banana to your post-workout shake. However, the ideal scenario is to workout in the afternoon and then have a carb-up dinner that swaps carbs for the usual fat.

NOTE: If you're practicing carb-ups for weight loss and following the Adapted Fat Burner or Full Keto profile, you may gain a little weight after a carb-up, but this practice should break a weight-loss plateau and allow you to keep losing weight. Just wait until you've dropped below your plateau weight before you do another carb-up.

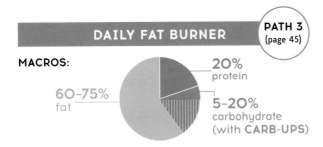

MACROS:

60–75% fat

20% protein

5–20% carbohydrate (with **CARB-UPS**)

With this profile, you'll start with evening carb-ups right away rather than wait until you're fully fat-adapted. You likely will not experience a ketogenic state in the traditional sense (outlined on pages 24 to 26)—that is, you will be priming your body for fat-burning, but you may not register ketones in the first couple of weeks, if ever. But fat adaptation should take hold as you adjust your evening carbs, beginning with a more-is-better approach and lowering the amount of carbohydrates as you go. You can time your carb-ups with anaerobic workouts if you like.

WHO IT'S GOOD FOR: Individuals with health imbalances (for example, thyroid imbalances or adrenal dysfunction), children, those who feel extremely restricted on the other profiles, vegans, and those with Candida (too much fat may cause a flare-up, so this profile offers an in-between option). It's also good if you're interested in pairing weight loss with body healing or you enjoy taking things day by day.

HOW TO EAT ON DAILY FAT BURNER: All of the recipes in this book will work for you. For carb-ups, look for recipes with carb-up instructions (see page 173). Because you are consuming carbs every night, you need only a touch.

CARBING UP: As soon as you switch to the keto diet, start carbing up every night. As long as you feel like having carbs, do it up! A good place to start is with ¼ gram of carbs for every pound (0.45 kg) that you weigh. You can reduce carbs from here—as your body becomes better at fat-burning, you may find that you don't need as many carbs as when you first started. If you go more than three or four days without having carbs at night, shift to the Adapted Fat Burner profile (page 48).

If you want to align your carb-ups with your workouts, just make sure that you carb up after a workout. However, the ideal scenario is to work out in the afternoon and then have a carb-up dinner that swaps carbs for the usual fat.

CARB-UP TIPS

- Do not add carbs to your meal without taking out the fats! Carbing up is about swapping the fats in your nightly meal for some carbs, not adding carbs to an already fatty meal. If you are not seeing results with your carb-up practice, it's likely that you're having too much fat in the carb-up meal and therefore overeating.

- For women, less is usually more. Begin with ¼ gram of carbs per pound of body weight and work your way up. A nice dinner with a bit of dessert action with fruit is a good place to start.

- This isn't about "eat more carbs at night and you'll be great." Carb-ups work because you are eating low-carb all day.

- Many of the recipes in this book include carb-up options to make adding carbs a cinch!

- Have a history of a disordered relationship with food? Don't plan your carb-ups! Take it day by day. If you feel like having carbs on a given evening, have them, and if you don't, don't.

FAT FUELED PROFILES

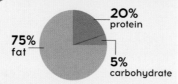 **PATH 1** (page 44) **CLASSIC KETO**

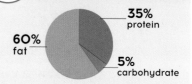 **PATH 2** (page 45) **PUMPED KETO**

CLASSIC KETO

- **20% protein**
- **75% fat**
- **5% carbohydrate**

LOW CARBOHYDRATE, MODERATE PROTEIN, HIGH FAT

Core of the keto diet and foundation of all the Fat Fueled Profiles

~~CARB-UPS~~

 IDEAL FOR:

- People who are not yet fat-adapted
- Sedentary individuals with health imbalances
- People with insulin resistance
- Aerobic athletes (more on page 74)
- People without hormonal imbalances
- Menopausal and post-menopausal women

 HOW TO EAT:

- **ck** Look for recipes marked with the Classic Keto symbol.
- **FAT** Consume lots of fat bombs; look for the Fat Bomb/Great for Adapting symbol.
- Enjoy a daily Rocket Fuel Latte (page 428).
- **+ ~~CARB-UP~~** Avoid recipes marked as Carb-Up Option.

PUMPED KETO

- **35% protein**
- **60% fat**
- **5% carbohydrate**

MODERATE FAT, HIGH PROTEIN, LOW CARBOHYDRATE

~~CARB-UPS~~

 IDEAL FOR:

- Individuals with hypo-glycemia or other blood sugar irregularities (see page 52) (this path may not be right for insulin-dependent diabetics)
- People who don't feel quite right on Classic Keto but are not interested in carb-ups
- People who are struggling with a weight-loss plateau

 HOW TO EAT:

- **pk** Look for recipes marked with the Pumped Keto symbol.
- Enjoy a daily Rocket Fuel Latte (page 428).
- Small meals may help keep insulin in check.

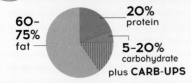 PATH 3 (page 45) **FULL KETO**	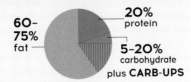 **ADAPTED FAT BURNER**	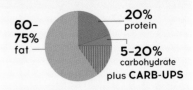 **DAILY FAT BURNER**

60–75% fat
20% protein
5–20% carbohydrate
plus **CARB-UPS**

Follow after you're
FULLY FAT-ADAPTED
(follow Path 1 or 2 first)

CARB-UPS
once a week,
always at night

60–75% fat
20% protein
5–20% carbohydrate
plus **CARB-UPS**

Follow after you're
FULLY FAT-ADAPTED
(follow Path 1 or 2 first)

CARB-UPS
2 to 3 times per week,
always at night

60–75% fat
20% protein
5–20% carbohydrate
plus **CARB-UPS**

Start carb-ups RIGHT AWAY
instead of waiting until
fully fat-adapted

CARB-UPS
every day,
always at night

 IDEAL FOR:

- Individuals with no health imbalances
- People with blood sugar irregularities (see page 52)
- Moderately active individuals (anaerobic activity 1–3 times per week)
- Sedentary individuals
- People who want to pair weight loss with physical training
- People who are struggling with a weight-loss plateau

 IDEAL FOR:

- Individuals with minor health imbalances (see page 31)
- Active individuals (anaerobic activity 3–7 times per week)
- People who want to pair weight loss with physical training
- People who are struggling with a weight-loss plateau

IDEAL FOR:

- Individuals with health imbalances (such as thyroid imbalances, adrenal dysfunction, or Candida)
- Children
- Vegans
- People who feel extremely restricted by other profiles
- People who want to pair weight loss with body healing
- People who want to take it day by day

HOW TO EAT:

ck For daily eats, look for recipes marked with the Classic Keto symbol.

FAT To boost fat intake, look for recipes marked with the Fat Bomb/Great for Adapting symbol.

+ CARB-UP Carb up once a week, always at night. Look for recipes marked as Carb-Up Option.

If desired, follow workouts with half a banana or a carb-up dinner.

1g Eat 1 g of carbs for every 1 lb (0.45 kg) of weight.

HOW TO EAT:

ck For daily eats, look for recipes marked with the Classic Keto symbol.

FAT To boost fat intake, look for recipes marked with the Fat Bomb/Great for Adapting symbol.

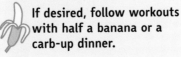 **+ CARB-UP** Carb up 2 to 3 times per week, always at night. Look for recipes marked as Carb-Up Option.

If desired, follow workouts with half a banana or a carb-up dinner.

½g Eat ½ g of carbs for every 1 lb (0.45 kg) of weight.

HOW TO EAT:

ck For daily eats, look for recipes marked with the Classic Keto symbol.

FAT To boost fat intake, look for recipes marked with the Fat Bomb/Great for Adapting symbol.

  + CARB-UP Carb up every day, always at night. Look for recipes marked as Carb-Up Option.

If desired, follow workouts with half a banana or a carb-up dinner.

¼g Eat ¼ g of carbs for every 1 lb (0.45 kg) of weight.

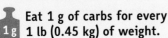 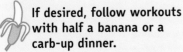

How to Determine Your Fat Fueled Profile

The following questions may help you get a sense of which Fat Fueled Profile would be best for your health status, relationship with food, hormone status, dietary preferences, and physical activity choices. If you answer "yes" to a question, place a check mark in all the blank boxes beside that question. At the end of each section (Health Status, Relationship with Food, etc.), total your score. At the end of the questionnaire, you should have an idea of which profile is the best fit for you in each section. If different Fat Fueled Profiles are recommended for different sections, remember that the higher the section is on the questionnaire, the more importance it has. For example, if you score a 5 for Daily Fat Burner in the Health Status section but a 6 for Classic Keto in the Hormone Status section, you may want to start with Daily Fat Burner and, once you feel great with some of the imbalances you're trying to get a handle on, consider switching to Classic Keto to address the Hormone Status concerns. The chart that follows the questionnaire further details which Fat Fueled Profiles are best for specific concerns, giving you more options.

NOTE: *You'll notice that weight loss is not part of the dietary preferences. This is because weight/fat loss is generally achieved when we have provided our bodies with the correct hormonal support and other aspects. Trust that the Fat Fueled Profile you determine is best for your body will take you to the place your body feels best. After correcting all of your health imbalances, you could try shifting to Classic Keto if you're not already there.*

ck = Classic Keto

pk = Pumped Keto

fk = Full Keto

afb = Adapted Fat Burner

dfb = Daily Fat Burner

	ck PATH 1	pk PATH 2	fk PATH 3	afb PATH 3	dfb PATH 3
HEALTH STATUS					
Are you in cancer recovery?	☐				
Have you been a chronic dieter, eating 1,200 calories off and on for years?	☐				☐
Did your health-care provider recommend that you go keto?	☐				☐
Are you breastfeeding?	☐				☐
Do you have digestive issues such as IBS, sensitivity to FODMAPs, or SIBO?	☐				
Do you have a history of anxiety or depression?					☐
Do you have a history of, or are you currently suffering from, Candida?					
Do you have an autoimmune condition such as Hashimoto's, arthritis, or lupus (not including autoimmune conditions that can make you incredibly tired, or type 1 diabetes)?	☐				
Do you have an autoimmune condition that can make you incredibly tired, such as MS, fibromyalgia, or chronic fatigue syndrome?					☐
Do you have heart health concerns such as high cholesterol and high blood pressure?	☐				
Do you have neurological health concerns such as Alzheimer's or Parkinson's disease?	☐				
Do you suffer from blood sugar irregularities such as dysglycemia, hypoglycemia, type 1 or 2 diabetes, or insulin resistance?	☐				
Has your gallbladder been removed? Or do you have fat absorption issues?	☐				
TOTAL	☐				

RELATIONSHIP WITH FOOD

	ck	pk	fk	afb	dfb
Are you easily triggered by weighing or measuring food?	▓	▓	▓	▓	
Do you have a history of an eating disorder?	▓	▓	▓	▓	
If you have yo-yo dieted, has it led to binges?	▓	▓	▓	▓	
TOTAL					

HORMONE STATUS

	ck	pk	fk	afb	dfb
Do you have adrenal dysfunction?	▓	▓	▓	▓	▓
Are you in menopause or post-menopausal?		▓	▓	▓	▓
Are you of reproductive age with no hormone concerns?	▓	▓	▓		▓
Are you of reproductive age with hormone concerns such as amenorrhea (lack of period), high estrogen, low progesterone, low DHEA, or low libido (everything except PCOS)?	▓	▓	▓		▓
Do you have PCOS?	▓	▓	▓	▓	▓
Do you have Hashimoto's (treated or untreated)?	▓	▓	▓	▓	▓
Do you have hyperthyroid (treated or untreated)?	▓	▓	▓	▓	▓
Do you have hypothyroid (treated or untreated)?	▓	▓		▓	▓
TOTAL					

DIETARY PREFERENCES

	ck	pk	fk	afb	dfb
Does eating too many Paleo-friendly carbs make you feel weird?		▓	▓	▓	▓
Do you feel better eating Paleo-friendly carbs than protein?	▓	▓		▓	▓
Do you feel better eating protein over fat or carbs?	▓		▓	▓	▓
If you've tried keto before or you're currently keto, have you felt/do you feel awful even after a couple of weeks?	▓	▓		▓	▓
If you've tried keto before or you're currently keto, have you felt/do you feel amazing?	▓		▓	▓	▓
Do you want to start slow, steadily reducing carb consumption day by day?	▓	▓	▓		
Are you vegan or vegetarian?	▓	▓	▓	▓	▓
TOTAL					

PHYSICAL ACTIVITY

	ck	pk	fk	afb	dfb
If you are already fat-adapted, do you primarily practice aerobic activities?		▓	▓	▓	▓
If you are already fat-adapted, do you primarily practice anaerobic* activities?		▓	▓	▓	▓
If this is your first attempt at keto, do you primarily practice aerobic activities?		▓	▓	▓	▓
If this is your first attempt at keto, do you primarily practice anaerobic* activities?	▓		▓	▓	▓
Are you pretty sedentary?		▓	▓	▓	▓
TOTAL					

*Anaerobic activity is high-intensity training such as HIIT, sprints, heavy weight training, or CrossFit.

Great if you have just one or two concerns that you wish to address with *The Keto Diet*.

| x | *First choice (equal if two or more are selected)* | x *Second choice* | x *Third choice* |

	ck PATH 1	pk PATH 2	fk PATH 3	afb PATH 3	dfb PATH 3
Adrenal dysfunction		X			X
Anxiety or depression			X	X	X
Autoimmune condition (such as Hashimoto's, arthritis, or lupus—not including autoimmune conditions that can make you incredibly tired, or type 1 diabetes)	X				
Autoimmune condition that can make you incredibly tired (such as multiple sclerosis, fibromyalgia, or chronic fatigue)			X	X	X
Blood sugar irregularities (such as dysglycemia, hypoglycemia, type 1 or 2 diabetes, or insulin resistance)	X	X	X		
Breastfeeding					X
Cancer recovery	X				
Candida					X
Cholesterol or high blood pressure concerns	X				
Chronic dieter			X	X	X
Digestive issues (such as IBS, FODMAP sensitivity, or SIBO)	X				
Hashimoto's (treated or untreated)	X				
Health-care provider recommended keto	X				
History with an eating disorder			X	X	X
Hyperthyroid (treated or untreated)	X				
Hypothyroid (treated or untreated)			X	X	X
Interested in starting slow			X	X	X
Menopause or post-menopausal	X				
Neurological concerns (such as Alzheimer's, intense brain fog, dementia, or Parkinson's)	X				
PCOS	X				
Removed gallbladder or fat absorption issues					X
Reproductive age, no hormone concerns			X	X	X
Reproductive age with hormone concerns (such as amenorrhea, high estrogen, low progesterone, low DHEA, or low libido—everything except PCOS)			X	X	X
Sedentary lifestyle	X				
Tried keto before, didn't feel right		X	X	X	X
Tried keto before, felt amazing	X	X			
Triggered by weighing/measuring food			X	X	X
Vegans and vegetarians			X	X	X
Workouts primarily aerobic (already fat-adapted)	X	X			
Workouts primarily anaerobic (already fat-adapted)	X	X	X	X	
Workouts primarily anaerobic (not fat-adapted)	X		X	X	
Yo-yo dieting leading to binges			X	X	X

I'm a twenty-six-year-old actress, writer, and YouTuber.

Before majoring in theater, I worked as a certified personal trainer. Having studied physical education and nutrition, I used to believe that a high-protein, high-carb, low-fat diet was the correct way of achieving physical fitness and health. And so, that was my lifestyle.

Years later, I was about 15 kg above my normal weight and full of health issues (food allergies and intolerances). After consulting with a nutritionist, I started to work out and diet so I could lose weight and regain my health. But it just didn't happen. I felt sleepy and tired all day. And not just regular tired, it was like my body was heavy. I could never focus. It felt like my brain didn't work. I had strange headaches and I was hungry all the time even though I ate six to eight meals a day, mostly lean protein and carbs. I was working out and dieting, and having little results. I was so tired I had a hard time getting out of bed in the morning. I felt like my body was broken. I told my nutritionist I felt horrible, but he said I had to focus more, and that it was all psychological.

One day, a friend of mine told me he was on a low-carb, high-fat diet. He told me he could feel his body healing, had so much energy during the day, and felt amazing. I wanted to give it a try, but I was afraid of eating fat, so I stuck to my regular diet and left it at that. A few months later, I was on YouTube and a video popped up. It was Leanne! Talking about a low-carb, high fat diet. I remembered what my friend said and decided to watch the video to the end. I remember Leanne saying, "If you're on a diet and you don't feel awesome, then it's not working for you." I thought about how awful I felt and decided to give keto a try. I watched all of Leanne's videos, read everything on HealthfulPursuit.com, and the next day, I ran to the supermarket, bought a ton of good fats and protein Leanne had suggested, and started a high-fat diet.

I felt awesome on the first day. I had so much energy, I was able to sleep better, I could focus, and for the first time in years, my body didn't feel heavy. I could feel my body healing and rebuilding itself. And the extra weight I had been trying to lose for so long finally started coming off. A few months later, I read Fat Fueled, Leanne's 30-day healing program. It was like saying "checkmate" to all my health problems.

I read about the keto flu, but I didn't have any symptoms at all. My body desperately needed fats, and once I was on keto, it just began to heal, and it's been healing until now, nonstop. I haven't had food allergy symptoms in a long time, and my digestive system works better than ever. And the hunger I used to feel disappeared. Now I only eat two to three meals a day and I'm almost never hungry between meals. I can work for hours without feeling tired.

Keto also affected me on a psychological level. I learned to love my body and I finally understood that my body wasn't broken, I just wasn't feeding it properly.

So thanks, Leanne! For inspiring me and so people around the globe to love ourselves and work with our bodies, instead of against them.

Thank you so much! Or, like we say in Portuguese: muito obrigada!

Luise
São Paulo, Brazil

CHAPTER 3

THE KETO EXPERIENCE

While I no longer rely on macro calculations and adherence to tracking, I know how important understanding macros is to the process of becoming fat-adapted. In the following pages, we'll run through the ins and outs of calculating and tracking your macros. Then we'll get into a mindfulness practice of stepping outside the tracking norm so that you have more time to do the things you love (like, anything other than tracking). Plus, if you're already wondering, "How the heck am I going to eat that much fat?" I'll provide you with some of my favorite fat-boosting strategies.

Let's dig in!

YOUR MACROS AND TRACKING

"Macro" is short for macronutrient—the carbohydrates, proteins, and fats you eat on a daily basis. The amounts of carbs, proteins, and fats you're aiming for are commonly referred as your macros. In the previous chapter, you may have noticed that the Fat Fueled paths and profiles refer to, for instance, 75 percent fat. This refers to the percentage of daily calorie intake that comes from fat.

So what exactly does "75 percent fat" mean? The answer requires a little bit of math, and the first step is knowing your total daily calories.

Pick a calorie goal that aligns with what you are doing right now, but know that you may be able to increase your calories later. When you're in ketosis, you may be able to eat more calories while still losing weight and improving your health.

There are 4 calories in a gram of carbohydrate, 4 calories in a gram of protein, and 9 calories in a gram of fat. That yields these equations for figuring out how many grams of each macro you can eat in a day:

Total daily calories x carb macro percentage = calories of carbs / 4 = grams of daily carbs

Total daily calories x protein macro percentage = calories of protein / 4 = grams of daily protein

Total daily calories x fat macro percentage = calories of fat / 9 = grams of daily fat

Here's an example. Let's say you're eating 2,000 calories a day and aim for a macro ratio of 5 percent carbs, 15 percent protein, and 80 percent fat.

First, calculate how many calories this allots for each macronutrient:

2,000 x 5% carbs = 100 calories of carbs

2,000 x 15% protein = 300 calories of protein

2,000 x 80% fat = 1600 calories of fat

Then calculate how many grams you get from that number of calories:

100 calories of carbs / 4 = 25 grams of daily carbs

300 calories of protein / 4 = 75 grams of daily protein

1,600 calories of fat / 9 = 178 grams of daily fat

It's somewhat important to know how to do the math, but I am here to make your life easier, so the table on the opposite page calculates the grams of fat, protein, and carbs for a wide range of calories per day and macro ratios.

CALORIES PER DAY

MACRO PERCENTAGES	1300	1400	1500	1600	1700	1800	1900	2000	2100	2200	2300	2400	2500	2600	2700	2800	2900	3000	3100	3200	3300	3400	3500
								CORRESPONDING INTAKE IN GRAMS															
CARBS																							
5%	16	18	19	20	21	23	24	25	26	28	29	30	31	33	34	35	36	38	39	40	41	43	44
10%	33	35	38	40	43	45	48	50	53	55	58	60	63	65	68	70	73	75	78	80	83	85	88
15%	49	53	56	60	64	68	71	75	79	83	86	90	94	98	101	105	109	113	116	120	124	128	131
20%	65	70	75	80	85	90	95	100	105	110	115	120	125	130	135	140	145	150	155	160	165	170	175
PROTEIN																							
10%	33	35	38	40	43	45	48	50	53	55	58	60	63	65	68	70	73	75	78	80	83	85	88
15%	49	53	56	60	64	68	71	75	79	83	86	90	94	98	101	105	109	113	116	120	124	128	131
20%	65	70	75	80	85	90	95	100	105	110	115	120	125	130	135	140	145	150	155	160	165	170	175
25%	81	88	94	100	106	113	119	125	131	138	144	150	156	163	169	175	181	188	194	200	206	213	219
30%	98	105	113	120	128	135	143	150	158	165	173	180	188	195	203	210	218	225	233	240	248	255	263
35%	114	123	131	140	149	158	166	175	184	193	201	210	219	228	236	245	254	263	271	280	289	298	306
FAT																							
55%	79	86	92	98	104	110	116	122	128	134	141	147	153	159	165	171	177	183	189	196	202	208	214
60%	87	93	100	107	113	120	127	133	140	147	153	160	167	173	180	187	193	200	207	213	220	227	233
65%	94	101	108	116	123	130	137	144	152	159	166	173	181	188	195	202	209	217	224	231	238	246	253
70%	101	109	117	124	132	140	148	156	163	171	179	187	194	202	210	218	226	233	241	249	257	264	272
75%	108	117	125	133	142	150	158	167	175	183	192	200	208	217	225	233	242	250	258	267	275	283	292
80%	116	124	133	142	151	160	169	178	187	196	204	213	222	231	240	249	258	267	276	284	293	302	311
85%	123	132	142	151	161	170	179	189	198	208	217	227	236	246	255	264	274	283	293	302	312	321	331

In the table, there are multiple percentage options for each macronutrient. The key is that your macros (carb percentage + protein percentage + fat percentage) always need to add up to 100 percent. The rest is up to you.

For example, if you choose 10 percent carbs and 20 percent protein, you will have to choose 70 percent fat because 10 + 20 + 70 = 100. Then check the table and you'll see that a daily intake of 1,300 calories with a 10/20/70 ratio will give you:

- **33 grams of carbohydrates**
- **65 grams of protein**
- **101 grams of fat**

Let's do another example. If you choose 5 percent carbs and 35 percent protein, you will have to choose 60 percent fat because 5 + 35 + 60 = 100. From there, you will see that a daily intake of 1,600 calories with a 5/35/60 ratio will give you:

- **20 grams of carbohydrates**
- **140 grams of protein**
- **107 grams of fat**

(Yes, even though you're eating 60 percent fat and 35 percent protein, you'll actually eat more grams of protein than grams of fat. This is because—as you'll recall—fat has more calories per gram than protein, and the percentage refers to the percentage of total daily calories from the macronutrient.)

There are a few ways to calculate your macros: you can do the math yourself using the equations on page 56; you can use the table above; or you can use an online calculator (search for "keto macro calculator" and a bunch will pop up).

Are you ready to start but prefer to dip a toe in rather than dive in all at once? Head to page 59 for steps to get into ketosis without the balls-to-the-wall mentality.

Four Ways to Track Your Macros

I've presented all these numbers to give you a general idea of how the macro ratios work out in practice. But you don't necessarily have to track every calorie or maintain a tight grip on your macros to make the keto diet work.

Personally, I'm not overly concerned about counting macros. I did it for a long time, and it made me crazy. Literally crazy. It was too easy to become obsessed with tracking my foods and counting calories. Now I choose not to, and I still do quite well with keto. And, dare I say it, most of us would be better off without all the tracking tools we've become so accustomed to.

But everyone is different and needs different things, so I'm going to introduce you to four strategies you could use to make sure you're getting the right amount of fat, protein, and carbs, whether you want to track macros or not. The key is finding a strategy that feels good to you.

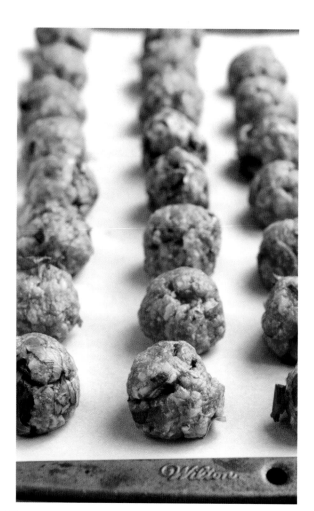

Tracking your intake the old-fashioned way can be beneficial when you're starting out on keto, especially so that you can keep track of your carbohydrates—if you've never been conscious of your carbohydrate intake, understanding the carbohydrate content of foods can take some getting used to. It's also the best way to really know all the details about the macros and calories you're consuming, which is particularly helpful if you find that you need to make some adjustments.

The downfall to tracking is that it can be overwhelming. If you do get overwhelmed, no worries—turn to the next page for other options. There are other ways to do this!

The important thing to remember about this method is that you have to know the calories, fat grams, protein grams, and carb grams in everything you eat. That spoonful of almond butter you ate? You need to know how many grams of fat, protein, and carbs it contained as well as how many calories, and you need to factor those numbers into your daily allotment for each macronutrient. So if you're aiming for 33 grams of carbs a day, after the almond butter at around 3 grams—assuming it was the first thing you ate today—you're down to 30 grams of carbs for the rest of the day. And so on with the remaining macros.

If you choose this option, tracking your intake with an application such as MyFitnessPal, FitBit Tracker, FatSecret App, My Macros+, Cronometer, or KetoDietApp is the way to go. With many of these apps, you can set your macro and/or calorie goals and input your daily eats while you're planning your meals for the week or while you're preparing a meal. Many app-based solutions come complete with verified nutrition data for foods, so when you input a food for a particular day, it will instantly update your daily macro and calorie intakes. You can also manually add recipes of your own, inputting nutrition information per serving, or develop the recipes and the corresponding nutrition information right there in the app.

Once you get in the swing of things, you can skip to option #4 on the next page, which is a fabulous strategy for someone who's learned how to sense when they're in ketosis and can feel the effect that an adjustment of macros has on their body. After eating this way for about thirty days, you should be in a place to trust your body and be able to skip to option #4.

OPTION #2: Delayed Tracking

Similar to option #1, but better if you don't want to track each morsel of food that enters your mouth but still want to see if you're hitting your macro targets exactly. Eat high-fat/low-carb (as best you can) for five days and write down everything you eat. After five days, enter what you ate meal by meal in a calorie-tracking app (find suggestions on page 59) that calculates daily macro percentages from those meals. After entering all the foods, you'll be able to see where you've landed on the macros. This will help you understand where your macro faults are, without the risk of obsessing about intake, tracking, and adherence to your "diet."

Once you get in the swing of things with delayed tracking, you can skip to option #4, which offers some of the same benefits without requiring you to write down everything you eat. Believe that your body knows what's best for you and trust the process.

OPTION #3: Follow a Meal Plan

Instead of following macro guidelines without question and worrying about hitting them every day, I encourage you to try out the meal plans, assess your hunger on a daily basis, and roll with it. You don't have to calculate anything—there are different plans for each Fat Fueled Profile, with all the work done for you. A huge benefit here, aside from not having to worry about figuring out what to eat and calculating macros, is that you can eat or not as you feel like it. Whether you enjoy the planned meal, delay it, or skip it depends entirely on whether you are hungry. This removes some of the anxiety that can be experienced when tracking—you have the flexibility to eat or not without worrying about whether you're hitting your day's macros.

The meal plans and shopping lists that begin on page 174 provide ample options so that you don't have to track when you first get started. Then, when you find a plan that works well for you—see page 63 for how to know when you're in nutritional ketosis—you'll know approximately which eating style feels best in your body.

OPTION #4: Use Daily Portion Plates

This option is great for those who don't respond well to tracking or have a somewhat solid idea of which foods are high in carbohydrates and how to switch them out for fats. The Daily Portion Plates help you achieve the benefits of nutritional ketosis without having to count, track, or go crazy over macros. The idea here is that you use your plate to visually estimate your macronutrients. Portion out your plate using your eyes, positioning protein on less than a quarter of the plate, with fat taking up the majority—imagine the tablespoons of fat you use to make your meal as lining up on the sides of your plate. The key to success with the Daily Portion Plates is to get out of your head and into your body. Try not to overthink it; if you need a visual, you can head to healthfulpursuit.com/plates to see a bunch of examples of my real-life portion plates.

Regardless of which option you choose, check in with yourself before you eat. Do you want to eat for emotional reasons? Are you actually thirsty? (It's amazing how often we get those signals confused.) Or are you truly hungry? These questions go a long way in helping you listen to your body so you can know when you're hungry, when you're full, and when you're seeking solace in food instead of meeting your emotional needs in another way. (There's a lot more on self-care and listening to your body starting on page 14.)

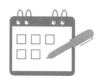

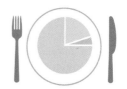

OPTION #1: Track Your Intake Meal to Meal	OPTION #2: Delayed Tracking	OPTION #3: Follow a Meal Plan	OPTION #4: Use Daily Portion Plates
Set your macro percentages and calorie goals yourself (see the equation on page 56), use the table on page 57, or use an online calculator	Set your macro percentages and calorie goals yourself (see equation on page 56), use the table on page 57, or use an online calculator	Follow a ketogenic meal plan (starting on page 174) that takes macros into account	Use your plate to visually estimate fat, protein, and carb intake
Track the macronutrient and calorie contents of everything you eat as you eat it (app recommendations are on page 59)	Eat high-fat/low-carb for 5 days and write down everything you eat in a notebook	➕ Allows you to assess your hunger and eat, delay, or skip a meal as needed	➕ Great for those who don't like tracking or already know how to swap carbs for fats
➕ Particularly useful when you're first starting out, especially for understanding carb consumption and identifying necessary adjustments	After 5 days, enter the food totals in an app that calculates macro percentages from the food you've consumed (app recommendations are on page 59)	➕ Less anxiety and more flexibility than tracking macros	See page 61 for more on Daily Portion Plates
❗ Can be overwhelming	Evaluate where you landed on the macros and adjust as needed		
	➕ Helps you know where your macro faults are without obsessing about intake and tracking		

DAILY PORTION PLATES

If macro counting makes you crazy, simply eyeing what's on your plate is a fabulous way to get things rolling in the right direction without totally stressing out about numbers.

Below you'll find the Daily Portion Plate for each meal in each profile. If you're following one of the profiles that call for carb-ups (Full Keto, Adapted Fat Burner, and Daily Fat Burner), use the plates from Classic Keto for breakfast and lunch every day and for dinner on the days when you're not doing a carb-up. Use the dinner plates for these profiles only on the days you eat a carb-up dinner.

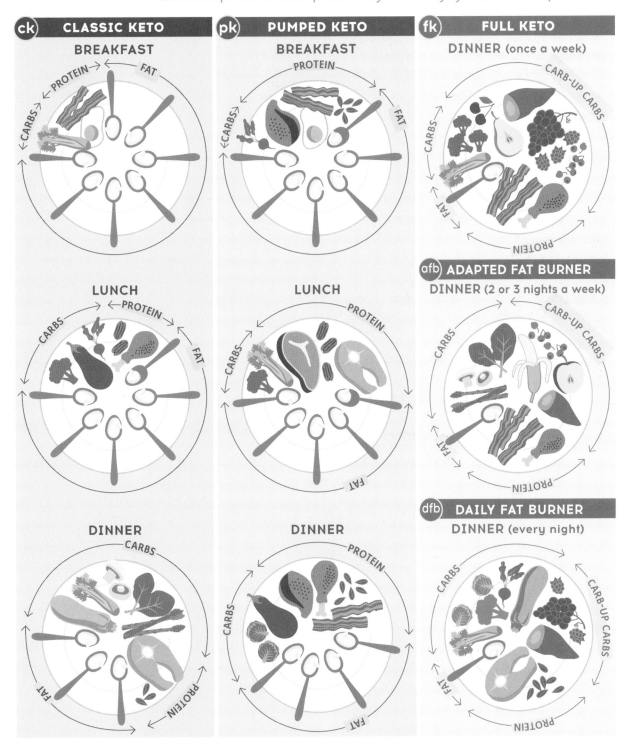

We know that the fewer carbs you eat, the faster you'll get into ketosis and start burning fat for fuel. However, there's a little caveat, and it's called fiber.

Fiber is a carb, but it doesn't spike blood glucose, and therefore insulin, as other carbs do. That's why many people who follow keto give fiber a hall pass, not worrying about how much they consume. They do so by subtracting the grams of fiber in a food from the total grams of carbohydrates. The result is what's called net carbohydrates.

TOTAL CARBS = all carbs, including fiber

NET CARBS = total carbs minus fiber

Personally, I like the net carbohydrate approach because it removes the stress that comes with wanting to maintain a healthy vegetable and fruit intake on keto. Once I started counting net carbs, I found it easier to feel okay about adding extra kale to my plate. Because in what world is eating more kale a bad thing?

But I also like paying attention to the amount of fiber I'm consuming—around 30 grams a day is where I feel best. I eat an additional 50 grams or so of carbohydrates on top of that, so my total carbs are 80 grams, but my net carbs are 50 grams.

Some people enjoy counting total carbs, and others do better counting net carbs. It's totally up to you. I find that those who don't thrive on a lot of vegetables and need a lower carbohydrate amount to get into ketosis often choose the total carbohydrate route. And those who love vegetables and can get into ketosis with higher carbohydrate amounts often choose to count net carbohydrates.

If you're having issues with the net carbohydrate approach, try removing low-carb dieting products. Companies often add loads of fiber to these products and then count only the net carbs—so even though an item is marketed as "low-carb," it could contain more than 30 grams of total carbohydrates per serving. Yes, technically this could still work on the net carbs theory, but my experience has been that these products can make your blood sugar go crazy. (And of course, avoiding packaged foods in general and focusing on whole food is a much better strategy for overall health.)

If you're already eating keto but haven't been focusing on whole food, on the Fat Fueled approach you may notice that you're eating more total carbs than you used to. In many cases, this is because you are increasing your fiber by eating whole foods, adding to your total carbohydrate amount. And this is okay. Adding fiber to your daily eats doesn't spike insulin, adds bulk to your stool, aids in digestive health (in most cases), and assists with the delicate balance and maintenance of your gut microbiome. However, the added fiber may kick some individuals out of ketosis, at least temporarily. You may be one of them! If you are, start counting total carbohydrates and you should be right as rain in a couple of days. Or simply avoid recipes that are loaded with flax seeds or chia seeds, and that should help calm things down.

If you've hit a weight-loss or ketosis plateau and you've tried different Fat Fueled Profiles, count your total and net carbs and see what the numbers tell you. You may find that you're choosing foods that are really low in fiber yet consuming too many total carbohydrates, which is throwing off your carbohydrate intake so you can't get into ketosis. If this is the case, the best approach I've found is upping your intake of fiber-rich vegetables to balance things out.

Head over to page 98 for a list of high-fiber foods.

HOW TO KNOW WHETHER YOU'RE IN KETOSIS

Nutritional ketosis is achieved when there are levels of ketones in the blood, breath, or urine. So it makes sense that measuring ketones is the standard way to figure out whether you're in ketosis. It's not the only way, though—which I'll get to in a moment.

But first, a quick clarification: although we often use the terms interchangeably, there's actually a difference between being fat-adapted and being in nutritional ketosis.

When you're fat-adapted, your body prefers fat to glucose. It has ramped up the enzymatic processes it needs to burn fat as energy and feel comfortable doing so. Once you're fat-adapted, it's possible to slip in and out of ketosis while remaining fat-adapted.

When you're in ketosis, your body is creating moderate levels of ketones by burning fat. So how can you be in ketosis without being fat-adapted? If your body isn't used to burning fat, it still prefers glucose as an energy source—even if there are ketones circulating in your blood because it has to burn fat. You're only fat-adapted once your body has made the switch to prefer fats. Here's one way to think of it: after eating ketogenic for three to five days, your body may be in ketosis, but it has yet to become fat-adapted. After three to five weeks, your body will be in ketosis and has probably become fat-adapted. Having a carb-up, for instance, may reduce the level of ketones in your blood for a brief period, but it won't change the fact that your body prefers burning fat to burning glucose.

As we discuss how to determine whether you're in ketosis, keep in mind that you don't have to worry about testing, monitoring, or tracking in order to achieve ketosis. If you're eating a lot of fats and few carbohydrates, you will likely get into ketosis just fine. But it can be helpful to know your numbers when you're working toward ketosis for the first time.

Stress can impact our ability to switch into fat-burning mode (see page 90 for more). This especially holds true when we're trying to get into ketosis, so during this period, try to reduce stress—see page 91 for tips.

Testing for Ketones

Ketone bodies can be found in your urine, breath, and blood, and there are instruments for measuring levels of ketones in each. Each tool measures a different type of ketone body.

Testing isn't strictly necessary, but it can be helpful. When I started out on keto, I tested my blood ketones multiple times a day at various times, recorded my results, and made a hypothesis each time about why my ketone level had increased or decreased. I did this for thirty days, which was enough to collect a bunch of ideas about what increased and decreased my ketone level. I don't test my ketones anymore because I know what nutritional ketosis feels like. When I'm on the mark, I'm good to go. When I don't feel it, I know where I fumbled and what to do to get it back—and I have all that information because I tested my blood for those first thirty days.

However, it's worth noting that more ketones doesn't necessarily equate to increased fat loss. Say, for example, you eat copious amounts of fat: enough that you're in ketosis and registering ketones, but too much to allow your body to burn its own fat stores. In this case, dietary fat is the energy source, not your body fat. The most important factors in natural fat loss are appetite balance, metabolic healing, and supporting yourself with positive behaviors.

Blood

Tests for: beta-hydroxybutyrate

Testing the blood for ketones is the most reliable and accurate approach. It's also the most expensive. The reusable meter costs about $28, and the one-use test strips range from $1 to $4 each. If you test twice daily, that's up to $240 a month just for test strips, not including the cost of the meter. My favorite blood ketone meter is the Precision Xtra Blood Glucose & Ketone Monitoring System from Abbott, available at most drugstores. It lets you test both your blood glucose and ketone levels at once.

When you measure your blood ketones, you're looking for a result of 0.5 to 3.0 mmol/l—any number in this range means that you're in ketosis. There is no need to go higher than 3.0 mmol/l; when my clients have a number higher than 3.0, it's often because they are not eating enough food or they're dehydrated. If you've tested in the morning, before eating, and your ketones have been above 3.0 mmol/l for a couple of days, please eat and/or drink more!

You know that you're in ketosis when your number is between 0.5 and 3.0 mmol/l. Your body is producing significant levels of ketones by burning fat. You know you're well on your way to becoming fat-adapted when your numbers have consistently been between 0.5 and 3.0 mmol/l for three to five days.

If you're interested in starting a carb-up practice, it's generally best to wait until either your ketones have registered between 0.5 and 3.0 mmol/l for five to seven days or you've been following the Classic Keto Fat Fueled Profile for ten to fifteen days, whichever happens later. Often these two things happen at around the same time.

Breath

Tests for: acetone (resulting from the breakdown of acetoacetate)

Testing the breath for ketones is reliable for most people, much more cost-effective than blood testing, and far more accurate than using urine strips. The best reusable ketone breath meter is made by a company called Ketonix. Their meter can be used multiple times and doesn't require extra strips; it's a one-time cost of $149 to $169, depending on the model you choose. To test, you simply breathe out naturally at a slow and steady pace for fifteen to thirty seconds. The tool will take a couple of moments to register a reading, flashing different colored lights.

The key to the success with the Ketonix meter is, when you first purchase it, to sit with it for about an hour and take a measurement every fifteen to twenty minutes, until the values are within the same range. This lets you work on your testing technique: how you blow into the device makes a difference in how the results are interpreted, so developing a technique and sticking to it will ensure that you're comparing apples to apples each time you test.

Note that your blood and breath ketones will likely not correlate because breath ketones can be influenced by many factors, such as water and alcohol intake.

A Ketonix Breath Ketone Analyzer indicates the level of ketones present by displaying a color: blue for no or very little ketones, green for trace amounts, yellow for moderate amounts, and red for high amounts. The newer models also indicate the level of ketones within each color by flashing from one to ten times. For example, it could flash ten times with a green light; that means you're at the high end of the trace group, one flash away from being in the yellow group (moderate amounts).

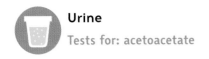

Urine

Tests for: acetoacetate

Testing the urine for ketones is the least accurate testing method. The problem is that it only detects excess ketone bodies that are excreted through the urine. As you continue to become keto-adapted, your body will likely become more efficient at using ketone bodies and therefore won't excrete as many into your urine. When this occurs, you may experience a drop in urine ketones, but if you measure blood or breath ketones, you'll see that you're still in ketosis.

If you decide to test your urine for ketones, the presence of ketones is indicated when the test strip changes color. The darker the color, the higher the ketones. The strips group levels together into trace, small, moderate, and large. The highest level you can test for with many ketone strips is "large" at 160 mg/dL, and this would result in a deep purple, eggplant color.

TESTING YOUR KETONES?
HERE ARE SOME TIPS:

• Do not take MCT oil directly before testing—it will throw off your results.

• Ketone concentrations are generally lower in the morning and higher in the evening.

• Ketone concentrations are usually higher directly following aerobic exercise.

• Ketone concentrations are usually lower directly following anaerobic exercise.

• Pick a time of day to test and be consistent.

• The status of your hormones and where you're at in your cycle may influence your ketone levels.

• When ketone levels are testing low, go for more fat bomb recipes.

An Alternative to Testing

If measuring your ketones isn't something you want to spend your time or money on, you can gauge where you are by looking at the signs that you're fat-adapted. This won't tell you how many ketones are circulating in your body, but it will tell you if your body is using fat as its preferred fuel—which is a good sign that you're in ketosis.

If you have three or more of the signs listed below, it's likely that you've made the switch and are fat-adapted:

- **You can skip meals without getting angry.**
- **It's easy to go three, four, or five hours without a snack.**
- **You don't get ravenous or crave carbs two to three hours after your last meal.**
- **You crave high-fat foods over high-carb foods.**
- **You don't need carbs to push through exercise plateaus.**
- **You experience steady energy throughout the day without afternoon crashes.**
- **Your thoughts seem clearer and more focused.**
- **You no longer experience keto flu.**

If you're interested in starting a carb-up practice, wait until you exhibit three or more of these signs. Generally, that happens after about ten to fifteen days on the Classic Keto Fat Fueled Profile. If you've started your journey with carb-ups right off the bat, say with the Daily Fat Burner Fat Fueled Profile, eliciting these signs can take thirty days or more.

WHAT TO EXPECT
WHEN YOU GO KETO

When I started out on keto, I found that I went through five phases of adjusting to the new eating style—and these phases seem to be pretty common for people making the switch. Of course, if you're concerned or unsure about anything you experience on keto, definitely chat with your health-care provider.

phase 1: CHANGE	Panic about eating fat	Find resources (like this book) to help you on your way	Research keto, feel good about it, but still panic a little	Try to eat high-fat/low-carb and realize that you're not eating enough fat	Discover fat bombs (see page 114); all becomes well with the world

phase 2: DEFINING	Try to understand macros	Get frustrated with macros and tracking	Use Daily Portion Plates (page 61) instead	Feel good	Play around with carbohydrate intake: How little can I eat? How many vegetables can I get away with?

phase 3: SYMPTOMS	Have acid reflux	Start taking digestive enzyme	Acid reflux gone	Get keto flu (page 94)	Start taking mineral drops and electrolyte powder	Start consuming Keto Lemonade (page 422), more greens, and avocados
	Muscle spasms gone	Take magnesium every night	Get muscle spasms	Brain fog gone	Eat more fats	Have brain fog	Keto flu gone

phase 4: BLISS	Intense hunger pains: gone	Digestion: smooth sailing	Energy: bursting	Weight: dropping	Mood: balanced

phase 5: REFINEMENT and EXPLORATION	Naturally fall into intermittent fasting (pages 68 to 72)	What keto foods do I enjoy most?	Play around with carbohydrate intake: Do I need carb-ups? How many per week? How much daily carbs can I get away with?	Switch around meal times to find optimal energy

HOW TO ADD MORE FAT

By now you're probably wondering, "How the heck do I eat that much fat?" I promise that after a couple of weeks of eating this way, you'll be creating strategies for fat consumption without even thinking about it. Until then, here are some tricks and shortcuts for adding more nourishing fats to the foods you love:

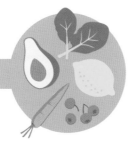

PRODUCE

Cook bacon for your salad, then add the drippings to the bowl.

Use steamed vegetables as a delivery system for coconut oil.

Snack on avocados drizzled with olive oil, salt, and chili powder.

Whip coconut cream with cacao powder and a touch of alcohol-free stevia for a high-fat delight. Top it with berries and you'll forget all about regular pudding.

Always use bacon grease to roast veggies.

Place MCT oil in a blender with tallow or lard and fresh spices. Blend, chill, and use as an herb butter on everything.

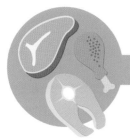

MEAT AND SEAFOOD

Dip cooked proteins in Kale Pâté (page 259).

Beef brisket has layers of natural golden fat. Once cooked, reheat slices in a pan with additional fat for crispy leftover brisket.

Grab a bag of pork rinds and enjoy with guacamole or avocado oil mayo.

Use coconut oil as a rub before roasting a whole chicken, then make gravy with the drippings.

Sauté everything in reserved bacon grease, tallow, lard, or duck fat.

Add 1 cup of olive oil or avocado oil to a jar with 3 tablespoons of spices. Allow to marinate for a week, then use as a salad dressing, dip, or marinade.

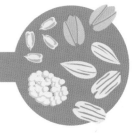

NUTS AND SEEDS

Top your salads and vegetable bowls with chia seeds, hulled hemp seeds, and/or sesame seeds.

Soak and roast your favorite nuts/seeds (see page 157 for instructions), then divide them into small packs for easy snacking. Add coconut oil and salt before eating!

Always have fat bombs (see page 114) on hand.

Spread nut, seed, or coconut butter on keto muffins (pages 238 and 239) and breads (pages 366 to 375).

EGGS

Save the yolks! If a recipe calls for egg whites only, freeze the yolks and use them in one large, bright scramble or add them (raw) to a Rocket Fuel Latte (page 428).

Scramble eggs with epic amounts of coconut oil, reserved bacon grease, or rendered fats (see page 159 for instructions or pages 167 to 171 for recommended brands).

Use avocado oil mayo to top eggs, chicken, salad, breads, fried vegetables, and more.

PANTRY ITEMS

Rocket Fuel Lattes (page 428) boost fat in the easiest way. Perfect for breakfast, snacks, or as a bedtime drink.

Combine a handful of chocolate chips with a spoonful of coconut butter or manna.

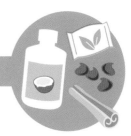

Mix tahini with ground cinnamon and a drop of alcohol-free stevia. Enjoy with a spoon.

FASTING AND KETOSIS: THE POWER COUPLE

Fasting is a scary word. I remember when my third-grade class collected pledges for a fast that we were going to perform at school in support of our class's sponsor child. The plan was to only drink water until we broke our fast at the end of the school day with a pizza party. All the kids did really well, except for me. I lasted until 9:35 a.m.—officially ten hours of fasting—when I dug some change out of my backpack and inconspicuously chose the richest possible treat out of the vending machine.

From then on, fasting scared me. I wouldn't have dreamed of skipping breakfast, let alone going a whole day without food. As a hypoglycemic, I thought I was one of those people who just couldn't go long periods without food, end of story. But looking back, my inability to fast was tied directly to the fact that I was an intense glucose-burner, relying heavily on six to eight meals a day to keep things balanced.

Don't let fasting fool you like it did me. It's not nearly as scary as you might think it is. In fact, it's downright awesome. Intermittent fasting (IF) is the practice of going sixteen to twenty-four hours without food, without struggling through it. When you're in ketosis, going sixteen to twenty-four hours without food is effortless. Your blood sugar is stable, which instantly reduces the need to eat every three to four hours. And without the ups and downs of blood sugar irregularities, the body isn't signaled to eat to make up for blood sugar lows.

It all boils down to the fact that when we're in nutritional ketosis, we have unlimited access to the energy stored in our body fat. Sure, our bodies will use dietary fat for fuel, too, but even when we don't eat, we're constantly being supplied with fuel that's stored on the body. Which means that fasting as a fat-burner is easy and natural—when you don't need extra fuel, you don't get hungry.

You also don't experience traditional hunger symptoms like anger, dizziness, light-headedness, or fatigue.

NOTE: *If you're in this for weight loss and planning to restrict calories as well as practice IF, please don't. It's one or the other. Combining calorie restriction with IF may cause health imbalances, can affect your body's ability to become fat-adapted, and will make you downright miserable.*

Fasting comes with tons of benefits:

- **Weight loss without slowed metabolism (which happens with calorie reduction dieting)**
- **Stable blood sugar**
- **Improved insulin sensitivity and lowered insulin levels**
- **Loss of body fat**
- **Lower blood pressure, cholesterol levels, and triglycerides**
- **Reduced inflammation**
- **Increased levels of ketones, which has a whole host of benefits (see page 26)**
- **Higher levels of human growth hormone, which aids muscle growth and fat-burning**
- **Reduced free-radical damage, which means slower aging**
- **Lowered risk of cancer when fasting is paired with a reduction in glucose, which fuels cancer cells**

NOTE: *Please, please don't think that the more and longer you fast, the better off you'll be. Fasting should be part of a balanced fat-fueled lifestyle. If fasting doesn't feel good or you're forcing yourself to fast, STOP, DROP, and LISTEN to your body.*

Interested in fasting? Head on over to page 428 for details on using Rocket Fuel Lattes to extend your fast.

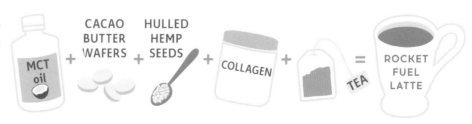

MCT oil + CACAO BUTTER WAFERS + HULLED HEMP SEEDS + COLLAGEN + TEA = ROCKET FUEL LATTE

My Anti-Fasting Message

I just told you how great a practice fasting is, and now I'm going to say the exact opposite. Why? Well, because we are all different. And not just different from one another—we're different from the people we were yesterday and the people we'll be tomorrow. There are days where fasting feels fabulous in my body, and there are days I can't go past 9 a.m. without a full keto breakfast.

I feel like many of us women have an all-or-nothing mentality. If we commit to fasting, gosh darn it, we're going to do it every day to cash in on the benefits, even if that means crappy sleep, endless hunger, reduced ketones (because of the stress we're putting on our bodies), less energy, imbalanced hormones, and more. If we read that it is good and we think we should be doing it, we do it, regardless of the price we have to pay.

So what do we do about this fasting thing? We listen to our bodies.

Don't feel like fasting today? Don't. Have breakfast—an RFL, a big-ass salad, bacon and eggs. Your body, your choice.

A Rocket Fuel Latte (page 428) doesn't count as food! Drink your morning RFL to give your body nutrients and fuel while continuing with your fast.

Continuing to drive ourselves into a fasted state, especially when our bodies are healing from hormonal imbalances (thyroid, adrenals, sex hormones, you name it) can make the situation worse. This was my experience, which is why I now fast only when it feels right. Today, I've been fasting for sixteen hours and I'm not even thinking about food. But yesterday was an all-out keto food fest, morning to night. It happens.

If you're implementing a ketogenic diet in hopes of healing your body from imbalances such as adrenal dysfunction, hypothyroidism, or low sex hormones, it may be best for you to skip the IF practices or, at most, practice a sixteen-hour fast when it's convenient and totally natural for you to do so.

It's also important to pay attention to your mental and emotional health during fasting. As someone with a history of disordered eating, following a strict intermittent fasting practice really didn't work for me. I found myself obsessing about my next meal, fantasizing about all the fabulous things I would eat and calculating when I could eat them. I calculated fasting hours so frequently that I started dreaming about it. Nightmares with clocks and fasting schedules became my reality at least three times a week. And when I finally did break the fast at the planned time, I ate until I was so full that I could barely move. Forget about listening to my body—I ruled what I ate, when, and how much.

If you, too, have a tense relationship with dieting or food restriction, or you have had an all-out war between your body and food at some point in your beautiful life, intermittent fasting may trigger something in you that you don't want to experience again.

I don't want to scare you away from fasting altogether—there are some great benefits to it. But keep in mind that you don't have to do it every day. Go with the flow. Listening to your body to create a keto intermittent fasting approach allows you to cash in on the IF benefits and use it as a tool to simplify your life, while also avoiding its potential pitfalls.

NOTE: *Some benefits of IF may be realized only during a twenty- to twenty-four-hour fast, but this may be true only for those not in ketosis. When a glucose-fueled person practices IF for twenty to twenty-four-hours, they experience the IF benefits as soon as their body starts creating ketones. The fat-adapted, whose bodies are already creating ketones, may start seeing benefits after just sixteen to eighteen hours.*

If you are on medication, have type 2 diabetes, or are pregnant, breastfeeding, or underweight, please chat with your health-care provider about whether IF is a good strategy for you before you go for it.

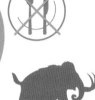

A BEGINNER'S GUIDE TO INTERMITTENT FASTING

16-HOUR FAST	24-HOUR FAST	CAVEMAN	UP AND DOWN
Practiced: 3–5 days a week	**Practiced:** 2–3 days a week	**Practiced:** 3–5 days a week	**Practiced:** 2–4 days a week
Format: Fast for 16 hours, eat for 8 hours. Example: Stop eating at 9 p.m. on day one, and start eating at 1 p.m. on day two.	**Format:** Fast for 24 hours. Example: Stop eating at 5 p.m. on day one and start eating at 5 p.m. on day two.	**Format:** Fast all day, eat one large meal at night.	**Format:** Restricted calories on day one, regular calories on day two.
Notes: This approach may not significantly limit calories, but it does give the body the needed time to increase ketones and gives the digestive system a nice break.	**Notes:** This reduces overall calorie intake without making you feel like you're going a full day without a meal.	**Notes:** Fasting during the day mimics the fight-or-flight response, helping to boost energy and stimulate fat-burning. Eating at night lays the groundwork for tissue repair and growth. (See page 41 for more on eating at night.)	**Notes:** On low-calorie days, total calories should be 20 percent of usual intake. For many people, this is about 400–500 calories for the whole day.
Natural Calorie Reduction: May be seen if you compare your daily intakes. Eat when you're hungry during the eight-hour window and don't worry too much about the calories you're consuming.	**Natural Calorie Reduction:** Can be seen if you look at your overall weekly intake. Eat when you're hungry during your eating window and don't worry too much about the calories you're consuming.	**Natural Calorie Reduction:** Can be seen if you compare your daily intakes. Eat during the eating window and don't worry too much about the calories you're consuming.	**Natural Calorie Reduction:** May be seen if you look at your overall weekly intake. On days where you are not restricting, eat when you're hungry and don't worry too much about the calories you're consuming.
Level of Difficulty: I	Level of Difficulty: III	Level of Difficulty: II	Level of Difficulty: III
Great as a daily practice, really easy to implement with little effort.	It's tempting to break the fast with an all-out gorge, but don't do it!	It's tempting to break the fast with an all-out gorge, but don't do it!	On low-calorie days, separate meals into two smaller meals and space them out throughout the day.

Breaking the fast with a carb-up meal is an awesome strategy for a lot of people.

If having just one meal a day sets you up for failure, approach the meal as a feast. A couple of hours after your first meal in the eating window, have a second. This strategy can be particularly helpful if having carbs after a long fast doesn't feel good in your body.

Ladies, Take Note: Fasting, Hormones, and Butter Coffee

When I first started an intermittent fasting practice, butter coffee was all the rage. If you aren't familiar with butter coffee, it's a blend of butter, MCT oil, and coffee that you consume in the morning instead of breakfast. The concept behind the fatty drink is that drinking it in the morning on a fasting day provides the body with the nourishing benefits of grass-fed butter and other healthy saturated fats while keeping blood sugar stable, reducing hunger, extending a fast, and generating a boost in ketone bodies. It's a way to practice IF without having to go oodles of hours without food.

I can't do butter, so I created a dairy-free mixture of coconut oil, MCT oil, and coffee. It was good, but after a couple of days of drinking it, I started getting the shakes. Each day after drinking the mixture, my mind began racing, I grew dizzy, and lethargy set in shortly thereafter. To top it off, my appetite slowly increased until the drink would hold me over for thirty minutes at most. This continued for weeks. I tried replacing the coffee with herbal tea and the fats with coconut-free options, but I saw no change in my symptoms.

My experience inspired me to create a video on butter coffee–based intermittent fasting, which is now one of the most popular videos on my YouTube channel, Healthful Pursuit. As soon as I shared my symptoms, women began speaking to me about it. Turns out, a lot of us were suffering.

So how do we get the benefits of fasting, enjoy butter coffee, and avoid the symptoms? The solution came when I realized that my symptoms were alleviated when I added a touch of whole-food protein and carbohydrate to my butter coffee. Instead of the message "Danger, only fat is coming in!" that the fat-only coffees had been sending my body, it sent my body the message "It's okay, we have fuel. Fat, protein, carbs—it's safe." And it did so without supplying so much fuel that my insulin levels spiked to process it, so I was able to keep fasting safely. Thus the Rocket Fuel Latte was born. (You'll find the recipe on page 428.)

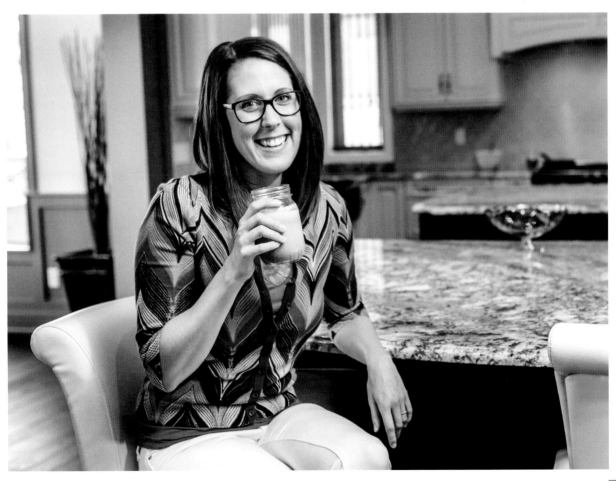

From that day forward, I started adding 3 grams of carbs and just under 10 grams of protein to my fatty coffees, and within a couple of days, I felt completely different. Within two weeks, I couldn't believe I'd gone that long with the standard fat-only drink and the misery that accompanied it.

Adding a touch of whole-food carbohydrates and proteins to butter coffee influences leptin, the hormone that makes you feel full. I think the fat-only experience may play around with leptin, making the body a bit confused. Remember how leptin sensitivity can change on a low-carb diet (see page 40)? My thought is that having a fat-only drink in the morning lowered the level of leptin in my body, so I wanted more food even though I was physically full. We know that a slight increase in carbohydrate intake can help us become more sensitive to leptin, making us feel satiated longer. While I'd love to jump in a lab and test my theory, it's not in the cards.

I, and so many in the Healthful Pursuit community, have had great experiences fasting with Rocket Fuel Lattes, and I hope you will, too! But I encourage you to test it for yourself. Try a fat-only drink in the morning—the classic coffee with grass-fed butter and MCT oil or, if you're sensitive to dairy, with cacao butter/oil or grass-fed ghee. Give that a try for a couple of days, then switch to a Rocket Fuel Latte. See how you feel—and if you test your blood glucose and ketones, watch those ketones increase and your blood glucose begin to fall!

I do believe that women may have a different experience with fasting than men. While there are studies that claim fasting doesn't have an effect on women's hormones, there are two reasons why those studies may not apply to women in everyday life.

The first is that a fourteen-day period of fasting—the most common in studies—is likely not going to make a large impact on a woman's overall hormonal balance. The longest-term fasting studies tend to look at those who fast during Ramadan, the month during which Muslims refrain from eating from sunrise to sunset. Studies would be more likely to catch changes in hormones if they looked at women who have been practicing intermittent fasting for at least three months.

The second is that many fasting studies are done on obese women. Fat cells create sex hormones, namely estrogen, and store these hormones and others. So when fat cells begin to shrink because fasting is causing these women to use body fat for fuel, the women in the studies become less able to produce estrogen. But at the same time, the shrinking fat cells are releasing stored hormones into the bloodstream to be discarded. It can take months for the process to level off, so, when these individuals receive blood tests throughout a study, the results show a false hormonal landscape. Testing for hormones even a month into a fasting period isn't likely to show the whole picture.

Given my experiences with butter coffee, it makes sense to me that some women may react negatively to having just fat in the morning. If a woman of reproductive age goes days having only fat in the morning, fasting through to the afternoon, and follows that fast with a calorie-restricted diet—ketogenic or otherwise—it could lead to imbalanced sex hormones and an interruption in fertility due to a lack of sustenance. After all, the female body is, from nature's perspective, a complex baby-making machine. Growing babies requires tons of nutrients and calories, and if the body believes there won't be enough to support a baby, the reproductive system can shut down as a protective mechanism. And while fat intake is critical for health, so is a balance of protein and carbohydrate.

While many women can go weeks, months, or even years practicing a protocol of butter coffee, fasting, and calorie restriction with absolutely no effect on their sex hormones, others are not so lucky. If you've recently adopted a butter coffee practice and have noticed symptoms quickly following, it could be a sign that your body doesn't like this approach. By switching to Rocket Fuel Latte (page 428) and adopting the IF strategies on page 70, which encourage you not to restrict calories while fasting, your body will receive signals that there are enough nutrients to go around, so it's safe to get pregnant. (Even if you don't want to get pregnant, it's important for your body to feel that it's safe to do so.)

WORKING OUT ON THE KETO DIET

Whether you're an aerobic or anaerobic athlete, the keto diet can be great for your workouts.

Aerobic exercise is essentially cardiovascular exercise—it's aimed at strengthening the heart and lungs. Anaerobic exercise primarily benefits other muscles to build strength and mass (although anyone who's done an anaerobic exercise like HIIT can vouch for its cardiovascular benefits). Each kind of workout demands the body use a different kind of fuel, which has implications for how we need to eat to get the most out of our workouts.

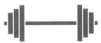

AEROBIC EXERCISE		ANAEROBIC EXERCISE
Distance running, cycling, dancing, cross-country skiing, swimming	**ACTIVITIES**	Sprinting (cycling or running), weight training, high-intensity interval training
Sustained for long periods	**DURATION**	Short, high-intensity sessions
Strengthens lungs and heart	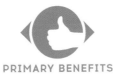 **PRIMARY BENEFITS**	Builds strength and muscle mass
Carbs (glucose/glycogen) or fat	**FUEL SOURCE**	Carbs (glucose/glycogen)
ck Classic Keto (page 47) or **pk** Pumped Keto (page 47)* *While some aerobic athletes thrive on Pumped Keto, others do not. Start with Classic Keto and, if you experience symptoms (see page 43 for signs that it's time to carb up), switch to Pumped Keto.*	**BEST FAT-FUELED PROFILE**	**ck** Classic Keto (page 47) or **fk** Full Keto (page 48) if you're active 1–3 days/week **afb** Adapted Fat Burner (page 48) if you're active 3–7 days/week
Can work, depending on your program (see page 68)	**FASTING**	Can work, depending on your program (see page 68)

Aerobic Athletes

An aerobic athlete has three fuel choices during activity:

**OPTION 1: Not fat-adapted.
Rely solely on glucose and frequent feeding with limited blood sugar control.**

- Carb-load before intense activity
- Constantly refuel during activity with glucose through gels, packs, and gummies
- Never switch to burning fat
- The fear of "bonking" or "hitting a wall" (experiencing sudden fatigue and loss of energy) dictates fuel choices before, during, and after exercise

**OPTION 2: Not fat-adapted.
Rely on glucose and fatty acids with blood sugar control.**

- Take a whole-food (likely Paleo) approach to nutrition
- Low blood sugar leads to quick mobilization of fatty acids, allowing the athlete to switch between fuel sources pretty efficiently
- May have to refuel during activity with Paleo-friendly carbohydrate sources
- As fatty acids are oxidized, glucose is spared, leaving some for recovery after the activity

**OPTION 3: Fat-adapted.
Rely solely on fatty acids with natural blood sugar control.**

- Follow a low-carb, high-fat diet
- Access fat stores 400 percent more efficiently than in option 1
- Can run on fat for hours with no need to refuel during exercise
- Best fuel choice for stamina and loss of body fat
- As fatty acids are oxidized, glucose supplied through gluconeogenesis is spared, leaving some for recovery after the activity

As you can see, options 1 and 2 aren't ideal—they don't result in efficient fat-burning, so the athlete is not using the stored energy most available, and blood sugar highs and lows can affect performance. With option 3, however, aerobic athletes can train their bodies to burn fat during exercise, which improves stamina, reduces body fat, and decreases post-exercise muscle damage.

Anaerobic Athletes

An anaerobic athlete has literally one choice when it comes to fuel for activity: glucose. Neither protein nor fat can be metabolized during anaerobic training, so all fuel needs to come from glucose. This poses a potential problem for low-carb athletes because they may not have the glycogen—stored glucose—they need to perform their anaerobic activity. While gluconeogenesis (see page 26) can help immensely with this process, the period of fat adaptation can be a tricky one for an anaerobic athlete.

Does this mean you can't be in ketosis and do anaerobic activities? Not at all. Once fat-adapted, gluconeogenesis should provide you with everything you need to crush your workouts. But in some cases it doesn't.

The traditional ketogenic diet and the high-protein ketogenic diet—in the Fat Fueled Profiles, these are Classic Keto and Pumped Keto (page 47)—may not work well for you while you're adapting and training; they decrease glycogen stores in the muscles, which means that on these profiles not enough glucose will be available for anaerobic training to be effective, at least until you adapt and gluconeogenesis can make up for the loss.

If you're new to keto and you don't want your training to take an initial hit (less energy, stamina, muscle power), the Full Keto or Daily Fat Burner profile (page 49) is the way to go.

If you're new to keto and don't mind your training taking an initial hit (less energy, stamina, muscle power), with potential long-term gain, Classic Keto (page 47) may be just the thing you're looking for.

If you're already keto and crushing your workouts, stay where you are!

If you're already keto and struggling on a Classic Keto (page 47) approach, some studies indicate that because protein can be converted to glucose when necessary, a high-protein ketogenic diet can work for anaerobic training. Personally, this didn't work for me whatsoever. But if you're interested in trying it, Pumped Keto (page 47) is the best option to roll with. But a better plan, in my view, is to adopt a carb-up practice. Note that this is not the same as carb loading. A high-fat diet with a carbohydrate load before anaerobic training has actually been shown to compromise performance during high-intensity activity. But a carb-up practice—incorporating carbs on a cyclical basis to build glycogen stores—has been shown to do marvelous things. (For how to do carb-ups right and more information about who might benefit from them, see pages 39 to 41.)

My personal experience using carb-ups to build epic muscle on an anaerobic-based exercise program is that it worked just as promised. I had a bunch of energy, built muscle easily, and felt on top of the world every six or seven days, when I loaded up my glycogen stores with carbs. For more on this strategy, check out pages 39 to 41.

Creating Positive Movement

There is beauty in sport, in growing muscle and training and adjusting strategies and protocols to lead to mega success. However, I've also seen the ugly side of this world.

While some individuals are able to maintain a workout schedule and training program that benefits their life, makes them feel good, and doesn't ruin their psyche, I am not one of those people. I was a junkie for marathon training, competitive swimming, cycling, heavy lifting, and dancing. If the activity promised to maintain my six-pack, I was there. I was also underweight, severely malnourished, depressed, without a period, and obsessed with food and exercise.

There came a time, after my tenth big race, when my body started to shut down. My energy was waning; my hips and knees were painful to the touch. I'll never forget the day I spent two hours on the bike with my coach and we had to cut it short because my knees were so inflamed that they'd started to lock up. I got off the bike, grabbed an exercise mat, and started doing core work. My coach told me to go home, but I refused. I had to keep training, couldn't miss a day. After all, the core workout didn't involve my knees, so what was the big deal?

After years of this destructive behavior, I finally learned to allow my body to just be. Part of the process of recovering from my workout obsession was stopping all training for a year. For six months, I stretched in the morning, walked when I felt like it, and slept a lot. In the six months following, I practiced hatha yoga a few days a week. And now I engage in positive movement.

I created a positive movement practice to lessen the stress and expectations I'd experienced while in the obsessive world of "working out." It's fabulous—it lets me do what I want to do and helps me maintain a body I feel good in without the self-loathing drill sergeant rules that a workout schedule and training program brought me.

My positive movement practice consists of doing things I enjoy doing that just happen to be "workouts." I don't have a training program. What I have is a calendar of all the activities going on in my area and a list of things I can do on my own time. What I do on any given day depends on how I'm feeling, what the weather's like, and how my workday is flowing.

For example, this Monday I went to a yoga class in the morning and in the evening took a one-hour walk to a coffee shop with my husband. On Tuesday morning, I drove to the largest hill in town and climbed it, drinking my chilled RFL when I reached the top. On Wednesday, my sister and I went stand-up paddleboarding for a couple of hours. On Thursday I was pretty tired, so I decided to hang out in the garden, pick weeds, and listen to music. Today is Friday, and I started the day with a thirty-minute walk and feel like I'll be in the mood for another come lunchtime. Tomorrow morning I'm headed to a dance class with a friend.

All the activities on my list are things I like, not things I think I should do. There is no running, cycling, or heavy lifting because I hate doing those things. Life is way too short to do things you don't want to do, with people you don't enjoy being with, for results that won't cure all the unhappiness you have about your body.

If you want to create a positive movement practice for yourself, here are a few tips to get started:

1. **Write down all the physical activities you like to do.**

2. **Next to each activity, write why you like it. For example: "I like stand-up paddleboarding because I get to be on the water. It makes me feel calm." Or "I like yoga because I get to interact with others in the studio. It makes me feel connected." Or "I like dancing because it helps me be aware of my body and makes me feel free."**

3. **From there, write down any caveats. Are there certain places you prefer to go for an activity? Certain people you enjoy doing them with?**

4. **Set the intention to practice one of these activities, perhaps on the weekend, and see how you feel!**

SUPPLEMENTS

SUPPORTIVE NUTRIENTS

For a long time, I was a proponent of using only whole foods to nourish my body. Problem was, it wasn't enough for me. I'd put my body through a lot, and many vital nutrient levels were dangerously low. So supplements had to take a seat at my healing table, and they may have to for you as well.

Foods   Recommended Brands

WHAT IT BENEFITS

whole body   digestive   immune   hormone   energy

anti-inflammatory   bone and joint   brain and neurological

TIME OF DAY

Breakfast **B**   Dinner **D**

Lunch **L**   Bed **C**

BONE STRENGTH

 greens, nuts and seeds, salmon, sardines

Protocol Bone Strength Formula

Contains vitamin C, vitamin D3, vitamin K2, thiamin, calcium, phosphorus, magnesium, zinc, copper, manganese, MCHA, glucosamine potassium sulfate complex, horsetail, and boron.

B **L**

CURCUMIN

 turmeric

Organika Curcumin

B **L** **D**

ENZYMES

 apple cider vinegar or lemon juice (before meals)

NOW Foods Super Enzymes

B **L** **D**

IODINE

 cod, cranberries, eggs, seaweed, strawberries, turkey

Pure Encapsulations Potassium Iodine

B

MAGNESIUM

 avocados, dark chocolate, dark leafy greens, fish, nuts and seeds

Viva Labs Magnesium Bisglycinate Chelate

Best to take before bed, but can be spread out if taking more than 1000 mg/day

MULTIVITAMIN

 vast array of real, whole foods

Pure Encapsulations Women's Nutrients

I don't love multis because the nutrient profiles are often imbalanced and the quality can be garbage.

B **L** **D**

NIACIN (VITAMIN B3)

 avocado, beef, chicken, liver, mushrooms, pork, salmon, turkey

Now Foods Flush-Free Niacin

When taking an individual B vitamin like niacin, it's best to supplement with a B complex also.

B **L** **D**

OMEGA 3

 beef, Brussels sprouts, cauliflower, flax seeds, salmon, sardines, shrimp, walnuts

Thorne Research Krill Oil OR (plant-based) Yes Parent Essential OR Barleans Omega Swirl Oils (great for kids)

B **L** **D**

PROBIOTICS

 fermented foods: kefir, kimchi, sauerkraut, sour pickles

NOW Foods Probiotic-10™ 50 Billion

I like taking my probiotics with a carb-up to aid in the uptake of the probiotic. You can take them on an empty stomach if that agrees with your body.

D **C**

But that doesn't mean you can't or shouldn't make whole foods your primary source for vital nutrients. That's how our bodies were designed to be nourished. Plus, eating certain foods together makes their nutrients more available than they would be when eaten alone or when obtained in supplements. For instance, the vitamins found in greens are absorbed better when they're consumed with olive oil because they're fat-soluble.

I need supplements for key nutrients in which I know I am deficient, but I also make sure I get those nutrients from the foods I eat every day. This is why the following chart lists food sources for each nutrient or supplement: so that you can create a balance all your own.

It's often best to work with a health-care practitioner to determine which supplements are best for your needs.

SELENIUM

beef, Brazil nuts, cod, chicken, lamb, oysters, salmon, sardines, scallops, sunflower seeds, turkey

NOW Foods Selenium (L-Selenomethionine)

VITAMIN A

cod liver oil, egg yolks, grass-fed butter, liver

Green Pastures Fermented Cod Liver Oil

Beta-carotene converts poorly to vitamin A, so it's not listed here.

VITAMIN B COMPLEX

chicken, dark leafy greens, seafood, spinach, turkey

NOW Foods Co-Enzyme B-Complex

VITAMIN B12

beef, crab, eggs, liver, mackerel, shellfish

Solgar Sublingual Methylcobalamin

For B12 injections, avoid cyanocobalamin and ask your doctor for methylcobalamin because it is better absorbed and retained.

VITAMIN C

bell peppers, broccoli, chiles, kale, strawberries, tomatoes

Pure Encapsulations Buffered Ascorbic Acid Capsules

Do not take directly after exercise as it can affect insulin sensitivity gained from exercise.

VITAMIN D

cod liver oil, egg yolks, liver, mushrooms, salmon, sardines

Metagenics D3 Liquid

The best source of vitamin D is the sun: expose as much skin as possible to sunlight for 10–20 minutes a day.

VITAMIN K2

broccoli, Brussels sprouts, cauliflower, chard, collards, kale, lettuce, parsley, spinach

Life Extension Super K with Advanced K2 Complex

VITEX

avocado, coconut, dark green vegetables, egg yolks, fermented foods, flax seeds, hemp, herbal teas, salmon, sardines, walnuts

Nature's Way Vitex Fruit (Chasteberry)

Consists of the herb chasteberry, so there are no foods that contain it, however I've listed foods that have similar properties in balancing hormones.

ZINC

beef, cashews, lamb, pumpkin seeds, sesame seeds, shrimp, turkey

NOW Foods Zinc Glycinate

Electrolytes

As glycogen stores are depleted as you become fat-adapted, the water that was stored with glycogen is excreted through the kidneys, causing an initial electrolyte imbalance. In addition, when your intake of carbohydrates is less than about 50 total grams a day, you need electrolytes in higher amounts in order to avoid keto flu (see page 94).

This is all to say that as you live as a strong, confident ketogenic warrior, you may find supplementing with electrolytes to be your saving grace, as it was mine. Electrolytes are a class of minerals that includes sodium, magnesium, and potassium. By managing your levels of these minerals, you can successfully avoid many of the side effects experienced with a low-carb diet. (More details about overcoming electrolyte imbalance are on page 95.)

NOTE: *Before increasing your electrolyte intake, be sure to chat with your health-care provider if you have kidney disease, are taking diuretics, take high blood pressure medication, have been told to avoid salt substitutes, or have heart failure.*

Let's start with sodium. The importance of sodium on a keto diet runs deep, insulin deep. We know that overall insulin requirements, and therefore insulin levels, are reduced on a ketogenic diet. When insulin is low, sodium is more easily extracted from the blood via the kidneys and excreted in the form of urine. You see where I'm going with this: a reduction in insulin levels (while totally awesome for overall health) impacts the availability of sodium, requiring you to eat more of the stuff. (See page 124 for information on the different kinds of salt.)

In the modern world, magnesium is one of the minerals in which we're most deficient. A combination of alcohol consumption, high stress, lack of nutrient-dense food, calcium supplement abuse, and digestive factors can cause a deficiency. Add a keto diet on top of that, and your body's in need of some mag, stat! Magnesium deficiency can be characterized by dizziness, fatigue, muscle cramps, high blood pressure, and weakness.

The factors that cause magnesium deficiency can also cause potassium deficiency. Signs of potassium deficiency can include constipation, depression, skin problems, and hypertension.

You could spend a bunch of money on electrolyte powders, or you could make a health-promoting electrolyte-rich drink that goes far beyond the benefits of a store-bought electrolyte mix. I'm a fan of my Keto Lemonade, which is higher in electrolytes than a powder and is made from real ingredients. See page 422 for the recipe.

In addition, the following foods are rich in electrolytes. If you incorporate these foods in your ketogenic diet, along with Keto Lemonade, you'll be set.

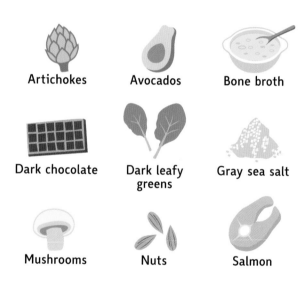

Artichokes	Avocados	Bone broth
Dark chocolate	Dark leafy greens	Gray sea salt
Mushrooms	Nuts	Salmon

It's no wonder that almost all of these foods are part of the Keto Power Foods List (page 111)!

KETO AT AND AWAY FROM HOME: BUYING GROCERIES, EATING OUT, AND TRAVELING

Whatever your budget, however many mouths you're intending to feed, and whatever stores you have access to, you can make keto work. This chapter offers tips and strategies for eating keto wherever you are, travel included!

THE PRICE OF GROCERIES

Our family of four, which includes Kevin and myself along with our two fur children, Lexy and Pebbles, spends $780 per month on groceries. I make the dogs' food, too, from basically the same things we eat, so this cost includes their food—and honestly, they often eat more than I do in a day.

This amount may seem like a lot, but according to the United States Department of Agriculture, a family of four with two young children on a low-cost food plan spends approximately $715.20 on groceries per month. Given that I'm feeding four with organic, non-GMO, quality-source foods at just $64.80 over the national average on the low-cost plan, I'd say this is cause for celebration.

I understand that money is often tight. Eating high-quality food means a great deal to Kevin and me, so we've cut down on things that mean less to us: for example, an unlimited gym membership, the cable TV we never watched, and a new car. Every time I get into my 2004 Ford Escape that has more than 186,000 miles on it, I think of how glorious my next grass-fed burger with avocado oil mayo and organic lettuce and tomato is going to taste.

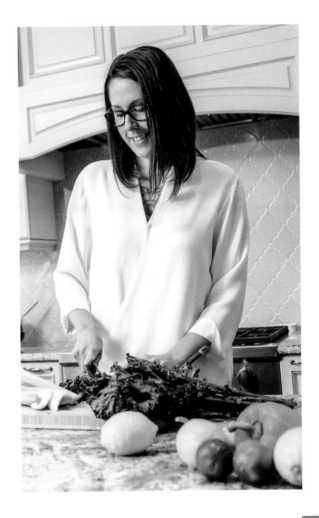

STICKING TO YOUR FOOD BUDGET

 Ferment your own vegetables. Use a starter culture like Caldwell Bio Fermentation or Body Ecology, which is good for over 24 pounds (12 kg) of vegetable fermentation action.

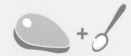 Grab lean cuts of meat and cook them in healthy fats (see page 67 for a list).

 Render your own fats (see page 159).

Use coconut oil in place of grass-fed butter, ghee, and cacao butter/oil.

 Stick to lower-cost nuts and seeds (see page 144).

 Find a friend who has hens and offer to take care of their children, mow their lawn, or walk their dog in exchange for a dozen eggs a week.

 Skip the prepackaged keto treats and make your own instead.

 Go for red meat instead of poultry.

 Stick to similar foods in your meal plans every week, at least as you're getting started, so that there's minimal waste and overwhelm.

 Be conscious of the food you're buying. Don't buy things you won't use.

 Stick to the perimeter of the grocery store. The middle is where the expensive things are.

 Swap your restaurant date night for a picnic at your favorite park.

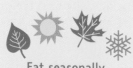 Eat seasonally. Produce that's in season is generally less expensive.

 Shop at farmers' markets. Many of them are not certified organic but use organic practices, which means a lower cost to you.

 Don't get distracted by bright, shiny things. Load up on full-fat proteins, low-carb vegetables, one cooking oil, and a couple of spices, and you'll be set.

 Make a list and stick to it!

GROCERY STORE GUIDE

Whether you're shopping for keto goods in store or online, this guide will give you an idea of which stores have the best value, align with what you're looking for, and are most convenient for your shopping needs. For both online and brick-and-mortar stores, I gathered the same items in my cart to determine the average grocery cost at each store. Then, after all was said and done, I rated each store based on shipping cost, accessibility, ease of use, and product cost.

Online Stores

THRIVE MARKET

RATING: ★★★★★

SHIPPING: Free on orders over $49

AVERAGE GROCERY COST: $ $ $

Least expensive of the online stores I looked at. Grocery cost was $84.40, with free shipping (because the order was over $49). However, there is a yearly membership fee of $59.95.

STRENGTHS

+ Significantly discounted prices (up to 50% off).
+ Easy to use—you can shop by certified gluten-free, certified kosher, certified organic, fair trade–certified, non-GMO-project certified, certified vegan, Paleo, dairy-free, grass-fed, low-glycemic, pasture-raised, locally sourced, and more.
+ When you sign up, you usually receive at least 1 month free, plus a discount on your first order, plus a free product.
+ Wide range of items, including food, health, babies & kids, home, and pets.
+ No annual fee for students.
+ Orders ship within 24 to 72 hours.

WEAKNESSES

− Requires an annual $59.95 fee.
− Not as wide a range of products as Amazon.
− Ships only to the contiguous U.S.; does not ship to Alaska, Hawaii, Puerto Rico, or Canada.

AMAZON

RATING: ★★★⯪☆

SHIPPING: Free shipping on eligible items with Prime membership. Otherwise, depends on the seller, product, and your location.

AVERAGE GROCERY COST: $ $ $

Most expensive of the online stores I looked at. Grocery cost was $119.79; shipping without Prime membership was $18; with Prime membership, $5 (not including the yearly membership fee of $99).

STRENGTHS

+ Wide range of products in more than 30 categories, including food, health, beauty, and cooking/kitchen.
+ Prime membership offers free two-day shipping on eligible items and further discounts for shopping Prime Pantry.
+ Students can get the first 6 months of their Prime membership free.
+ Occasional discounts for buying in bulk.
+ Amazon-verified purchase reviews are available, so you know that the reviewer actually bought the item.
+ If your cart totals $49 or more, small "add-on" items, such as silicone molds, olives, spices, and other inexpensive items, can be added to your order at no additional shipping cost. Note that the product needs to be sold directly by Amazon.
+ When you search for a food item, you can search by fat calories per serving, specialty food type (organic, kosher, GMO-free, gluten-free, etc.), brand, certification (organic, non-GMO, kosher, gluten-free, etc.), price, nutrition facts per serving, international shipping eligibility, and many other specifications.

WEAKNESSES

− Prime membership costs $99 per year or $10.99 per month (but membership is not required to shop Amazon).
− Not all products are sold directly by Amazon or another dependable source. Do your research before purchasing from an independent seller.

iHERB

RATING: ★★★★☆

SHIPPING: Discounted on orders of $40 or more; actual cost depends on where you live.

AVERAGE GROCERY COST: $$$

Mid-range. Grocery cost was $105.67; no membership fee.

STRENGTHS

+ Features supplements, herbs, bath, beauty, grocery, baby, and sports categories.

+ No annual fee or membership required.

+ For every purchase, a credit of 10% of the order total (excluding shipping) is applied to your next order.

+ Uses 100% post-consumer recycled paper for 90% of all shipping boxes. Bubble wrap is 40% recyclable.

+ Accepts over 45 international currencies.

+ When you search for a food item, you can search by brand, specialty (chemical-free, B corp, Halal, egg-free, peanut- and tree nut–free, etc.), price, rating, and more.

+ Lots of choices for quality nuts, seeds, and nut/seed butters.

WEAKNESSES

− Smaller grocery/food selection than Amazon or Thrive Market.

− Fewer big-name brands.

For grass-fed, pastured, wild-caught, and free-range proteins that can be ordered online and delivered right to your door, I highly recommend ButcherBox.

COSTCO

RATING: ★★★★★

AVERAGE GROCERY COST: $$$

Mid-range. Grocery cost was $2.68/oz. However, there is a yearly membership fee of $55 to $110.

STRENGTHS

+ Low prices.

+ Cooking oils, like coconut oil, avocado oil, and olive oil, are priced better than you'll find anywhere else.

+ Wide range of organic products.

+ Wide range of wild seafood and pasture-raised meats.

+ Carries a wide range of products, from grocery to home to clothing.

WEAKNESSES

− Requires a yearly membership fee of $55 to $110.

− Everything is sold in bulk, so if you have a smaller family, your groceries may go bad before you can use them up.

− Very busy on weekends, with long lines.

− Large store, so it can take a long time to complete your shopping trip.

− Not a wide range of specialty products (e.g., no cocoa butter or Primal Kitchen mayo).

− Easy to overspend because the carts are huge and there's a lot of random stuff in the aisles.

PICK-UP-AND-GO OPTIONS

· Hot dog without the bun, topped with sauerkraut, mustard, and onions (order at the counter).

· Caesar salad (order at the counter or pick up in the refrigerated section; ask for no croutons).

· Rotisserie chicken (in the meats section).

· Ceviche shrimp (in the meats section).

KROGER

RATING: ★ ★ ★ ☆ ☆

AVERAGE GROCERY COST: $ $ $
Mid-range at $3.19/oz.

STRENGTHS

+ Smaller stores make for quicker shopping trips.
+ Modest assortment of organic products and pasture-raised meats.

WEAKNESSES

− Few specialty products (e.g., no cocoa butter or Primal Kitchen mayo).

PICK-UP-AND-GO OPTIONS

· Made-to-order sandwich counter: skip the bread and choose a lettuce wrap filled with mayonnaise, meats, avocado, tomato, cucumber, onions, etc. instead.
· Prepared guacamole from the deli or produce aisle and precut packaged veggies like celery and cucumber.

WALMART

RATING: ★ ★ ★ ☆ ☆

AVERAGE GROCERY COST: $ $ $
Least expensive store at $2.53/oz.

STRENGTHS

+ Lowest prices.
+ Wide range of products, from grocery to home items to clothing.

WEAKNESSES

− Few organic products or pasture-raised meats.
− Few raw nut/seed options.
− Store is fairly large and usually has long lines, so it may take you longer to complete your shopping trip.

PICK-UP-AND-GO OPTIONS

· Premade salads: If you can't tolerate dairy, skip the provided dressing and top with an avocado, olive oil, vinegar/lemon juice, sea salt, and black pepper.
· Many stores have Subway restaurants inside. Order a salad topped with bacon, avocado, meats, egg, and oil and vinegar.

WHOLE FOODS

RATING: ★ ★ ★ ★ ☆

AVERAGE GROCERY COST: $ $ $
Most expensive at $4.43/oz.

STRENGTHS

+ Wide range of specialty products (like cocoa butter and Primal Kitchen mayo).
+ Save money by purchasing nuts and seeds from bulk bins.
+ Many great to-go/quick options.
+ Wide range of organic, fair-trade, pasture-raised products. Everything in the produce section is labeled with its origins, and most of it is labeled by growing method (organic, conventional, no-spray, etc.).
+ Smaller stores make for quicker shopping trips.

WEAKNESSES

− Most expensive of all in-person options.

PICK-UP-AND-GO OPTIONS

· Hot food bar with Paleo-friendly and keto-friendly options. Choose meats, low-carb veggies, and healthy fats.
· Salad bar: Choose meats, low-carb veggies, and healthy fats.
· Deli: Make your own sandwich. Go for lettuce-wrapped or choose a keto-friendly premade item, like chicken salad or grilled salmon and low-carb veggies.
· Sushi wrapped in greens instead of rice and stuffed with veggies. Swap the provided sugary peanut sauce for coconut aminos or a mayo-based sauce.
· EPIC Bars: Great for a keto-friendly snack, available in flavors like chicken Sriracha, salmon with sea salt and black pepper, and bacon.

Looking for full keto-friendly shopping lists for these seven stores? Go to healthfulpursuit.com/grocerystore

TRAVEL GUIDES

The epitome of practical actions is making an eating style work for you when you're traveling or on the go or you just don't want to make dinner. By the end of this section, you'll have every tool you need to feel supported, no matter where you are.

Traveling with Your Rocket Fuel Latte

There isn't a vacation I've gone on without bringing the ingredients necessary to make a Rocket Fuel Latte (page 428) on the go.

NOTE: *Do you have travel Rocket Fuel Latte strategies? Share them online using the hashtag #rocketfuellatte so that everyone can see them!*

Assuming that you can get hot liquid, such as coffee or tea, where you're going, here's what you'll need:

Mixer for combining the ingredients together (choose one)

- Electric handheld milk frother (see page 166)
- Heat-safe shaker bottle
- Airtight travel mug (I like S'well water bottles for this)

Fat (choose one)

- MCT oil, either in a travel container or as capsules
- Coconut oil
- Cacao butter/oil wafers (pack in a little baggie)

Sweetener (choose one)

- Alcohol-free liquid stevia
- Stevia packets

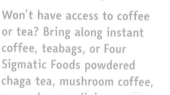

Won't have access to coffee or tea? Bring along instant coffee, teabags, or Four Sigmatic Foods powdered chaga tea, mushroom coffee, or mushroom elixirs. Just add hot water and go!

Protein (choose one)

- Collagen peptides stick packs from Vital Proteins
- Protein powder, in single-serve baggies or in one large container with a scoop. (If your protein powder comes in single-serve packets, that's a bonus!) If you choose protein powder, you likely won't need stevia if it's already sweetened.

Carb

- Nut or seed butter packets (I like coconut butter, smooth almond butter, and sunflower seed butter packets)

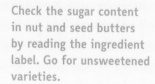

Check the sugar content in nut and seed butters by reading the ingredient label. Go for unsweetened varieties.

To make your RFL:
Simply place all the RFL ingredients in a mug. If you're using a milk frother, froth until combined. If you're using a shaker bottle or travel mug, shake until combined. Be careful when opening an airtight travel mug, as shaking hot liquids can cause an explosion of RFL all over your clean shirt.

KETO TRAVEL STRATEGIES

Whether you're traveling by plane, train, or automobile, I have you covered with these travel strategies so that you'll always have a keto-supporting solution for your next adventure!

AIRPLANE: DESTINATION TO HOME

HOTEL OR CRUISE SHIP (no access to kitchen)

CONDO RENTAL OR FRIEND/ FAMILY VISIT

CAMPING (access to cooking equipment)

SNACKS

DAILY EATS

TRAVELING HOME FROM A PLACE WITH A KITCHEN

NON-PERISHABLE SNACKS

- EPIC brand bars or bites
- Plastic baggies of collagen peptides for adding to drinks
- Packets of almond butter or coconut butter
- Macadamia nuts
- Pork rinds
- Dark chocolate bar
- Tea and/or coffee packets
- Canned salmon
- Roasted almonds
- Raw cookies
- Paleo granola
- Flax crackers
- Seaweed chips
- Freeze-dried berries
- Mixed nuts
- Pumpkin seeds

TRAVEL-SAFE MEALS

- Ultra-crispy bacon wrapped in a paper towel
- Fat bombs (refer to the chart on pages 432 to 434)
- Celery sticks with almond butter or tahini
- Shredded coconut with fresh berries and whipped coconut milk
- Easy travel meals (such as Allspice Muffins, page 238; Chicken Crisps, page 248; and Cracked-Up Ham Salad Sandwiches, page 324)

WITHOUT A KITCHEN

- Travel-ready RFL ingredients (page 84)
- Single-serve packets of coconut oil for warm vegetables
- MCT oil, olive oil, or avocado oil for salads, vegetables, and just about everything else
- Snack packs of olives to add to meals or snacks
- Collagen peptides to add to cold drinks—shake and go for quick protein
- Hulled hemp seeds for salads, vegetables, nut butter, and more

WITH A KITCHEN

+ ACCESS TO GROCERY STORE

- Flaxseed focaccia mix (page 372) in a resealable plastic bag; add wet ingredients at your destination
- 5 favorite spices in mini containers
- Olive oil
- Coconut oil or grass-fed tallow in a glass jar, (placed in a resealable plastic bag just in case)
- Apple cider vinegar

NO ACCESS TO GROCERY STORE

- One heat-stable oil (e.g., coconut oil) and one salad-friendly oil (e.g., olive oil)
- Vegetables that will hold up well in a cooler, like kale, zucchini, cucumbers, and radishes (greens in plastic clamshells fill with cooler water and get mushy)
- Meats divided into single-serve packets and frozen individually
- Carb-ups that travel well, like plantain chips, potatoes, and sweet potatoes

- No matter where you're headed, an insulated bottle that keeps liquids hot or cold is as versatile as they come. I love my S'well water bottle!

- If you can't find travel items at your local health food store, many of them can be ordered online.

- Packets of tea and coffee are great for plane travel. When the cart comes by, ask for hot water and you're all set! The packets are also super helpful when you arrive at your destination so that you can make your RFL.

- Depending on how long you'll be traveling, consider fasting from home to your destination.

- I love packing airplane food in my stainless-steel bento box from ECOlunchbox. It holds up to 8 cups of food, perfect for my hubby and me.

- If you don't have access to a kitchen and therefore will have most of your food prepared for you, you may find it difficult to get enough fat to feel satiated. Bringing fats to add to your meals, like avocado oil, coconut oil, MCT oil, olive oil, and olives, can help.

- If you have access to a kitchen, swing by a health food store when you arrive at your destination to pick up fresh vegetables, meats, and a couple of carb-up items.

- Remember to pack your milk frother or a resealable cup for shaking up your morning RFL.

KETO, RESTAURANT STYLE

When I first started eating keto, I was traveling all summer long. I ate at restaurants a lot and got along fabulously well at creating keto meals on the go, no matter where I was or what I was up to.

I've never had an issue ordering a keto-friendly meal at a restaurant. (Okay, except for the time we went to a premade-sandwich shop. That was impossible, for obvious reasons.) Rest assured, eating out doesn't have to mean frustration or complexity. In fact, it's quite enjoyable. Here are some tips for your next restaurant visit.

General Tips

- The nicer the restaurant, the easier it is to make substitutions.

- Look for restaurants that have a gluten-free menu and swap the sugars for fats.

- Choose meat and veggie dishes without grains.

- Add fat! Ask for avocado, bacon, fried eggs, mayo, olive oil, or olives.

- Try bringing fat with you. Coconut oil is my top choice.

- Watch the sauces and dressings! Many are loaded with sugar.

- Opt for water with your meal, or choose from one of the low-carb drink options on page 117.

- For breakfast, if the restaurant serves eggs and bacon, you're usually set! Omelets: total win.

Meal Tips

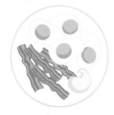 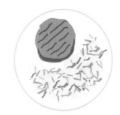 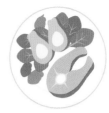

BREAKFAST: 4 eggs sunny side up with 2 sides of bacon and house-made mayonnaise (if it's made with olive oil) or olive oil

LUNCH: The highest-fat burger on the menu with a double order of coleslaw (usually made with dairy-free ingredients) or a spinach-based side salad if the coleslaw contains a bunch of sugar

DINNER: The highest-fat steak on the menu (see below), grilled salmon, or dark meat covered in olive oil, with a side of avocado and greens

Specific Restaurant Dishes

PASTA: Swap the pasta for a bed of vegetables (such as arugula, spinach, or zucchini). Watch for sugar added to tomato-based sauces.

SALADS: Ask for extra avocado and bacon as a replacement for fruit, dried fruit, or grains. For dressing, your best bet is oil and vinegar. Cobb salad is always a winner; simply ask for it without corn or cheese (if you're dairy-free) and you're good to go.

PROTEINS: Choose fatty proteins like salmon, duck, lamb, or pork short ribs. Fat is where toxins are stored, so if the meat quality is questionable, opt for lean meats and add plant-based fats like avocado oil or olive oil instead.

STEAK: The fattiest steaks are filet mignon, New York strip, T-bone, and rib-eye steaks. Dairy allergy? Ask for veggies without butter on the side.

SUSHI: Get anything without rice! They will roll up all the ingredients and, if you ask, will include additional avocado in place of rice. (P.S.: Sushi is great for carb-ups!)

BURGERS: Check that the patty is just meat (no oats, wheat germ, or other fillers), then ask that the bun be replaced with a lettuce wrap. Swap the fries for a side salad.

CHICKEN: Choose grilled, broiled, or roasted.

WINGS: Make sure they're not breaded or coated in rice flour, potato starch, or the like. If you're trying to avoid vegetable oils, skip the wings unless you find a restaurant that uses tallow in its fryers.

MEXICAN: Ask for any dish without the tortillas, rice, or beans. Guacamole can be served with raw vegetables, and meat platters are always a great option. Enchiladas are generally a no-go, as they are cooked in the tortillas and can't be separated. Try taco fillings served over a bed of romaine lettuce.

INDIAN: Ask for curry options that are not thickened with flour. Replace bread and rice with fresh vegetable sticks. Watch vegetable-based curries, as they're often packed with high-carb ingredients. Try cauliflower or mushroom bhaji, chicken korma (contains dairy), shahi paneer (contains dairy), or chicken shorba.

CHINESE: Chinese food is tricky, as everything has sauce and likely sugar. I ask for dry meat (duck is always safe), sautéed and served over raw bean sprouts or a fresh salad.

TAPAS: Generally a win, as tapas dishes are usually pretty low in carbohydrates and more meat-based. Avoid bread-based dishes and look for plates made up of meat and vegetables.

CAFÉS: Ask if the café has unsweetened coconut milk or almond milk or unsweetened brewed tea (hot or cold). My favorite: a decaf Americano misto made with coconut milk. (At least that's how we Canadians order a coffee with only a touch of milk.) As for food, I've never had any luck in a café. Wouldn't it be crazy if the café you went to tomorrow sold fat bombs?!

Leanne's work has been an amazing resource for me. I found Leanne after doing the Bulletproof diet for several weeks. There are certainly a lot of resources out there for those wanting to follow keto, but the majority of them are focused on men.

What I love about Leanne's protocols is that they are for women. My favorite of her teachings are the ones she does on body image and the ketogenic diet because they've taught me to not stress out about calories, macros, and the little things that cause added stress. I can focus on how my plate is supposed to look instead of calculating everything down to the drop.

Leanne's approach is one of freedom and normalcy. Her recipes are incredible, simple, and super easy to follow. I think a lot of people living a ketogenic lifestyle tend to eat the same foods over and over, probably because it is easier, but Leanne gives us so many recipes, options, and choices, which makes eating so much more fun and enjoyable...and I LOVE to eat!

I feel great, my obsessing over what to eat or not to eat is gone, and most importantly, I have learned to listen to what my body needs and doesn't need, and that it is all a work in progress. I am forever grateful to Leanne, her vast knowledge, her fun outlook on life, and her "no judgment zone" attitude towards this awesome lifestyle!

Annette
Missouri

I am sitting writing this with tears streaming down my face. I finished Fat Fueled, *Leanne's second how-to guide on ketogenic living, and I feel, perhaps for the first time, understood.*

I have struggled with my weight my whole life, going from compulsive eating to compulsive dieting and back again. I was put on my first low-fat diet by my mother when I was four years old, participated in group diets with my friends in primary school, had lap-band surgery (and complications), yo-yo dieted between 80 and 120 kg (176 and 264 pounds), was hospitalized with depression, had suicidal tendencies, and was ruled by my broken relationship to food.

Finding you and your books—crying again—has been like finding a friend in a sea of strangers.

Leanne, I want to say thank you for being a virtual hand to hold. For caring enough to share your struggles, your insights, your mistakes, your successes, and, perhaps most importantly, your loving philosophy. Your kind recognition that every body is different (I seem to need to keep my carbs to under 15g to lose weight) and needs gentle experimentation to find the right balance, is so important because it doesn't make me feel defective for not being able to eat the same as everyone else in order to get the same results.

I am so grateful for you, and the tools you have put in my hands that can truly help me "love myself thin"—and not just thin but healthy, vital, and optimistic for the first time in my life.

Thank you.

Kim
Sydney, Australia

CHAPTER 5 TROUBLESHOOTING

When you change the way you're doing something, you often face new challenges. Keto is no different. In this chapter, I've outlined some common issues that may arise when you start eating more fat.

This isn't to deter you from change; you know why you want to shift toward a high-fat lifestyle, and the benefits far outweigh the potential challenges. Rather, it's to equip you with the tools and information you need so that if something happens, you'll have a better understanding of why it's occurring and what to do about it.

The cool thing about all this is that every challenge has the potential to bring you closer to health in a holistic way, creating positive behaviors for the betterment of your life. Keto isn't just about losing weight; it's about getting to know your body and learning to listen to it. When you open up to the idea that your body knows best, you develop a primal knowledge of what your body needs—even, or maybe especially, when things aren't going right.

If you are concerned about any symptoms you experience on keto, please speak with your health-care provider so that you can come up with a plan that suits your needs.

CAN'T ADAPT OR OVERCOME A WEIGHT PLATEAU

CAN'T ADAPT

HIT WEIGHT PLATEAU

So often I hear from women who have reduced their calories to low, low levels, yet after six weeks of a 1,200-calories-a-day diet that's 85 percent fat, they're still stuck in the same place, just more frustrated.

Despite what you may have been told, success on the keto diet isn't always determined by how much fat you're eating, whether you're eating too many carbs, or how many ketones you're registering. While these factors are pivotal for becoming fat-adapted on the keto diet, they're not the only things to look at when you're running into issues. The culprit could be a number of other things.

Stress

  The largest of the culprits that may be standing between you and fat adaptation is stress, so we'll start there. Becoming fat-adapted requires you to be a chill human being with the ability to cope with stress naturally, without letting the little things consume you.

Are you stressed? If there's anyone who understands what a high-stress lifestyle will do to your ability to lose weight, get into ketosis, or maintain weight loss, it's me. In 2014, I lost twenty pounds of hormone-related weight by eating keto, and I maintained that weight loss quite effortlessly for two years. Then, in early 2016, loads of stress came into my life, and boom, those twenty pounds were back on like the NKOTBSB world tour (New Kids on the Block / Backstreet Boys—please tell me you didn't skip that one).

I hadn't changed anything in my diet, but the weight piled on fiercely. When I tested my ketones, they barely registered. However, on a day when I wasn't surrounded by stress, eating the same things I had for weeks, even months prior, my ketones measured much higher. All that had changed was my environment. Interestingly, as soon as the stressful period ended, the weight came down without my having to do anything, and a state of ketosis, and fat-burning, came effortlessly.

Stress's impact on weight gain, or the inability to lose weight, is real. And an abundance of stress, whether it is mental (you're worrying about what others may think of you, preparing for a big presentation, getting the kids to soccer practice on time) or physical (you're being chased by a tiger or crushing it a little too hard at the gym), will affect your ability to become fat-adapted and stay in fat-burning mode.

If you haven't become fully fat-adapted because you're chronically stressed, no amount of switching Fat Fueled Profiles, reducing calories, or playing with macros is going to help. The problem is cortisol, a hormone that's created during stress. Cortisol causes blood glucose to spike so that your muscles have the fuel to outrun that tiger. While this works well for a short time to help you get away from the tiger, a chronic elevation of cortisol causes an increase in insulin output to manage chronically high blood glucose. Constant overuse of this system makes cells insulin-resistant, so glucose doesn't get stored but stays available in the bloodstream. Good luck getting or staying fat-adapted in this state.

Why does that affect the ability to become fat-adapted? Remember, insulin tells the body not to burn stored fat. So when chronic stress is causing your insulin levels to increase, your body isn't getting the message to switch to burning fat instead of glucose.

Creating a calm environment that doesn't spike cortisol can be especially challenging for us ladies—we often live in a state of chronic stress, leading to constant peaks and valleys of insulin that prevent us from tapping into our fat stores. But we need to tap into those stores in the first ten days of eating keto-style so that we can become efficient at using fat as our primary fuel.

Cortisol also comes into play if we're not getting enough protein. Remember our friend gluconeogenesis, the process that uses protein to create adequate glucose for the functions of the body that need them? (See page 26 for more.) When we're not eating enough protein, amino acids from our own muscles can be used instead. Cortisol is what's used to break down muscle mass for gluconeogenesis, so without enough dietary protein, cortisol can go up, too. This is an instance where what we're eating and how we're approaching the ketogenic diet can make it next to impossible for us to feel good and get the results we want. If you want to be in a fat-burning state (and something tells me you do), it's important to eat enough protein to avoid this unnecessary increase in cortisol and breakdown of muscle.

Another contributor to stress is dietary stress. In the case of keto, it can be the stress that you impose on yourself by forcing yourself to fast rather than doing it when it comes naturally. Find more on why you shouldn't force your body to fast on page 69.

A big part of cutting stress can be, counterintuitively, cutting back on workouts. If you're reducing calories, intermittent fasting, and working out and you're feeling like it's impossible to become fat-adapted, it's likely that all the physical stress you're putting on your body is resulting in an imbalance of cortisol on top of everyday stress. Not only is that affecting your ability to become fat-adapted, but you've probably also noted that you're not gaining muscle. That's cortisol again—it reduces protein synthesis, so all those workouts aren't building muscle.

Here are my suggestions for reducing stress:

1. Stop working out—it's counterproductive if you're chronically stressed, placing more stress on your body and not getting you the results you're looking for.

2. Take up a self-care practice (see page 14).

3. Reduce insulin by continuing to follow the keto diet and perhaps following an intermittent fasting practice (see pages 68 to 72).

4. If you decide to follow Step 3, look to putting an end to calorie restriction—eat when you're hungry and allow your body to guide the way.

5. Reduce dietary stress by following the Daily Fat Burner profile (page 49)—after thirty days, switch to Classic Keto (page 47) and see if you're able to become fat-adapted.

By reducing both mental and physical stress, you're improving your cortisol response, which lowers your insulin and indirectly improves gluconeogenesis pathways. It will make becoming—and staying—fat-adapted a mega reality for you.

Trying Too Hard and Letting Calories Run the Show

 Closely related to the mental and physical stress described above is dietary stress. On page 18 we chatted about what happens when your calorie intake decreases to the point that it slows your metabolism. This is often what has happened in the case of weight-loss plateaus. With a slower metabolism, your body needs less fuel just to keep the basic processes running—instead of needing, say, 2,000 calories a day, it needs only 1,800. That means that while you were once able to lose weight on 1,800 calories a day, you'd now need to cut back to 1,600—but eventually your metabolism would slow even further. It's a vicious cycle.

Being hard on yourself may be keeping you from moving forward. Maybe your life has revolved around dieting, counting, tracking, and worrying about food for eons. You may be thinking, "Here's another diet that I suck at...." Let's change the conversation, yes?

Try becoming part of a group or community that has nothing to do with health, nutrition, dieting, or your body. You could join a knitting group, take a class in a foreign language, or join a book club—you get the idea. You may be surprised at how much stress is taken off your food choices when you have something to look forward to other than your next meal.

Ignoring Your Body's Signals

 What *your* body needs is different from what my body needs or what Sally's body needs. And Joe over there? It's a whole different ball game with that guy. To assume that following a single diet perfectly will lead to abundant success for everyone is ludicrous. You have to do what's right for *you*. And where a lot of people run into issues with any diet—the keto diet is no exception—is that they don't listen to their bodies.

Maybe fasting is great for you, or maybe it's not. Maybe having an RFL in the morning feels awesome, or maybe it doesn't. Maybe having one meal a day works wonders, or maybe it's torture.

Here are the most common body signals that I see people struggle with, along with some suggestions for handling them:

- **Constant hunger.** *Try bulking up your meals with vegetables. My favorites for this purpose are kale, cabbage, Brussels sprouts, and romaine lettuce. By filling your belly with low-carb vegetables, you'll be less likely to get that empty feeling that can come with a classic ketogenic meal, which, while high in fat and great for energy, is often low in volume.*

- **No hunger at all, ever.** *This is great for weight loss and often starts right before you become fully fat-adapted, at about the seven- to ten-day mark. But if you don't have much weight to lose, you know that intermittent fasting doesn't feel good in your body, or you're concerned about overall nutrient intake, try switching to a Fat Fueled Profile that includes carb-ups (pages 48 and 49). While the carb-up itself shouldn't lead to intense hunger the following day, it may help reset your appetite.*

The most important thing is to pay attention to what your body is telling you.

Calorie Counting and Fasting

It's really either/or with these two strategies: practicing both at the same time can wreak havoc on your health, leading to weight-loss plateaus, nutrient deficiencies, imbalanced hormones, and more. My vote is for fasting because it's a lot easier and way less stressful. (See pages 68 to 72 for more about fasting.)

Lack of Belief

 Most of us grew up "knowing" that fat makes you fat, calories must be counted, our bodies can't be trusted, and margarine is the only safe fat. It's hard to break through these beliefs when the same messages continue to be at the forefront of most health advice to this day. When you start eating ketogenic, these beliefs are challenged, and that can lead to a deep skepticism that prevents you from fully engaging in the process.

Your mind is a powerful thing. If you believe that something won't work, it probably won't. I'm hoping that reading through these pages has helped you become ready to give up the old beliefs and behaviors that are disrupting your success.

One thing you may want to try is a mantra practice. Traditionally, mantras are words or sounds that are repeated to aid concentration in a state of meditation, but they can also be used to change thought patterns. While that may sound a little woo-woo, there are studies on mantras that prove their validity. Here are a couple of mantras that I used when I was trying to break free of past beliefs surrounding fat intake, weight loss, calories, and exercise:

May I be worthy

May I be peaceful

May I be nourished

May I be free to do what my body feels

May I be happy

May I be safe

May I be healthy

May I be free of mental suffering or distress

May I be open to opportunities

Try repeating some of these throughout the day—I like to do it in the shower, while I'm eating, or during a walk. It's quite a phenomenal practice!

No Support Network

  Feeling alone and turning to social media for a sense of worth, only to compare your actions to others and feel worse about yourself, can affect your inflammatory response and metabolism in a negative way, to the point that it can keep you from becoming fat-adapted or losing weight. Finding an in-person support system can be a big help.

I'm not recommending that you go out and find the latest and greatest diet group that will encourage you to engage in negative behavior. Instead, try getting together with friends and nurturing your relationships with people who will support you in doing what's best for your body. Having strong, positive relationships and feeling supported in our efforts to improve our health can lower inflammation, boost metabolism, and reduce stress!

Unrealistic Goals

After the initial twenty-pound weight loss that I experienced on the keto diet, I decided twenty pounds wasn't enough and set my sights on another twenty. When I was just five pounds away from my goal, my weight loss slowed nearly to a stop. I would get down to two pounds and then jump up by five pounds quicker than you can say "dieting sucks."

I had made up my goal weight in my head, not yet accepting that every body is different and that losing the extra five pounds wouldn't make me any happier or healthier. In fact, I had to do a lot of unhealthy things to get to my coveted goal weight, and once I got there, it was incredibly challenging to stay there. One hour of training a day became two, 1,200 calories became 1,000, I fasted, I supplemented—it was horrible.

There are many things my body can do. I can grow the most insane quads you've ever seen. I can dance like no one's business, grow hair faster than most human beings, and even balance on my head for more than a minute. But I can't go under a size seven without surgically removing one of my hip bones, develop visible six-pack abs (those damn genes), or win a marathon.

There are things that *your* body is really good at, too, and things that are next to impossible. If you're frustrated that the scale won't budge, even after trying all the strategies in this book for busting through a plateau and speaking with a health-care professional about your hormone balance, it may be time to assess whether your goal weight is realistic.

Maybe your goal weight or desired body composition simply isn't in the cards for you, and it's time to accept that. You may want to try beginning a daily gratitude practice and listing five things that you're grateful for, whether in your life or about your body. Perhaps your body has done one of these awesome things today:

- **Gotten stronger**
- **Learned a new physical skill**
- **Taken you to the top of a hill**
- **Fought off an infection**
- **Healed a wound**
- **Given you sexual pleasure**
- **Allowed you to hear your favorite music**

By focusing on these things, you can begin to appreciate your body where it is right now.

The Wrong Foods

   The standard ketogenic diet can be packed with dairy, refined oils, conventionally raised animal proteins, artificial colors, flavors, and sweeteners, bars, boxed food, and the like. All of which can keep you from becoming fat-adapted, increase inflammation, and/or make your body hold on to weight that would otherwise be easy to drop.

If your approach has included dairy (including butter, sad face), sweeteners (even stevia can affect some people), deli meats, or food bars and supplements marketed as low in net carbs (see page 62 for the difference between net carbs and total carbs), you may want to try going a couple of weeks without them.

The good news? Everything in *The Keto Diet* will help you overcome this hurdle by showing you how to eat keto with whole foods!

Or perhaps you're dealing with food allergies and sensitivities without knowing it. When our bodies are inflamed because we've ingested foods that we're sensitive to, the last priority is making sure we're on track for weight loss. And unless we're pretty in tune with our bodies, many food sensitivities can go unnoticed for a long time, if they're ever discovered at all. They can show up as acne, stomach pain, acid reflux, heartburn, constipation, menstrual irregularities, dry eyes, headaches—the list goes on. When we're hit with these sorts of symptoms, we don't often think that the food we're eating might be the culprit.

If you're not sure whether a food is causing you grief, try removing the common culprits—nuts, seeds, eggs, dairy, fish, shellfish, and peanuts—for six to eight weeks, then reintroduce one of these foods every couple of days to see what happens. If a recipe in this book contains a common allergen, it's highlighted on the page, so it's easy to find recipes that resonate with your current health and food sensitivity status.

You could also ask your doctor to send you for an immunoglobulin E (IgE) blood test. It checks for antibodies associated with allergic reactions, so it can show you whether allergies and sensitivities are a problem for you. It may also be helpful to test your hs-CRP, a protein found in the blood that is directly influenced by the level of inflammation in the body. When it's high, inflammation is increased. When it's low, inflammation isn't a concern.

Your Body Doesn't Know What Time It Is

 Having a balanced circadian rhythm is really important for regulating metabolic processes, which helps with weight loss and overall health. This is something I personally struggle with if I'm not careful, so here are the many things I do to encourage my body to fall asleep easily come bedtime, wake up refreshed, and have adequate energy all day long:

- **Get sunshine (real or from a full-spectrum lamp) when you first wake up.**
- **Because the blue light from electronic screens can disrupt circadian rhythms when you use a device after sunset, install an app like f.lux that adapts the color of your display to the time of day.**
- **For the same reason, get blue-blocking glasses if you're going to watch TV after the sun sets.**
- **Don't bring your phone into the bedroom with you.**
- **Meditate before bed.**
- **Try not to chow down on chocolate before bed.**

There's an Imbalance in the Way

 If your thyroid is performing suboptimally or your adrenal glands have had enough, no amount of dieting is going to help your weight situation—it may be time to see a health-care professional. That said, as you eat keto, many health imbalances might begin to mend themselves, leading you toward an easier path to weight loss.

There's nothing wrong with working one-on-one with a health-care professional to support the part of your body that needs supporting while also following the keto diet. Think of it as a double whammy!

And if you have a known health imbalance and want to understand how to adjust the keto diet to support it, my Fat Fueled program (healthfulpursuit.com/fatfueled) is a pretty good resource.

KETO FLU

Most of us have spent our entire lives fueling our bodies with carbohydrates that our entire system—from cells to organs to brain and nervous system—has ramped up enzymatic processes and adjusted hormonal responses to deal with. When we switch up the process, asking our bodies to fuel with fat, it can take time for them to adjust. Another way of looking at this is to think of it as carbohydrate withdrawal.

For some, this adjustment period comes with mild to intense symptoms, collectively called "keto flu." (Others transition quite effortlessly without symptoms—lucky!)

Many people who experience keto flu, myself included, initially blame the diet. Ironically, one of the common theories about why some individuals experience keto flu and others do not is that it depends on how carb-dependent you were before going keto. The more carbs you're used to relying on, the worse the symptoms. As someone who's gone through the fat adaptation process twice, I can say that the second time was leaps and bounds easier than the first. Because I never went back to the sheer amount of carbohydrates I used to consume, it wasn't such an adjustment to make the switch again.

There are other possible reasons that some people experience keto flu: primarily stress, imbalanced intake of vitamins and minerals, or deficiency in electrolytes and dehydration. (Glycogen has a lot of water stored with it; as your glycogen stores get used up, that water is released, and with the water go electrolytes.)

As you embark on the keto diet for the first time, it's important to be ahead of the game when it comes to the keto flu. Do these things and you should be all set:

- **Reduce stress (see pages 90 and 91).**
- **Take nutritional supplements (see page 76).**
- **Understand the important of electrolytes (see page 78).**
- **Drink Keto Lemonade (page 422).**
- **Consume at least 1 teaspoon of gray sea salt every day.**
- **Drink lots of water.**
- **Be extra mindful if the sport you're engaged in makes you sweat a lot.**
  - *Drink Rocket Fuel Bone Broth (page 426).*
  - *Eat electrolyte-rich foods (see the list on page 78).*

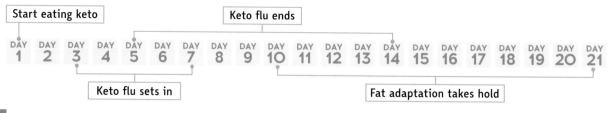

Start eating keto — DAY 1

Keto flu sets in — DAY 3

Keto flu ends — DAY 10

Fat adaptation takes hold — DAY 14–21

DAY 1 DAY 2 DAY 3 DAY 4 DAY 5 DAY 6 DAY 7 DAY 8 DAY 9 DAY 10 DAY 11 DAY 12 DAY 13 DAY 14 DAY 15 DAY 16 DAY 17 DAY 18 DAY 19 DAY 20 DAY 21

CRUSHING THE KETO FLU

SYMPTOMS OF KETO-FLU

BRAIN FOG

HEADACHES
H_2O

DIZZINESS
K	Mg
Na	Ca
P	Cl

IRRITABILITY

INSOMNIA

NAUSEA

HEART PALPITATIONS*
H_2O
K	Mg
Na	Ca
P	Cl

CARB CRAVINGS/ HYPOGLYCEMIA

DIARRHEA
K	Mg
Na	Ca
P	Cl

FATIGUE/ WEAKNESS/ POOR ATHLETIC PERFORMANCE
Mg
K	Mg
Na	Ca
P	Cl

MUSCLE CRAMPS
H_2O Mg
K

Above all, patience is required... and water!

ACTIONS:

 MORE WATER
Drink water, drink water, drink water!

 ELECTROLYTES (SEE PAGE 78)
Drink Keto Lemonade (page 422) and Rocket Fuel Bone Broth (page 426), and consume at least 1 teaspoon of gray sea salt every day.

 ELECTROLYTE-RICH FOODS
Potassium: avocados, nuts, dark leafy greens, salmon, mushrooms

Magnesium: nuts, dark chocolate, artichokes, fish, spinach

Sodium: salt, bone broth, bacon, pickles, fermented vegetables

Calcium: dark leafy greens, almonds, sardines

Phosphorus: nuts, seeds, dark chocolate

Chloride: olives, seaweed, salt, low-carb veggies

 MORE FAT!
Power through and eat more fat to encourage your body to become fat-adapted. Go for the fat bomb recipes (refer to the chart on pages 432 to 434).

 MOVEMENT
Any movement you can handle during the transition will be helpful. If symptoms are intense, walking and gentle yoga are fabulous!

 MAGNESIUM
Eat the magnesium-rich foods listed listed above and supplement with magnesium.* I like Natural CALM powdered magnesium.

 POTASSIUM
Supplement with potassium and eat the potassium-rich foods listed above.

 INCREASE DIGESTIVE POWER!
Take an ox bile supplement,* probiotics, and fermented foods.

*Can be discontinued once symptoms have cleared up, if desired

*IMPORTANT: If you are diabetic or on high blood pressure medication, heart palpitations could be a sign that your medications need to be adjusted. (Diabetics must test their blood sugar regularly while adapting to keto to ensure they do not experience low blood sugar.) Talk to your health-care provider if you experience symptoms.

PHYSIOLOGICAL INSULIN RESISTANCE

While it doesn't happen to everyone, you could experience physiological insulin resistance after going low-carb. What happens is that your peripheral tissues enter into an insulin-resistant state to preserve glucose for the parts of your body that require it. So even if there's glucose floating around, certain tissues in the body (that would have normally used the glucose happily) become insulin resistant in order to allow certain cells to grab it. You may recall from Chapter 1 that with pathological insulin resistance, cells stop responding to insulin's signals because glucose is constantly high, causing insulin to be constantly high also—like the villagers in the tale of the boy who cried wolf, cells stop paying attention to insulin's frequent signals. Physiological insulin resistance is different: the body is conserving glucose for the parts of the body that absolutely require it. This is a normal biological reaction to a lack of carbohydrates in the diet and gluconeogenesis (see page 26) at work. Think of it as adaptive glucose sparing, or as the opposite of diabetes.

The classic sign that you're experiencing physiological insulin resistance is that your fasting blood glucose (as measured with a glucometer) frequently rises above 100 mg/dl.

It took me about six months of full-time ketogenic eating before I experienced it, but some of my clients have had it in as little as two to three weeks.

Nine times out of ten, the only symptom people with physiological insulin resistance experience is raised glucose levels in the morning, and most medical professionals will tell you that it's totally normal and harmless. Those who are symptom-free are usually in need of the weight loss that comes from a ketogenic diet. In these cases, insulin sensitivity is improved and all is well with the world.

But when a low-carb diet is coupled with calorie reduction, lack of protein (which affects gluconeogenesis; see page 26), and forced intermittent fasting (see pages 68 to 72) in a body that is pretty lean already, insulin sensitivity is reduced and physiological insulin resistance can feel not so awesome. I personally felt like garbage when I began experiencing it, and incorporating a carb-up practice reset things and helped immensely. If you experience physiological insulin resistance and find that you feel fine, there's nothing wrong with continuing your journey without carb-ups.

Why do carb-ups help with physiological insulin resistance? Unlike pathological insulin resistance, the only reason physiological insulin resistance is doing its thing is because dietary carbohydrate is so low. Once you practice a small carb-up, your body has a touch more glucose to play with, and, if you were experiencing symptoms, they should dissipate quickly.

ACNE

You may find that your skin drastically improves on keto—or gets worse. If you're in the clear-skin camp, hurrah! Many specialists recommend a keto diet to clear up acne, so you're one of the lucky ones.

If you're the victim of cystic acne that appears overnight or small pimples that spread across your chin and jawline, let's talk.

There are a couple of reasons for acne on keto. One is directly related to the keto diet itself, either because of the foods you eat or the process of becoming fat-adapted, and the other is a result of the weight you're losing. Either way, there's no need to panic: I come with solutions! The chart below will help you understand what's going on and give you some tips for mitigating your skin's reaction.

SKIN DOS AND DON'TS

❌ DO NOT

- Pick blemishes
- Use harsh chemical-based cleansers
- Assume that only external forces will help—food matters, too
- Clean your face more than twice a day (three times if working out)

✅ DO

- Use gentle cleansers
- Exfoliate regularly
- Use charcoal or mud face masks
- Spot-treat with tea tree oil
- Tone with 1 part apple cider vinegar to 3 parts water
- Try acupuncture

REASON
DIET CHANGE
Oil production changes with diet, and this can lead to acne.

WHAT TO DO

- Use a natural face moisturizer
- Get facials
- Drink water
- Drink Tulsi tea
- Get out in the sunshine
- Supplement with zinc
- Supplement with vitamin A
- Supplement with holy basil

REASON
USING FAT FOR FUEL
Running off your stored body fat releases the toxins and estrogen housed in fat cells. Meanwhile, in men and those on keto for necessary weight loss, androgen levels may increase with keto, which causes acne.

WHAT TO DO

- Supplement with chlorella
- Doctors may recommend birth control pills, but ask about bioidentical hormones first (for more on this, check out healthfulpursuit.com/podcast)

REASON
DETOXIFICATION PROCESS
Release of toxins causes acne.

WHAT TO DO

- Supplement with probiotics
- Supplement with milk thistle
- Try a far-infrared sauna to help eliminate toxins (SaunaSpace is my favorite; use coupon code HEALTHFUL for 5% off)

REASON
FOOD SENSITIVITIES
Increases overall inflammation, leading to acne. Usually related to gut health.

WHAT TO DO

- Remove common allergens like nuts, seeds, eggs, dairy, fish, shellfish, and peanuts
- Remove nightshades
- Avoid corn-based products, such as the sweetener erythritol
- Supplement with fish oil and probiotics
- Get gelatin from bone broth or by adding a supplement to hot drinks

CONSTIPATION

When I shifted overnight from a vegan diet to Paleo, I had the worst constipation known to man. But after a couple of weeks, my body sorted things out and I was back to normal. Heck, I was *better* than normal!

Any dietary change is often met with a change in digestive function. There's nothing to be concerned about; it's just a bit annoying.

Here are some things you can do to ease symptoms during the transition:

- Drink Keto Lemonade (page 422)
- Consume fermented foods such as sauerkraut, kimchi, water kefir, and pickles (fermented, unpasteurized)
- Have at least 2 tablespoons of MCT oil in the morning
- Eat chia pudding in the morning
- Drink lots of water, especially when you first wake up
- Supplement with magnesium throughout the day, and take magnesium oxide in the evening before bed
- Supplement with vitamin C
- Supplement with probiotics

Although constipation may just be a part of the transition to keto, some keto foods are constipation triggers. If you're concerned about particular foods, try the following:

- Go a couple of days without nuts, seeds, or nut/seed butters.
- If you've switched from a low-fiber diet (standard American diet), increase vegetables slowly so as not to aggravate your system.
- If you've switched from a fiber-rich diet (whole-food vegan diet), focus on filling your keto diet with loads of fibrous foods such as avocado, flax, chia, coconut, collards, mustard greens, and endive.
- Practice a dairy-free keto protocol (see page 145 for more on quitting dairy).
- To see if you have food sensitivities, such as to nuts, seeds, eggs, dairy, fish, shellfish, or peanuts, try removing them from your diet for six to eight weeks, then reintroduce one every couple of days to see what happens. You may find that you need to avoid some of these foods completely in order to stay regular.

Many of these actions will help your bowels do their thing as your body adapts to being fueled by fats.

DRAGON BREATH

Not everyone will experience a change in the smell of his or her breath on keto, but if you do, you'll notice…or your husband will tell you about it nicely. Don't worry, it's a temporary effect that will last just a week or two as you become fat-adapted.

When your body starts producing ketones on a low-carb diet, one ketone body, acetone, is exhaled. You'll know that you've fallen victim if your breath becomes fruity and smells a bit like nail polish. Acetone may also result in a change in body odor.

If after two weeks you're still experiencing the breath of the dragon, *Game of Thrones* style (unfortunately, it doesn't come with Daenerys Targaryen's gorgeous hair), here are some practices and actions to alleviate the symptoms:

- Ensure that you're hydrated and drink Keto Lemonade (page 422).

- Maintain oral hygiene. While keto breath comes from the lungs, it doesn't hurt to keep your mouth fresh! Use a tongue cleaner, floss, and brush your teeth after eating.

- Chew on fresh mint leaves or place a drop of peppermint essential oil on your tongue if you're self-conscious about it.

- Drink 2 tablespoons of apple cider vinegar with ½ cup (120 ml) of water in the mornings.

- Switch to the Daily Fat Burner (page 49), Adapted Fat Burner (page 48), or Pumped Keto (page 47) profile to stay in fat-burning mode yet potentially reduce the amount of ketones your body is producing. If you want to maintain the benefits of the ketogenic diet, you could increase your intermittent fasting practice to offset the change.

SCALP ISSUES: DANDRUFF, ITCHINESS…

Like constipation, there can be two causes of scalp issues on the keto diet. The first possible cause is the changes you've made to your diet—if this is the case, as your body adapts, the symptoms should dissipate.

If they don't, or you feel that what you're experiencing isn't because of the changes to your diet, there are a couple of things you can look at as well as do to mitigate the annoyance of scalp itchiness and the embarrassment that comes along with snow on your shoulders:

- Keep your house at a moderate temperature, not too hot.

- Keep your head warm and covered from cold winter air.

- Supplement with garlic and grapefruit seed extract.

- Use tea tree oil products directly on the scalp.

- Reduce inflammation by beginning a yoga practice. (It's best to avoid hot yoga when scalp issues arise.)

- Clean your hairbrushes and other hair tools regularly.

- Consume 2 tablespoons apple cider vinegar with ½ cup (120 ml) water in the mornings.

- Create a honey mask for your hair by combining 9 parts honey to 1 part water. Apply to the affected areas once a day.

As someone who has battled psoriasis, a chronic autoimmune disease, and tried every medical shampoo on the market, I can tell you that the keto diet has completely vanquished all of my symptoms. The only time my psoriasis returns is when I eat foods that I know I'm sensitive to: nuts, seeds, grains, or dairy.

In case food sensitivities are also an issue for you, take a look at what you're eating:

- Go a couple of days without nuts, seeds, or nut/seed butters.

- Practice a dairy-free keto protocol (see page 145 for more on quitting dairy).

- To see if you have any food sensitivities, such as nuts, eggs, dairy, seeds, fish, shellfish, and peanuts, try removing them from your diet for six to eight weeks, then reintroduce one every couple of days to see what happens.

- Remove any grain products and their derivatives.

- If you drink alcohol, discontinue for two weeks to see if symptoms improve.

- If nothing works, Candida might be the culprit. *While a ketogenic diet is generally quite Candida-friendly and can help reduce flare-ups, the amount of fat you're eating can also trigger a flare because Candida is stimulated by both sugar and ketones. If your body is creating too many ketones, you may want to reduce your fat intake for a couple of days (the easiest way is to swap your RFL for a solid meal or intermittent fast without a fatty drink), and see if your symptoms improve. If it's improved, the Daily Fat Burner Fat Fueled Profile (page 49) may be best for you.*

LOWERED ALCOHOL TOLERANCE

Major heads-up on this one: when you're eating keto, your alcohol tolerance goes way, way down. It's like the first time you ever had a drink (when you were of legal age, of course).

It's unclear why alcohol tolerance is reduced, usually by about half, while on the ketogenic diet. There really isn't any way to change it, so just think of it as a good sign that you're in ketosis.

For more about alcohol on the keto diet, see page 119.

ELEVATED CHOLESTEROL

If you have any concerns about elevated cholesterol, see page 32 for more information.

HAIR LOSS

During my first attempt in ketosis, my protocol was to eat as little as possible, go to bed hungry as often as I could, intermittent fast no matter how much I wanted food, workout for up to three hours a day, and eat less than 20 grams of carbohydrates and 50 grams of protein every day, without exception. Six months into the diet, I was losing hair by the handful. Every morning, my pillow looked like Cousin It had visited and left half of himself on my pillow. This continued for six months no matter what supplement concoction I tried.

As soon as I incorporated a carb-up practice, switching from a Classic Keto to an Adapted Fat Burner Fat Fueled Profile, my hair loss stopped in a matter of days, and all of my hair was back to normal in a couple of months.

Looking back, I can see an alternative to carb-ups: I could have eaten enough, stopped forcing myself to intermittent fast when I was hungry, reduced strenuous workouts, and allowed more flexibility with my carbohydrate and protein intake while staying on the Classic Keto Fat Fueled Profile (page 47).

Currently, I'm following the Full Keto profile (page 48), eating enough, and practicing movement that feels good, and I have no hair loss to report.

On a ketogenic diet, hair loss can be caused by intense and rapid weight loss, a massive reduction in calories, or could be a temporary symptom of switching to keto. Most hair loss is noticed three to six months after the event that causes it. For example, when you change to a low-carb diet, you may notice hair loss at month 3. Because there are multiple reasons for hair loss on keto, there are also multiple solutions—different people may find that some work better than others.

REASON
CALORIE RESTRICTION

DURATION
Until you do something about it

WHAT TO DO

- Eat enough that you're satisfied throughout the day
- Discontinue forced intermittent fasting

REASON
WEIGHT LOSS

DURATION
About 3 months

WHAT TO DO

- Follow the steps for hair loss due to low carbs, below
- Follow the steps for hair loss due to nutrient deficiencies section, below

REASON
DEMANDING EXERCISE

DURATION
Until you do something about it

WHAT TO DO

- Live with it
- Switch to Pumped Keto (page 47), Full Keto (page 48), Adapted Fat Burner (page 48), or Daily Fat Burner (page 49)

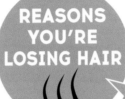

REASONS YOU'RE LOSING HAIR

(AND WHAT TO DO ABOUT IT)

REASON
LOW CARBS

DURATION
About 3 months, at which time baby hairs will be noticeable in the places where you lost hair

WHAT TO DO

- Be patient
- Switch to Pumped Keto (page 47), Full Keto (page 48), Adapted Fat Burner (page 48), or Daily Fat Burner (page 49)
- Support your diet with biotin and collagen supplements to make hair stronger
- Consume bone broth

REASON
HEALTH IMBALANCE

DURATION
Until you do something about it

WHAT TO DO

- Seek medical support
- Determine which Fat Fueled Profile will support you best (see pages 52 to 54)

REASON
PSYCHOLOGICAL STRESS

DURATION
Until you do something about it

WHAT TO DO

- De-stress following the steps on page 91
- Seek medical support
- Switch to Pumped Keto (page 47) or Daily Fat Burner (page 49)

REASON
NUTRIENT DEFICIENCIES

DURATION
Until you do something about it

WHAT TO DO

- Follow the meal plans and recipes in this book, beginning on page 174
- Switch to Pumped Keto (page 47), Full Keto (page 48), Adapted Fat Burner (page 48), or Daily Fat Burner (page 49)
- Ask your doctor to do a blood test to see where you're lacking
- Eat enough that you're satisfied throughout the day
- Discontinue intermittent fasting
- Ensure you're eating enough protein

INSOMNIA

If your sleep has never been better, awesome! However, a few people, myself included, experience insomnia when they start eating low-carb.

In my case, I have to avoid the Classic Keto Fat Fueled Profile (page 47) and follow the Full Keto (page 47), Adapted Fat Burner (page 48), or Daily Fat Burner (page 49) Profile in order to maintain healthful sleep. Second, I have to make sure that I am eating enough. Those two things work wonders for my sleep!

Here are some solutions that may improve your symptoms:

- **Reduce caffeine consumption.** *On keto, you may be consuming more caffeine than you're used to in the form of fatty coffees, sugar-free chocolates, or cacao powder. Make your RFL with herbal tea or decaf coffee and limit chocolate consumption to the morning or for occasional treats.*

- **Have a hot bath or shower an hour before bed.**

- **Avoid evening workouts.**

- **Take magnesium with every meal.**

- **Take melatonin.** *However, it's best to treat this as a temporary solution and not take it for extended periods. Also, many individuals may find that they are allergic to melatonin. If you're going to experiment, it's best to do it at home (not on a plane for the first time!) and in small doses at first.*

- **Make sure you're eating enough!** *If you're going to bed hungry or forcing intermittent fasting, this could be leading to insomnia.*

- **Practice the circadian rhythm tips on page 93.**

- **Switch to Pumped Keto (page 47), Full Keto (page 48), Adapted Fat Burner (page 48), or Daily Fat Burner (page 49).** *Certain bodily processes need glucose, especially thyroid hormone conversion and red blood cell glycolysis. When we don't consume enough carbohydrates (how much is enough varies from person to person), the body can create glucose from protein (see page 26 for more on gluconeogenesis). However, the process involves a spike in cortisol if not enough protein is consumed, which may lead to sleepless nights, inability to lose weight, and other symptoms.*

KETO RASH

Some people can follow a keto diet for years and never experience keto rash. Thankfully, the rash affects only a handful of individuals—but that doesn't help you if you're one of the unlucky few!

Keto rash, also known as prurigo pigmentosa, begins as itchy red bumps that can merge and form larger bumps that are sometimes filled with a small amount of fluid; eventually there can be fully developed lesions on top of the bumps. The rash can be exacerbated by hot weather or exercise and is instantly alleviated when carbohydrates are increased. (There are ways to treat it other than quitting keto: keep reading!)

Sadly, there isn't much research on why keto rash happens or why only some people experience it. Many of the suspected causes are related to the creation of ketones, such as being on a standard ketogenic diet, fasting, losing weight, being pregnant (pregnant women often dip into ketosis while sleeping, even when not on the keto diet), being anorexic—the list goes on. But since we're focused on rashes caused by the keto diet, let's narrow our discussion to that.

Time and time again, when I meet with a client who has keto rash and we go through his or her symptoms, health status, and imbalances, more often than not there's a clear connection between the onset of the rash and the following:

- **Candida die-off**

- **Fungal infections**

- **Imbalanced gut bacteria**

- *H. pylori* **infection**

- **Fasting (therefore, deep ketosis)**

I'm unsure whether the symptoms are aggravated by a ketogenic diet more than any other diet or whether it's simply that these events occur more often on a keto diet.

On the flip side, we could be looking at the keto rash conundrum all wrong. We know that on a ketogenic diet, the ketone body acetone can be excreted from the skin in the form of sweat. If you're a highly active person, it's very possible that the ketone body excretion is what's causing the rash, but that's just a guess.

Whatever the cause, if left alone, the rash usually dissipates in a couple of weeks. If you can't wait for it to clear on its own, here are some things you can try:

- **Avoid drastic temperature changes.**
- **Wear comfortable clothing.**
- **Choose exercise that does not cause excessive sweating (preferably none at all). If you sweat, take a shower directly afterward and use a natural soap such as Dr. Bronner's castile soap.**
- **Switch from the Classic Keto Fat Fueled Profile (page 47) to Pumped Keto (page 47) or Full Keto (page 48).**
- **Stop intermittent fasting.**

Your doctor is likely to recommend antibiotics, antifungals, or antihistamines, but studies show that once you stop taking the medication, the rash will come back.

I'm crossing my fingers and toes that, in a couple of weeks, the rash will be a thing of the past and you can go on living your keto life, confidently!

ADAPTED BUT STILL NOT FEELING RIGHT

Many of the symptoms and side effects discussed in this chapter occur when you're in the process of becoming fat-adapted, in the first, say, thirty days of your keto experience. But what if you start to feel unwell after two months, four months, or six months?

If you are experiencing any of the symptoms in this chapter, please read over the suggestions for overcoming the hurdle. It's very possible that some of these suggestions will help. However, if they don't, I have one last message for you. And I'm hoping it resonates because it's the last trick in my bag, aside from meeting up with you at your favorite coffee shop and enjoying fatty coffees while chatting about your health for hours on end. (I would love that, but alas, it's impossible to meet with everyone, a sad realization I had to come to early on in my work.)

If what you're doing isn't working, you owe yourself to change, just as you did when you found the keto diet, desperate for something to help you lose weight, heal your body, or free you from a broken relationship with food. If you feel that something isn't right, you should honor that feeling. No amount of reading books, browsing blogs, or speaking with gurus is going to give you the answer.

I don't have the answer for you. Your friend doesn't have the answer for you. That other book about ketosis doesn't have the answer for you. This isn't meant to make you feel alone but rather empowered. *You* have the answer for you.

If you've been eating Classic Keto for six months and your hair is falling out, you're tired, and your performance sucks, one person may tell you to keep going, and someone else may tell you to change your Fat Fueled Profile. But what do *you* feel like doing? If there's anything I hope you take away from this book, it's that only you know what's right for your body. By eating all the fats over the last couple of months, you've likely developed a stronger connection to what your body needs and when. This is great! Tap into that and see what's up!

Maybe you need something completely unrelated to your diet—a date night, a girls' night out, a spa day, a solo walk in the park, more music in your life, more creativity, less noise, more connection, more free time, a good housecleaning, time away, time in, a good book, a new look, a fresh coat of paint....

You can change Fat Fueled Profiles, work out less, eat more, stop counting calories, surround yourself with body positivity (I highly recommend this one), stop putting yourself to high standards, accept your body, feel gratitude for the awesomeness in your life, stop counting macros, delete your calorie-tracking app, or listen to my podcast for inspiration (healthfulpursuit.com/podcast). You can decide to stick it to society and quit your diet mentality (like, yesterday), grab a bag of your favorite treats and go somewhere special to enjoy each one, have water balloon fights with your kids....

You can do anything you'd like to do with the body you have. I truly believe that the keto diet has the potential to change everything for you, but if you're not feeling it, it's not that you aren't trying hard enough or that there's something wrong with you. It could be that it's not working because you're not bending to what your body really needs (see page 14).

Take the time to work *with* your body instead of against it, and I know you'll land somewhere perfect.

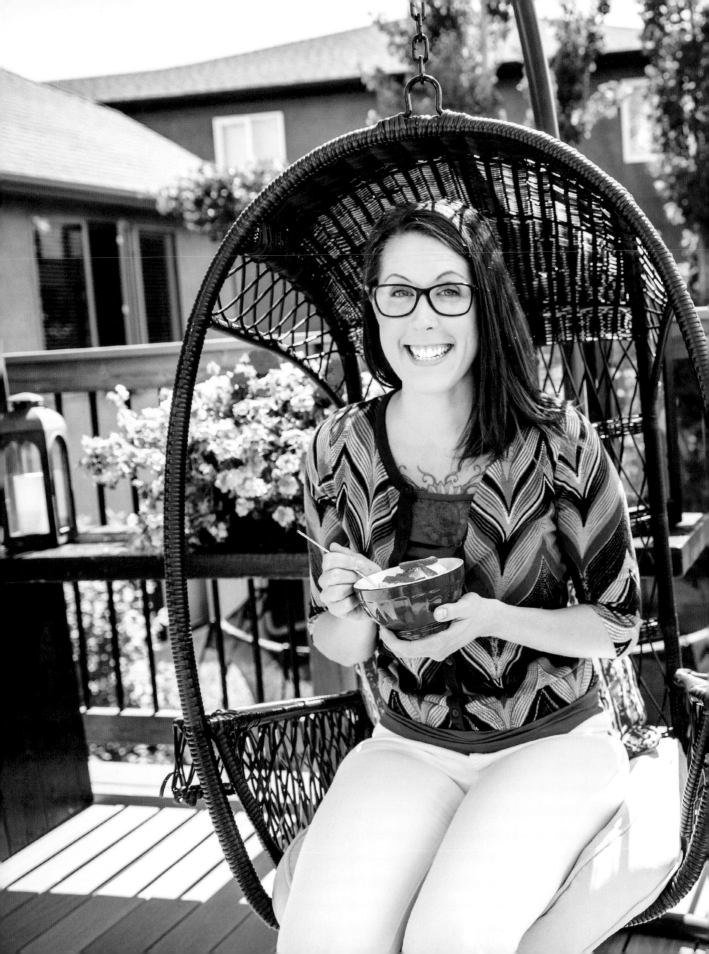

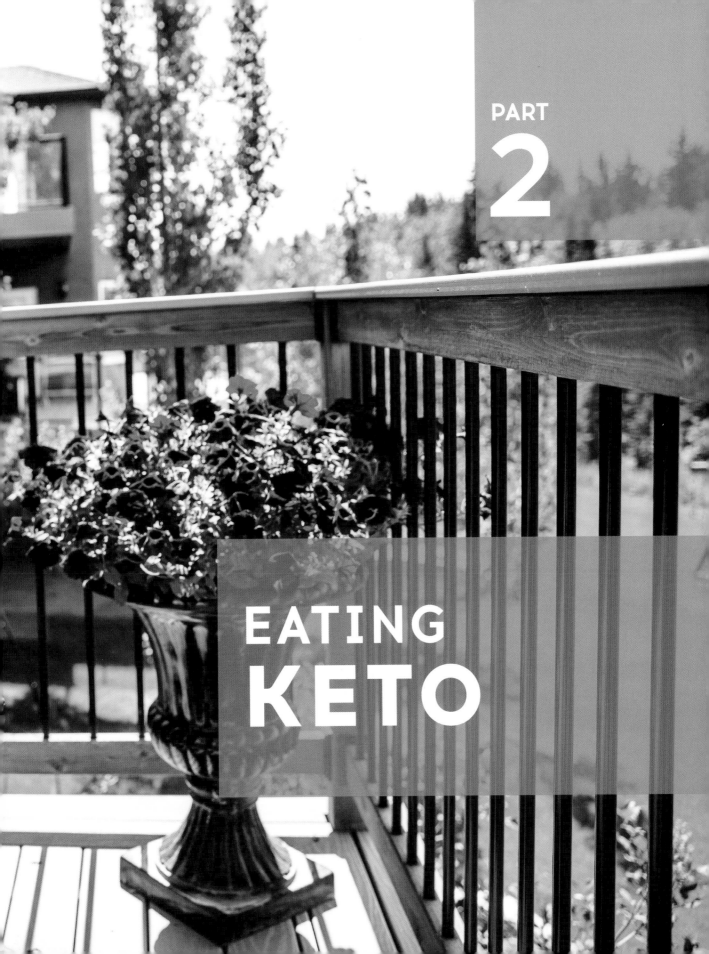

PART
2

EATING KETO

CHAPTER 6 FOOD: THE GOOD, THE BAD, AND THE UGLY

Unless you live a life free from all media (in which case I'm so jealous), over the years you've likely gathered information from various sources on the foods you should and should not eat.

Eat low-fat, low-carb, high-protein; eat whole grains, avoid sugar, go Paleo...and now you're being told to eat more fat than ever before. What gives?

From Chapter 1, you know just how phenomenal fat is for your body. And perhaps you've seen firsthand just how wonderful it's been for a friend or family member. But it may be less clear exactly which foods are the best to eat on keto and which you'll want to avoid—especially when it comes to foods that we've been traditionally told are healthy, like dairy, legumes, and grains. In this chapter, we'll talk about specific foods and how to tailor what you eat to give you the best results on the keto diet.

But this is about creating your keto eating style. It needs to be something you feel isn't restrictive, so you can follow it forever and not have yucky feelings about it.

WHAT YOU'LL BE EATING, AND NOT EATING

I like to think of the body as a cup. Every day you eat food to fill your cup, but there's only so much food that will fit into the cup. Now, imagine that at the end of the day, all of the less-nourishing foods were removed from your full-to-the-brim cup. Now it's only half full. Instead of providing your body with a full cup of nutrients, you've only supplied it with half of what it needs. And if you're only getting half of what you need, over time your body will begin to display symptoms of lack. If the cup isn't full of nutrients, the body has to prioritize processes and cut corners to maintain status quo—that can mean reducing digestive processes, muscle building, hormone regulation, and more.

Our goal, then, is to get rid of less-nourishing food to make space in our cups for foods that count, that will nourish our bodies so they stay balanced, happy, and whole. Those less-nourishing foods are grains, sugars, processed foods, dairy, legumes, starches (in excess), and fruit (in excess). (Whoa, did she just put sugar and dairy in the same bucket? Yeah, I did. More on that later.)

Viewing my body as a cup has helped me immensely in comprehending how important it is to eat whole foods that nourish my body. A "healthy" chocolate cake made with almond flour, cacao powder, and natural sweeteners doesn't have much in the way of nutrients, and it takes up just as much space in my cup as a huge portion of grass-fed ground beef, greens, and crushed almonds. When I assess whether the cake is worth it, I envision 30 percent of the cake staying in my cup and 100 percent of the beef mixture staying in my cup. I'll be the first to say that I enjoy treats and will choose the cake when I actually feel like the cake. Life is about balance. But staying mindful of what fills my cup with the most nutrients helps me be honest with myself about how I'm nourishing my body.

This is why my approach to eating keto is all about whole-food awesomeness—because I want your cup to be filled to the brim as much as possible.

If decoding how your body responds to food is confusing to you and makes no logical sense, stick to foods from the "yes" group and a small amount from the "sometimes" group.

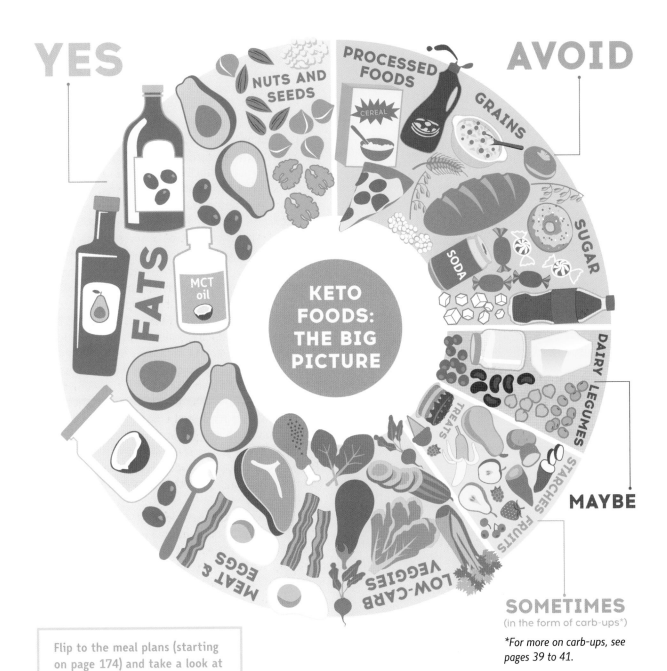

YES

NUTS AND SEEDS

FATS

MCT oil

PROCESSED FOODS

CEREAL

GRAINS

SUGAR

SODA

AVOID

KETO FOODS: THE BIG PICTURE

DAIRY

LEGUMES

STARCHES

TREATS

FRUITS

MAYBE

LOW-CARB VEGGIES

MEAT & EGGS

SOMETIMES
(in the form of carb-ups*)

*For more on carb-ups, see pages 39 to 41.

Flip to the meal plans (starting on page 174) and take a look at the kinds of foods you can eat every day. Then look through the recipes, starting on page 216.

Making Sense of "Maybe" and "No" Foods

There are foods we won't be eating too much of with the Fat Fueled approach to keto. Remember from Chapter 1 that this approach combines Paleo and keto, which means that we're focusing on real, whole foods that nourish the body and avoiding those that are less-nourishing.

Dairy
Cheese, milk, ice cream, yogurt

So many people are allergic or sensitive to lactose, whey, or casein that it's worth avoiding all dairy products for a month—that will give you time to heal, and if you want to try reintroducing it after thirty days, you'll be able to see its effects clearly. But even if you aren't sensitive to dairy, you may want to fill your cup with more-nourishing items.

Milk from cows was meant to nourish calves, not humans. Despite popular belief, it doesn't increase bone strength on its own—it mostly lacks vitamin D (there are trace amounts in whole milk), which the body needs to absorb calcium. In fact, in some cases it can increase the risk of fractures because to digest dairy, the body needs to use essential nutrients and minerals that would otherwise be used to build bone. Dairy is also linked to an increased risk of prostate cancer, ovarian cancer, type 1 diabetes, and multiple sclerosis. There are many possible reasons for this:

- **Whey proteins raise our insulin levels, causing imbalances in blood sugar.**

- **Casein proteins increase insulin growth factor (IGF-1), which affects the placenta of pregnant women, speeds the growth of cancer cells, causes acne, and more.**

- **Dairy products can increase inflammation in the body and affect immune system response.**

- **Natural hormones in milk (designed to stimulate the calf's growth) can lead to unnecessary weight gain.**

- **Depending on the quality, dairy may affect hormone balance and fertility. Hormones found in dairy products include prolactin, melatonin, growth hormone, thyroid stimulating hormone, estrogens, progesterone, and more.**

But not all dairy is created equal. Head to page 147 to learn more about the benefits of grass-fed ghee and butter and its role in your ketogenic life.

Legumes
Beans, lentils, peanuts, soy, peas

Eating a few servings of legumes a week is fine as long you tolerate them well. As with dairy, try removing them entirely for thirty days to give yourself time to heal, then you can try reintroducing them slowly. Be sure to select fermented forms, when available, and non-GMO options.

But again, also as with dairy, there are several reasons to avoid them even if you do tolerate them well. For starters, there are a plethora of foods that are far more nutrient-dense than legumes. Legumes are generally quite high in carbs (although you can find a list of lower-carb legumes quite easily with a quick Google search). They're also rich in lectins, a type of protein that can bind to cell membranes and interfere with digestive function, impair growth, damage the lining of the small intestine, and wreak havoc on skeletal muscle. (However, it's been shown that much of the lectins in legumes are removed upon cooking.) Peanut lectin, whether cooked or raw, contains high levels of toxic mold that affect the way that cells reproduce, increase inflammation, damage organs (among other things), and may increase risk of atherosclerosis, liver disease, cancer, digestive issues, autoimmune conditions, and more.

Phytic acid is an antinutrient found in many legumes that makes the absorption of key nutrients a lot harder (more on this on page 155). Our guts produce an enzyme that aids in the breakdown of phytic acid, so it may be less of a concern than we're often told. But if your gut bacteria are compromised, you may not have enough of this enzyme, so phytic acid may have more of an effect. If you do choose to include legumes in your keto life, try soaking them first to eliminate 30 to 70 percent of the phytic acid—see page 157 for general soaking instructions.

And finally, legumes contain FODMAPs (fermentable oligosaccharides, disaccharides, monosaccharides and polyols), which can impact digestive function. Making legumes a regular part of your diet can significantly contribute to gut irritation.

Grains

Corn, quinoa, wheat, oats, rice, breads

On a keto diet, the first problem with grains is that they're quite high in carbs and will likely kick you out of ketosis. They also contain gluten, a protein that can cause digestive problems. Those with celiac disease cannot tolerate any amount of gluten, but even among those without celiac disease, 29 percent have an antibody called anti-gliadin IgA. This antibody is dispatched by the gut to ward off gliadin, a component of gluten—so even in those without celiac disease, the body may respond to gluten as a threat.

> My IBS symptoms completely went away when I stopped eating grains. Like, 100 percent.

The benefits of fiber from grains may not be all it's cracked up to be. When fiber is ingested, it bashes up against cells, rupturing the cells. Sounds...dangerous. And though grains do contain vitamins and minerals, you can easily get these from other sources, like keto-friendly vegetables!

Like legumes, many grains contain toxic mold and lectins, which are only decreased during the soaking and sprouting process. I've had people ask me if sprouted/fermented bread, with grains, is okay on a Fat Fueled diet. I think it can be, as long as it feels really good in your body. If this is you, perhaps try adding it to your carb-up practice and see how you do.

Sugar

Table sugar, agave nectar, high-fructose corn syrup, brown sugar, and items that contain them

All kinds of sugar are quite high in carbs and will likely kick you out of ketosis. There's really no silver lining to sugar: it contains minimal essential nutrients, affects insulin and blood sugar regulation, easily converts to fat, can cause nonalcoholic fatty liver disease, and drastically increases cancer risk (cancer cells thrive on sugar).

Maple syrup and honey can have a place in your keto diet if you're practicing carb-ups (see pages 39 to 41). However, I highly recommend that you reserve them for special occasions, as they can be very triggering—once you have a spot of sugar, you want more!

Processed Foods

Artificial sweeteners such as aspartame, conventionally prepared cakes and cookies, packaged snacks like granola bars, chips, protein bars, meal replacements (shakes or otherwise), and crackers

Processed foods are quite high in carbs and will likely kick you out of ketosis. They often contain refined grains, which may lead to weight gain, obesity, heart disease, and type 2 diabetes. They also frequently contain health-damaging trans fats (see page 133) and high amounts of the wrong kind of salt (see page 124). High amounts of high-fructose corn syrup or agave, which are common in processed foods, also affect insulin and blood sugar. In fact, just take a look at the problems listed above for grains and sugar—all that applies in abundance to processed foods. Processed foods also contain minimal essential nutrients and are easy to overconsume.

While there are low-carb processed food options out there that may comply with a low-carb approach, many of the problems mentioned above apply for these foods. They're often devoid of nutrients, lack the ability to satiate, are extremely expensive, and will likely kick you out of ketosis due to their high level of carbohydrates, which are mitigated with copious amounts of insoluble fiber to lower net carbs (see page 62), but can still affect your ability to stay fat-adapted.

FOOD QUALITY

It's not just the kinds of foods you eat that are important. It matters how those foods were raised or grown, too. Let's take a quick look at the options that are out there and which are best for your overall health.

Organic Produce

Organic produce is free of pesticides, chemical fertilizers, industrial solvents, irradiation, and genetic modification. This affects some produce more than others: if you eat the peel or skin of an item, it's generally better to purchase organic because of the heightened level of pesticides. Produce that you may want to purchase organic includes:

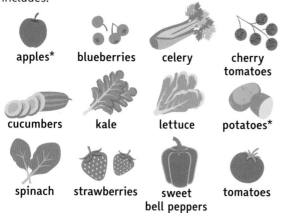

apples*	blueberries	celery	cherry tomatoes
cucumbers	kale	lettuce	potatoes*
spinach	strawberries	sweet bell peppers	tomatoes

Higher in carbohydrates; generally used during optional carb-ups

Grass-Fed/Pastured/Free-Range/ Organic Animal Products

Since you'll be eating quite a lot of animal fat on keto, it's important to ensure that it's high-quality. The biggest sign of quality is that the animals are free to roam and eat their natural diet—in the case of cattle, that's grass and other vegetation; in the case of poultry, it's insects and vegetation.

Conventionally raised steers spend the first few months of their lives on pasture and then are sent to feedlots where they are fed enormous quantities of corn, soy-based protein supplements, antibiotics, and other drugs, including growth hormones. This makes sense economically: the goal is to grow a calf to 1,200 pounds as quickly as possible, then slaughter it and make room for more. Sadly, the grain-based diet is incompatible with their digestive system—cattle evolved on a diet of grass and other vegetation, not grains. Their grain-based diet can lead to inflamed organs and imbalanced gut bacteria, which can lead to issues of *E. coli*. With the combination of the drugs they're given and the environment they're in, all of these toxins are held in the fat of the animal.

Conventionally raised poultry are kept in cages and fed a diet of grains. They're often treated with antibiotics, but the FDA prohibits treating poultry with growth hormones. Because they're kept in cages, they get no exercise and are not able to eat their natural diet of insects and vegetation.

Like chickens, pigs cannot legally be treated with hormones, but conventionally raised pigs may be treated with antibiotics or fed products that are grain-based (often genetically modified) and contain waste products, chemical additives, and other dangerous ingredients. They are also kept in cramped pens.

There are several alternatives to conventionally raised animals. "Free-range," "cage-free," "all-natural," "pastured," "organic"—they're all labels that can mean different things, but the FDA only regulates the use of "free-range" and "organic."

To be certified free-range, poultry must have access to the outdoors (there's no minimum amount of time they must be outside, though, and having access to the outdoors does not mean having access to vegetation).

To be certified organic, animals must have access to the outdoors, cannot be treated with antibiotics or hormones, and must be fed organic feed (which means it can't include genetically engineered products or be grown using pesticides). It doesn't necessarily mean that cattle are grass-fed or grass-finished—and just because cattle are grass-fed doesn't necessarily mean that they're organic.

Although they're not regulated labels, the terms "pasture-raised" and "humanely raised" are worth looking for.

Given what I've seen at feedlots and read about conventionally raised meats, I choose grass-fed organic beef, pastured organic chicken and eggs, and pasture-raised pork from ranchers that I know, are local, and treat their animals well. Grass-fed fatty acids are higher in omega-3s, conjugated linoleic acids (which may assist in a number of health problems, from cancer to asthma to cardiovascular disease), and saturated and monounsaturated fats (see page 132). Their antioxidant profile is richer and nutrient composition fuller.

But organic and grass-fed meats are often more expensive, and if purchasing top-of-the-line animal products isn't in the budget, that's fine. Purchase the leaner versions to avoid the toxins that may be stored in the fat and add your own plant-based fats, such as coconut or avocado oil.

Stick to a low-carb, high-fat diet by picking up some items outlined on the food lists beginning on page 115, opt for whole-food sources and glorious greens, and you should be just fine!

In the case of seafood, I prefer wild-caught over farm-raised because farm-raised fish have less vitamin D; higher levels of omega-6 (see page 133), which may lead to excess inflammation, which in turn is linked to diabetes, cardiovascular disease, and Alzheimer's; and far less omega-3.

KETO POWER FOODS

I call them power foods, and I try to incorporate at least two to three servings into my day. These foods are keto-supporting, fat-burning powerhouses that'll boost energy, aid in balancing hormones, and increase nutrient intake, all without breaking the bank—a triple threat!

Apple Cider Vinegar, raw and unfiltered

WHY IT'S AWESOME: Improves insulin sensitivity. Aids in fat loss.

HOW TO USE IT: Sauté some veggies, add a splash of vinegar. Make salad dressing with it. Pour it over a bowl of ground beef and sautéed vegetables.

FAVORITE BRAND: Bragg

Avocados

WHY IT'S AWESOME: Lowers cardiovascular risk factors. Reduces inflammation.

HOW TO USE IT: Slice, sprinkle with salt and chili powder, and enjoy with a spoon. Blend with coconut milk, coconut oil, and a spoonful of cacao powder. Mash and add lemon and a touch of stevia.

Blueberries (best for carb-ups)

WHY IT'S AWESOME: Protect against free radical damage. Lowers LDL oxidation.

HOW TO USE IT: Add to a grilled chicken salad for an easy carb-up dinner. Stir into a glass of coconut milk with a splash of vanilla extract. Blend with nut or seed milk, collagen, and a drop of stevia.

Bone Broth (page 151)

WHY IT'S AWESOME: Reduces inflammation. Improves sleep.

HOW TO USE IT: Freeze in silicone ice cube trays for quick use—either drop in a mug and heat up, or add to a recipe. Add to sautéed vegetables. Use to cook your evening carb-ups (see pages 39 to 41).

FAVORITE BRAND: If you don't have time to make bone broth, enjoy the associated health benefits by adding gelatin to hot drinks or making gummies (page 406). My favorite brand is Vital Proteins collagen protein beef gelatin.

Broccoli

WHY IT'S AWESOME: Lowers cholesterol. Reduces cancer risk.

HOW TO USE IT: Chop and sauté with ground beef and fresh herbs. Try it raw, smothered in mayonnaise with a touch of apple cider vinegar.

NOTE: *Broccoli is goitrogenic, meaning it may harm your thyroid gland. If you're concerned about metabolic health, it's best to cook your broccoli before eating it.*

Coconut Oil

WHY IT'S AWESOME: Increases metabolism. Reduces hunger and cravings.

HOW TO USE IT: Blend it into your nighttime tea with collagen. Heat with dried herbs and place in a container to chill, then use it as an herb butter.

FAVORITE BRAND: Now Foods and Chosen Foods coconut oil spray

Dark Chocolate
(100% raw cacao and/or free from sugar)

WHY IT'S AWESOME: Rich in antioxidants. Reduces cardiovascular risks.

HOW TO USE IT: Enjoy with a dollop of coconut butter. Shave over a bowl of fresh berries. Add to a batch of fat bombs (see page 114).

FAVORITE BRANDS: Giddy YoYo HUNDO bars and Lily's Sweets sugar-free chocolate chips

Egg Yolks

WHY IT'S AWESOME: Most nutritious food on the planet. Promotes healthful cholesterol levels.

HOW TO USE IT: Cook like scrambled eggs for the brightest scramble you've ever had! Make hollandaise sauce and drizzle it over your veggies. Add to your next Rocket Fuel Latte (page 428).

Fermented Foods

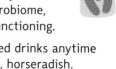

WHY IT'S AWESOME: Promotes eye health. Encourages a balanced gut microbiome, which can improve digestive functioning.

HOW TO USE IT: Drink fermented drinks anytime during the day. Add sauerkraut, horseradish, kimchi, or pickles to salads or burgers, or place on top of one-pan meals.

FAVORITE BRANDS: Bubbies sauerkraut, GT's kombucha, Wildbrine kimchi, and Kevita water kefir

NOTE: *Go for unpasteurized sauerkraut and kimchi. You want the live bacteria!*

Flax Seeds

WHY IT'S AWESOME: Balances digestive function. Reduces hunger and cravings.

HOW TO USE IT: Prepare a batch of Flaxseed Cinnamon Bun Muffins (page 239) or Classic Flaxseed Focaccia (page 373).

FAVORITE BRAND: Bob's Red Mill

NOTES: *Flax seeds contain substances that bind with sulfur compounds that could be harmful to the thyroid gland. If you're trying to improve the health of your thyroid, enjoy flax as a treat every once in a while. Also, a couple of tablespoons a day goes a long way. If you've never had flax before, start small and work your way up.*

Garlic

WHY IT'S AWESOME: Boosts immune system. Antifungal and great in a Candida protocol. Balances blood sugar. Reduces oxidative stress related to hypertension.

HOW TO USE IT: Cook everything with it.

Grass-Fed Beef Tallow

WHY IT'S AWESOME: Aids in fat loss. Provides copious amounts of antioxidants.

HOW TO USE IT: Make Roasted Brussels Sprouts with Walnut "Cheese" (page 388), Steak with Tallow Herb Butter (page 306), Mind-Blowing Burgers (page 308), or Bombay Sloppy Jolenes (page 302).

FAVORITE BRAND: EPIC

Kale

WHY IT'S AWESOME: Rich in vitamin C, which helps synthesize collagen. Aids in the development of strong bones.

HOW TO USE IT: Sauté with bone broth (page 151) and chill until ready to eat. Make it the base of a salad. Drizzle with olive oil, apple cider vinegar, and salt and bake in a 300°F oven for 10 to 15 minutes for kale chips. Never consume raw: cook lightly by running under hot water for 20 to 30 seconds before preparing in salads, smoothies, or other recipes where raw kale is called for. Add a handful to a Keto Milkshake (page 423).

Liver

WHY IT'S AWESOME: Aids in eye health. Supports metabolism. Extremely nutrient-dense.

HOW TO USE IT: Make The Only Way I'll Eat Liver (page 274) or add to a food processor, grind, then add to raw ground beef before sautéing.

FAVORITE BRAND: Not a fan of eating liver? Pick up a bottle of Vital Proteins beef liver capsules instead for the benefits of liver without the taste.

Raw Coconut Meat

WHY IT'S AWESOME: Supports healthy digestion. Supports balanced glucose tolerance.

HOW TO USE IT: Eat it straight from the coconut. Blend with water for thick coconut milk. Chop up and sauté with vegetables. Add to a salad.

Resistant Starches (carb-ups only)

WHY IT'S AWESOME: Unlike common starches, resistant starches (RS) do just that—resist digestion, making them less likely to spike blood glucose or insulin. RS feed gut bacteria, helping maintain a diverse gut microflora, which has been linked to improvements in anxiety, IBD, depression, obesity, and more. Low in calories and doesn't affect insulin or glucose.

HOW TO USE IT: There are many forms of resistant starch. My favorite is cooked and cooled potatoes or rice.

NOTE: *The items can be reheated but must not reach temperatures of 130°F (55°C) or more. Best option: make salads with them!*

Sardines

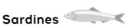

WHY IT'S AWESOME: Promotes bone health. Rich in components that support heart health.

HOW TO USE IT: Prepare Sardine Fritter Wraps (page 362), mix with mayo as you would tuna salad, or fry in your favorite oil and serve with Verde Caesar Salad with Crispy Capers (page 289).

Seaweed

WHY IT'S AWESOME: Promotes digestive health. Maintains thyroid health.

HOW TO USE IT: Crumbled over cauliflower rice (page 364). Wrap fresh veggies like sushi rolls. Use as a wrap for your favorite sandwich fillings.

NOTE: *Too much seaweed can overload your system with potassium, causing issues with your kidneys. Just don't add platefuls of seaweed to your daily meals and you should do great.*

Wild-Caught Pacific Salmon

WHY IT'S AWESOME: Aids in bone and joint health. Promotes brain health.

HOW TO USE IT: Make Crispy Salmon Steaks with Sweet Cabbage (page 356), Shaved Cucumber and Smoked Salmon Salad (page 297), or Salmon Cakes with Dill Cream Sauce (page 360).

NOTE: *Wild-caught salmon has less inflammatory omega-6, fewer calories, fewer contaminants, more magnesium, and more potassium than farmed salmon.*

My twenty-five-year-old self, who was afraid of fat and terrified to see it coupled with the word *bomb*, is shaking her fist at me. Previous self, chill out; this is awesome.

FAT

So what the heck's a fat bomb? It's an extremely high-fat, low-carb, moderate-protein snack. In fact, it's so high in fat that over 85 percent of its calories come from fat.

Fat bombs can be sweet or savory. Sweet fat bombs are usually made from items such as coconut, chocolate, nut butter, seed butter, ghee, cacao butter, or coconut oil, combined with some sort of natural sweetener, such as erythritol or stevia. Many savory fat bombs are made from ingredients such as tallow, lard, bacon, avocado, or chicken skin and spices.

Fat bombs come in numerous forms, from soups to bark, balls, cookies, bars, chunks—you name it. Sweet fat bombs are often prepared in silicone molds. While these molds are fun because they come in different shapes and sizes, they're not necessary. Any fat bomb recipe that calls for a silicone mold can be made into a bark: instead of pouring it into a mold, transfer it to a baking pan, allow it to set, and break it into pieces after it hardens.

Fat bombs can be a lifesaver, especially when you're just starting out on your keto journey. These little powerhouses feel like indulgent treats, yet they're packed with nourishing and satisfying fats. They're particularly handy when you're on the go. Take a couple of these bad boys with you and you'll be good to go!

Refer to the chart on pages 432 to 434 for fat bomb recipes, perfect for any occasion. Prepare them as appetizers at your next gathering and see what happens. My friends and family love them—they always ask me to bring "those fatty things" with me.

QUICK SNACKS

Ten years ago, my favorite snacks were saltine crackers with margarine, Jujubes, and extra-large soda slushies, so I'm pretty proud of this list of twenty quick keto-friendly snacks. Each has less than a handful of common ingredients that are just thrown together in a bowl—and most of them require no cooking.

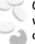 Avocado halves drizzled with olive oil, salt, and pepper

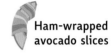 Ham-wrapped avocado slices

 Jicama fries with avocado oil mayo

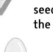 Ants on a log (celery, sesame seeds, nut or seed butter—or skip the sesame seeds)

 Cacao butter wafers with nut or seed butter

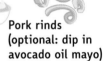 Hard-boiled eggs

 Almonds sprinkled with cacao powder, salt, and stevia

 Pork rinds (optional: dip in avocado oil mayo)

 Bacon-wrapped cucumber sticks

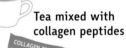 Tea mixed with collagen peptides

COLLAGEN PEPTIDES

 Cucumber slices dipped in tahini

 Smoked oysters

 Olives

 Walnuts sprinkled with nutritional yeast, MCT oil, and salt

 Beef jerky with macadamia nuts

 Pickles

 Coconut cream with berries

 Sunflower seeds

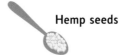 Hemp seeds

Almond butter with chia seeds

FOOD LISTS

Let's get thinking about food gathering. I've compiled this hefty list to provide you with a ton of options, so that restriction on the keto diet path is as incomprehensible as flying pigs.

FATS

Power Foods

Avocados (see page 111)

Beef tallow

Coconut oil

Dark chocolate (100% raw cacao and/or sugar-free)

Flax seeds

Oils

Almond oil ❄

Avocado oil ❄ (see page 135)

Butter, grass-fed **DAIRY**

Cacao butter/oil

Canola oil **PUFA** ❄

Chicken fat (schmaltz), free-range

Coconut oil

Duck fat, free-range

Flaxseed oil **PUFA** ❄

Ghee, grass-fed **DAIRY**

Goose fat, free-range

Hazelnut oil ❄

Hemp seed oil **PUFA** ❄

Lard, pasture-raised

Macadamia nut oil ❄

MCT oil

Olive oil ❄

Palm fruit oil ❄

Palm kernel oil ❄

Tallow/suet, grass-fed

Walnut oil **PUFA** ❄

Nuts/Seeds*

Almonds

Brazil nuts

Cashews **CARBS**

Chia seeds

Coconut

Hazelnuts

Hemp seeds

Macadamia nuts

Pecans

Pine nuts **CARBS**

Pistachios **CARBS**

Pumpkin seeds **CARBS**

Sesame seeds **CARBS**

Sunflower seeds **CARBS**

Walnuts

Other Whole Foods

Avocados

Bacon

Olives

Nut or Seed Butters ❗

Almond butter

Brazil nut butter

Coconut butter

Hazelnut butter

Hemp seed butter

Macadamia nut butter

Pecan butter

Sunflower seed butter **CARBS**

Tahini **CARBS**

Walnut butter

NOTE: *Many of the animal-based protein options will also be good sources of fat.*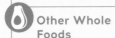

PUFA *Best used sparingly; higher in PUFAs (see page 133)*

CARBS *Best used sparingly; higher in carbs*

DAIRY *If you are sensitive to dairy, this may not be the best choice*

❄ *Ideally cold-pressed*

❗ *Watch for sugar, gluten, preservatives, and dairy!*

*As well as their flour and milk varieties. Nuts and seeds are best soaked and then roasted at 150°F (65°C); see page 157.

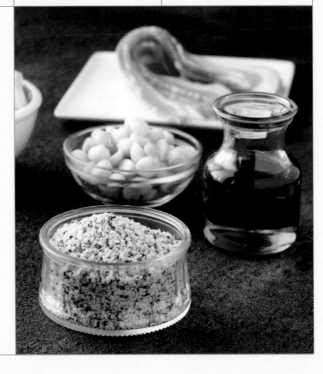

PROTEINS

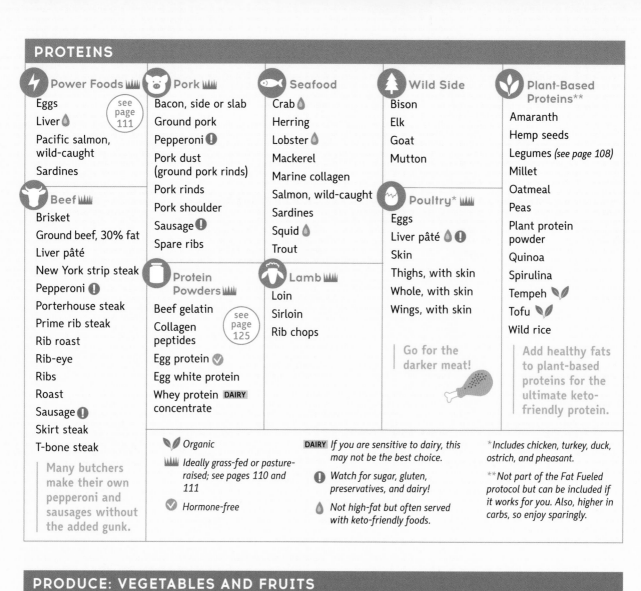

Power Foods
- Eggs
- Liver ◊ _(see page 111)_
- Pacific salmon, wild-caught
- Sardines

Beef
- Brisket
- Ground beef, 30% fat
- Liver pâté
- New York strip steak
- Pepperoni ❶
- Porterhouse steak
- Prime rib steak
- Rib roast
- Rib-eye
- Ribs
- Roast
- Sausage ❶
- Skirt steak
- T-bone steak

Many butchers make their own pepperoni and sausages without the added gunk.

Pork
- Bacon, side or slab
- Ground pork
- Pepperoni ❶
- Pork dust (ground pork rinds)
- Pork rinds
- Pork shoulder
- Sausage ❶
- Spare ribs

Protein Powders
- Beef gelatin
- Collagen peptides _(see page 125)_
- Egg protein ✓
- Egg white protein
- Whey protein **DAIRY** concentrate

Seafood
- Crab ◊
- Herring
- Lobster ◊
- Mackerel
- Marine collagen
- Salmon, wild-caught
- Sardines
- Squid ◊
- Trout

Lamb
- Loin
- Sirloin
- Rib chops

Wild Side
- Bison
- Elk
- Goat
- Mutton

Poultry*
- Eggs
- Liver pâté ◊ ❶
- Skin
- Thighs, with skin
- Whole, with skin
- Wings, with skin

Go for the darker meat!

Plant-Based Proteins**
- Amaranth
- Hemp seeds
- Legumes _(see page 108)_
- Millet
- Oatmeal
- Peas
- Plant protein powder
- Quinoa
- Spirulina
- Tempeh 🌱
- Tofu 🌱
- Wild rice

Add healthy fats to plant-based proteins for the ultimate keto-friendly protein.

🌱 Organic

〰 Ideally grass-fed or pasture-raised; see pages 110 and 111

✓ Hormone-free

DAIRY If you are sensitive to dairy, this may not be the best choice.

❶ Watch for sugar, gluten, preservatives, and dairy!

◊ Not high-fat but often served with keto-friendly foods.

* Includes chicken, turkey, duck, ostrich, and pheasant.

** Not part of the Fat Fueled protocol but can be included if it works for you. Also, higher in carbs, so enjoy sparingly.

PRODUCE: VEGETABLES AND FRUITS

Organized from lowest in carbs to highest. Remember, if it feels good to you, you don't have to count your kale to have success on keto!

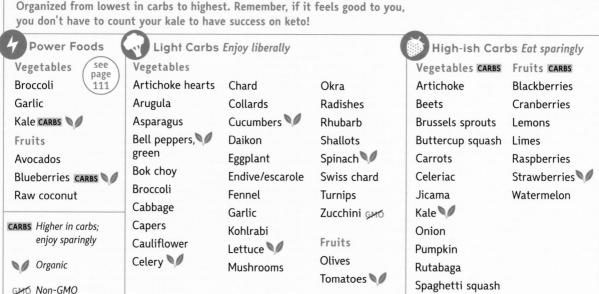

Power Foods
Vegetables _(see page 111)_
- Broccoli
- Garlic
- Kale **CARBS** 🌱

Fruits
- Avocados
- Blueberries **CARBS** 🌱
- Raw coconut

CARBS _Higher in carbs; enjoy sparingly_

🌱 _Organic_

GMO _Non-GMO_

Light Carbs _Enjoy liberally_
Vegetables
- Artichoke hearts
- Arugula
- Asparagus
- Bell peppers, green 🌱
- Bok choy
- Broccoli
- Cabbage
- Capers
- Cauliflower
- Celery 🌱

- Chard
- Collards
- Cucumbers 🌱
- Daikon
- Eggplant
- Endive/escarole
- Fennel
- Garlic
- Kohlrabi
- Lettuce 🌱
- Mushrooms

- Okra
- Radishes
- Rhubarb
- Shallots
- Spinach 🌱
- Swiss chard
- Turnips
- Zucchini GMO

Fruits
- Olives
- Tomatoes 🌱

High-ish Carbs _Eat sparingly_
Vegetables **CARBS**
- Artichoke
- Beets
- Brussels sprouts
- Buttercup squash
- Carrots
- Celeriac
- Jicama
- Kale 🌱
- Onion
- Pumpkin
- Rutabaga
- Spaghetti squash

Fruits **CARBS**
- Blackberries
- Cranberries
- Lemons
- Limes
- Raspberries
- Strawberries 🌱
- Watermelon

OPTIONAL CARB-UPS

For even more carb-up ideas and food prep instructions, visit healthfulpursuit.com/carbup to download the complimentary PDF "Carb-Up Recipes."

 ### Starches

Acorn squash
Arrowroot
Cassava flour
Cassava/yuca root/ manioc
Delicata squash
Green banana flour
Green plantains

Kabocha squash
Parsnips
Potatoes
Sweet potatoes
Tapioca starch
White rice*
Yams

 ### Fruits

Apples 🌱
Apricots
Bananas
Cherries

Dates
Figs
Grapes
Kiwifruit

Melon
Oranges
Pears

Sweeteners

Coconut sugar
Honey, unpasteurized
Maple syrup
Yacón syrup

Not part of the Fat Fueled protocol but can be included if it works for you. 🌱 *Organic*

EXTRAS

 ### Power Foods *(see page 111)*

Apple cider vinegar
Bone broth *(page 151)*
Fermented foods (kimchi, sauerkraut, kombucha, water kefir)
Seaweed

 ### Drinks

Almond milk
Coconut milk, light or full-fat
Coffee
Soda sweetened with stevia
Sparkling water
Tea

Pantry Items

Cacao nibs
Cacao powder
Chocolate chips, stevia-sweetened
Kelp noodles
Lemon extract
Lemon juice
Nutritional yeast
Vanilla extract

 ### Snacks

See also page 114

Coconut chips, unsweetened
Dark chocolate (100% raw cacao and/or free from sugar)
Kale chips CARBS
Meat sticks, Paleovalley
Nut and seed butters, unsweetened
Pickles ❗
Pork rinds, cooked in acceptable fat
Seaweed chips ❗
Sugar-free jerky, EPIC bars and bites

 ### Spices

Allspice powder
Bay leaves
Black pepper, ground
Cajun seasoning *(page 232)*
Cardamom
Cayenne pepper
Chili powder
Chinese CARBS five-spice
Cinnamon, CARBS ground
Cloves, ground
Coriander, ground
Cumin

Curry powder *(page 235)*
Garlic powder CARBS
Ginger powder
Gray sea salt or Himalayan rock salt
Nutmeg, ground
Onion powder CARBS
Red pepper flakes
Seasoned salt *(page 117)*
Smoked paprika
Turmeric
Vanilla powder

 ### Dairy*

Butter, grass-fed
Ghee, grass-fed
(see page 147)

Sweeteners**

Erythritol
Monk fruit extract/ lo han guo
Stevia, alcohol-free
Xylitol

Fresh Herbs

Basil
Chives
Cilantro
Dill

Mint
Oregano
Parsley
Rosemary

Sage
Tarragon
Thyme

Condiments

Avocado oil mayo
Balsamic vinegar CARBS
Coconut aminos
Fish sauce
Horseradish
Hot sauce
Mustard
Tomato sauce ❗
White wine vinegar

CARBS *Best to use sparingly; larger quantities can pack a lot of carbs.*

❗ *Watch for sugar, gluten, preservatives, and dairy!*

* *Not part of the Fat Fueled protocol but can be included if it works for you. Choose high-quality, grass-fed/finished products.*

** *Liquid forms are best: they're free of carb-heavy maltodextrin and dextrose.*

SWEETENERS

Before we talk about different kinds of sweeteners, I want to chat with you about going sugar-free. If you've been rockin' a high-fat, low-carb life for a while, you've probably noticed that you don't seek out sugary foods as much as you used to, especially if you are at the point where you're listening to your body. If you're coming here from the other end of the spectrum, though—eating every sugary thing that isn't nailed down or going out to restaurants daily—removing all sugar from your life immediately isn't a realistic goal. And we have to be real here.

If you're new to the world of keto, take it slow and figure out what works for you. I still have sugar once in a while. In fact, as I am writing this, it's 11 p.m., I am sitting on the floor cross-legged with my blue light blockers on, and there's a tall herbal chai latte beside me, homemade and sweetened with maple syrup. The key is that I know I'm in a good place to have a bit of carbs: it's late, the carbs will help me sleep well, and it's been a couple of days since I've had a load of carbohydrates. (For more on eating carbs at night and the benefits of carb-ups, see Chapter 2.)

The sweeteners listed below are all keto-friendly and can help you enjoy some treats in your life, especially as you adjust to the keto lifestyle. That said, you'll be far better off creating a life for yourself that doesn't revolve around sweetened goodies, even if they contain the "keto safe" stuff. If you're craving a little sweetness, try a fresh bowl of berries or a sliced kiwi with some shredded coconut. In my experience, sweeter whole foods will always, always surpass treats made with the sweeteners listed below. The fewer sweet things you incorporate into your life, the less you'll crave sweetness.

If you're at a bakery and wondering which conventional sweetener is best, stick to brown rice syrup (if you're not sensitive to grains), dextrose (if you're not sensitive to corn), and maple syrup. These sweeteners have very little fructose, which in excess may cause liver damage, increase the risk of developing insulin resistance, speed up aging, encourage inflammation, and cause an overgrowth of bacteria in the gut. And maple syrup boasts some minerals and nutrients.

Okay, let's review some keto-friendly sweeteners, so you'll have enough information to make the best choice for you. These are natural sweeteners, and the only ones that might affect blood sugar are xylitol and maltitol. Overall, though, all of these sweeteners, even xylitol and maltitol, have much less impact on blood sugar than other sweeteners such as white sugar, agave nectar, and the like.

Erythritol

RATING: ★★★★☆

Unlike other sugar alcohols, erythritol is broken down in the small intestine; since it doesn't reach the colon, it doesn't cause the digestive problems that can occur with other sugar alcohols. This makes it a potentially great option for those with digestive imbalances. A word of caution: if you have kidney problems, check with your health-care provider before consuming erythritol. Also, if you are sensitive to corn, you may want to move on to another sweetener, as this one is derived from corn.

Inulin

RATING: ★★★★☆

Generally extracted from chicory root. Be careful if you're sensitive to FODMAPs (see page 128). What I like about inulin is that it caramelizes like sugar, making it fun for baking. It can have a laxative effect, so it's best diluted by mixing it with other sweeteners such as stevia. Inulin is often used in stevia baking blends.

Maltitol

RATING: ★☆☆☆☆

Tastes very similar to sugar, which is why you see it in many sugar-free products on the market. It's commonly linked to digestive issues such as bloating, diarrhea, and abdominal pain. I'll never forget the time that I bought Red Vines licorice before a movie thinking it was regular licorice—I ate the entire bag during the movie and finally, after barely making it to the bathroom for the fourth time, realized that I had bought the diabetic (maltitol-sweetened) licorice by accident. Never again. Of all the options listed here, maltitol is the most likely to boost your blood sugar. That, combined with the poo-tastic effects, makes me not even want to put it on this list.

Monk Fruit

RATING: ★★★★★

Also called luo han guo. It can be difficult to find, but Asian markets are a good bet. Pure is best; otherwise, it can be mixed with a bunch of other ingredients that you don't want.

Stevia

RATING: ★★★★★

Has been shown to reduce blood pressure and inflammation, although there aren't many studies to support this just yet. You can use 100 percent pure stevia or get it mixed with other sweeteners. I enjoy the alcohol-free drops or the crushed stevia leaf, which is unprocessed.

Xylitol

RATING: ★★★☆☆

A sugar alcohol like erythritol that doesn't raise blood sugar. If you experience gut pain the first time you try xylitol, it's likely because you ate too much of it at first—our bodies have an enzyme that breaks down xylitol, but if it isn't in use, it takes time to build it up, and if you don't have enough of the enzyme, you'll have some stomach pain. It's also possible that it was a low-quality xylitol. Look for birch-sourced, North American xylitol or pumpkin-based xylitol (if you have a birch allergy), as these will be free from corn. Note to pet owners: Xylitol is very toxic to dogs. Make sure they don't eat any of it!

You'll notice that sucralose, aspartame, and saccharin didn't make it onto this list. They are as synthetic as synthetic gets, and I'm pretty sure synthetic sweeteners aren't going to help us heal and be awesome. If you've landed on a bunch of low-carb goodies that use sucralose, that's a winning sign that the product should be avoided.

ALCOHOL

Alcohol is good for you in moderation. Having a drink every now and then may help reduce the risk of:

- **Coronary heart disease**
- **Type 2 diabetes**
- **Bone atrophy**
- **Cognitive impairment**
- **Erectile dysfunction**

But notice that I said "every now and then" and "may." I wouldn't plan a bender with your pals in the name of strengthening your bones. And all of alcohol's health benefits—and then some—can also be achieved by following a high-fat ketogenic eating style.

Also, if you have weight to lose or are trying to become fat-adapted, drinking alcohol may limit your progress. And when I say "may," I mean "will." Here's why: Alcohol is the first fuel your body burns, before carbohydrates or fat. This does not completely stop fat-burning, but it does pause it until the alcohol is used up. So once the alcohol is burned through, you will immediately go back to burning fat, or continue to work toward becoming fat-adapted. For some people, however, drinking alcohol can stall weight loss for days—or jump-start it in other cases!

If you're the type of person who doesn't respond well to alcohol or doesn't know when to stop, or if you're attempting to switch into fat-burning mode, I'd avoid alcohol. I personally have for a very long time.

CHOOSING ALCOHOL MINDFULLY

Enjoy a drink with friends now and again? Here are the most popular drinks to choose from and the impact they'll have on your high-fat, low-carb ketogenic life.

Because there are so many choices to brands and types of drinks, sometimes a range of calories, carb counts, and sugar amounts are listed. Also, many companies are resistant to sharing nutritional information about their products. The ranges were prepared with the information available, but some brands may fall outside these ranges.

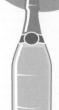

CHAMPAGNE
SERVING AMOUNT: 4 fl. oz. (120 ml)
CALORIES: 90
CARB COUNT: 1.6 g
SUGAR: 0.8 g
BEST CHOICES: brut natural, brut

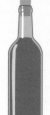

RED WINE
SERVING AMOUNT: 5 fl. oz. (150 ml)
CALORIES: 125
CARB COUNT: 3.8 g
SUGAR: 0.9 g
BEST CHOICE: Cabernet Sauvignon, Merlot, Pinot Noir

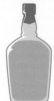

WHISKY, BOURBON, BRANDY, SCOTCH, COGNAC
based on 80 proof (40% alcohol)
SERVING AMOUNT: 1 fl. oz. (30 ml)
CALORIES: 64
CARB COUNT: 0 g
SUGAR: 0 g

Research has found antioxidant activity in bourbon, Armagnac brandy, and cognac.

BEST CHOICE: on the rocks; whisky with Zevia cola; brandy with apple cider vinegar, water, and stevia; scotch with Zevia ginger ale and lime juice; cognac with water, lemon juice, and stevia

See page 121 for more low-sugar mixers

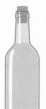

WHITE WINE
SERVING AMOUNT: 5 fl. oz. (150 ml)
CALORIES: 120
CARB COUNT: 3.8 g
SUGAR: 1.4 g
BEST CHOICE: Chardonnay, Pinot Grigio, Sauvignon Blanc

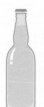

LIGHT BEER
SERVING AMOUNT: 12 fl. oz. (350 ml)
CALORIES: 104
CARB COUNT: 6 g
SUGAR: 0.3 g
BEST CHOICE: Beck's Premier Light, Bud Select, Coors Light, Michelob Ultra, Michelob Ultra, MGD

VODKA, GIN, CLEAR/DARK RUM
based on 80 proof (40% alcohol)
SERVING AMOUNT: 1 fl. oz. (30ml)
CALORIES: 64
CARB COUNT: 0 g
SUGAR: 0 g
BEST CHOICES: on the rocks, herb-infused vodka and water, gin with mineral water and lemon slices, rum and Zevia cola

HARD CIDER
SERVING AMOUNT: 12 fl. oz. (350 ml)
CALORIES: 99–200
CARB COUNT: 1–30 g
SUGAR: 1–24 g
BEST CHOICES: Bulmer's Original, Mercury Dry, Strongbow Low Carb

REGULAR BEER
Craft beers and IPAs have been omitted because they pack a lot of carbohydrates.
SERVING AMOUNT: 12 fl. oz. (350 ml)
CALORIES: 150
CARB COUNT: 9–13 g
SUGAR: 0–10 g
BEST CHOICE: Rhinebecker Extra, San Miguel

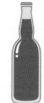

STOUT
SERVING AMOUNT: 12 fl. oz. (350 ml)
CALORIES: 200
CARB COUNT: 20–25 g
SUGAR: 10–15 g
BEST CHOICE: Brooklyn Dry Irish Stout, Guinness Draught

UMBRELLA DRINKS
Included so that you can see the sugar… so much sugar!
SERVING AMOUNT: 12 fl. oz. (350 ml)
CALORIES: 300–780
CARB COUNT: 30–90 g
SUGAR: 13–85 g

- Do you find dry champagne too dry? Try adding a drop of alcohol-free stevia. It sweetens it up, sugar-free style.

- Alcohol is dehydrating, so be sure to drink extra water before your drink, while you're drinking, or immediately after.

- If you've been on a high-fat/low-carb ketogenic diet for some time, remember, you're now a lightweight! Be careful the first time you drink after becoming fat-adapted, as your body can't handle as much alcohol as you're used to.

- Organic red wine boasts higher antioxidant content with less toxic mold—meaning it's a better-for-you beverage.

- Low-sugar mixers for whisky, bourbon, brandy, scotch, cognac, vodka, gin, and rum: water kefir, kombucha, Zevia stevia-sweetened soda, mineral water, citrus essential oils, lemon juice, lime juice, soda water, unsweetened cranberry juice, coconut milk, seltzer water, cucumber juice, watermelon slices. You can also infuse these alcohols with fresh herbs, or add stevia drops to flavor and sweeten more naturally.

- White wine is lower in phenols and antioxidants than red wine.

- What makes a light beer? It's the alcohol content. Anything under 5 percent alcohol is considered "light."

- Light beer has the same lower phenol and antioxidant activity as white wine.

- Most beer and stouts contain gluten! If you're avoiding gluten or you're celiac, try hard cider instead.

- Hard cider offers an impressive antioxidant boost, but watch for the "dry" ciders that contain a considerable amount of sugar.

- A common belief is that the lighter the color of beer, the fewer the carbs. Sadly, the color of the beer you're drinking doesn't always equate to the carb count.

COCONUT PRODUCTS

When I first began investigating coconut products as replacements for nuts, dairy, and the like, I was confused by all the options. What's the difference between coconut oil and coconut butter? What is coconut manna? What is coconut milk? What's the difference between coconut milk and coconut oil? I'm laying it all down.

Coconut has saved my dairy-free keto life numerous times. Now I hope it can do the same for you.

Coconut Milk
This creamy milk is made from blended and strained coconut meat. Much of the oil is removed. Full-fat coconut milk is great for recipes that call for 2 percent or whole milk, while light coconut milk is great for recipes that call for skim or 1 percent milk. Substitute coconut milk for dairy milk on a 1:1 ratio.

Coconut Butter/Manna
Solid at room temperature and mildly fibrous, coconut butter is made from ground coconut meat. Coconut butter is to coconuts as peanut butter is to peanuts. It's a great replacement for white chocolate.

Coconut Water

Coconut water is what you get when you open up a coconut: it's the "plasma" of the coconut, the water contained in the nut. Slightly high in carbohydrates and low in fat, it's a great base for smoothies, and its high electrolyte content makes it a fabulous replacement for sports drinks. But watch the carbohydrate and sugar content!

Coconut Cream

This high-fat, thick, whipping-cream-like product is made from blended and strained coconut meat, like coconut milk, but much of the oil is retained to thicken it. It can be used 1:1 in place of cream in just about any recipe. Although you can buy coconut cream, you can also get it from a can of full-fat coconut milk: chill for at least twenty-four hours and the cream will thicken at the top; all you have to do is scoop it out!

Shredded Coconut

Just what it sounds like: the shredded and dried meat of the coconut. Finely shredded coconut can be used in place of flour in my recipes, while long shredded coconut is great as a base for homemade granola (page 246) and snacks.

Coconut Flour

Made from coconut meat that's been dehydrated and ground, this is an extra-dry, grain-free, low-carb flour. Because it's so dry, baking and cooking with coconut flour can be challenging. The key is to make sure you're using enough eggs (or egg-free replacements). The light coconut flavor allows coconut flour to blend seamlessly into sweet or savory baked goods, and it makes a wonderful coating for chicken, fish, or other proteins.

Coconut Oil

Solid at room temperature, coconut oil is fat that's been extracted from the meat of the coconut. Coconut oil is to coconuts as olive oil is to olives. Use it in place of butter at a 1:1 ratio.

MCT Oil

MCT stands for "medium-chain triglycerides," a kind of fat the oil contains in abundance. Sourced from coconut and palm oils, this odorless, translucent liquid is often used to boost ketone production. Use it in homemade salad dressing, drizzle it over cooked dishes, or add it to your Rocket Fuel Latte (page 428). It's suitable for cooking at temperatures below 320°F (160°C).

COCONUT MILK
- Creamy
- Made from blended and strained coconut meat with oil removed

COCONUT CREAM
- Thick cream–like whipped cream
- Blended and strained coconut meat with oil kept in

COCONUT OIL
- Solid at room temperature
- Coconut oil is to coconut as olive oil is to olives

COCONUT BUTTER
- Solid at room temperature
- Made from ground coconut meat

SHREDDED COCONUT
- Bits of coconut meat
- Coconut meat, shredded and dried

COCONUT FLOUR
- Extra-dry flour alternative
- Coconut meat, ground and dried

COCONUT WATER
- Liquid
- The plasma of coconut

FERMENTED FOODS

Think of fermented foods as your ticket to long-lasting gut health: they feed the good gut bacteria we need for a balanced microflora. And the health of your gut dictates, in many ways, the health of your entire body. Having a healthy gut, supported by regular fermented foods and a keto diet, has the following benefits:

- **Stabilizes behavior and mood**
- **Encourages a positive, disease-free life**
- **Controls blood sugar**
- **Reduces the risk of obesity**

Fermented foods are filled with nutrients: they're rich in B vitamins and vitamin K2 (which reduces arterial plaque). They help to protect against infection (great during cold and flu season!), inhibit the growth of Candida and other yeasts, keep you regular, and help detoxify the body, drawing out heavy metals and other toxins. Fermentation also lowers the allergenic qualities of whatever food is fermented—so, for example, yogurt may be easier to digest for those who don't tolerate dairy well. And if you eat fermented foods at every meal, they can replace a probiotic supplement, saving you money.

> If you've never eaten fermented foods before, start small with a tablespoon and work your way up to as much as ½ cup (120 ml) with every meal.

Just about anything can be fermented, from vegetables to teas, water, or milk. If you're purchasing fermented foods from the store, look for keywords like "unpasteurized," "fermented," "raw," and "organic." You can also ferment your own foods using guides from sites such as wikiHow, Cultures for Health, or Nourishing Days. Store-bought fermented foods and starter cultures for homemade ferments can vary widely in quality, so it's important to find a high-quality source. My favorite brands are Caldwell Bio Fermentation and Body Ecology.

> Much of the sugar used in fermentation is eaten up in the process, but there is still some sugar in the final product. If you're purchasing fermented foods, be sure to read the labels. If you're making your own, you won't know exactly how much sugar is in the final result, but the longer you ferment, the less sugar the food will contain.

FERMENTATION The process of fermentation preserves food naturally while also boosting its health benefits.

ACETIC FERMENTATION—Bacteria consumes alcohol and leaves behind fermented liquid.
Example: vinegar

LACTIC ACID FERMENTATION—Uses lactic acid bacteria, which is found in all things grown in the earth/soil, as well as strains naturally present in dairy milk.
Examples: kimchi, sauerkraut, pickles (not the conventional stuff), yogurt*, cheese*

SYMBIOTIC FERMENTATION—Bacteria and yeast feed off sugar and make alcohol.
Examples: water kefir, kombucha

YEAST FERMENTATION—Yeast eat sugar to create CO_2, which makes the product fizzy depending on how long it ferments.
Examples: beer, wine, sourdough bread* *

FOODS THAT CAN BE FERMENTED

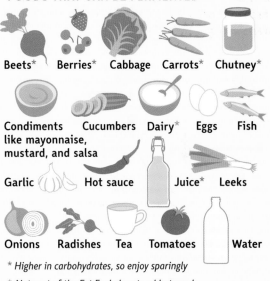

Beets*   Berries*   Cabbage   Carrots*   Chutney*

Condiments like mayonnaise, mustard, and salsa   Cucumbers   Dairy*   Eggs   Fish

Garlic   Hot sauce   Juice*   Leeks

Onions   Radishes   Tea   Tomatoes   Water

* Higher in carbohydrates, so enjoy sparingly

* Not part of the Fat Fueled protocol but can be included if it works for you

BENEFITS OF FERMENTED FOODS

- **Feed good gut bacteria for a healthy gut**
- **Healthy gut = good digestion, stable mood, controlled blood sugar, lowered risk of obesity**
- **Rich in B vitamins and vitamin K2**
- **Less allergenic than the unfermented food**
- **Help to protect against infection**
- **Inhibit Candida**

SALT

It's time to get over your fear of salt! Our bodies need salt to function—to pass nutrients through cells, regulate blood pressure, maintain balanced blood sugar, and more. And now that you're eating whole foods, the absence of processed foods can mean you're getting less salt than you need. You can and should add salt to your meals—even when I think there's enough salt on my food, I add more. Heck, I even add it to my water, tea, and coffee.

But wait! Not all salt is created equal.

Table Salt

Heavily processed to eliminate most of the good things you need from salt. It's generally bleached and heated and contains calcium silicate to prevent clumping. Avoid it.

Iodized table salt has added iodine, a mineral your body needs. But there are gray sea salts that are rich in iodine and much less processed than table salt.

For every gram of table salt you consume, your body uses 23 times the amount of cell water to neutralize the salt as it would for sea salt, causing excess fluid in your body tissues, which can result in kidney issues, gallstones, arthritis, gout, and cellulite. The lesson? When you buy store-bought products, purchase those with no added sodium and add your own healthy salt. Same goes for eating out at restaurants. Many restaurants can prepare your chosen meal without the use of salt so you can add your own.

Kosher Salt

Slightly less processed than table salt but yields a similar nutrition profile. Many use it instead of sea salt for meats because sea salt has a strong sodium flavor. But overall, the benefits aren't there for this one. I avoid it.

Sea Salt

Harvested directly from evaporated seawater or underground salt mine resources, sea salt is usually minimally processed. Best used after cooking to maintain its unique flavor. My concern with sea salt is that our oceans are getting more and more polluted, so I'm not 100 percent confident in the purity of sea salt. However, it's a much safer and healthier option than table salt.

In my own recipes, including those in this book, I use gray sea salt. It is rich in minerals and contains few impurities.

Himalayan Salt

Packed with minerals often not found in any other form of salt, Himalayan rock salt is known for its light pink color, and it's growing in popularity by the hour. It is over 250 million years old, which means that it's absolutely free from toxins and pollutants.

Himalayan rock salt was my go-to salt until I learned that, due to processing practices, some sources are higher in fluoride than others. We don't want fluoride in our system because it can counteract iodine and suppress the thyroid, slowing down our metabolism and affecting sex hormone balance. However, I haven't been able to find much detail on the fluoride rating of everyday Himalayan rock salt. So I've continued to use Himalayan salt from San Francisco Salt Company in my daily Keto Lemonade (page 422).

Think of Himalayan rock salt as a bioidentical supplement that your body is able to instantly recognize and utilize. That's why it's a main ingredient in the Keto Lemonade!

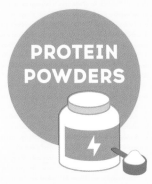

PROTEIN POWDERS

POW! WITH PROTEIN POWDER

If you've embraced the power of balanced protein intake (and if you haven't, please go back and read pages 36 and 37!), it's time to talk about protein powders and their place in the equation.

Protein powder is a valid option when:

- **You need more protein daily than you can possibly eat in salmon, grass-fed beef, and the like.**

- **You feel good on a higher protein amount but can't stomach the cost of buying all grass-fed all the time.**

- **Your digestive functions, such as stomach acid or bile production, are impaired.**

- **You're on the go a lot and having a balanced meal isn't always an option.**

- **You enjoy traveling but know that the food options will leave you yearning for more.**

- **You're looking for a protein option that boosts health overall—a double whammy!**

What I'm not saying here is that you can replace all your protein sources with protein powder. So often, I see people replacing quality foods with subpar protein powders, without thinking of quality, or they rely too heavily on protein powders (high-quality or otherwise) when they would benefit from consuming whole-food sources of protein instead, like good ol' grass-fed beef. Quality is everything, especially when it comes to protein powders. Sure, you could use a chalky powder that provides nothing but protein. Or you could choose a protein powder that not only offers protein but also boasts health with a balance of vitamins, minerals, and essential nutrients. For more on protein powders and the best selection for your needs, head on over to healthfulpursuit.com/proteinpowder, where I've prepared an epic free resource that goes through it all for you.

- **Add to a smoothie or a Keto Milkshake (page 423).**

- **Add to a shaker cup with coconut milk, MCT oil, and alcohol-free stevia.**

- **Stir into cold or hot tea.**

- **Use as a replacement for one-quarter of the flour called for in a recipe.**

- **Add to your next batch of avocado pudding (page 146).**

- **Stir into a batch of fat bombs.**

- **Make a blended "ice cream" treat! Combine ¾ cup (180 ml) of almond milk, 15 ice cubes, 1 scoop of vanilla protein powder, 2 tablespoons of unsweetened cocoa powder, 2 teaspoons of chia seeds, and 1 to 2 drops of alcohol-free stevia. Blend and enjoy.**

- **Use instead of collagen in your next Rocket Fuel Latte (page 428). Just be sure it doesn't exceed 10 grams of protein or it will break your fast!**

If you care about hitting your protein goals, especially in the case of Pumped Keto (page 47), you will probably rely on a protein powder at some point. Instead of aimlessly scavenging the shelves at your local supplement shop, go there equipped with the facts you need to make a solid choice based on your requirements, preferences, and budget with the epic resource I've prepared for you over at healthfulpursuit.com/proteinpowder.

All protein powders fall in the "supplements" category, and therefore the government's regulation of their contents is very limited. Because of that, it's especially important to know where your protein powder is coming from in order to avoid toxic ingredients, like anabolic steroids, mercury, lead, or arsenic. In my book, the labels "grass-fed" and "hormone-free" go a long way toward indicating a quality protein powder, but check out the reputation of the company itself.

Collagen is a protein found in the connective tissues of your body. It's a form of fibrous protein that provides a supportive structure for our body tissues such as our muscles, bones, and ligaments. As we age, we produce less and less collagen, leading to wrinkles and folds in our skin.

Collagen peptides, often referred to as "collagen," can be added to cold or hot beverages and will not gel in cold liquids or alter the texture in any way. Whereas gelatin—which contains collagen—will become gel-like in cold liquids, making it great for hot keto drinks (like Rocket Fuel Lattes, page 428) or made into gummies (like Iced Tea Lemonade Gummies, page 406).

Regardless of what form you choose, each kind is comprised of peptides—short-chain amino acids. These natural peptides are highly bioavailable, digestible, and soluble in cold water. Think: the most powerful, nourishing, digestive-supportive protein powder out there...that has zero taste. The only difference is that the gelatin product "gels" and the collagen-only product doesn't.

Using collagen may encourage:

- **Strong bones and joints. It's a source of proline and glycine, two building blocks of cartilage that are essential for refueling after exercise and sports.**

- **Bright (wrinkle-free) skin. Boosts hydration, prevents deep wrinkles, and maintains the health of skin.**

- **Weight loss. Consists of 97 percent pure, keto-friendly protein, keeping you full and satiated. You can use it as a replacement for protein powder!**

- **Restful sleep, by stimulating growth hormone release.**

My favorite brand of both collagen and gelatin is Vital Proteins.

With minimal amounts of carbohydrates and a blank canvas when it comes to fat, egg protein powder is a low-carber's dream! It's dairy-free as well, making it a prime choice for those who are allergic to whey (see page 127).

Sadly, it can prove challenging to find whole-egg protein powder that has both white and yolk, making it more nutritionally dense. However, egg white protein powder from free-range eggs still has higher amounts of vitamins A, B, D, and E than its conventional counterparts made with eggs from hens who lived their lives in battery cages.

I suppose if someone were to enjoy heaps of egg protein powder every day, she or he could display symptoms of a biotin deficiency—things like hair loss, depression, and complexion issues—because raw egg whites contain a protein that interferes with your body's ability to use biotin. And there are some risks to using factory farm-sourced eggs, such as the potential for salmonella, use of antibiotics, and more. But overall, egg protein is a great source for protein powder.

My favorite egg protein powders are from Paleo Pro and NOW Foods. For more on why they're my top picks, including the health benefits and features compared with other protein powder choices, head to healthfulpursuit.com/proteinpowder.

For the moment, let's skip right over how much protein is in plants and pretend that broccoli actually has more protein than steak. Just because it has more protein doesn't mean that our bodies can use all of it.

There are eight essential amino acids that your body cannot create and therefore needs to get from foods. Most plant sources of protein are relatively low in, or completely lack, those essential amino acids. But let's say that the protein powder you've chosen contains all essential amino acids. The first thing to check is the balance of those amino acids—there should be a table listing them on the label. We want to see leucine, lysine, and tyrosine, followed by isoleucine, cysteine, threonine, and valine. The smallest amount should be tryptophan. If all these are listed in this order, you know that the protein powder is at least providing the amino acids your body needs on a daily basis in the amounts you need. (If you're also eating animal proteins, this isn't such a concern—you'll likely reach your essential amino acid requirements quite easily.)

So your plant-based protein powder has all of the essential amino acids, in a ratio that works well. But sadly, it's still going to have lower bioavailability than other protein powder options like whey, collagen, and egg. That means the body isn't able to actively use every bit of what you're ingesting; some of it goes to waste, and you don't get the full amount that the label indicates.

The following table represents the percentage of the protein in a source that our bodies can put to use (1 = 100 percent).

PROTEIN	PDCAAS*
Eggs	1.00
Casein	1.00
Whey protein	1.00
Soy protein	1.00
Pea protein concentrate	0.89
Vegetables	0.73
Legumes	0.70
Rice	0.50

*protein digestibility corrected amino acid score

That PDCAAS number is a way to measure the bioavailability of protein from a given source. However, it was calculated for the amino acid requirements of children, as they have the highest need for a balance of amino acids. Seniors are less able to extract necessary elements from a protein (due to the changes in gut microbiome, among other things), so they'll get less than the PDCAAS number might indicate.

As you can see from the table, animal-based proteins, except for soy protein, outperform plant-based proteins when it comes to bioavailability. Much of this is because plants contain anti-nutrients, which affect nutrient absorption. (See page 155 for more.) However, soaking nuts and seeds or sprouting or fermenting grains can reduce their antinutrient load, making their protein more bioavailable.

So if you're going to consume a plant-based protein, first make sure it has all the essential amino acids in the right amounts, then look at how the grains, nuts, or seeds are processed. If they're processed without first being soaked, sprouted, or fermented, it may have an impact on the protein bioavailability—and it could do harm to your gut over the long term.

My favorite brand for those that opt-in to plant-based protein powder is Genuine Health fermented vegan proteins+. For more on why you may not see your favorite brand of plant protein powder here, head to **healthfulpursuit.com/ proteinpowder**.

 Whey protein is found in milk, so as someone who's dairy-free with an allergy to casein, lactose, and whey, whey protein powder is totally out of the question for me. (It's whey too much dairy! Sorry, had to do it.) But my husband, who has a lactose allergy, can handle whey isolate just fine. If you can't tolerate dairy products or find that they spike cravings, I'd skip the whey. And because whey can increase insulin and blood glucose, I don't recommend it for those adjusting to the keto diet.

However, if you tolerate dairy well and it feels good in your body, whey protein powders may be great for you. For more details on what protein powder may be right for you, I've prepared a who's who of whey protein and other protein powders at **healthfulpursuit.com/proteinpowders**.

ADJUSTMENTS FOR SPECIAL DIETS

If you're wondering how to adjust the keto diet to meet your needs as it relates to fructose malabsorption, an autoimmune protocol, nightshade intolerance, or a vegan lifestyle, you've come to the right place.

FODMAPs

FODMAP stands for Fermentable Oligosaccharides, Disaccharides, Monosaccharides, and Polyols. In some people, these carbohydrates and sugar alcohols can trigger symptoms of irritable bowel syndrome, including abdominal pain, nausea, diarrhea or constipation, and bloating. Some of the keto foods/carb-up foods that contain FODMAPs are: garlic, onions, asparagus, cauliflower, celery, seaweed, mushrooms, shallots, avocados, processed meats, pickles, sweeteners (see page 118), carb-up sweeteners (maple syrup, honey), tahini, flax seeds, chia seeds, and almond milk.

Any of the five Fat Fueled Profiles outlined on pages 47 to 49 can be used alongside your avoidance of FODMAP-rich foods. All you have to do is plug the low-FODMAP foods into your Daily Portion Plate (see page 61) and you're good to go. Think greens, meats, and fats three times per day. If you're looking for a dependable FODMAP resource, I enjoy the information shared on ibsdiets.org.

AIP

The Autoimmune Protocol was developed by Dr. Loren Cordain and Robb Wolf, and it outlines that certain foods have the propensity to trigger inflammation in people with autoimmune conditions. These foods include dairy, eggs, nightshades, nuts, and seeds. The keto diet is quite AIP-friendly with a couple of exceptions.

Eggs
In recipes that call for eggs, like cookies, cakes, or baked goods, try using a gelatin egg (equal to one egg). To prepare a gelatin egg, place ¼ cup (60 ml) water in a small saucepan. Sprinkle 1 tablespoon of gelatin over the entire surface of the water. Let the saucepan sit untouched for 5 minutes. After 5 minutes, turn the burner on low and whisk for 1 minute, or until the texture is smooth. Use the mixture in the cake, batch of cookies, or baked good that you're making. If it's a dish that is served with an egg, simply omit the egg. For egg-free mayonnaise, go to page 220.

Nuts and Seeds
Coconut in various forms is a great replacement for nuts and seeds in recipes. Be careful of recipes that are entirely flax-based!

Nightshades
Check the suggestions on the next page.

Fructose
If practicing carb-ups, limit intake to no more than 20 grams of fructose (the sugar found in fruit) a day.

Sweeteners
You may have issues with the sweeteners used in the recipes in this book and in any keto diet: xylitol, erythritol, and stevia. If you're already eating AIP-friendly, you probably have a pretty good handle on using light sweeteners, if any. So the sugar-free portion of going keto may be a breeze!

Nightshades

Nightshades are a family of plants, the vast majority of which are inedible or poisonous, but many of which are common vegetables. Of the keto/carb-up ones we eat or supplement with, there's ashwagana, bell peppers, bush tomato, eggplant, hot peppers, paprika, pepinos, pimentos, potatoes, tamarillos, tomatillos, and tomatoes. For some, consuming these items can cause excess inflammation in the body. Here are a couple of substitution strategies:

Bell Peppers
You could omit them and add a handful of kale at the end of cooking. If you're making a stuffed vegetable dish and bell peppers are the star of the show, try substituting a hollowed-out zucchini.

Eggplant
Zucchini is the perfect replacement. It slices thin just like eggplant and holds up similarly in many recipes.

Hot Peppers
These include cayenne pepper, paprika, and other spices made from dried peppers. For spices, I omit those listed and replace them with cumin, turmeric, and/or oregano. For hot sauce in recipes, horseradish is a good alternative.

Potatoes
Radishes work beautifully as replacements for roasted potatoes. Mashed cauliflower works as mashed potatoes, and potato salad is fabulous when made with rutabaga instead.

Tomatoes

There's no perfect substitute for tomatoes, so I've found that it's best at first to look for recipes that don't have tomatoes in them, so you're not eating your salsa sans tomato and thinking, "This really sucks." Once you're accustomed to not eating tomatoes, you can go back to a recipe that calls for it and omit it without feeling like you're missing out. I simply omit tomatoes from sauces and stews and go for more vegetables and more bone stock. For curries, I use coconut milk as the base instead.

Vegan

I was vegan for a very long time, and it didn't do my body any good. (The story of why I stopped is on my website, healthfulpursuit.com/stoppedvegan.) Given my experience and what I've seen in my nutrition practice, I think there are bodies that respond well to the vegan lifestyle and bodies that don't. Mine is one that doesn't.

It is possible, though not always easy, to stay vegan on the keto diet. The key to success with transitioning to being a keto vegan, I've found, is in understanding and coming to terms with what is best for your body. If you're truly "supposed" to be vegan, your carb tolerance will be a lot higher than most, meaning you can eat more carbohydrates than most people and slide into ketosis quite effortlessly.

If you're carbohydrate sensitive, as I am, eating a relatively high amount of carbohydrates (high for a ketogenic diet) while trying to get into ketosis may be next to impossible. And being vegan may not be the best option for you, period. (I feel like I have a right to say that because I was vegan for so long and I totally understand how frustrating, challenging, and scary it is to admit that the vegan lifestyle isn't right for you.)

But let's assume that you've never felt better as a vegan, and you want to give keto a whirl as one. Here are some steps to help you adjust:

1. **Get friendly with low-carb vegetables (see page 116).**
2. **Get to know your fats.** *Just about everything is game for you, minus the animal fats.*
3. **Source your low-carb proteins.** *Keto is not a high-protein approach, so keto-friendly foods like almonds, non-GMO soy, broccoli, asparagus, garlic, turnip greens, spinach, tomatoes, chickpeas, lentils, navy beans, and black beans may work well for you.*
4. **Give up the grains.** *Quinoa, a pseudo-grain, is often great on keto—it's more like a seed than a grain—but if you're sensitive to grains, you may find that you're also sensitive to quinoa. Amaranth is a great keto option, too.*
5. **Ditch the packaged food.** *Bread, corn chips, potato chips, protein bars, pretzels, crackers, pasta, baked goods, and popcorn are to be avoided. Instead, make a couple of batches of focaccia (page 372) and Italian Zucchini Rounds (page 250) to snack on.*
6. **Bake with hemp protein or pumpkin seed protein.** *Both are nearly net-neutral in the carbohydrate department, meaning that they have just as much fiber as they do carbohydrate. (See page 62 for more on net versus total carbs.)*

I never really had weight or body image issues growing up. I ate whatever I wanted, whenever I wanted, and I loved food. I didn't have a very active lifestyle—never played sports or anything like that—but my senior year of high school I got really into weightlifting. I had a half-day in school and started eating out a lot (lots of fast food), so I started gaining weight. That's when I started going to the gym, and the weight came off no problem. Actually, it would be more accurate to say the fat came off no problem—I gained a bunch of muscle, so the scale went up, but my body fat went down to 18 percent, and I loved it.

When I went to college I kept this lifestyle and it worked, but in my second year, I was put on Adderall. In the year and a half I was on the medication my weight dropped from 150 to 115 lbs.

I only ate one meal a week.

I only slept once a week.

I smoked a pack of cigarettes every five hours.

I knew this wasn't healthy, but I loved the feeling of being unstoppable while I was on the medication.

What I didn't love was that I was weak, to the point that I couldn't walk from my class to my car without throwing up. For a girl who was once strong, this was unacceptable. So I stopped taking the medication.

During the first 26 days I was off the medication, I gained 23 lbs. This was in 2008. Today, I weigh 209 lbs, the heaviest I've ever been. My body has never recovered from that period of time.

I tried keto for the first time this past fall at the recommendation of a friend (a male friend, who had great results) and I lost about six pounds in the first week. But then life happened and I fell back to my old eating habits.

I decided to get back into a ketogenic way of eating and found Leanne's blog, HealthfulPursuit. com. Since then, I've looked at losing weight in a whole new light. I did terrible, terrible damage to my body when I was on that medication. And I think I still need to heal from that and that it might take a considerable amount of time.

So I put my scale into storage and I started a food journal. As a child, I loved eating the fat off steak, so I feel like, in a way, I was always meant to eat like this. And I feel great. I have more energy, I fast naturally, and I sleep better if I have a little carb-up before bed (which Leanne taught me is totally okay and actually nourishing for my body). My relationship with my food is now more mindful, and I have Leanne to thank for that—not only has she provided the keto community with incredible resources, but the support system she's created with the HealthfulPursuit.com readers is unmatched.

I've read The Keto Beginning and I'm working through Fat Fueled now. I listen to her podcast so much that I'm picking up a Canadian accent…not even kidding.

Thank you, Leanne, for your work, for having the strength to endure your own personal struggle, and for being generous enough to share it as well as your time with the rest of us.

Erica
West Virginia

CHAPTER 7

FATS TO LOVE, FATS TO HATE, FATS TO RUN AWAY FROM

It's no secret that you're going to be eating a lot of fat, so it only makes sense to truly understand what's behind the goods—the keywords to watch for, the ones to avoid, the marketing gimmicks, all of it.

Many companies use flashy words to grab our attention, which makes us think that their product is better than it actually is. Case in point: olive oil. Did you know that there was a time when 70 percent of extra-virgin olive oil sold was cut with cheaper oils? Although the space has improved in the last couple of years, many olive oils could still contain canola oil or various other oils that aren't olive. After other oils are added, the concoction is chemically deodorized, colored, and sometimes even flavored—and sold as "extra-virgin" oil. Yikes!

One of the things that make a fat or oil safe or unsafe is whether it's become rancid, or oxidized. When a fatty substance has been exposed to more heat, oxygen, or light than it can withstand, it goes rancid. And once rancid, these fats may have an effect on our overall health by increasing inflammation. Oxidization can occur in the processing of a fat or oil: if it's overprocessed using methods that go beyond what it can handle or methods that are not safe for the oil, or if it's not stored properly.

Let's make solid, educated decisions for ourselves. Knowledge is power, so let's get started.

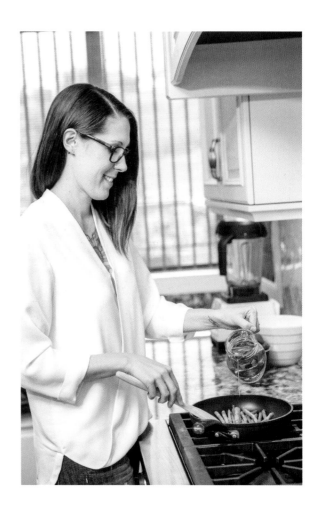

SATURATED FATS

CONSUME OFTEN. Saturated fats are stable, solid at room temperature, and great for cooking. They've gotten a bad rap over the years, but they're actually awesome for our health. They're great for the heart, liver, brain, nervous system, and more—check out the list of health benefits on page 134.

The common fear that saturated fat raises cholesterol is completely unfounded. In fact, focusing on a carbohydrate-rich diet rather than a saturated-fat-rich diet increases the risk of coronary heart disease by lowering HDL cholesterol and increasing small-particle LDL (see pages 31 to 33 for more on cholesterol). In other words, it's not saturated fat or dietary cholesterol that increases the amount of small, dense LDL cholesterol in our bodies—it's an overconsumption of carbohydrates. And despite the popularity of low-fat diets, the increase in the prevalence of diabetes and obesity in the U.S. occurred with an increase in the consumption of carbohydrates, not saturated fat.

EXAMPLES OF SATURATED FATS:

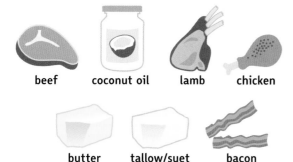

| beef | coconut oil | lamb | chicken |

| butter | tallow/suet | bacon |

MONOUNSATURATED FATS (MUFAs)

CONSUME OFTEN. Typically liquid at room temperature and solid when chilled, monounsaturated fats are moderately stable and good for light cooking, between 320°F (160°C) and 350°F (177°C). As long as the oils you're consuming are minimally processed—look for keywords like "cold-pressed," "centrifuge-extracted," and "expeller-pressed"—there's little chance of consuming oxidized fats, which can cause cell damage.

Monounsaturated fats offer several health benefits, especially when they're used instead of trans fats—check out the list on page 134.

> Conventional grain-fed meats are higher in omega-6 and lower in omega-3 than grass-fed meats. Can't access grass-fed meats? Go for the leaner varieties and add your own healthy fats.

EXAMPLES OF MONOUNSATURATED FATS:

 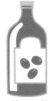

| avocado oil | olive oil | almond oil |

| macadamia nuts | avocados | hazelnuts |

POLYUNSATURATED FATS (PUFAs)

USE SPARINGLY. Polyunsaturated fats are always liquid. They're more likely to become oxidized during heating, so they're not good for cooking unless they are naturally refined and bear a label defining that they are "cold-pressed," "centrifuge-extracted," or "expeller-pressed." Seek out minimally processed or naturally refined oils, which are less likely to be oxidized.

Foods containing these oils, such as salmon, trout, hemp seeds, chia seeds, and flax seeds, should be minimally heated, just until cooked.

Two polyunsaturated fats, omega-3 and omega-6, are considered essential fatty acids: the body cannot produce them, yet they're required for normal body functions, so they must be obtained through food (or supplements). Consuming an unbalanced ratio of omega-3 to omega-6—in the standard American diet, that means too much omega-6—is associated with an increase in inflammatory diseases such as metabolic syndrome, autoimmune disorders, irritable bowel syndrome, inflammatory bowel disease, rheumatoid arthritis, cancer, and psychiatric disorders. The ideal ratio of omega-6 to omega-3 is 1:1; the typical ratio in the standard American diet is between 10:1 and 25:1. A ketogenic diet that's high in saturated fat and low in processed oils is naturally balanced in omega-3 and omega-6.

Soybean oil and corn oil are two of the top "heart-healthy" polyunsaturated oils recommended by health-care organizations, but their ratios of omega-6 to omega-3 are 7:1 and 46:1, respectively. And the processing of these fats causes them to become oxidized, contributing to free-radical formation and inflammation. Safer polyunsaturated fats are hemp seed oil, walnut oil, flaxseed oil, and canola oil, assuming that they are minimally processed and cold pressed. These oils should not be heated.

Plant-based omega-3s are more difficult for the body to convert to the forms it can use, EPA and DHA, so it's better to go with animal-based forms, such as fish. EPA and DHA are essential for fetal development, regulated immune response, reduction in inflammation, and improved cardiovascular function.

TRANS FATS

AVOID Trans fats are found primarily in man-made fats, particularly those that are hydrogenated or partially hydrogenated. If you see the words "trans fat" on a box, bottle, or bag, drop it and walk in the opposite direction.

Naturally occurring trans fats are found in small amounts in dairy products and meat from grass-fed animals, and these trans fats actually are beneficial: they can reduce body fat, increase muscle mass, and potentially curtail the formation of breast cancer.

Man-made trans fats are created when hydrogen is added to vegetable oils to make them solid at room temperature. The body doesn't recognize these hydrogenated, fully transformed fats and doesn't know how to eliminate them from cells. They're harmful for health in many ways, from contributing to heart disease to increasing the risk of type 2 diabetes—see the full list on page 134.

The recognized dangers of trans fats has led to their elimination from many consumer goods. Interesterified fat, which is created through an oil refinement process that chemically alters and molecularly rearranges fats, has gained popularity in its place. But this fat promises to raise blood glucose and depress insulin production.

Avoid scary fats by opting for fresh ingredients instead of donuts, cookies, buttery spreads, store-bought salad dressings, and conventional mayonnaise.

FATS EXPLAINED

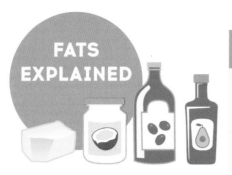

MONOUNSATURATED FAT (MUFA)

Seek out minimally processed oils that are less likely to have oxidized fats. Consume often.

HEALTH EFFECTS

CAUTION REQUIRED ⚠

- Encourages weight loss when used in place of trans fats and rancid polyunsaturated fats
- Reduces pain and stiffness from rheumatoid arthritis
- Decreases risk of breast cancer
- Lowers risk of heart disease and stroke
- Reduces belly fat when carbs are reduced and fats are added in their place
- Improves blood sugar control

CASE AGAINST/FOR

➕ More stable than polyunsaturated fats

➕ Safe to heat when naturally contain saturated fats

POLYUNSATURATED FAT (PUFA)

Seek out minimally processed oils that are less likely to have oxidized fats. Consume occasionally.

HEALTH EFFECTS

CAUTION REQUIRED ⚠

- Omega-3s improve bone strength and reduce the production of inflammatory substances.
- Omega-6s are essential for brain and muscle development, support the nervous system, and contribute to the production of hormone-like messengers that impact mood, the immune system, and fluid balance.
- A 1:1 ratio of omega-6 to omega-3 is beneficial against inflammatory diseases, but too much omega-6 is associated with inflammatory diseases, from autoimmune disorders to cancer.

CASE AGAINST/FOR

➕ Balance of omega-6 to omega-3 is essential for health

➖ Some polyunsaturated fats, like soybean oil and corn oil, have unhealthy ratios of omega-6 to omega-3

➖ More prone to oxidization when highly processed

➖ Heating causes oxidization, so not good for cooking

CASE AGAINST/FOR

➖ Extremely damaging to health

(Does not apply to naturally occurring trans fats such as those found in a grass-fed/finished steak)

SATURATED FAT

Two thumbs up. Consume regularly.

USE LIBERALLY 👍

HEALTH EFFECTS

- Is the preferred fuel for your heart
- Increases HDL cholesterol see page 32
- Increases uptake of calcium so it can be effectively incorporated into bone
- Protects the liver from toxins and free radical damage
- Reverses inflammatory changes brought on by alcohol abuse
- Coats the spaces in our lungs to protect us from getting sick
- Provides the brain with the raw materials it needs to function optimally
- Boosts metabolism by improving nerve signaling throughout the body
- Provider of and carrier for fat-soluble vitamins A, D, E, and K
- Strengthens the immune system by boosting cells' ability to destroy viruses, bacteria, and fungi

CASE AGAINST/FOR:

➕ Doesn't raise cholesterol or increase risk of heart disease

➕ Doesn't make you fat

➕ Stable fat that isn't easily oxidized (which can cause cell damage)

TRANS FAT

All bad things. Never consume.

HEALTH EFFECTS

- Increases risk of type 2 diabetes
- Causes a redistribution of fat tissue into the abdomen, which is associated with an increased risk of heart disease
- Sparks insulin resistance
- Contributes to the occurrence of coronary heart disease
- Associated with systemic inflammation, which can affect many bodily processes, including digestion
- Damages memory
- May cause asthma in children

AVOID ☠

PRACTICAL OIL GUIDE

Since I started my ketogenic journey, I've stuck primarily to tallow for cooking and avocado oil for salads. Nothing much else needed! I'm a one-trick pony; simple is the way I roll. But then I went out for coffee with a girlfriend and she started asking me about oils and their PUFA content, and I realized that if she was asking, perhaps some of you would, too.

I know I can't be the only one who sticks to her favorite oils. But what if your go-to oil makes you prone to inflammation brought on by an onslaught of free radical damage? If your fat consumption rises to ketogenic levels and the fat you're consuming is poor quality, you're in for a not-so-fun ride.

I've tried to present as many relevant data points as possible so that you can make informed decisions for yourself. And what you decide may differ from what the person next door decides. I hope that this information will make it easier for you to pinpoint the qualities you're looking for. And I've given feedback and guidelines based on my personal opinions, what I choose to consume, and why.

Components That Make Up a Good Cooking Oil

There are three things to watch for when it comes to oils. Think of them as the pillars of oil quality:

- EXTRACTION AND PROCESSING METHOD: *The method used to extract the oil can affect whether the oil supports or damages our health. Was it extracted with chemicals? If toxic chemical solvents such as hexane are involved, trace amounts of chemical residue are left in the final product. Was it extracted with high heat? If so, was the source of the oil meant to withstand those temperatures? If not, the oil can become oxidized and is likely refined further to remove the smell of rancidity. See page 137 for more information on extraction and processing methods.*

- RATIO OF OMEGA-6 TO OMEGA-3: *The balance of omega-6 to omega-3 is important for overall health and wellness (see page 133 for more). We want a ratio as close to 1:1 as possible. If an oil is too high in omega-6 and too low in omega-3, it can spark an onslaught of inflammation. Note: This applies only to oils high in PUFA to begin with. If an oil has an imbalanced ratio of omega-6 to omega-3 but has only 10 percent PUFA, it's not as big a deal as an oil that contains, say, 50 percent PUFA. See page 138 for a ranking of omega-6 to omega-3 ratios in various oils.*

- SMOKE POINT: *Defines an oil's ability to withstand heat while remaining stable. If you're baking a cake at 350°F (177°C) and use an unstable oil such as walnut oil, the baking process is going to oxidize the fat, and the oil will go rancid right there in the cake. You'll be left with one yucky-tasting cake at the end. But that same oil will thrive when used in a raw nut or seed pâté. See page 138 for a ranking of the smoke points of various oils.*

Here are a few other things to consider when choosing a cooking oil:

- **Check the expiration date and choose an oil that's close to harvest date or at least six months from expiration.**

- **Oil deteriorates faster in a clear bottle. While plastic bottles protect from light, there is concern that the plastic may dissolve into the oil over time. It's best to choose oils in dark glass containers.**

- **Your pots and pans can make a difference! Metals like iron and copper can encourage oxidation, speeding up rancidity.**

Smoke Point
Like extraction and processing methods, smoke point defines the line between a health-promoting oil and a health-destructing oil. The less processed an oil is, the higher the nutrient content, and therefore the less likely it is to want to play with high heat.

The more saturated fats and monounsaturated fats an oil contains, the more stable it is. Conversely, the more polyunsaturated fats an oil contains, the more unstable it is at high temperatures—it's prone to oxidation, which encourages inflammation.

When heated past its smoke point, fat begins to break down and release free radicals, harmful compounds that damage cells, and acrolein, the chemical that gives foods a scorched aroma and flavor. If the oil smokes in the pan, discard it, clean the pan, and start over at a lower temperature. While those pancakes may look really good, when the oil is smoking it has become damaged, and potentially cancer-causing properties have formed.

The chart on the opposite page focuses on unrefined oils unless otherwise noted. Refined oils are lower in nutrients, so it's best to limit your consumption, but they're great for occasional cooking and baking when you need a heat-stable fat and a bit of variety.

> If you are sensitive to dairy, ghee and butter may not be the best choices for you. Ghee is naturally whey-free, but depending on how it is processed, most ghee contains varying amounts of casein and lactose. If you're looking for a high-quality ghee, Tin Star Foods tests each batch to ensure that it's extremely low in casein and lactose. Fourth & Heart brand ghee is fabulous, too.

> If you're wary of your oils, give them a sniff. If they smell a bit off, don't use them!

Canola Oil

I know what many of you are thinking: *Wait, what? Did she just put canola oil on the list of safe cooking oils? No way is this woman sane.*

I know. It blew me away, too. But with the right selection, canola oil is safer than many other oils out there. The omega-6 to omega-3 ratio of canola oil is on point—the distribution of SFAs to MUFAs and PUFAs is fabulous, and you can source cold-pressed versions, no problem. So the standard checks are in place.

So why did canola oil get a bad reputation? It's generally assumed that all canola oil is refined, solvent-extracted, and processed to the nth degree. In addition, there's a ton of genetically modified canola oil on the market today—about 90 percent of the world's canola crop is genetically modified.

But let's say we could get a non-GMO, organic, cold-pressed, and unrefined or chemical-free/low-heat-refined canola oil, which we can. What then? Keeping in mind what makes a good cooking oil (see page 135), let's take a look at how canola stacks up to other oils.

Both flaxseed oil and hemp seed oil are touted as health-promoting oils for the very components that canola oil contains, and in many cases canola oil does it better. The PUFA content of unrefined canola oil is 32 percent, hemp seed oil is 80 percent, and flaxseed oil is 66 percent. From this information, we can draw the conclusion that canola oil is naturally more stable than hemp or flax. I'll put that in the "win" column. Looking now to the omega-6 to omega-3 ratio, canola sits at 2:1, hemp seed at 3:1, and flaxseed at 4:1. We know that the closer the ratio is to 1:1, the better off we'll be. Again, "win" column.

I'd say canola oil is doing pretty well for itself. But let's dig a little deeper into its past to understand what went wrong and how we can find a good source of the stuff.

Canola was bred from rapeseed, which thirty years ago contained elevated levels of erucic acid, a monounsaturated omega-9 fatty acid considered harmful to humans. Canola has been bred over the years to have less erucic acid; today's canola oil contains less than 2 percent. (Note that breeding plant varieties for certain qualities is very different from genetically modifying it—the former has been done for thousands of years, while genetic modification is a very recent development.)

Yes, a lot of canola oil is produced from genetically modified rapeseed. But there are non-GMO brands out there. A representative from the Non-GMO Project writes:

> If a product has our Non-GMO Project Verified seal, you can be sure that it was produced using industry best standards for GMO avoidance.
>
> We offer non-GMO verification for canola oil produced from rapeseed that has not been genetically modified. Natural cross-breeding techniques that have been used by farmers for thousands of years are not considered genetic engineering under our Standard.

Is the ultra-refined, heat-processed, chemically extracted, genetically modified canola oil bad? You bet it is. Do I plan on drowning myself in non-GMO, organic, cold-pressed, unrefined, or chemical-free/low-heat refined canola oil? No. Just like I don't plan to do the same with hemp seed, walnut, and flaxseed oils anytime soon because of their PUFA content (more on page 133).

But I won't go around shaming canola oil anymore. If you look for the same markers of quality used to evaluate any high-PUFA oil, it's just as good.

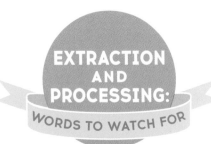

EXTRACTION AND PROCESSING: WORDS TO WATCH FOR

INGREDIENT QUALITY

★ = recommended

NON-ORGANIC:		ORGANIC:		NON-GMO:		GRASS-FED:		FREE-RANGE:
Pesticides and other environmental toxins used in growing the source ingredient are concentrated in the oil.	vs	No pesticides or chemical fertilizers are used.	vs	No genetically modified crops are used to make the oil. Important to watch for in canola oil, corn oil, cottonseed oil, salmon oil, and soy oil.	vs	Grass-fed animal-based fats are higher in nutrients than their grain-fed counterparts. (See page 110 for details.) Applies to tallow/suet, butter, and ghee.	vs	Free-range animal-based fats are higher in nutrients than their "cage-free" counterparts. (See page 110 for details.) Applies to chicken fat, duck fat, and goose fat.

EXTRACTION METHOD

EXPELLER-PRESSED:		COLD-PRESSED:		CENTRIFUGE-EXTRACTED:		SOLVENT: ☠
Squeezed or milled without external heat or chemicals. Much flavor and nutrients are kept intact, but there is a risk of oxidation due to heat from friction.	vs	Expeller-pressed in a temperature-controlled setting; product never rises above 120°F (49°C). Flavors and nutrients are kept intact and there is minimal oxidation.	vs	Pressed, then separated through centrifugal force. Flavors and nutrients are kept intact; considered raw, and no oxidation takes place.	vs	Heated to 500°F (260°C) and treated with hexane, a chemical solvent, then treated again to remove the solvent. Minimal taste and very few nutrients; may be rancid due to high heat. Shelf life of three to four years. If you don't see "expeller-pressed," "cold-pressed," or "centrifuge-extracted" on the label, you can just about bet that it's solvent-extracted.

❗ CAUTION when used on highly unstable fats

PRESSING (refers to part of the extraction method for coconut oil, olive oil, or avocado oil)

VIRGIN:		EXTRA-VIRGIN:
Unrefined and mechanically extracted. In the case of olive oil, more acidity than extra-virgin but less than 2 percent.	vs	Unrefined, mechanically extracted. In the case of olive oil, contains no more than 0.8 percent acidity and means the same thing as "first cold pressed."

There aren't any studies that prove GMO crops are bad for consumption, but there aren't any that prove they're safe, either.

PROCESSING*

CHEMICALLY PROCESSED ☠

UNREFINED:		REFINED:
Immediately bottled after being expeller-pressed, cold-pressed, or centrifuge-extracted, with no additional steps. Milky appearance and superior in taste, quality, and nutrient density. Shorter shelf life and lower smoke point than refined oils.	vs	Look for oils that are naturally refined with low temperature and natural agents. They lack nutrients but are fun to cook with at times. Usually treated with chemicals and heated to over 500°F (260°C), but naturally refined oils use low temperature and natural agents such as citric acid. Bleached or deodorized after extraction to remove impurities, making them more stable, especially for higher-temperature cooking. Clear in appearance; reduced flavor and nutrients. "Pure" indicates a mix of refined and unrefined oils; "light" indicates refined oil with a light taste.

You're better off using naturally heat-stable fats that are high in nutrients for high-heat cooking and reserving refined (chemically or not) oils for special occasions. You'll be eating lots of fat with keto, so it's nice to have a variety!

*Although the terms refined and unrefined are standard, not all terms are. A product might be labeled "extra-virgin" because it has been processed with minimal extraction, whether mechanically or chemically pressed. Unsure of what process is behind an oil? Call the company and ask!

OMEGA AND SMOKE POINT: Rank Them Oils

These oils are organized by their smoke point and PUFA content, which dictate where they sit on the chart. The higher the oil on the chart, the better it is for cooking.

INGREDIENT QUALITY:
Organic = 🌿
Non-GMO = GMO
Grass-fed = ⋙
Free-range = FREE
Ethical standards = ✓***
Pasture-raised = ▬

EXTRACTION:
Cold pressed = ❄
Centrifuge extracted = ⟲
Expeller pressed = 💧

PRESSING:
Extra-virgin = EV
Virgin = V

PROCESSING:
Unrefined = Ø
Naturally refined = R

AWESOME—USE REGULARLY 👍

Name	Smoke Point	Cooking Method	Storage	Omega-6 to -3 ratio	SFA %	MUFA %	PUFA %	Look For...
Avocado oil, refined	520°F (271°C)	Baking/ Roasting and Frying	6–12 months | Dark bottle | Cool place out of direct sunlight	N/A*	20	70	10	🌿 ❄ or ⟲ EV or V | R
Olive oil, refined	465°F (240°C)	Baking/ Roasting and Frying	6–12 months | Dark bottle | Cool place out of direct sunlight	N/A*	14	74	8	💧 | R *referred to as "light" or "pure"*
Ghee*	450°F (232°C)	Baking/ Roasting and Frying	12–24 months | Unrefrigerated | Extend life by storing excess in the freezer	N/A*	51	23	3	⋙
Palm kernel oil	450°F (232°C)	Baking/ Roasting and Frying	12–24 months | Unrefrigerated | Extend life by storing excess in the freezer	N/A*	82	11	1	🌿 ✓ | ❄ or ⟲ or 💧 Ø or R
Red palm oil	450°F (232°C)	Baking/ Roasting and Frying	12–24 months | Unrefrigerated or on the counter | Extend life by storing excess in the freezer	N/A*	49	37	9	🌿 ✓ | ❄ or ⟲ or 💧 Ø or R
Hazelnut oil	430°F (221°C)	Baking/ Roasting and Frying	6–12 months | Dark bottle | Cool place out of direct sunlight	N/A*	7	78	10	🌿 | ❄ or ⟲ or 💧 | R
Tallow/Suet	400°F (205°C)	Baking/ Roasting and Frying	12–24 months | Unrefrigerated | Extend life by storing excess in the freezer	N/A*	50	42	4	⋙
Macadamia nut oil	390°F (198°C)	Baking/ Roasting and Frying	6–12 months | Dark bottle | Cool place out of direct sunlight	N/A*	12	71	12	🌿 | ❄ or ⟲ or 💧 | R
Chicken fat (schmaltz)	375°F (190°C)	Baking/ Roasting and Frying	12–24 months | Unrefrigerated | Extend life by storing excess in the freezer	N/A*	32	46	22	FREE or ▬
Duck fat	375°F (190°C)	Baking/ Roasting and Frying	12–24 months | Unrefrigerated | Extend life by storing excess in the freezer	N/A*	37	50	13	FREE or ▬
Goose fat	375°F (190°C)	Baking/ Roasting and Frying	12–24 months | Unrefrigerated | Extend life by storing excess in the freezer	N/A*	32	55	10	FREE or ▬
Cacao butter/oil	370°F (188°C)	Baking	12–24 months | Unrefrigerated | Extend life by storing excess in the freezer	N/A*	60	33	3	🌿 | Ø or R
Lard/ Bacon grease	370°F (188°C)	Baking	12–24 months | Unrefrigerated | Extend life by storing excess in the freezer	N/A*	39	45	11	FREE or ▬
Butter*	350°F (177°C)	Baking	12–24 months | Unrefrigerated | Extend life by storing excess in the freezer	N/A*	51	23	3	⋙
Coconut oil	350°F (177°C)	Baking	12–24 months | Unrefrigerated | Extend life by storing excess in the freezer	N/A*	87	6	2	🌿 | ❄ or ⟲ or 💧 EV or V | Ø or R
Avocado oil	350°F (177°C)	Salads/ Baking	6–12 months | Dark bottle | Cool place out of direct sunlight	N/A*	20	70	10	🌿 | ❄ or ⟲ EV or V | Ø

Name	Smoke Point	Cooking Method	Storage	Omega-6 to -3 ratio	SFA %	MUFA %	PUFA %	Look For...
Olive oil, virgin	320°F (160°C)	Salads/Light Finishing	6-12 months | Dark bottle | Cool place out of direct sunlight	N/A*	14	74	8	🌿 | ❄ | EV | Ø
Olive oil, extra-virgin	320°F (160°C)	Salads/Light Finishing	6-12 months | Dark bottle | Cool place out of direct sunlight	N/A*	14	74	8	🌿 | ❄ | EV | Ø
Almond oil	320°F (160°C)	Salads/Light Finishing	6-12 months | Dark bottle | Cool place out of direct sunlight	N/A*	8	70	17	🌿 | ❄ | Ø
MCT oil	320°F (160°C)	Salads/Light Finishing	6-12 months | Dark bottle | Cool place out of direct sunlight	N/A*	97	0	0	See page 140 for a guide to MCT oil.

see note on PUFA, page 140

CAUTION— CHOOSE TOP-QUALITY AND USE SPARINGLY ⚠

Name	Smoke Point	Cooking Method	Storage	Omega-6 to -3 ratio	SFA %	MUFA %	PUFA %	Look For...
Canola oil, refined	400°F (205°C)	Baking/ Roasting and Frying	2-6 months | Dark bottle | In the fridge	3:1	7	56	32	🌿 GMO ❄ or ⊙ | R
Hemp seed oil	330°F (165°C)	Salads/Light Finishing	2-6 months | Dark bottle | In the fridge	3:1	8	12	80	🌿 | ❄ | Ø
Walnut oil	320°F (160°C)	Salads/Light Finishing	2-6 months | Dark bottle | In the fridge	5:1	9	23	63	🌿 | ❄ | Ø
Canola oil (see page 136)	225°F (108°C)	Salads	2-6 months | Dark bottle | In the fridge	2:1	7	56	32	🌿 GMO | ❄ | Ø
Flaxseed oil	225°F (108°C)	Salads	2-6 months | Dark bottle | In the fridge	4:1	9	20	66	🌿 GMO | ❄ | Ø

AVOID ☠

Name	Omega-6 to -3 ratio	SFA %	MUFA %	PUFA %	Concern/Comment
Soybean oil	8:1	14	23	58	Safer than most if non-GMO and not heat- or chemical-processed. Not Fat Fueled approved because sourced from a legume.
Rice bran oil	21:1	25	38	37	High omega-6 to omega-3 ratio. Not Fat Fueled approved because sourced from a grain.
Wheat germ oil	8:1	19	15	62	Safer than most if not heat- or chemical-processed. Not Fat Fueled approved because sourced from a grain.
Peanut oil	32:1	17	46	32	Safer than most. Not Fat Fueled approved because sourced from a legume.
Sesame oil	138:1	14	40	42	High omega-6 to omega-3 ratio. PUFA a concern. Can be used sparingly as a drizzle on once-in-a-while recipes.
Corn oil, unrefined	83:1	13	24	59	High omega-6 to omega-3 ratio. Highly GMO. PUFA a concern. Not Fat Fueled approved because sourced from a grain.
Grapeseed oil	676:1	10	16	70	High omega-6 to omega-3 ratio. PUFA a concern.
Corn oil	46:1	13	24	59	High omega-6 to omega-3 ratio. PUFA a concern. Highly GMO. Not Fat Fueled approved because sourced from a grain.
Sunflower oil, unrefined	40:1	10	45	40	High omega-6 to omega-3 ratio. PUFA a concern.
Cottonseed oil	256:1	26	18	52	High omega-6 to omega-3 ratio. PUFA a concern. Highly GMO.
Safflower oil, unrefined	133:1	9	12	75	High omega-6 to omega-3 ratio. PUFA a concern.
Vegetable shortening	8:1	18	44	34	Quality of ingredients and processing methods scare me.**
Margarine, soft	3:1	20	47	33	Quality of ingredients and processing methods scare me.**
Vegan spreads	3:1	20	47	33	Quality of ingredients and processing methods scare me.**

*Minimal amount of PUFAs, so omega-6 to omega-3 ratio is not a concern

**Although the omega-6 to omega-3 ratio is good, the way in which it's processed, additional ingredients such as "buttermilk powder 1 percent" or "natural flavors," and dearth of non-GMO options put it on my avoid list.

***Palm fruit oil and palm kernel oil are a bit controversial because their production may cause deforestation and endanger orangutan populations. Look for sustainably sourced palm oil products.

EVERYTHING MCT OIL

MCT stands for "medium-chain triglyceride." MCTs are great on a keto diet because they are converted to ketones quicker than other saturated fats.

MCTs offer several health benefits:

- Encourage ketone body development
- Improve blood sugar regulation
- Improve cognition and memory
- Reduce cravings
- Help prevent the development of metabolic syndrome
- Encourage weight loss
- Improve gut health and absorption of nutrients

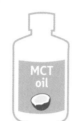

HIGH-PUFA OILS **CANOLA, HEMP SEED, WALNUT, AND FLAXSEED OILS**

While their ratio of omega-6 to omega-3 is pretty good, canola, hemp seed, walnut, and flaxseed oils contain a high amount of PUFAs. And while omega fatty acids are good for overall health (see page 133), an excess of PUFAs is just that: an excess. This is why they've been listed in the caution section—not because they're bad, but because they're not as essential as highly saturated fat, which can be consumed on a regular basis.

In all, it's about incorporating PUFAs in a small way, not a substantial way. Add a little here and there throughout the week, but allow MUFAs and SFAs to take center stage.

Also, the processing of these oils is very important, especially when they contain 50 percent PUFAs or higher, because oxidation begins the moment the components are extracted and exposed to heat, air, or light. Even if the oil is cold pressed, standard processing exposes it to air and light. Please, be sure you know your oil source and the processing it underwent. This is your best bet for reducing your consumption of unstable and rancid fats.

There are several kinds of MCTs. In a highly saturated fat like coconut oil, you're going to find:

- **C6 (caproic acid):** Quickly converted to ketones but can upset the gut
- **C8 (caprylic acid):** Quickly converted to ketones; has antimicrobial properties, which promote a healthy gut; doesn't need liver processing to get ketone generation firing
- **C10 (capric acid):** Slower to turn into energy than C8
- **C12 (lauric acid):** Has to be broken down in the liver, making ketone production fairly slow; more of a long-chain triglyceride than a medium-chain triglyceride
- **C14:** Found mostly in saturated fats; the long-chain fatty acids in coconut oil

A high percentage of the saturated fat in coconut oil is C12 (lauric acid), an SFA that has been shown to improve cholesterol levels, reduce symptoms of acne, and have a positive influence on hormone levels. However, because it's more similar to a long-chain fatty acid, it doesn't provide as many of the MCT benefits outlined above.

So for encouraging ketone production and all-around keto support, MCT oil, rather than coconut oil, is considered the gold standard. C8 (caprylic acid) is the "best" form of MCT for keto—it helps generate ketones, has antimicrobial properties, and doesn't require liver action to get the party started.

It's not about removing coconut oil completely and consuming only "the best" MCT oil—it's about using a combination on your journey to keto awesomeness! Because MCT oil is a refined oil in that it lacks nutrients found in unrefined coconut oil and palm oil, I incorporate the unrefined versions of these oils into my keto diet to balance things out. For example, I like to cook and bake with coconut oil and use C8 MCT oil in salad dressings, chilled sauces, and my daily RFL.

USING KETO FATS AND OILS

For best-pick qualities for these cooking oils, turn to page 138.

If you just want to know what to cook with and how to do it, this section gives you the tools you need.

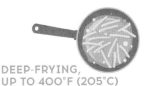

DEEP-FRYING, UP TO 400°F (205°C)
· Avocado oil, refined
· Canola oil, refined**
· Tallow/Suet

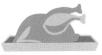

ROASTING, UP TO 375°F (190°C)
· Avocado oil, refined
· Chicken fat (schmaltz)
· Duck fat
· Ghee*, grass-fed
· Goose fat
· Hazelnut oil
· Palm fruit oil
· Tallow/Suet

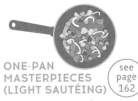

ONE-PAN MASTERPIECES (LIGHT SAUTÉING) see page 162
· Avocado oil, refined
· Chicken fat (schmaltz)
· Duck fat
· Ghee*
· Goose fat
· Hazelnut oil
· Lard/Bacon grease
· Palm fruit oil
· Tallow/Suet

BAKING: SOLID FATS
· Butter*
· Cacao butter/oil
· Coconut oil
· Ghee*
· Lard

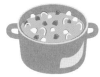
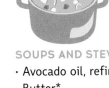

BAKING: NOT-SO-SOLID FATS
· Avocado oil, refined
· Canola oil, refined**
· Hazelnut oil
· Olive oil, refined
· Palm kernel oil

SOUPS AND STEWS
· Avocado oil, refined
· Butter*
· Chicken fat (schmaltz)
· Coconut oil
· Duck fat
· Ghee*
· Goose fat
· Lard/Bacon grease
· Palm fruit oil
· Tallow/Suet

WARMED SAUCES
· Avocado oil, refined
· Butter*
· Chicken fat (schmaltz)
· Coconut oil
· Duck fat
· Ghee*
· Goose fat
· Lard/Bacon grease
· MCT oil
· Palm kernel oil
· Tallow/Suet

ROCKET FUEL LATTE
· Almond oil
· Butter*
· Cacao butter/oil
· Coconut oil
· Hazelnut oil
· Macadamia nut oil
· MCT oil
· Palm kernel oil

see page 428

SAVORY FAT BOMBS
· Butter*
· Chicken fat (schmaltz)
· Coconut oil
· Duck fat
· Ghee*
· Goose fat
· Tallow/Suet

SWEET FAT BOMBS
· Butter*
· Cacao butter/oil
· Coconut oil
· Ghee*

MAYONNAISE
· Avocado oil, refined
· Bacon grease
· Canola oil**
· Hazelnut oil
· Macadamia nut oil
· MCT oil
· Olive oil, refined

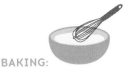

NUT AND SEED PÂTÉS
· Almond oil
· Avocado oil, refined
· Canola oil**
· Hazelnut oil
· Hemp seed oil**
· Macadamia nut oil
· MCT oil
· Olive oil, extra-virgin
· Olive oil, virgin
· Palm kernel oil
· Walnut oil**

SALAD DRESSINGS
· Almond oil
· Avocado oil, refined
· Canola oil**
· Flaxseed oil**
· Hazelnut oil
· Hemp seed oil
· Macadamia nut oil
· MCT oil
· Olive oil, extra-virgin
· Olive oil, virgin
· Palm kernel oil
· Walnut oil**

*If you are sensitive to dairy, this fat/oil may not be the best for you. For example, ghee is naturally whey-free, but depending on processing, most ghee contains varying amounts of casein and lactose.

**Consume smaller amounts due to higher PUFA content, as outlined on page 136.

WHOLE-FOOD FATS

When I say fats, you think bacon! Fats, bacon! Fats, bacon! When I first went keto, I thought fats and immediately thought oils. But there's a lot more than oils out there to boost your keto awesome.

In addition to oils, whole-food sources of fats include avocados, olives, nuts (almonds, macadamia nuts, pecans, etc.), seeds (hemp, sesame, sunflower, etc.), side bacon, pork shoulder, egg yolks, chicken thighs, salmon, sardines, beef brisket, steak, and more. All of my favorite whole-food fats can be found in the list on page 115.

Nuts and Seeds

Let's dig a little deeper into nuts and seeds because they're amazing whole-food fats. They're a fabulous way to bulk up the fat content of your day, increase protein (especially if you're vegan), and boost your intake of fiber. But some nuts and seeds pack a pretty mean carbohydrate punch and should be saved for special occasions. One serving may be a small handful, who's ever eaten a small handful of nuts or seeds? Having two to three handfuls of high-carbohydrate nuts or seeds can make it extremely difficult for you to become fat-adapted. And we don't want that!

> Soaking and roasting is the healthiest (and tastiest) way to prepare nuts and seeds. Check out why on page 155.

You'll find extensive data on nuts and seeds in the chart on page 144. Following is an explanation of the various categories in that chart, which also serves as a general overview of what to think about when choosing nuts and seeds.

A note on one conspicuous absence in the chart: peanuts are legumes and not keto-friendly. (But if you're wondering about coconut, which *is* included in the chart: it's technically a kind of fruit known as a drupe, though the USDA classifies it as a tree nut—but most people with tree nut allergies can tolerate coconut.)

Cost

If you're a nut monster like myself, nothing motivates you more than knowing exactly how much money you're eating—literally. The cost in the chart on page 144 is per serving, so you can see exactly how much those four handfuls of almonds are costing you. Brazil nuts, coconut, flax seeds, sesame seeds, and sunflower seeds for the win!

Calories

If you haven't caught on already, I'm not a huge supporter of calorie counting or tracking to lose weight or manage health. So much more goes into a successful weight-loss journey than calories. But I know how much people love the c-word, so I've included it here. The real takeaway for calories? Just because an item is "low-calorie" doesn't mean that it meets your requirements. Take, for example, pumpkin seeds. You may think, *It's fatty, it's low-calorie, double bonus!* Think again, my friend. Check out that net carb amount: 10. A couple of handfuls of those "low-calorie" seeds and you'll be cursing my name, wondering why fat adaptation is so easy for everyone but you. On the other side of the coin are Brazil nuts, seemingly "bad" because they are high in calories, but check out the net carbs: 2! That means you can enjoy six Brazil nuts (straight from the freezer is the tastiest way) and count only 2 net carbs toward your total carbohydrates for the day. I call that a #win.

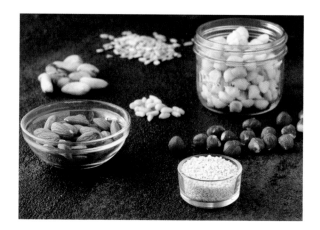

Fat

If you're fearful of the high amounts of fat in nuts and seeds and wondering how eating them is going to help you lose the fat on your body, regulate your metabolism, and feel good, backtrack to page 33 and give it another read-through. I totally understand what you're going through—when I first started eating keto, I was overwhelmed by the amount of fat I was consuming. But after thirty days of a life transformation, I decided that fat wasn't so bad. Macadamia nuts pack an intense fat punch and are a perfect companion for a busy high-fat lifestyle.

Net Carbs

Remember on page 62 where I outlined why net carbs are the bomb-diggity? They're especially important when it comes to vegetables, fruits, condiments, nuts, and seeds. And while it can be pretty easy to guesstimate whether a vegetable, fruit, or condiment is low-carb, it gets a bit tricky when it comes to nuts and seeds. For example, you'd think that if a sunflower seed is relatively low-carb, then a pumpkin seed would be, too, right? Wrong! The crème de la crème of low-carb nuts/seeds, based on net carbs, are almonds, Brazil nuts, hazelnuts, macadamia nuts, pecans, walnuts, flax seeds, chia seeds, and hemp seeds.

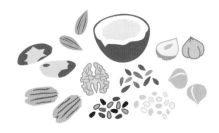

Protein

We know that reducing carbohydrates allows us to slide into a ketogenic, fat-burning state, but protein also plays a valuable role in getting us there. Eating too much protein can affect our ability to adapt to fat-burning mode (see pages 36 and 37 for more). When looking at nuts and seeds, it's important to take note of their protein content. Most nuts and seeds contain a similar amount of protein per serving (except hemp—wowza!).

Ratio (Fat:Net Carbs:Protein)

Ratios are helpful for determining whether a food matches your eating style. Let's say your macros have you at around 70 percent fat, 20 percent protein, and 10 percent carbs. This works out to a ratio of 7:2:1, fat to net carbs to protein. So eating nuts/seeds that have a similar ratio will work fabulously for you. Say, for example, almonds: they're a bit higher in protein than you need, but their ratio of 7:3:1 is pretty darn close. The only ones that really aren't close to the ratio you're shooting for are cashews, pistachios, and pumpkin seeds. Then there are sesame and sunflower seeds, which aren't horrible but are lower in fat than other options compared to the carbohydrates they come with. I like to combine sesame and sunflower seeds with additional fat when cooking with them.

Now go out there and nut up your life!

KETO NUTS AND SEEDS

Item	Serving Size (28 g)	Cost Per Serving	Calories	Fat (g)	Total Carbs (g)	Net Carbs (g)	Protein (g)	Ratio (Fat: Net Carbs: Protein)
ALMONDS*	25	$0.92	163	14	6	2	6	7:1:3
WALNUTS*	13 halves	$1.05	185	18	4	2	4	9:1:2
BRAZIL NUTS**	11	$0.74	186	19	4	2	4	10:1:2
PINE NUTS*	3 tbsp	$1.23	191	19	4	3	4	6:1:1
CASHEWS*	19	$0.80	157	12	9	8	5	2:2:1
PUMPKIN SEEDS*	3 tbsp	$0.49	126	5	15	10	5	1:2:1
COCONUT**	¼ cup	$0.37	100	10	4	1	1	10:1:1
FLAX SEEDS**	3 tbsp	$0.31	151	12	8	1	5	12:1:5
HAZELNUTS*	25	$1.23	178	17	5	2	4	9:1:2
CHIA SEEDS**	3 tbsp	$0.62	138	9	12	2	5	5:1:3
MACADAMIA NUTS**	12	$1.54	204	21	4	2	2	11:1:1
HEMP SEEDS**	3 tbsp	$1.05	170	13	3	1	10	13:1:10
PECANS*	19 halves	$1.11	196	20	4	2	3	10:1:2
SESAME SEEDS*	3 tbsp	$0.31	160	14	6	3	5	5:1:2
PISTACHIOS*	49	$1.54	159	13	8	5	6	3:1:1
SUNFLOWER SEEDS**	3 tbsp	$0.31	163	14	6	3	6	5:1:2

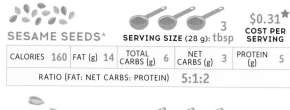

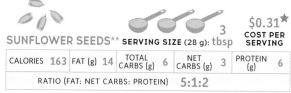

*Dry-roasted organic   **Raw organic

QUITTING GRAINS AND DAIRY

I know, it sounds daunting, doesn't it? But dropping grains and dairy may be the best thing you ever do for yourself. Think: smooth-running digestion, clear complexion, reduced cravings, no more brain fog, energy in the early-morning hours...you get the idea.

It's clear that grains don't belong on a Fat Fueled keto diet. The fact that they're carbohydrate bombs is enough for some people, but for me, it's their inability to fill up my nutrients cup (see page 106) and the fact that they make me feel mental that have had me grain-free for more than five years.

Dairy is where things get a little gray. Some people thrive on it, while other people don't do so well. If you're part of the latter crew, continue on.

Do you want to add a cheesy flavor to your recipes without using actual cheese? Try nutritional yeast, a natural-food product made from a single-celled organism that grows on molasses. Once harvested, it's washed and dried with heat to deactivate it. It tastes like cheese and is low-carb and delicious. But it doesn't melt like cheese. I like to use it as a Parmesan cheese replacement.

GOING DAIRY-FREE: ALL YOUR OPTIONS

Dairy: It gives me acne, a bloated stomach, headaches, and clogged sinuses. It's not pleasant. Do you experience similar effects?

For many of us, going dairy-free is the right choice for our bodies. But maintaining excitement about dairy-free meals can be a challenge. No cheese on pizza, sad face. No lasagna ever again, triple sad face. But I found a way to have all these things without letting my dairy allergy stop me from enjoying the flavors of life.

The following guides, tricks, and quick recipe tips will have you saying, "Dairy? Dairy who?" in no time. Well, that's sort of a lie. You may pine for dairy for a while. Three months, to be exact. Did you know that there is a protein in cheese that mimics proteins in breast milk, instilling a sense of calmness, belonging, and love? If you were breast-fed, those feelings you had with your mom during those tender first months are the same ones you have when you're consuming cheese. No wonder so many of us can't ditch the stuff!

I promise, though, that if you give this dairy-free thing a try and you start to feel better without it, you'll want it less often. And when you do eat it, you may be reminded just how horrible it makes you feel. But hey, if dairy makes you feel great and you love it, why remove it? It's all about listening to your body.

Make dairy-free versions of your favorites and skip the mucus, inflammation, and tummy pain. Your acne will thank you for it!

HOW TO MAKE THINGS DAIRY-FREE

MAKE

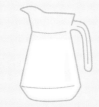

MILK

See page 156 for a guide to making your own nut milks.

SOUR CREAM

Makes: 1 cup (240 ml)

Soak 1 cup (155 g) raw cashews in water for 6 hours. Using a fine-mesh strainer, drain and rinse. Place in a high-powered blender with ½ cup (120 ml) fresh water, ⅓ cup (80 ml) lemon juice, ¼ cup (40 g) raw macadamia nuts, 1 tablespoon nutritional yeast, ¾ teaspoon gray sea salt, and ½ teaspoon ground white pepper. Blend until creamy.

CREAM CHEESE

Makes: 1 cup (240 ml)

Soak 1½ cups (235 g) raw cashews in water for 12 to 24 hours. Using a fine-mesh strainer, drain and rinse. Place in a high-powered blender with 2 tablespoons apple cider vinegar, 2 tablespoons lemon juice, and 2 tablespoons fresh water. Blend until smooth. Transfer to a piece of cheesecloth, wrap with twine, hang over a bowl, and let drain overnight.

PUDDING

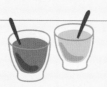

Makes: 1 cup (240 ml)

In a blender, puree the flesh of 3 Hass avocados, ½ teaspoon vanilla extract, ⅛ teaspoon gray sea salt, 4 drops liquid stevia, and either ⅓ cup (80 ml) lemon juice or ¼ cup cacao powder.

BUY

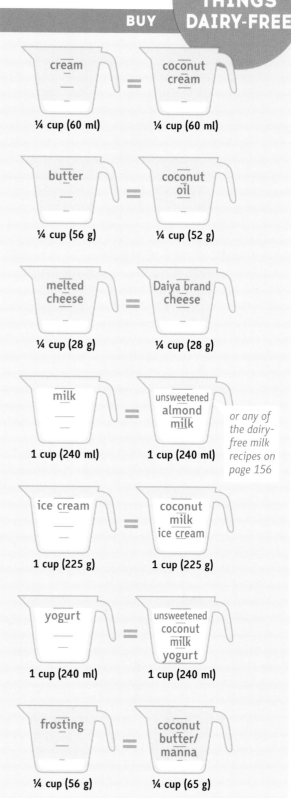

cream
¼ cup (60 ml)
= coconut cream
¼ cup (60 ml)

butter
¼ cup (56 g)
= coconut oil
¼ cup (52 g)

melted cheese
¼ cup (28 g)
= Daiya brand cheese
¼ cup (28 g)

milk
1 cup (240 ml)
= unsweetened almond milk
1 cup (240 ml)
or any of the dairy-free milk recipes on page 156

ice cream
1 cup (225 g)
= coconut milk ice cream
1 cup (225 g)

yogurt
1 cup (240 ml)
= unsweetened coconut milk yogurt
1 cup (240 ml)

frosting
¼ cup (56 g)
= coconut butter/ manna
¼ cup (65 g)

DAIRY THAT MAY BE OKAY FOR YOU

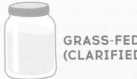

GRASS-FED GHEE (CLARIFIED BUTTER)

- Great for high-temperature cooking; has a smoke point of 450°F (232°C)
- Naturally whey-free; should also be free of casein and lactose
- Rich, buttery, nutty flavor
- Stable at room temperature for up to three months

- ⊕ Rich in fat-soluble vitamins A, D, E, and K, which support skeletal, immune, neurological, and cardiovascular systems
- ⊕ Rich in short-chain fatty acids that nourish the cells of the digestive tract
- ⊕ High in CLA, which aids in the reduction of body fat and inflammation and in the maintenance of balanced cholesterol

GRASS-FED BUTTER

- Awesome for light cooking and baking; has a smoke point of 350°F (177°C)
- Easily accessible; can be purchased from almost any grocery store
- Must be refrigerated

- ⊕ Rich source of short-chain fatty acids that reduce inflammation
- ⊕ Vitamin K2 helps decalcify arteries
- ⊕ Saturated fat lowers risk of heart disease and improves HDL to LDL balance and LDL particle size

GOING GRAIN-FREE

If you're transitioning to a high-fat eating style from the world of Paleo, you're already well versed in the ways of grain-free living. But if you had toast for breakfast, a rice stir-fry for lunch, and quinoa pilaf for dinner, we have a ways to go together. I won't sugarcoat it: the transition will be an adjustment as you trade old habits for new, but I'm here for you!

NOTE: *Whole grains contain all parts of the seed, while refined grains often have the bran or germ removed, leaving just the highly starchy endosperm. We're often told that whole grains are healthy, but they're just as damaging as refined grains.*

The best advice I can give you is to take it slow and remember that Rome wasn't built in a day. If you go off grains cold turkey and end up feeling restricted because too much has been eliminated from your diet in an extremely short period, you'll be less likely to stick with this way of eating long-term. But if your transition to keto feels like a natural progression of learning what feels good in your body, it'll be easier to stay with it.

When you're invited to a dinner party and your host asks you what you do and don't eat, tell them that you love vegetables and meats instead of explaining all the things you can't have. It's much simpler this way.

The challenges that arise from removing something from your diet aren't exclusive to keto. Any eating style change that involves removing a staple item from your eating arsenal is going to be difficult because it forces you to change your way of doing things. And any alteration to your normal day-to-day is going to be frustrating at first—simple as that.

There are two things that make removing something from your diet simpler and more doable. The first is substitutions, and that's something I can help you with. The second is passion, and that's something I can help you with indirectly.

Substitutions are easy. I've included a how-to guide in the following pages that provides the solutions you need to swap out grains for their inexpensive grain-free counterparts.

But passion is a trickier beast. You have to *want* to try something new based on your desire to feel better. Really, it comes down to that. I can tell you that I've felt better since going grain-free and that it's eliminated the inflammation in my body characterized by tight joints, irregular digestion, foggy brain, uncontrollable appetite, and nutrient deficiencies…but whether that motivates you to really get behind eliminating grains depends on what you care about.

> When you're at a restaurant, order from the gluten-free menu or opt for a full-sized entree that generally include things like roasted chicken or steak with steamed vegetables or salads. (See page 86 for more on eating keto at restaurants.)

Here's a list that I refer to when I forget just how horrible I felt on grains. Your version of grain-free may include white rice, the occasional bowl of sprouted quinoa, or fresh sourdough. And that's okay; everyone's approach will be slightly different.

With any change, there's a period of overwhelm as we sink our feet into the sand and familiarize ourselves with the new landscape around us. I'm hoping that, by sharing tools, tips, and facts, I can help you feel supported with solutions and passion-driving information.

> Whole-grain or not, don't be fooled by tricky product marketing. If the product contains any of these items, it's not grain-free.

> If you do consume grains on occasion, sprouting and fermenting them makes their nutrients more accessible.

Before we get to the opting out part, let's run through what grains are and why we're removing them.

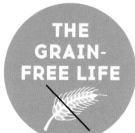

THE GRAIN-FREE LIFE

GRAINS TO DITCH

BR BARLEY	**BG** BULGUR	**EK** EINKORN	**FO** FARRO	**GN** GRANO
KT KAMUT	**RE** RYE	**SP** SPELT	**TR** TRITICALE	**WE** WHEAT
AA (GF) AMARANTH	**BW** (GF) BUCKWHEAT	**CN** (GF) CORN	**KW** (GF) KANIWA	**ML** (GF) MILLET
OT (GF) OATS	**QN** (GF) QUINOA	**RC** (GF) RICE	**SR** (GF) SORGHUM	**TE** (GF) TEFF
WR (GF) WILD RICE				

GRAIN-FREE ALTERNATIVES

			AL ALMONDS	**AS** APPLESAUCE
CL CAULIFLOWER	**CI** CHIA	**CO** COCONUT	**CF** CRICKET FLOUR	**FL** FLAX
HM HEMP	**PW** PROTEIN POWDER	**PU** PUMPKIN PUREE	**SQ** SQUASH	**SF** SUNFLOWER

(GF) *Gluten-free*

GRAIN-RELATED SYMPTOMS

Amenorrhea (absence of menstruation)
Autoimmune diseases
Blisters
Brain fog
Constipation
Cravings
Dental enamel defects
Depression
Diabetes
Diarrhea
Dry skin
Eczema
Fatigue
Feeling faint
Food sensitivities

Gut inflammation
High blood pressure
Increased cholesterol
Insulin resistance
Lack of appetite
Liver disease
Memory loss
Muscle pain
Muscle wasting
Night blindness
Psoriasis
Rashes
Restless sleep
Rheumatoid arthritis
Slow growth in children
Weight gain

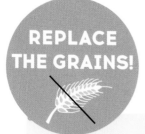

REPLACE THE GRAINS!

The tricks and recipes you need to shift to grain-free.

 =

WHITE OR BROWN RICE = CAULIFLOWER RICE

2 cups (390 g) cooked rice

1 batch Cauliflower Rice (364)

Best used in recipes that call for a sprinkle of cooked quinoa, like salads

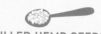

QUINOA = HULLED HEMP SEEDS

1 tablespoon cooked quinoa

1 tablespoon hulled hemp seeds

CAKE BATTER = BLANCHED ALMOND FLOUR OR COCONUT FLOUR

CRACKERS = CRISPY MEATS OR DEHYDRATED LOW-CARB VEGETABLES

 396 / 398

Carrot Cake

St. Louis Gooey "Butter" Cake

 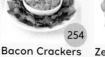

254 / 252 / 248

Bacon Crackers

Zesty Nacho Cabbage Chips

Chicken Crisps

NOODLES = SPIRAL-SLICED VEGETABLES

See page 154 for more on spiral slicing.

Use a spiral slicer to turn zucchini, radishes, turnips, cucumbers, broccoli stems, or daikon into fabulous noodle replacements. During a carb-up, starchy veggies such as jicama, carrots, potatoes, beets, parsnips, and sweet potatoes are fun, too.

 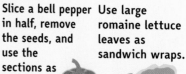 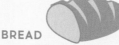

BREAD

Use cucumber or pickle slices as mini sandwich bread pieces.

Slice a bell pepper in half, remove the seeds, and use the sections as bread.

Use large romaine lettuce leaves as sandwich wraps.

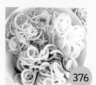

376 / 381 / 276

Zoodles and Doodles

Pesto Zoodles

Chicken Noodle Soup

302 / 366 / 362

Bombay Sloppy Jolenes

Crusty Sandwich Bread

Sardine Fritter Wraps

PIZZA = USE MEAT AS THE BASE

 312

Michael's Pepperoni Meatzza

ROLLED OATS = HULLED HEMP SEEDS

1 cup (100 g) rolled oats

1 cup (150 g) hulled hemp seeds

 244

Grain-Free Hemp Seed Porridge

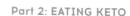

KETO IN THE KITCHEN

KETO FUNDAMENTALS

Let's get to the implementation strategies—how to make the keto diet work in the kitchen to save you time, energy, and money. In this chapter, I'm sharing with you the tips, tricks, strategies, and techniques I use to prepare keto classics such as nut butters, bone broths, rendered fats, and more.

BONE BROTH

Bone broth is a reduction of the minerals and healing components of animal bones in a delicious, drinkable form. The bones are boiled in water over a long period to allow their nutrients to seep into the water. The bones are then strained, and you're left with bone broth.

While you can purchase bone broth, making your own will help you stick to a budget and ensures that you're in control of the quality of ingredients used. Bone broth has minimal fat, moderate carbohydrate, and a good helping of protein, making it a fabulous meal replacement either plain or boosted with power ingredients like ginger, garlic, fresh herbs, MCT oil, coconut oil, or your favorite fat. I also love cooking with bone broth—nothing makes me quite as happy in the kitchen as grabbing a couple of frozen cubes of homemade broth to use in a batch of fried cauliflower rice, fried cabbage, or rich stew.

If you cook with bone broth in a slow cooker or pressure cooker, reserve all the cooking liquid when you're done and use it in your cooking throughout the week. It will be a mixture of fat, gelatin, and spices—perfect for sautéing meats, eggs, and vegetables.

Why It's Good for You

Think of bone broth as a magic elixir that's filled with all the minerals your body needs to be the best version of itself. When I was studying nutrition, if an exam asked us to list foods that were rich in a certain mineral, I would always list bone broth—and it was always correct. (I never went wrong with avocado or liver, either. These three are the epitome of nutrient-dense, nature-infused foods that everyone should include in their diets. For more on keto power foods, see page 111.)

Here are some of the things that bone broth can do for you:

- **Reduce cellulite**
- **Improve connective tissue for healthy range of motion and improved athletic ability**
- **Improve hair strength and increase growth**
- **Balance digestive system**
- **Remineralize teeth, preventing tooth decay**
- **Boost immune system**
- **Regulate blood sugar levels**
- **Boost antioxidants, slowing aging and preventing cell damage**
- **Promote the creation of new muscle cells**
- **Reduce intestinal inflammation**
- **Improve gut lining to reduce food sensitivities**

Quality Ingredients Are Key

Because bone broth is a nutrient-dense cocktail, it's important to use high-quality, nutrient-dense ingredients to create it. (For more on sourcing, see page 110.) Here are the keywords to look for when buying bones for stock:

- **Beef, bison, or lamb bones:** grass-fed, grass-finished
- **Chicken, duck, or goose bones:** corn-free, soy-free, free-range
- **Fish bones and/or heads:** wild-caught
- **Pork bones:** pasture-raised

The easiest way to acquire bones is to save them from the meals you're preparing. I always have four large freezer-safe bags of bones in the freezer—one for pork, one for beef, one for chicken, and one for fish. Whenever I use bone-in meat for a meal, I place the leftover bones in the appropriate bag. Once the bag is full, it's time to make broth!

If saving bones isn't your jam or you want to get a head start on creating bone broth, your best bet is to do a quick internet search for "grass-fed butcher [your city]." The search results should display local ranches, shops, and cooperatives that are associated with grass-fed cattle. Call and ask if they sell bones, using the keywords listed earlier as guidelines. You may also be able to find high-quality bones in the freezer section of your favorite health food store, but that can get expensive.

> If you need a boost of fat for the day, try blending MCT oil with your bone broth in a blender!

HOW TO MAKE BONE BROTH

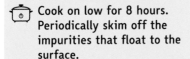

PICK YOUR BASE 2 pounds (910 g):

Beef bones
Chicken bones
Oxtail
Duck bones

Pork bones
Lamb bones
Goose bones
Bison bones

Fish bones and/or heads, gills removed; all bones are fair game
Shellfish

BOOST THE GELATIN (optional)

Beef knuckle (for beef broth)

Chicken feet (for chicken broth)

CHOOSE A COOKING TOOL

Pressure cooker   Slow cooker   Stockpot

COVER WITH WATER

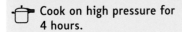

COOK!

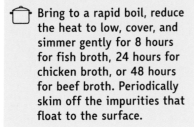

Cook on high pressure for 4 hours.

Cook on low for 8 hours. Periodically skim off the impurities that float to the surface.

Bring to a rapid boil, reduce the heat to low, cover, and simmer gently for 8 hours for fish broth, 24 hours for chicken broth, or 48 hours for beef broth. Periodically skim off the impurities that float to the surface.

GET FANCY WITH IT (optional)

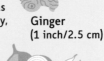

Fish sauce (2 teaspoons), for chicken broth

Black peppercorns (1 teaspoon)

Fresh herbs (handful), such as parsley, rosemary, or thyme

Ginger (1 inch/2.5 cm)

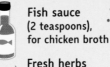

Carrots (2)   Celery stalks (2)   Onion (1)   Garlic cloves (2)

ADD MUST-HAVES

Apple cider vinegar (2 tablespoons)

Finely ground gray sea salt (1 teaspoon)

> Adding apple cider vinegar helps break down the bones.

CHILL OUT

Remove from heat and strain into a heatproof bowl. Discard the solids.

Allow the broth to cool completely.

Remove the top layer of fat and share with your dog or discard, optional.

Store in an airtight container in the fridge for up to 3 days or in the freezer for up to 6 months.

> Store your broth so it's easy to cook with later! Pour it into silicone ice cube trays, freeze, and transfer the cubes to a freezer-safe bag. Use the cubes in your cooking. Each cube is about 2 tablespoons of broth.

Using bones from conventionally raised sources, such as grain-fed cattle? The slow cooker and stockpot options are best, as you can remove the lid during cooking and skim off the impurities that float to the surface.

NOTE: *A good broth is gelatinous when completely cooled. If your batch is less firm than Jell-O but still quite gelatinous, you've cooked it long enough and with the right ingredients! If not, it's still delicious and nutritious. To boost the nutrients, you can add unflavored gelatin or collagen peptides while it's still hot.*

YOUR LOW-CARB NOODLE HOUSE

Spiral slicing is the art of transforming vegetables and fruits into noodles, either with a vegetable peeler or with a spiral slicer, an inexpensive tool specifically designed to make noodles. Spiral slicers come in all sorts of shapes and sizes; see page 165 for more information.

Because these noodles are made entirely of plants, they're completely gluten-free, grain-free, dairy-free, low-carb (in most cases), Paleo, and vegan. If you can eat the plant, you can eat the noodle.

Spiral-sliced noodles:

- Lower the carb count of your favorite pasta dishes
- Quickly boost your vegetable intake
- Are super fun for kids; you can create different-colored noodles from different vegetables
- Eliminate the need to purchase low-carb noodles, which can be quite costly
- Make eating seasonally a lot easier
- Are ready much quicker than your average noodles, often with no cooking required

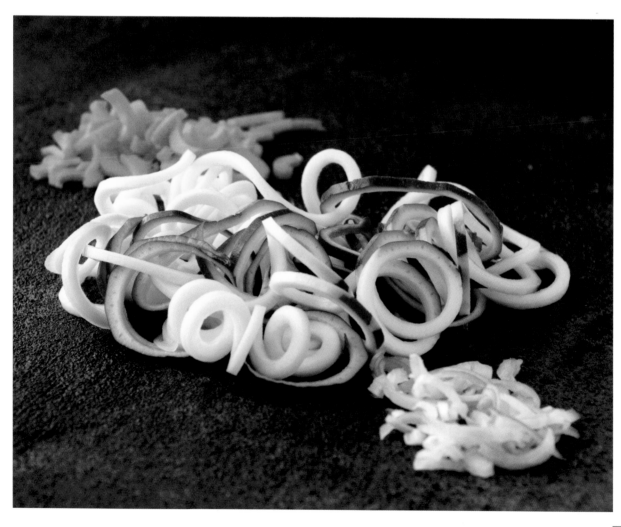

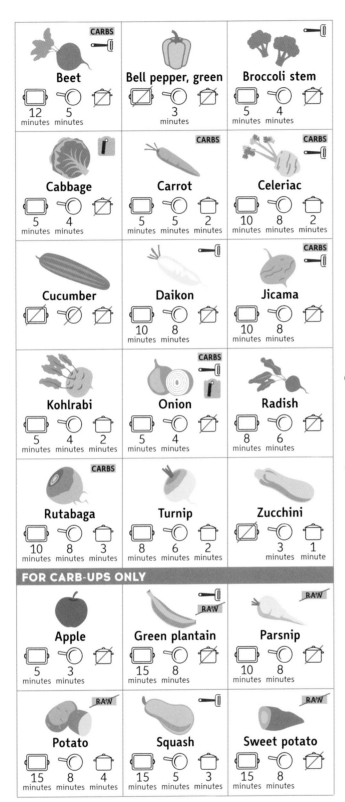

Produce	Notes	Roast	Sauté	Boil
Beet	CARBS, peel before spiral slicing	12 minutes	5 minutes	—
Bell pepper, green	peel before spiral slicing	—	3 minutes	—
Broccoli stem	peel before spiral slicing	5 minutes	4 minutes	—
Cabbage	use a flat blade	5 minutes	4 minutes	—
Carrot	CARBS	5 minutes	5 minutes	2 minutes
Celeriac	CARBS, peel before spiral slicing	10 minutes	8 minutes	2 minutes
Cucumber		—	—	—
Daikon	peel before spiral slicing	10 minutes	8 minutes	—
Jicama	CARBS, peel before spiral slicing	10 minutes	8 minutes	—
Kohlrabi		5 minutes	4 minutes	2 minutes
Onion	CARBS, peel before spiral slicing, use a flat blade	5 minutes	4 minutes	—
Radish		8 minutes	6 minutes	—
Rutabaga	CARBS	10 minutes	8 minutes	3 minutes
Turnip		8 minutes	6 minutes	2 minutes
Zucchini		—	3 minutes	1 minute

FOR CARB-UPS ONLY

Produce	Notes	Roast	Sauté	Boil
Apple	peel before spiral slicing	5 minutes	3 minutes	—
Green plantain	RAW, peel before spiral slicing	15 minutes	8 minutes	—
Parsnip	RAW	10 minutes	8 minutes	—
Potato	RAW	15 minutes	8 minutes	4 minutes
Squash	peel before spiral slicing	15 minutes	5 minutes	3 minutes
Sweet potato	RAW	15 minutes	8 minutes	—

CARBS *High-ish in carbs, so eat sparingly outside of carb-ups.*

Peel before spiral slicing.

Use a flat blade.

RAW *Do not consume raw.*

WHAT TO SPIRAL SLICE

This page shows some of my favorite produce to turn into noodles, but you can go beyond my recommendations and play with your local produce. Follow these simple guidelines when choosing a vegetable or fruit to spiral slice:

- Choose produce that's firm and solid rather than squishy or juicy.
- Avoid produce that has seeds throughout, is hollow, or has a pit.
- Choose produce that is more than 2 inches long.
- Look for fairly straight produce. Anything that's weirdly shaped will wobble in the spiralizer and make your life difficult.

HOW TO SPIRAL SLICE (AND BE AWESOME)

COOKING YOUR NOODLES

ROAST: Toss the noodles in melted tallow or refined avocado oil, spread evenly on a lined baking sheet, and cook at 400°F (205°C) for the amount of time listed. Sprinkle with finely ground gray sea salt and enjoy.

SAUTÉ: Place melted tallow or refined avocado oil in a frying pan. Add the noodles and toss to coat. Cook over medium heat for the amount of time listed.

BOIL: Bring a pot of salted water to a boil. Add the noodles and cook for the amount of time listed. Drain, rinse, and serve hot, or pat dry and chill.

WAYS TO USE LOW-CARB NOODLES

- In place of pasta (as in Chicken Alfredo, page 342, or Pesto Zoodles, page 381)
- In a breakfast scramble
- In pasta salad
- In a green salad
- As a wrap filling
- In soup (like Chicken Noodle Soup, page 276)

MAKE YOUR OWN MEAL

Top noodles with sauce.

Add a protein.

Drizzle with fat.

Done!

PREPARING NUTS AND SEEDS

Think of your favorite animal and its natural defense mechanism. For instance, skunks have their foul-smelling spray, hairy frogs can break their own bones to hide from predators, and porcupine quills detach easily. Defense mechanisms like these aren't seen only in the animal kingdom. Plants also have defense mechanisms, and they're called antinutrients. Remember, plants reproduce through nuts and seeds, so when we eat them, we prevent the plant from reproducing. Antinutrients help a plant reproduce by making the consumption of nuts and seeds less beneficial and eventually even harmful. Although plants contain a handful of different antinutrients, I'm going to focus on phytic acid because it poses the greatest risk to digestive health and mineral balance.

Phytic acid is found in the hulls of nuts and seeds. When consumed, it can block the absorption of magnesium, copper, zinc, iron, and calcium. Although this doesn't have an immediate health effect, long-term consumption of foods rich in phytic acid can have lasting effects on health, including tooth decay, bone loss, and psychological imbalance.

I know, I sound all doom and gloom here, but there's an easy fix. Soaking and roasting nuts and seeds helps neutralize antinutrients like phytic acid. Your gut will love you for it. (While sprouting and fermenting would be on the table if we were speaking about grains or legumes, these steps may not decrease the phytic acid in nuts and seeds.) Nut and seed milks are generally good options because the nuts and seeds are soaked in the process of making them. The same goes for homemade nut and seed butters and flours—the nuts and seeds are soaked and roasted in the process.

However, if you notice digestive upset when you consume raw nuts or seeds but not when you consume soaked or roasted nuts or seeds (or items made from them), it's highly advisable to limit your intake of store-bought nut and seed products, including flours, butters, milks, and treats made with them. Store-bought products likely have not been prepared in a manner that removes phytic acid. (By the way, none of this applies to coconut. Eat it any which way and you'll be good.)

WHEN ARE NUTS AND SEEDS SAFE?

RAW—Usually okay if the nuts/seeds will be used in cooking. This includes flax seeds and nut/seed flour (the baking process will roast the seeds, removing phytic acid).

SOAKED—A step that makes nut/seed milks, butters, and flours safe.

ROASTED—A step that makes nut/seed butters and flours safe; also good for snacking.

Nut and Seed Milks

Nut/seed milks are nondairy milks made from a combination of filtered water and the nuts or seeds of your choice. They often make a great substitute for dairy milk without the damaging effects of dairy. These dairy-free alternatives taste great, are easier on digestion, and are super affordable.

A serving of nuts/seeds has about the same amount of carbohydrates as a serving of homemade nut/seed milk. Check out the chart on page 144 for a rundown of the macronutrients in a wide variety of nuts and seeds.

All your favorite low-carb nuts/seeds are great for making milk, except flax seeds and chia seeds. I've tried to make flax milk and chia milk, and they both tasted gross—not good enough to share by any means!

Put That Pulp to Use

After Step 5, you'll have a nut milk bag filled with pulp. Instead of throwing the goodness away, here are some ways to use the pulp:

- **Make flour.** Spread the pulp on a dehydrator sheet or lined baking sheet and dehydrate or bake at 150°F (65°C) for three to four hours, until completely dry. If the flour can be pinched together easily, like a snowball, it's not ready yet.

- Stir it into a bowl of Grain-Free Hemp Seed Porridge (page 244).

- Add it to your next keto smoothie (pages 424 and 425).

HOW TO MAKE NUT/SEED MILKS

STEP 1. FILL

Place 2 cups (475 ml) warm filtered water in a large bowl.

Add ½ teaspoon salt. Stir until dissolved.

NOTE: *Coconut and hemp seeds do not need to be soaked; for these, go straight to Step 4.*

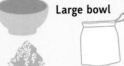

Large bowl

Finely ground gray sea salt or Himalayan rock salt

Nut milk bag or unused nylon stocking with no reinforced toe

Blender

 Mason jar

STEP 2. ADD

Add the nuts/seeds of your choice, in the quantity specified below. Make sure that the water completely covers the nuts/seeds.

STEP 3. SOAK AND RINSE

Cover the bowl with a towel and let the nuts/seeds soak on the counter. After soaking, drain the liquid and rinse the nuts/seeds under cold running water.

STEP 4. BLEND

Place the rinsed nuts/seeds in a blender with the following amounts of filtered water. Blend on high for about 1 minute, until smooth and creamy.

STEP 5. STRAIN

Pour the contents of the blender through a nut milk bag and into the bowl, straining the pulp. Lightly squeeze to remove excess liquid. Transfer the milk to a mason jar or other fridge-safe container. It will keep in the fridge for 2 to 3 days.

For added nutrients, skip Step 5, leaving your nut milk filled with fibrous pulp. This makes a great addition to Rocket Fuel Lattes (page 428), homemade granola (page 246), or smoothies. It's not so good in baking recipes, however, as it can change the fiber profile of the dish.

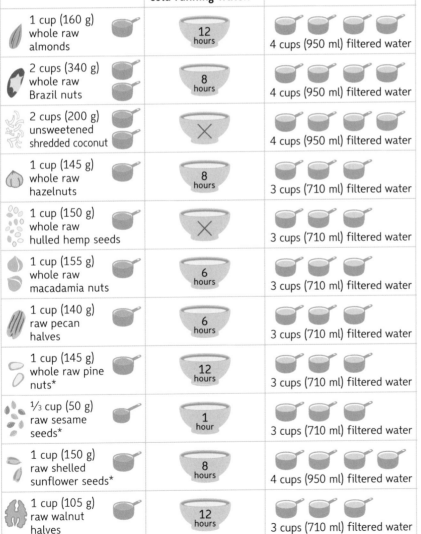

Nuts/seeds	Soak	Blend water
1 cup (160 g) whole raw almonds	12 hours	4 cups (950 ml) filtered water
2 cups (340 g) whole raw Brazil nuts	8 hours	4 cups (950 ml) filtered water
2 cups (200 g) unsweetened shredded coconut	✕	4 cups (950 ml) filtered water
1 cup (145 g) whole raw hazelnuts	8 hours	3 cups (710 ml) filtered water
1 cup (150 g) whole raw hulled hemp seeds	✕	3 cups (710 ml) filtered water
1 cup (155 g) whole raw macadamia nuts	6 hours	3 cups (710 ml) filtered water
1 cup (140 g) raw pecan halves	6 hours	3 cups (710 ml) filtered water
1 cup (145 g) whole raw pine nuts*	12 hours	3 cups (710 ml) filtered water
⅓ cup (50 g) raw sesame seeds*	1 hour	3 cups (710 ml) filtered water
1 cup (150 g) raw shelled sunflower seeds*	8 hours	4 cups (950 ml) filtered water
1 cup (105 g) raw walnut halves	12 hours	3 cups (710 ml) filtered water

MIX IT UP!

After straining, clean out the blender and return the strained milk to it. Then have fun adding flavors! I like to add:

- Alcohol-free stevia
- Cacao powder
- Finely ground gray sea salt
- Ground cinnamon
- Ground turmeric
- MCT oil
- Pumpkin pie spice
- Vanilla powder

These nuts/seeds are a bit too high in carbs for regular snacking, but when made into nut/seed milk and consumed sparingly, they can be a great addition to a ketogenic diet.

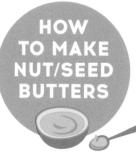

HOW TO MAKE NUT/SEED BUTTERS

STEP 1. FILL
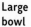

Place 2 cups (475 ml) warm filtered water in a large bowl.

Add ½ teaspoon salt. Stir until dissolved.

NOTE: *Coconut (shredded and whole) does not need to be soaked; go straight to Step 4.*

STEP 2. ADD

Add the nuts/seeds of your choice, in the quantity specified below. Make sure that the water completely covers the nuts/seeds.

STEP 3. SOAK & RINSE

Cover the bowl with a towel and let the nuts/seeds soak on the counter. After soaking, drain the liquid and rinse the nuts/seeds under cold running water.

STEP 4. ROAST

Set your dehydrator to 150°F (65°C) or oven to 275°F (135°C). Spread the nuts/seeds on a dehydrator sheet or bare rimmed baking sheet and dry for...

STEP 5. BLEND

Transfer the roasted nuts/seeds to a food processor fitted with the "S" blade or to a high-powered blender and process until smooth. Add your favorite oil if desired for smoothness and to increase the fat content. MCT oil is my personal favorite for nut/seed butter!

	SOAK	DEHYDRATOR	OVEN	BLEND
1 cup (160 g) whole raw almonds	12 hours	12 to 24 hours	20 to 30 minutes, rotating every 10 minutes, until fragrant	2 tablespoons oil
2 cups (340 g) whole raw Brazil nuts	8 hours	18 to 24 hours	30 to 40 minutes, rotating every 10 minutes, until fragrant	¼ cup (60 ml) oil
2 cups (200 g) unsweetened shredded coconut	✕		10 to 20 minutes, rotating every 5 minutes, until fragrant	¼ cup (60 ml) oil
Flesh from one whole coconut (600 g), sliced thin	✕	12 to 24 hours	20 to 30 minutes, rotating every 5 minutes, until fragrant	¾ cup (180 ml) oil
1 cup (145 g) whole raw hazelnuts	8 hours	12 to 24 hours	20 to 30 minutes, rotating every 10 minutes, until fragrant	2 tablespoons oil
1 cup (155 g) whole raw macadamia nuts	6 hours	12 to 24 hours	15 to 20 minutes, rotating every 5 minutes, until fragrant	2 tablespoons oil
1 cup (140 g) raw pecan halves	6 hours	12 to 24 hours	20 to 30 minutes, rotating every 5 minutes, until fragrant	2 tablespoons oil
⅓ cup (50 g) raw sesame seeds*	1 hour	8 to 12 hours	10 to 15 minutes, rotating every 5 minutes, until fragrant	1 teaspoon oil
1 cup (150 g) raw shelled sunflower seeds*	8 hours	8 to 12 hours	15 to 20 minutes, rotating every 10 minutes, until fragrant	2 tablespoons oil
1 cup (105 g) raw walnut halves	12 hours	12 to 24 hours	20 to 30 minutes, rotating every 5 minutes, until fragrant	2 tablespoons oil

*These seeds are a bit too high in carbs for regular snacking; they're best used in dressings, where only a tablespoon or so is used at a time.

 Hemp seeds make a great seed butter, but they don't need to be soaked or roasted—just put them in the blender! You can also add them to any of the nuts/seeds above just before blending.

Nut and Seed Butters

While you can purchase butters made from nuts and seeds, you can save a lot of money by making them yourself, and you'll know that they're free from added sugar and preservatives.

Because it's easy to consume a ton of nut/seed butter, it's important to make it from lower-carb nuts and seeds. The chart on page 144 gives the macronutrient information for a range of nuts and seeds.

Flax seeds and chia seeds don't do well on their own in a butter, but they make great additions to butters made from other seeds or nuts! Simply add 1 to 3 tablespoons of flax/chia seeds to your nut/seed butter just before blending.

HOW TO RENDER FATS (AND WHY YOU'D WANT TO)

Beef tallow, pure lard, leaf lard, duck fat—these are all rendered fats. Rendered fats are fabulous for high-heat cooking and baking, wonderful as replacements for butter, amazing on roasted veggies, and will add jaw-dropping richness to your favorite cookie recipe.

The act of rendering is, essentially, cooking down animal fat to a consumable state. I like to compare it to cooking bacon. Bacon comes complete with protein (the pink stripes) and fat (the white stripes). When you cook it, the protein remains, some of the fat gets crispy, and the rest of the fat renders into bacon grease—a rendered fat. When rendering fats, you're collecting the fats cooked down from bacon-like pieces of various animals, which can range from containing quite a lot of protein to having barely any or none at all.

You can purchase rendered fats from your favorite Paleo-friendly retailer, but you can also render them on your own. You're probably thinking, *Render my own fats? Leanne, are you insane?* It sounds complicated, and it took me over a year of eating keto to even become curious about rendering my own fats. Surprisingly, though, there isn't much to it. The hardest thing is finding high-quality fats to render. Once you've located a good source, it's a breeze.

NOTE: *Rendered animal fats are primarily saturated fats. For more on saturated fats, go to page 132.*

Rendered animal fats are best for cooking; they're not so great for cold uses, like salads.

Doing the Math

Saving money encourages me to do just about anything. In the case of rendered fats, there are big savings to be had, especially if you're on the path to boosting your fat intake.

The cost to render 14 ounces (360 g) of lard at home is $2.61. To purchase this amount already rendered costs around $11.44. The same is true for rendered tallow: to make 14 ounces (360 g) costs $3.07, while the purchase price for the same amount is $11.44.

Ready to save nearly 75 percent by rendering your own fats? When I say it like that, you really can't say no, can you?

Where to Find the Fat

This is the only piece of the fat-rendering puzzle that can get a little tricky. Your experience with locating a source of unrendered (raw) fat depends largely on your location.

You're looking for quality-conscious farmers, butchers, and suppliers who, ideally, don't care about the fat they throw away and will simply gift it to you, or at least sell it to you cheap. Your best bet is to do a quick internet search for "grass-fed butcher [your city]." The search should return the names of ranches, shops, and local cooperatives that are associated with grass-fed products.

Why should you care about the quality of the fat? Because toxins such as pesticides, hormones, and environmental pollutants are stored in fat cells, and these can affect your health. If you're going to be consuming a large amount of animal fat, it's important to know that it doesn't contain any dangerous compounds.

Here are some questions you can ask to determine whether the source you've contacted is the right fit for you. If they say "yes" or "not sure" to any of the following, it may be a sign that they're not the best option:

- **Are there GMO seeds in the animals' feed?**
- **Do you use antibiotics on any of the livestock?**
- **Do you use hormones on any of the livestock?**

Here are the keywords I use to find the highest-quality fats for rendering:

- **Lard:** *pasture-raised*
- **Beef or lamb fat:** *grass-fed, grass-finished*
- **Chicken or duck fat:** *corn-free, soy-free, free-range*

If you find a good source and they ask how they should prepare the fat for you, ask them to remove as much of the protein as possible. If they can make the pieces small, too, that will also help!

Use the rendered fat on roasted vegetables or meats or in stews, soups, or stir-fries.

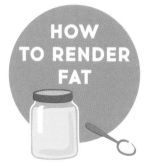

HOW TO RENDER FAT

There are two ways to render fat: the dry way and the wet way. I'm not a huge proponent of wet rendering, where water is added to the fat during the rendering process. I find that adding water dilutes the flavor of the end product, and if not done correctly, it can cause the fat to become rancid more quickly. The following tutorial is for the dry method.

Rendering fats can stink up your house. That's why I love using my pressure cooker for the job: it contains the smell during the rendering process.

CHOOSE 1 TO 2 POUNDS OF FAT → PREP THE FAT

Leaf lard	Lamb suet	Cut off all the protein.
Fatback (pure) lard	Schmaltz (chicken skin and fat)	Chop the fat into small pieces, ¼-inch (6 mm) or so.
Beef fat (preferably suet for the mildest flavor)	Duck fat	

RENDER

 PRESSURE COOKER: Place the fat pieces in the pressure cooker, lock the lid in place, and set to "slow cooker" mode, low setting if there's an option. Cook for 4 hours, or until the fat pieces rest in a layer at the bottom of the cooker and have turned golden to dark brown. Stir every hour or so.

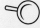 **SLOW COOKER:** Place the fat pieces in the slow cooker, add ¼ cup (60 ml) water, cover, and cook on low for 4 hours, or until the fat pieces rest in a layer at the bottom of the cooker and have turned golden to dark brown. Stir every hour or so.

 STOVETOP: In a large saucepan or frying pan, cook the fat pieces over medium-low heat for 1 to 2 hours, until crisp, rotating frequently.

OVEN: Preheat the oven to 250°F (120°C). Place the fat pieces on a lined rimmed baking sheet and cook for 1 to 2 hours, until crisp, rotating frequently.

STRAIN

Set a mesh strainer over a heatproof bowl.

Pour the rendered fat and crispy bits through the strainer into the bowl. This will strain the crispy bits from the rendered fat.

Allow the fat to cool slightly, but do not let it harden. Transfer the rendered fat to mason jars.

Allow the fat to cool completely, then cover. Store in the fridge for up to several weeks or in the freezer for up to 6 months.

I can't express how blessed I feel to have come across Leanne's website, HealthfulPursuit.com, and her books, especially Fat Fueled, *at the very beginning of my keto journey. The abundant information helped so much with making sure I embarked on this lifestyle in the most healthful, caring, and balanced way, keeping my health at the forefront of my actions.*

I was quite overweight and lost about 25–30 kg from eating a super healthy diet and training regimen. I started competing in bikini fitness competitions, lost my period, and became obsessed with prepping my meals and counting my macros. At the time, I was scared to eat out or socialize, and missing a prepped meal stressed me out. I haven't completely let go of tracking my macros, but I know I'm well on my way and feel so free being able to go hours without eating and stressing out, feeling full and satisfied, and being able to eat out and choose fat-fueled food easily. I'm so glad I read Fat Fueled *so I didn't let myself go to extremes and made sure I would carb up, eat when I was hungry, and not overdo fasting.*

Leanne, thank you so much. I can only imagine how hard it is to give every piece of knowledge to us in such a thorough, careful, and loving way. I love to listen to your audio books and podcasts whilst driving, cooking, and eating dinner instead of watching television. It makes me more aware of what I'm eating and helps me appreciate my food.

Zoe
Victoria, Australia

Leanne's programs have seriously changed my life. Before finding Leanne, I struggled for two years with general imbalanced health. I had brain fog, I couldn't concentrate, I started to gain weight that I couldn't get off, and I was tired all of the time. A doctor diagnosed me with ADD and I started medical treatment.

After two years of not feeling better, even on the medication, I found Leanne's YouTube channel and online programs, Fat Fueled *and* The Keto Beginning. *I began with* The Keto Beginning *and started to feel better, but something still wasn't right. This is when I purchased* Fat Fueled *and finally found myself a doctor who would listen.*

I was diagnosed with Hashimoto's thyroiditis, and although that's not the best news to receive, I knew exactly how to support it through Leanne's programs and information. I knew that I would be able to thrive with this disease.

A month after beginning the Fat Fueled program, I am feeling better than I have in a very long, long time. I can't thank Leanne enough.

Ashley
Arizona

CHAPTER 10
COOKING KETO: TIPS, TRICKS, AND STRATEGIES

No one believes me when I tell them that I don't enjoy cooking. Sure, I've created a successful business around cooking and meal prepping, but that doesn't mean I enjoy spending oodles of hours in the kitchen, especially in the summer, on weekends, after a long workday, on my birthday, when my toes are cold, when I have other plans...you get the idea. Basically, I would rather do anything other than waste away in my kitchen while everyone else is out doing fun things.

Once you've prepared a couple of the recipes in this book, you'll find that I cut corners, don't follow the rules, and use the path of least resistance to get us to the table and chowing down quickly. In this chapter, you'll find my best tips and tricks to help you do the same.

ONE-PAN MEALS

If there are days when you can't bear to follow a recipe or think of grocery shopping and you're fresh out of inspiration, I have a strategy to share with you. I call it the one-pan strategy, and I use it every day. If you follow me on Instagram (@healthfulpursuit), you know exactly what I mean.

This strategy is simple: throw everything in a bowl/pot/frying pan, wait ten to fifteen minutes, and you're eating. Ready to go through the basics? Let's do it.

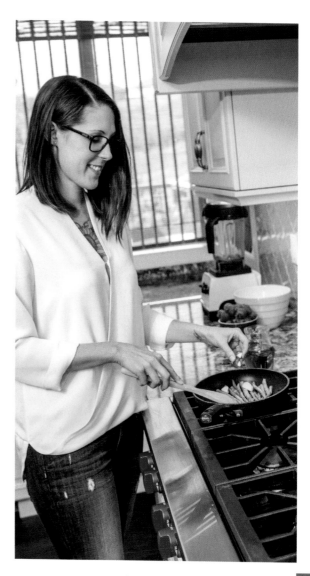

COOL BOWL	LEFTOVER PAN	WARM BOWL	GROUND PAN	ROASTED PAN
	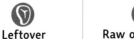			
Leftover cooked meat	Leftover cooked meat	Raw or cooked meat of any kind	Raw ground meat (defrosted if frozen)	Chicken thighs, chicken wings, fish fillets, or pork tenderloin
Raw or leftover cooked greens or low-carb vegetables	Fresh or frozen low-carb vegetables	Fresh or frozen low-carb vegetables	Fresh or frozen low-carb vegetables	Roasting-friendly vegetables, such as broccoli, cauliflower, carrots, radishes, or zucchini
Such as olive oil, avocado oil, nut oil, seed oil, nuts, or seeds	Heat-stable fat, such as lard, tallow, coconut oil, palm oil, or avocado oil	Heat-stable fat, such as lard, tallow, coconut oil, palm oil, or avocado oil	Heat-stable fat, such as lard, tallow, coconut oil, palm oil, or avocado oil	Melted heat-stable fat, such as lard, tallow, coconut oil, palm oil, or avocado oil
Such as vinegar, mayo, lemon juice, or your favorite herbs/spices	Your favorite herbs/spices	Bone broth or coconut milk (great for curry dishes), your favorite herbs/spices	Your favorite herbs/spices, vinegar, or lemon juice	Your favorite herbs/spices
Place everything in a bowl. Toss to combine and serve.	*Combine everything in a sauté pan or skillet. Cover and cook over medium heat for 10 minutes, until heated through.*	*Combine everything in a saucepan. Cover and bring to a boil over medium heat. Reduce the heat and simmer for 10 minutes, or until any raw meat is cooked through.*	*Cook the ground meat in a sauté pan or skillet over medium heat until only lightly pink. Add the vegetables, fat, and spices and cook for another 10 minutes, until the meat is fully cooked through.*	*Preheat the oven to 400°F (205°C). Toss the veggies in the melted fat and coat the meat with the spices. Place both veggies and meat in a cast-iron skillet and roast in the oven for 25 to 30 minutes, until the meat is cooked through.*
WINNING COMBO:	**WINNING COMBO:**	**WINNING COMBO:**	**WINNING COMBO:**	**WINNING COMBO:**
Chilled roasted chicken, mixed greens, leftover roasted broccoli, roasted walnuts, mayonnaise, lemon juice	*Chopped leftover burger patties, sliced cabbage, lard, salt, and pepper*	*Leftover cooked duck breast, Zoodles (page 376), chopped green onion, duck fat, chicken bone broth*	*Ground turkey, cremini mushrooms, celery, carrots, coconut oil, ground thyme, rosemary, sage*	*Chicken thighs coated in salt and pepper, carrots and cauliflower florets tossed in tallow*
Add sauerkraut or pickles to the mix! Have leftover vegetables? Add them, too.	Add freshness by making a cool bed for the heated mixture: Chop up your favorite low-carb vegetable (cucumbers are great) and toss with olive oil and vinegar. Serve the cooked mixture on top.	Anything goes! Have favorite salads or more complex dishes? Throw those ingredients in the pot and let the dish come to life.	Ground beef and horseradish: an awesome combination. You can thank me later.	Roasted Pans are delicious served with a large dollop of avocado oil mayo, either homemade (page 220) or store-bought (my favorite is from Primal Kitchen).

 Protein   *Veg*   *Fat*   *Extras*

TRICKS AND SHORTCUTS

I'm no master chef. I cut corners to save time, I refuse to fill my cupboards with kitchen paraphernalia I'll only use once, and I omit ingredients if they're too expensive. I hate spending more than thirty minutes (max!) on a recipe.

So, to meet all my requirements, I've developed some kitchen tricks. Now, I'm sure you've done some of these things, too—great minds—but I'm hoping some of these tips will light a bulb over your head and a fire in your belly!

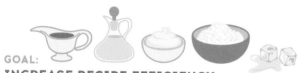

GOAL:
INCREASE RECIPE EFFICIENCY

ACTION:

Always have the following prepped and stored in the fridge or pantry to make preparing keto meals quick and easy!

- Mayonnaise (page 220)
- Infused Oil (page 228)
- Kickin' Ketchup (page 223)
- Cauliflower Rice (page 364)
- Chopped low-carb veggies *(Separate your veggies into what you like to cook and what you like to eat raw. I have one container filled with chopped veggies for salads and another with chopped veggies for stir-fries.)*
- Bone broth (page 151)

GOAL:
ADD MORE PROTEIN TO RECIPES

ACTION:

Stir in some collagen or gelatin.

Throw in an egg or three, or some ground chicken.

GOAL:
HEAT FOODS FAST

ACTION:

The verdict is out on whether microwaves are healthy or dangerous. But if I have a choice between using a microwave to heat my food and not eating because I don't have time to heat things up, you better believe I'll be using a microwave.

If you're reheating a liquid and you have a high-powered blender, you can heat it up in the blender! Just blend on high for about 2 minutes.

GOAL:
MAKE FAT BOMBS WITHOUT A FANCY SILICONE MOLD

ACTION:

Any fat bomb that requires chilling can be poured onto a silicone- or parchment paper–lined rimmed baking sheet—after it sets, just break it apart into serving-size pieces. Or you can use a silicone steaming dish, silicone ice cube tray, or silicone muffin mold.

GOAL:
MAKE RICED CAULIFLOWER

ACTION:

Break the head of cauliflower into florets. Run the florets through a handheld cheese grater or the grater attachment of your food processor. Store in the fridge or freezer.

GOAL:
SKIP THE MEAT THERMOMETER

ACTION:

For steak, use the touch test. (There are lots of comparisons out there; my favorite can be found at http://lifehacker.com/267250/determine-the-doneness-of-a-steak.)

For chicken, poke the thickest piece with a knife. If it's undercooked, the knife will come out wet and the juices will be pinkish; if it's cooked, the knife will come out only slightly damp. If it's very dry, it's overcooked. Nothing a little fat can't help!

GOAL:
END THE ONION TEARS

ACTION:

Stick a spoon in your mouth, keep your mouth open as you cut, or dice the onion in a bowl of water.

GOAL:
FIND A VINEGAR SUBSTITUTE

ACTION:

The juice from unpasteurized sauerkraut works great!

GOAL:
MAKE HARD-BOILED EGGS EASY TO PEEL

ACTION:

Add a splash of vinegar to the pot before boiling the water.

GOAL:
FIND CHEAP AIRTIGHT CONTAINERS

ACTION:

Use mason jars!

GOAL:
STOP THROWING AWAY MOLDY PRODUCE

ACTION:

GARLIC: Peel and freeze individual cloves, then mince directly from the freezer when ready to use.

GINGER AND TURMERIC: Freeze after purchase, then grate directly from the freezer when ready to use.

CUCUMBER: Slice and freeze. Flavor water by transferring it to a water bottle directly from the freezer.

GOAL:
SAVE TIME DURING FOOD PREP

ACTION:

Cut everything with scissors! This is especially handy for meat.

GOAL:
ROAST NUTS AND SEEDS FAST

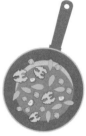

ACTION:

Place the nuts or seeds in a frying pan over medium heat and cook, rotating often, until they turn light golden.

GOAL:
MAKE ICED TEA FAST

ACTION:

Use half the amount of hot water you normally would. Let the tea steep for the prescribed time in a large heatproof jar. Add ice at 125 percent of the volume of water missing. For example, if you need another 1 cup (240 ml) of water, add 1¼ cups (175 g) of ice. Allow to melt and use in your favorite recipes, like Iced Omega Tea (page 420).

GOAL:
MAKE ROCKET FUEL LATTES LICKETY-SPLIT

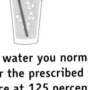

ACTION:

Once you've discovered your favorite way to enjoy an RFL (page 428), mix together all the ingredients but the coffee/tea in little jars or silicone molds. For the jars, refrigerate and scoop when ready to use. For the molds, freeze so that the mixture can pop out like an ice cube. When ready to make your drink, transfer the premixed ingredients to a blender along with the coffee/tea and blend!

CHAPTER 11 USING THE RECIPES

If you're new to keto, some of the ingredients used in the recipes in this book may seem foreign. But don't fret: while the ingredients may sound like they come from a far-off land, I can just about guarantee that you won't have trouble finding them, especially after reading the following pages. In this chapter, I'll guide you through the tools and ingredients used in the recipes. Let's go!

KITCHEN APPLIANCES AND TOOLS

The first kitchen tools I owned were a set of six pots and pans that my parents had received as a wedding gift eighteen years prior. It was one of those lead-filled enamel-coated sets. Hey, a girl's got to cook in something!

Funny enough, I still have about the same number of tools in my kitchen. I'm a minimalist when it comes to just about everything (except crafting supplies—I'm crazy about crafting supplies), but I've found that a handful of helpful tools make whole food–based ketogenic living that much sweeter. These tools aren't required, though. If you have a plate, a heat source, and a place to keep things cold, you'll be just fine. In fact, most nights all I use is a cutting board (and sometimes I skip that and cut right on the counter, which my husband loves), a knife, and my cast-iron pan. So you don't have to go all out, because I sure don't.

These are my favorite kitchen tools for making a healthful ketogenic life just a bit easier. But I've also included recommendations and strategies on making do without these tools, to save money and space in your kitchen.

⭐ - highly recommended

SPIRAL SLICER ⭐
Create delicious noodles from vegetables and fruits, from carrots to turnips to apples and everything in between.

COST:	GOING WITHOUT:
$$	Vegetable peeler

OPTIONS

KitchenAid stand mixer spiral slicer attachment: Place the produce in the prongs, turn on your mixer, and walk away.

COST:	TIME:	WASTE:	NOODLE SIZE/SHAPE:
$$$	Quickest	Minimal	Various

Inspiralizer: Place the produce in the machine and crank with your hand.

COST:	TIME:	WASTE:	NOODLE SIZE/SHAPE:
$$	Quick	Minimal	Various

Julienne peeler: Similar to a peeler, but with little teeth along the blade. Drag along the produce to create noodles.

COST:	TIME:	WASTE:	NOODLE SIZE/SHAPE:
$	Slow	Moderate	One option, creating slender, short noodles

Vegetable peeler: Grab the produce and start peeling!

COST:	TIME:	WASTE:	NOODLE SIZE/SHAPE:
$	Slowest	Moderate	One option, creates flat, wide noodles

Not mentioned, because they frustrate me and others: handheld spiral slicer and top-down spiral slicer.

Wondering which low-carb vegetables and fruit make the best noodles? Or how to use noodles in meals? Turn back to page 154!

NUT MILK BAG
For making your own nut and seed milks.

COST:	GOING WITHOUT:
$	A square of Swiss voile fabric or an unused nylon stocking (without a reinforced toe)

SILICONE MOLDS AND ICE CUBE TRAYS

Make a batch of bone broth and freeze it in cubes for fast access. Or make your favorite fat bomb in a fun heart-, star-, or flower-shaped silicone mold.

COST:	GOING WITHOUT:
$$$$	Instead of pouring the mixture into a silicone mold to harden/freeze, pour it into a rimmed baking sheet lined with parchment paper or a silicone mat.

CAST-IRON PAN ⭐

My cast-iron pan is my go-to cooking tool. Anything you want to cook, heat, or make crispy, cast iron will do it—and it can go straight into the oven!

COST:	GOING WITHOUT:
$$$$	Any pan will do; it just won't have the same crisp-ability and versatility.

Older cast iron is smoother and generally well seasoned. Look for used cast iron at thrift shops or garage sales; any kitchen supply store will sell new cast-iron pans.

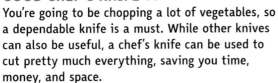

Keep your pan seasoned longer by cleaning it with coarse salt or a microfiber cloth instead of soap. Some people say that you can wash a well-seasoned cast-iron pan with soap without problems. If that's you, well done.

GOOD CHEF'S KNIFE ⭐

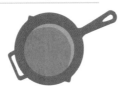

You're going to be chopping a lot of vegetables, so a dependable knife is a must. While other knives can also be useful, a chef's knife can be used to cut pretty much everything, saving you time, money, and space.

COST:	GOING WITHOUT:
$$$$	Any knife will do; just be careful, as dull blades aren't fun to cut with and can cause a disaster if you cut yourself (take it from someone who lost the tip of her thumb in a dull-knife accident).

ELECTRIC HANDHELD MILK FROTHER

For a frothy Rocket Fuel Latte (page 428) no matter where you are.

COST:	GOING WITHOUT: Heat-safe shaker
$$$$	bottle or airtight travel mug

NOTE: *Traveling is probably the only time you'll use your milk frother. See page 84 for tips on making RFLs while traveling.*

IMMERSION BLENDER

For making the perfect batch of homemade mayo (page 220). Also fabulous for a smooth RFL (page 428).

COST:	GOING WITHOUT:
$$$$	Whisk, high-powered blender, or food processor

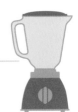

HIGH-POWERED BLENDER ⭐

For making salad dressing (pages 224 to 227), pâté (pages 258 and 259), and smooth RFL (page 428). Less messy and higher-capacity than a regular blender.

COST:	GOING WITHOUT:
$$$$	Whisk, immersion blender, standard blender, or food processor

If you add whole nuts or seeds to your RFL, a high-powered blender makes the final mixture perfectly smooth.

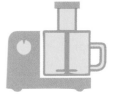

FOOD PROCESSOR

Make the smoothest nut butter, grate cauliflower with ease, and pulse soaked/roasted nuts and seeds into flour.

COST:	GOING WITHOUT:
$$$$	High-powered blender or hand grater

If you have a food processor, there is no need for a mandoline! Many food processors come with attachments that perform many of the same tasks.

If you have a high-powered blender, you may not need a food processor. The only time you'll struggle is when you want to make epic batches of grated cauliflower for cauliflower rice (page 364), but a hand grater will do the trick, and it's a good workout, too!

MULTI-COOKER ⭐

It sautés, it pressure-cooks, it slow-cooks, and it can create a meal in under 20 minutes. Plus, rendering fats is a cinch! Sometimes these are called pressure cookers; look for one that has multiple settings.

COST:	GOING WITHOUT:
$$$$	Slow cooker (or just cook on the stovetop)

INGREDIENTS

If you're wondering which brands of ingredients I used in the recipes in this book, or you need some tips on working with unfamiliar ingredients, the following pages are for you.

ALMOND BUTTER: I enjoy using almond butter as a base for sauces, dressings, and dips. It's also a fabulous replacement for flour in baked goods, like my Crusty Sandwich Bread (page 366). My favorite brands are Artisana, Barney Butter, Justin's, and Kirkland. If a recipe specifically calls for smooth almond butter, Barney Butter Bare Smooth is my go-to.

ALMOND FLOUR: Blanched and finely ground. My favorite brands are Barney Butter, Bob's Red Mill, and JK Gourmet.

APPLE CIDER VINEGAR: Purchase the raw/unpasteurized, unfiltered version. My favorite is from Bragg.

AVOCADO: A large Hass avocado with skin and pit weighs about 8 ounces (225 g). With the skin and pit removed, the flesh of one avocado measures 6 ounces (170 g); this is what I used in all my recipes.

AVOCADO OIL: Best for cooking with high heat while adding minimal flavor. My favorite is from Primal Kitchen. While you can purchase unrefined avocado oil, I dislike the flavor, so I choose not to prepare recipes with it. For information about heat stability, see page 138.

BACON: Uncured, sugar-free bacon is the best! Purchase it at any health food store. If you can't find uncured and sugar-free bacon, look for hormone-free bacon with as little sugar/carbs as possible.

BACON GREASE: After cooking bacon, simply drain the fat into a heatproof jar and store it on the counter for a couple of days. For information about heat stability, see page 138.

BEEF: Purchase grass-fed and grass-finished beef. My favorite place to get high-quality animal proteins is ButcherBox. (For more on meat quality, see page 110.) For the recipes in this book, I used ground beef with a fat content of 25 percent. If you want to replicate the nutritional information cited for a recipe exactly, you can ask your butcher to prepare ground beef for you that has exactly 25 percent fat. Otherwise, look for the fat content on the label.

BONE BROTH: Homemade bone broth is best (see page 151), but if you don't have the time or energy to make it yourself, my favorite store-bought brands are EPIC, Kettle & Fire, Osso Bueno, and Pacific Natural Foods. I used unsalted broth in all the recipes in this book.

CACAO BUTTER: The fat from chocolate, perfect for fat bombs. My favorites are from Divine Organics, Earth Circle Organics, Giddy YoYo, Healthworks, Sunfood, and Wild Foods Co. For information about heat stability, see page 138.

CACAO NIBS: Little pieces of cacao beans that have been dried, fermented, roasted, or a combination of the three. Their texture is similar to that of coffee beans, and the chocolate flavor is very strong. I enjoy sprinkling cacao nibs on Coconut Whipped Cream (page 414). My favorite brands are Earth Circle, Healthworks, and Wild Foods Co.

CACAO POWDER: A raw form of cocoa powder that has a lot more flavor. You can find it at most grocery stores. My favorite brands are Earth Circle Organics, Giddy YoYo, Healthworks, Thrive Market, and Wild Foods Co.

CANNED SEAFOOD (anchovies, sardines, oysters, and salmon): The thing to watch out for with canned seafood products is what they're packed in. Opt for seafood packed in extra-virgin or virgin olive oil, not highly processed oils such as sunflower or safflower oil. My favorite brands are Crown Prince, Safe Catch, Sea Fare Pacific, and Wild Planet.

CANOLA OIL: For details on why it's safe to consume organic, cold-pressed, unrefined canola oil—though only sparingly—see page 136. My favorite brand is Maison Orphée.

CAULIFLOWER: A large head of cauliflower measures about 1¾ pounds (780 g) in all my recipes. If the cauliflower is further broken up into florets or riced, both the weight and the volume are listed. Some of the recipes in this book call for riced cauliflower, florets that have been grated to resemble rice. Many stores, such as Trader Joe's, sell bags of frozen riced cauliflower. Alternatively, you can make your own: see page 163.

CHIA SEEDS, WHOLE AND GROUND: Black or white seeds that are rich in omega-3 fatty acids. When using them in cooking, do not expose them to temperatures higher than 350°F (177°C). They can be purchased whole and then ground in a blender, food processor, or spice/coffee grinder. Alternatively, you can buy them ground for baking. Whole chia seeds are great for making chia pudding. My favorite whole chia seeds are from Bob's Red Mill and Navitas Naturals.

CHICKEN FAT (SCHMALTZ): My favorite is from Fatworks. To render chicken fat at home, see page 159. For info about heat stability, see page 138.

CHOCOLATE BARS / CHOCOLATE CHIPS / BAKING CHOCOLATE: For your baking pursuits, use chocolate that's unsweetened or sweetened with a mixture of stevia or erythritol. My favorites are Ghirardelli Baking Bar and Lily's Sweets Baking Chips and Baking Bars.

COCONUT AMINOS: A tasty soy sauce replacement! My favorite brand is Coconut Secret.

COCONUT BUTTER: Coconut butter is to coconuts as peanut butter is to peanuts; it's ground coconut meat. You can find it at many grocery stores in the ethnic or natural foods section. My favorite is from Artisana.

COCONUT CREAM: Purchase in cans labeled "coconut cream"; if you can't find these, purchase a can of full-fat coconut milk and place it in the fridge for at least 24 hours. Then flip the can upside down, open it halfway, and let the liquid drain out. Use the remaining coconut cream in your recipe. My favorite brand is Aroy-D.

COCONUT FLOUR: Dehydrated and finely ground coconut. My favorites are from Bob's Red Mill and Let's Do Organic.

COCONUT MILK, FULL-FAT AND LITE: Full-fat is where it's at! But sometimes you want a little less fat so that the milk is more versatile—say, in a bowl of granola (page 246). Both products can be found in cans or Tetra Pak cartons, often in the nondairy milk, ethnic, or natural foods section of the grocery store. For full-fat, my favorite brands are Aroy-D, Native Forest, and Real Thai, and for lite, Aroy-D.

COCONUT OIL: Coconut oil is to coconuts as olive oil is to olives; it's oil that is pressed from coconut meat. Opt for unrefined versions from the first cold-pressing of organic coconuts. My favorite brands are Healthworks, Kirkland Organic, NOW Foods, Nutiva, and Thrive Market. For info on heat stability, see page 138. Some of my recipes call for butter-infused coconut oil, which is coconut oil that's infused with all-natural, vegan, keto-friendly plants and extracts to mimic the taste of butter. My favorite brand of butter-infused coconut oil is Ellyndale Organics. And for coconut oil spray that's free from chemical propellants and other harmful ingredients, I prefer Chosen Foods brand.

COCONUT, SHREDDED: Always go for the unsweetened variety. I like the longer shreds because they are more versatile: if you need smaller shreds, you can simply grind the coconut in a spice/coffee grinder, blender, or food processor. My favorite brands are Bob's Red Mill and Thrive Market.

COLLAGEN PEPTIDES: The most abundant protein in the body and a natural, high-quality supplement for every day. It's a white powder that dissolves completely into hot or cold liquids. My favorite brand is Vital Proteins.

CUCUMBER: I use English cucumbers. Unless otherwise specified, use large ones, which weigh about 15 ounces (430 g).

DUCK FAT: Rendered duck fat can be found at most health food stores. My favorite is from EPIC. For rendering duck fat at home, see page 159. For information about heat stability, see page 138.

EGGS: Some recipes call for the use of raw eggs, which does carry some risk of salmonella. If you're not down with that plan—and if you're pregnant or children will be eating the dish, there's extra reason to be cautious—please skip the recipe or omit the raw eggs. I purchase my eggs locally, and they're from free-range hens that are fed no corn or soy, and I've had no problems consuming these eggs raw.

ERYTHRITOL: A sugar alcohol with a taste that is bang-on to table sugar. My favorite erythritol is from Swerve. I use the confectioners' style because it's smooth, which works beautifully in fat bombs, and it's versatile for making baked treats. (For more on sweeteners, see page 118.) However, if you have a corn allergy or are FODMAP sensitive, it's better to use stevia.

FERMENTED FOODS (kimchi, sauerkraut, kefir, and more): As great as homemade fermented foods are, you'll never see me making my own—I just don't have the time! My favorite brands are Bubbies for pickles and sauerkraut, Wildbrine for kimchi, and KeVita for water kefir. If you're looking to ferment your own vegetables, the word on the street is that Body Ecology and Caldwell Bio Fermentation have great fermentation starters.

FLAX SEEDS, WHOLE AND GROUND: Brown or golden seeds that are high in omega-3 fatty acids. For baking, do not exceed 350°F (177°C). Flax seeds can be purchased whole and then ground in a blender, food processor, or spice/coffee grinder. Alternatively, you can buy them ground. I rarely use flax seeds in their whole form, but I like to purchase them whole and grind them myself because preground have a risk of oxidation. My favorite brands are Bob's Red Mill and NOW Foods.

GELATIN, UNFLAVORED: Similar to collagen but even better for gut health. This white powder can be added to hot liquids; if you want to use it in a chilled liquid, it needs to be added while the liquid is still hot (see, for instance, the Iced Tea Lemonade Gummies on page 406). My favorite brand is Vital Proteins.

GHEE: Clarified butter with the milk solids removed. Ghee is naturally whey-free and should be casein- and lactose-free as well—but, depending on how it's processed, most ghee contains some casein and lactose. If you are sensitive to dairy or react to histamines, it may be better to steer clear. My favorite allergy-friendly ghee brands are Fourth & Heart and Tin Star Foods.

HEMP SEEDS, HULLED: Also known as hemp hearts, these are my favorite low-carb, vegan-friendly protein. My favorites are from Manitoba Harvest, which you can find at most grocery stores.

LAMB: Opt for pasture-raised lamb. For more on meat quality, see page 110.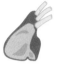

LARD: Rendered pork fat. Lard can be purchased at many health food stores; my favorite is from EPIC. You can also make it at home; see page 159. For information about heat stability, see page 138.

LEMON JUICE: I like to use freshly squeezed lemon juice, but you can use store-bought if you prefer. If you're out of lemon juice, an equal amount of apple cider vinegar is often a good alternative.

MAYONNAISE: You can make your own mayo (see page 220) or purchase avocado oil mayonnaise, which is rich in health-promoting fats. Stay away from vegetable oil–based mayonnaise. My favorite avocado oil mayonnaise is from Primal Kitchen.

MCT OIL: A healthy ketone-boosting oil—for details, see page 140. Bulletproof Brain Octane is 100 percent C8 MCT oil, which converts to ketones faster, making it my all-time favorite MCT oil. However, it's also expensive, and NOW Foods MCT is a great alternative, although it contains a combination of C8 and C10 MCTs. For information about heat stability, see page 139. While coconut oil is not as powerful for boosting ketones, it can be used in place of MCT oil.

MUSTARD, DIJON: Surprisingly, many mustards contain sugar, alcohol, and other odd ingredients. Check the labels to find one without these ingredients—my favorite brand is Annie's Naturals. If you're following a low-FODMAP diet, mixing ground mustard seeds with a bit of water is the best way to go.

NONDAIRY MILK: Not milk in the traditional sense; these products are made by combining nuts, seeds, or coconut with water to produce a milk-like beverage. (See page 155 for how to make your own nut/seed milks.) When a recipe calls for nondairy milk, go for an unsweetened, unflavored milk, such as almond milk or lite coconut milk. My favorites are almond milk from MALK and New Barn and lite coconut milk from Aroy-D.

NONDAIRY YOGURT: Yogurt made from nondairy sources. Coyo brand yogurt is hands down the tastiest yogurt, and it just so happens to be dairy-free and keto-friendly.

NUTRITIONAL YEAST: Deactivated yeast that has a strong nutty, cheesy flavor, perfect for making dairy-free "cheese" sauce! It can be found at most grocery stores and health food stores. My favorite brands are Bob's Red Mill and NOW Foods.

NUT BUTTER (Brazil nut, cashew, macadamia, pecan, walnut, etc.): *See also* almond butter. A wonderful accompaniment for a keto diet, and great on a spoon straight from the jar. My favorite brands are Artisana and Dastony Organics. See page 157 for how to make nut and seed butters.

NUTS (almonds, Brazil nuts, cashews, pecans, pine nuts, walnuts, etc.): For health reasons, it's best to soak and/or roast nuts before consuming them (see page 157). My favorite brands of raw nuts are Barney Butter, Kirkland, NOW Foods, and Thrive Market.

OLIVE OIL: I use extra-virgin olive oil in most recipes where a light flavor is preferred (or at least is compatible with the recipe). The only time I use refined olive oil is to make mayonnaise (page 220). For an explanation of the different terms used to describe olive oil, see page 137. For information about heat stability, see page 139. A few of my recipes call for butter-infused olive oil, which is olive oil that's been infused with all-natural, vegan, gluten-free, keto-friendly plants and extracts to mimic the taste of butter. It can be found at most oil bars and specialty shops. My favorite olive oils are from Kasandrinos.

OLIVES: The best olives are packed in extra-virgin or virgin olive oil, or in water with a touch of salt. That's it! My favorite brands are Lindsay Olives and Mario Camacho Foods.

PALM OIL: There are two forms of palm oil: red palm oil and palm kernel oil. Red palm oil is extracted from the fruit of the oil palm tree and is rich in vitamins A and E. Palm kernel oil comes from the seed of the palm tree, does not have the same nutrient profile, and contains far more saturated fat. I recommend red palm oil for its nutrients. When purchasing, look for ethically sourced, organic red palm oil, and be wary of oils produced in Southeast Asia, where there is a higher likelihood that the production of palm oil may disrupt orangutan habitats. My favorite brand of red palm oil is Nutiva.

PEPPERONI/SAUSAGE: Finding dairy-free, gluten-free pepperoni that doesn't contain added gunk or artificial junk and actually tastes good is a difficult feat. My favorite carb-free, grass-fed, fully cooked sausages, which can be used in place of pepperoni in recipes, are from Paleovalley.

PORK: Choose pasture-raised pork. My favorite is from ButcherBox. For more on meat quality, see page 110.

PORK RINDS: Fried pork skin. There are a lot of poor-quality pork rinds made with questionable oils, so read labels and choose your brand carefully. My favorite is Bacon's Heir.

POULTRY: Purchase soy-free, corn-free, free-range poultry. My favorite is from ButcherBox. For more on meat quality, see page 110.

PROTEIN POWDER: See pages 125 to 127 for details on protein powder. For drink recipes that call for protein powder, I recommend using collagen in cold drinks and gelatin in hot beverages. Bone broth protein also mixes well into liquids, but it does lend a taste to the finished drink.

SALAD DRESSINGS: Homemade dressing is always best (see the recipes on pages 224 to 227), but for store-bought, my go-to brand of keto-friendly dressings is Primal Kitchen.

SEAFOOD: Look for ethically sourced fish—read more on page 111.

SEA SALT, FINELY GROUND GRAY: In most of my recipes, I use finely ground gray sea salt; my favorites are from Real Salt and San Francisco Salt Company. However, I like to use Himalayan rock salt (also referred to as pink salt) in drinks because it has a milder flavor.

SEED BUTTER (hemp, pumpkin, sunflower, etc.): If you're baking with seed butter, look for smooth varieties with no added sugar or vegetable oils. My favorite brands are Dastony Organics, Maranatha, and SunButter. See page 157 for how to make your own nut and seed butters.

SEEDS (pumpkin, sesame, sunflower, etc.): For health reasons, it's best to soak and/ or roast seeds before consuming them (see page 157). My favorite brand of seeds is NOW Foods.

SPICES AND SPICE BLENDS: Combine individual spices and herbs to make your own spice blends (see pages 232 to 235), or purchase the mixes. My favorite brand is Simply Organic.

STEVIA, LIQUID: There are a lot of nasty-tasting stevia products out there, but I've found high-quality ones that make a great replacement for xylitol or erythritol in low-carb baking if you're sensitive to FODMAPs. My favorite is stevia glycerite from NOW Foods. It's alcohol-free and doesn't have a metallic aftertaste like other stevia products. For more on sweeteners, see page 118.

TAHINI: This sesame seed paste is a staple in my kitchen for its versatility and ease of use. My favorite brands are Artisana and Once Again.

TALLOW: Rendered beef fat. It can be purchased at many health food stores; my favorite is from EPIC. You can also make it at home; see page 159. For information about heat stability, see page 138.

VANILLA EXTRACT OR POWDER: These two forms of vanilla can be used interchangeably, in equal amounts. In no-bake goods, I like to use alcohol-free vanilla extract so it doesn't lend a taste of alcohol. My favorite brand of extract is Simply Organic. Vanilla powder is simply ground vanilla beans, and its flavor is pure and delicious! My favorite powder is from Wild Foods.

WINE, RED OR WHITE: Wine is optional, but it adds flavor with minimal carbohydrates, as most of the alcohol burns off during cooking.

XYLITOL: A sugar alcohol generally sourced from birch, although you can also find xylitol made from squash. If you're sensitive to FODMAPs, you may do better with stevia. Unlike stevia and erythritol, xylitol contributes to the carbohydrate content of a dish. It can be found at most grocery stores. My favorite brands are NOW Foods (birch), Xyla (birch), and Pumpkin Pure (kabocha squash). For more on sweeteners, see page 118.

ZUCCHINI: A medium zucchini measures 7 ounces (200 g) in the recipes in the book.

MAKING SENSE OF THE RECIPES

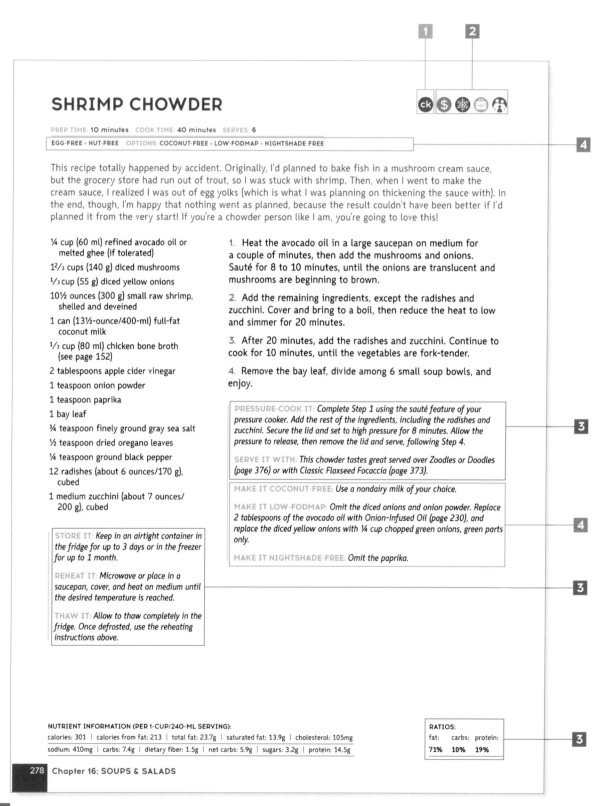

SHRIMP CHOWDER

PREP TIME: **10 minutes**   COOK TIME: **40 minutes**   SERVES: **6**

EGG-FREE • NUT-FREE   OPTIONS: COCONUT-FREE • LOW-FODMAP • NIGHTSHADE-FREE

This recipe totally happened by accident. Originally, I'd planned to bake fish in a mushroom cream sauce, but the grocery store had run out of trout, so I was stuck with shrimp. Then, when I went to make the cream sauce, I realized I was out of egg yolks (which is what I was planning on thickening the sauce with). In the end, though, I'm happy that nothing went as planned, because the result couldn't have been better if I'd planned it from the very start! If you're a chowder person like I am, you're going to love this!

¼ cup (60 ml) refined avocado oil or melted ghee (if tolerated)

1²⁄₃ cups (140 g) diced mushrooms

⅓ cup (55 g) diced yellow onions

10½ ounces (300 g) small raw shrimp, shelled and deveined

1 can (13½-ounce/400-ml) full-fat coconut milk

⅓ cup (80 ml) chicken bone broth (see page 152)

2 tablespoons apple cider vinegar

1 teaspoon onion powder

1 teaspoon paprika

1 bay leaf

¾ teaspoon finely ground gray sea salt

½ teaspoon dried oregano leaves

¼ teaspoon ground black pepper

12 radishes (about 6 ounces/170 g), cubed

1 medium zucchini (about 7 ounces/ 200 g), cubed

1. Heat the avocado oil in a large saucepan on medium for a couple of minutes, then add the mushrooms and onions. Sauté for 8 to 10 minutes, until the onions are translucent and mushrooms are beginning to brown.

2. Add the remaining ingredients, except the radishes and zucchini. Cover and bring to a boil, then reduce the heat to low and simmer for 20 minutes.

3. After 20 minutes, add the radishes and zucchini. Continue to cook for 10 minutes, until the vegetables are fork-tender.

4. Remove the bay leaf, divide among 6 small soup bowls, and enjoy.

PRESSURE-COOK IT: *Complete Step 1 using the sauté feature of your pressure cooker. Add the rest of the ingredients, including the radishes and zucchini. Secure the lid and set to high pressure for 8 minutes. Allow the pressure to release, then remove the lid and serve, following Step 4.*

SERVE IT WITH: *This chowder tastes great served over Zoodles or Doodles (page 376) or with Classic Flaxseed Focaccia (page 373).*

MAKE IT COCONUT-FREE: *Use a nondairy milk of your choice.*

MAKE IT LOW-FODMAP: *Omit the diced onions and onion powder. Replace 2 tablespoons of the avocado oil with Onion-Infused Oil (page 230), and replace the diced yellow onions with ¼ cup chopped green onions, green parts only.*

MAKE IT NIGHTSHADE-FREE: *Omit the paprika.*

STORE IT: *Keep in an airtight container in the fridge for up to 3 days or in the freezer for up to 1 month.*

REHEAT IT: *Microwave or place in a saucepan, cover, and heat on medium until the desired temperature is reached.*

THAW IT: *Allow to thaw completely in the fridge. Once defrosted, use the reheating instructions above.*

NUTRIENT INFORMATION (PER 1-CUP/240-ML SERVING):
calories: 301 | calories from fat: 213 | total fat: 23.7g | saturated fat: 13.9g | cholesterol: 105mg
sodium: 410mg | carbs: 7.4g | dietary fiber: 1.5g | net carbs: 5.9g | sugars: 3.2g | protein: 14.5g

RATIOS:
fat:	carbs:	protein:
71%	10%	19%

278 Chapter 16: SOUPS & SALADS

1. FAT FUELED PROFILES

Indicates which Fat Fueled Profiles the recipe falls under.

 CLASSIC KETO:
Contains at least 65 percent fat and has 10 percent carbs or less.

 PUMPED KETO:
Contains at least 30 percent protein.

 FAT BOMB/GREAT FOR ADAPTING:
Contains at least 85 percent fat.

3. INSTRUCTIONS

• **STORE IT:**
Info on how to store the dish in the fridge, in the freezer (if applicable), or on the counter.

• **THAW IT:**
Info on how to thaw a freezer-safe dish or prepare it from its frozen state.

• **REHEAT IT:**
Info on how to reheat the dish, if applicable.

• **PREP AHEAD:**
Tips for reducing prep time by planning ahead.

• **PRESSURE-COOK IT:**
Instructions for preparing the recipe in a pressure cooker.

• **SERVE IT WITH:**
Suggestions for making the recipe a complete meal by pairing it with a couple of easy additions or other recipes from this book.

• **RATIOS:**
The ratio of fat, carbs, and protein, using total (not net) carbohydrate count.

 MAKE IT A CARB-UP:
Instructions for adapting the recipe for a Full Keto, Adapted Fat Burner, or Daily Fat Burner carb-up. When carbs are introduced to a recipe, fat is reduced accordingly, which will change the flavor of the dish. Carb-up suggestions can be found on page 117.

MEASURING PRODUCE

In the ingredient lists of the recipes, weight isn't usually listed for whole produce. Instead, I've provided size descriptors to help with shopping. However, if the item is chopped or the weight can vary from country to country, I've included the weight of the item to assist with recipe preparation.

2. FEATURES

Outlines important features of the recipe.

 BUDGET-FRIENDLY:
Costs less than $3 per serving.

 FREEZER-SAFE:
Can be made and stored in the freezer for later use.

LUNCH-FRIENDLY:
Won't get soggy and can be enjoyed lukewarm or cold. Best stored in a thermal lunch kit. Store warm drinks in a Thermos or S'well water bottle.

 FAMILY-FRIENDLY:
Makes at least four servings.

 QUICKIES:
Ready in ten minutes or less, from start to delicious finish.

4. DIETARY

Info for those with food sensitivities and allergy concerns. If a recipe can be made without a particular ingredient, it will be listed after the word option, *and details about how to adapt the recipe will appear at the bottom of the page.*

• **COCONUT-FREE:**
Does not contain coconut or its derivatives.

• **EGG-FREE:**
Does not contain eggs.

• **NIGHTSHADE-FREE:**
Does not contain nightshades.

• **NUT-FREE:**
Does not contain nuts. (Coconut is not considered a nut.)

• **LOW-FODMAP:**
Is low in FODMAPs. However, if you are severely sensitive to FODMAPs, look over the recipe carefully, as items such as coconut milk have been placed in the "safe" category if ½ cup (120 ml) or less is consumed per serving. The FODMAP rating for nutritional yeast is unknown, so it is marked as safe in this book, and avocado is considered safe at ⅛ avocado per serving.

• **VEGETARIAN:**
Is lacto-ovo vegetarian.

• **VEGAN:**
Is free of all animal products.

When I began eating keto, not only was I clueless about how to add more fat to recipes (I've got you covered there with the recipes in this book), but I also couldn't figure out how to eat enough fat or plan my meals efficiently. More often than not, I found myself slathering mayo on chicken thighs and calling it lunch and dinner. Boring! Had I been given a meal plan, figuring out how to make keto work for me would have been a lot less painful and a bunch more enjoyable.

THE FAT FUELED PROFILES

The five different meal plans take you through 28 days of each of the five Fat Fueled Profiles.

The **Classic Keto** plan (used to become fat-adapted) is different from the **Full Keto** and **Adapted Fat Burner** plans, meaning that once you're adapted, you can switch to Full Keto (one carb-up a week) or Adapted Fat Burner (about two carb-ups a week) without repeating meals for another 28 days.

The **Classic Keto** (no carb-ups) and **Daily Fat Burner** (daily carb-ups) plans are similar, so if you're working to become fat-adapted with the Classic Keto plan and decide that following a plan that excludes carb-ups doesn't work for your body, you can switch to a plan that has carb-ups without having to do a massive amount of shopping.

The **Pumped Keto** plan is in a league of its own, showing you how to make a higher-protein keto plan work from day to day.

After you've followed the plans for a while, remember that your body is in the driver's seat and will tell you if it needs more food, is getting too much food, doesn't like certain aspects of the plan, and so on. Listen to your body! These meal plans

are templates to get you in the groove, but you don't have to follow them to achieve "success."

LEFTOVERS

I've set up these meal plans to make things as easy as possible for you. They make generous use of leftovers, for example; recipes marked as *"Leftover"* aren't being made from scratch. You'll find numbered notes at the bottom of the plans telling you to freeze or refrigerate servings for use later in the plan.

A handful of the recipes used as leftovers call for perishable ingredients that can't be frozen, such as endive for the Bombay Sloppy Jolenes. For those recipes, the amount of perishables called for in the weekly shopping list has been reduced to just what's needed for that week. And there are some recipes that yield extra leftovers not used in the plan, which you'll find listed at the end of the plan. These leftover meals are great to share with loved ones, when you need extra food throughout your week, or to help you create your week 5 plan.

FOOD INTAKE AND TIMING

Each plan is meant to feed one person. If you have more mouths to feed, simply multiply the recipes and shopping lists by the number of people eating.

To help you avoid plateaus, macros and calorie intake vary from day to day. When you first start eating keto, you may find that you're overly hungry. Many of the plans compensate with a higher food intake when you first get started, decreasing it as your body adjusts.

If you need to add more food to your day, the first page of each meal plan comes complete with notes on how to add more food easily and effortlessly.

If you're not hungry for a meal, simply freeze that portion, offer it to a friend, or move that meal to the next day. The nutrition information and macro calculations are based on the assumption that all of the meals planned for the day, including snacks, are eaten.

If you prefer to eat only two meals per day, you can easily combine the day's meals as you like (although there are days that call for only two meals; see pages 68 to 72 for more on the practice of intermittent fasting).

KETO DRINKS

Keto Lemonade (page 422) has been sprinkled throughout some of the plans. If you are new to the keto diet, it's highly advisable that you prepare this recipe daily and have it on hand as you go through the adaption process. **Rocket Fuel Lattes** make frequent appearances as well; when RFL is called for in the plan, it is assumed that you will consume the full 16 fl. oz./475 ml as one serving. I highly doubt you'll have a hard time chugging it down.

SHOPPING LISTS

The shopping lists are arranged by category: fresh produce; meat, eggs, and broth; fats and oils; dried herbs and spices; and pantry items, such as flours and vinegars. **Salt and pepper** are not included since most people have these essential ingredients on hand at all times. I have assumed that you will be buying **bone broth and mayonnaise** for use in the meal plans; if you prefer to make these recipe components at home, you'll need to visit the recipe page and add those ingredients to your shopping list for the week. I've also assumed that you will either purchase **spice mixes** like Italian seasoning or have them prepared in advance, since they keep in the pantry for a long time.

For the sake of simplicity, when a recipe gives alternate ingredient choices, such as "3 tablespoons avocado oil or extra-virgin olive oil," the shopping lists include just the most common option (usually the first choice listed). To view alternate choices, visit the recipe page.

Finally, remember that if you have **food sensitivites,** you will need to adjust the shopping lists to accommodate any modifications made to the recipes.

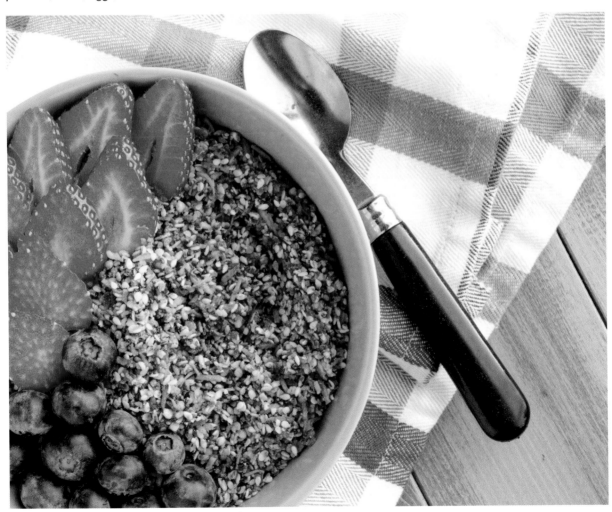

ck

WEEK 1

PATH 1
CLASSIC KETO

This plan is for the Classic Keto Fat Fueled Profile (find out more on page 47). Whether you're new to keto or an avid veteran, this plan will provide you with some variety in your high-fat life. Follow this plan until you're fat-adapted (see pages 63 to 65 for more on how to tell whether you are fat-adapted) before switching to the Full Keto or Adapted Fat Burner meal plan.

Not enough food for you? The simplest way to add bulk to the meals without having to worry about affecting your macros is to increase the fat in your Rocket Fuel Latte (RFL), whip up a fat bomb (see the chart beginning on page 432) and enjoy it after a meal, or double up on serving sizes, doubling the recipes as needed.

SHOPPING LIST FOR WEEK 1

FRESH PRODUCE

arugula, 2½ oz. (70 g)
avocado, Hass, 1 large
basil, ½ small bunch
cauliflower, 1 large head
celery, 1 small stalk
chives, 1 small bunch
cilantro, 1 small bunch
dill, ¾ tsp finely chopped
garlic, 1 clove
ginger root, 1½-inch (3.75-cm) piece
lemons, 9, plus 5 optional *(for lemonade and Hamburger Dinner)*
lime, 1
mint, 4 sprigs *(optional, for lemonade)*
onion, white, ¼
onions, green, 4
parsley, 1 small bunch
spinach, 5 oz. (140 g)
turmeric root, 9-inch (23-cm) piece

MEAT, EGGS, AND BROTH

anchovy fillets, 2 (0.4 oz./13 g)
bacon, 13 oz. (370 g)
bacon, preferably thick-cut, 13 oz. (370 g)
beef broth, ½ cup plus 2 Tbsp (5 fl. oz./ 150 ml) *(If making homemade broth, see page 152 for ingredients.)*
chicken thighs, boneless, skinless, ¾ lb (340 g)
eggs, 1 dozen large
ground beef, 20% to 30% fat, 1 lb (455 g)
pork shoulder blade chops (aka shoulder chops, blade steaks, or pork shoulder steaks), bone-in, about ½ inch (1.25 cm) thick, 1¼ lbs (600 g)

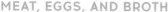

FATS AND OILS

avocado oil, refined, 4½ Tbsp
cacao butter, ½ cup (120 g)
coconut oil, ½ cup (105 g)
lard, 2 Tbsp, plus more for the pans
mayonnaise, made with avocado oil, ¼ cup plus 1 Tbsp (65 g) *(If making homemade mayo, see page 220 for ingredients.)*
MCT oil, 1 cup plus 2 Tbsp (270 ml)

DRIED HERBS AND SPICES

Cajun Seasoning (page 232), 2½ tsp
cayenne pepper, ½ tsp
cinnamon, ground, 2 Tbsp plus 2 tsp
cloves, ground, ¼ tsp
Italian Seasoning (page 234), 1 Tbsp plus 1 tsp
nutmeg, ground, ⅛ tsp
oregano leaves, 1 Tbsp plus 1 tsp
thyme leaves, 1 Tbsp plus 1½ tsp

PANTRY ITEMS

almond butter, unsweetened smooth, 1 Tbsp
almond flour, blanched, 2 cups (220 g)
aloe vera juice, from the inner fillet, ¼ to ½ cup (60 to 150 ml) *(optional, for lemonade)*
apple cider vinegar, 2 Tbsp plus 1¾ tsp
baking powder, 1 Tbsp plus ¼ tsp

cacao powder, ¼ cup (20 g)
capers, 1 Tbsp
coconut milk, full-fat, 1 (13½-oz./400-ml) can plus cup (4 fl. oz./120 ml)
coconut, unsweetened shredded, ½ cup (50 g)
coffee, ground, ¾ cup (65 g), or tea of choice, ⅓ cup (10 g) loose tea or 8 bags
collagen peptides, ½ cup (80 g)
Dijon mustard, 1 tsp
erythritol, confectioners'-style, ⅓ cup plus 3 Tbsp (85 g)
flax seeds, whole, 1½ cups (264 g)
gelatin, unflavored, 1 Tbsp
hemp seeds, hulled, ¼ cup plus 2 Tbsp (56 g)
nondairy milk, 4½ cups (37 fl. oz./1.1 L)
nutritional yeast, ½ cup plus 2 Tbsp (42 g)
pork rinds, unseasoned, 1.4 oz. (40 g)
stevia, liquid, ¾ tsp *(optional, for drinks)*
tea of choice, 2 tsp loose tea or 2 bags
vanilla extract, 1 Tbsp plus 1¾ tsp
white wine, such as Pinot Grigio, Sauvignon Blanc, or unoaked Chardonnay, 2 Tbsp plus 2 tsp

Finely ground gray sea salt and ground black pepper will be needed for many of the recipes. Purchase once and use throughout the plan.

	MEAL 1	MEAL 2	MEAL 3	SNACKS	DAY MACROS/TOTALS	
DAY 1	FLAXSEED CINNAMON BUN MUFFINS[1] ½ ❄ P239 AND ROCKET FUEL LATTE P428	SPINACH SALAD WITH BREADED CHICKEN STRIPS ½ P284	ONE-POT HAMBURGER DINNER P310	BACON FUDGE[2] ❄ P394 AND KETO LEMONADE P422	fat 75% carbs 7% protein 18% calories 2039 total fat 171 sat. fat 84.9	chol. 358 sodium 1818 carbs 34.7 fiber 19.5 net carbs 12.5 protein 89.8
DAY 2	ROCKET FUEL LATTE P428	*Leftover* One-Pot Hamburger Dinner	SHOULDER CHOPS WITH LEMON-THYME GRAVY ½ P332	BACON CRACKERS[3] ½ ❄ P254 *dipped in* MCT GUACAMOLE *(eat 2 servings)* P260	fat 76% carbs 5% protein 19% calories 1897 total fat 161 sat. fat 83.3	chol. 262 sodium 2427 carbs 24.7 fiber 15.8 net carbs 8.9 protein 87.9
DAY 3	FAT-BURNING GOLDEN MILKSHAKE P416	*Leftover* Spinach Salad with Breaded Chicken Strips	*Leftover* One-Pot Hamburger Dinner *topped with leftover* MCT Guacamole *(eat 2 servings)*	KETO LEMONADE P422	fat 74% carbs 9% protein 17% calories 1866 total fat 154 sat. fat 93.8	chol. 254 sodium 1836 carbs 41.1 fiber 22.5 net carbs 15.9 protein 78.2
DAY 4	*Leftover* Flaxseed Cinnamon Bun Muffins AND ROCKET FUEL LATTE *with 2 Tbsp. additional collagen* P428	*Leftover* Bacon Fudge	*Leftover* Shoulder Chops with Lemon-Thyme Gravy	KETO LEMONADE P422	fat 80% carbs 4% protein 16% calories 1517 total fat 134 sat. fat 68.9	chol. 222 sodium 1143 carbs 17.5 fiber 9 net carbs 5.8 protein 59.8
DAY 5	FAT-BURNING GOLDEN MILKSHAKE *with 2 Tbsp. collagen blended in* P416	*Leftover* Bacon Crackers *dipped in leftover* MCT Guacamole *(eat 2 servings)*	*Leftover* Shoulder Chops with Lemon-Thyme Gravy	KETO LEMONADE P422	fat 80% carbs 6% protein 14% calories 1602 total fat 142 sat. fat 86.1	chol. 161 sodium 1575 carbs 24.7 fiber 12 net carbs 10 protein 56.1
DAY 6	PANCAKES ½ P236	*Leftover* One-Pot Hamburger Dinner *topped with leftover* MCT Guacamole	FAT-BURNING GOLDEN MILKSHAKE P416	KETO LEMONADE P422	fat 73% carbs 7% protein 20% calories 1832 total fat 149 sat. fat 101	chol. 443 sodium 2133 carbs 32.2 fiber 14.1 net carbs 15.4 protein 91.5
DAY 7	*Leftover* Flaxseed Cinnamon Bun Muffins AND ROCKET FUEL LATTE P428	BACON LOVERS' QUICHE[4] ❄ P240 AND VERDE CAESAR SALAD WITH CRISPY CAPERS[5] ½ ❄ P289		ACV ICED TEA P418	fat 79% carbs 7% protein 14% calories 1262 total fat 111 sat. fat 53.9	chol. 223 sodium 1217 carbs 22.9 fiber 14.4 net carbs 8.5 protein 44

½ HALF BATCH
❄ FREEZE
UPPERCASE RECIPES are to be made fresh.

[1]Freeze 1 muffin for week 2, 1 for week 3, and 1 to enjoy after the plan.
[2]Freeze half of the fudge for use in week 2.
[3]Freeze 1 serving of crackers for use in week 2.
[4]Freeze 1 quiche for use in week 2, 2 quiches for use in week 3, and ½ quiche for use in week 4. (Each quiche is 2 servings.)
[5]Refrigerate half of the Verde Caesar Salad for use in week 2.

SHOPPING LIST FOR WEEK 2

FRESH PRODUCE

asparagus, ½ bunch (about
6½ oz./185 g)
berries, ½ pint (6 oz./170 g)
(optional, for porridge)
butter lettuce, 1 small head
cilantro, ½ bunch (about ¾ oz./25 g)
garlic, 6 cloves
ginger root, 2-inch (5-cm) piece
kale, 5 oz. (140 g)
lemon, 1 large
limes, 3 small
mint, 4 or 5 sprigs
mushrooms, white, 4 (about 2 oz./57 g)
onions, green, 2 bunches
parsley, 5 or 6 sprigs
radishes, 16 (1 large bunch)
zucchini, 4 medium

MEAT, EGGS, AND BROTH

bacon, regular (not thick-cut), 5 strips
bone broth, 1⅓ cups (10⅔ fl. oz./315 ml)
*(If making homemade broth, see page 152 for
ingredients.)*
beef brisket or chuck roast, 1½ lbs (680 g)
beef chuck roast, 1 lb (455 g)
eggs, 2 large
ground beef, 20% to 30% fat, 1 lb
(455 g)
pepperoni, 3¾ oz. (105 g)
pork belly, side of, ½ lb (225 g)
turkey thighs, bone-in, skin-on,
1¼ lbs (600 g)

FATS AND OILS

avocado oil, refined,
1½ cups (350 ml), plus
more for general use
cacao butter, 3 Tbsp
coconut oil, ⅓ cup (80 ml)
coconut oil, butter-infused, ¼ cup
(60 ml)
mayonnaise, made with avocado oil,
1 cup plus 1 Tbsp (220 g)
*(If making homemade mayo, see page 220 for
ingredients.)*
MCT oil or coconut oil, 3 Tbsp

DRIED HERBS AND SPICES

Cajun Seasoning (page 232), 2¼ tsp
cinnamon, ground, 1 tsp
cloves, ground, ⅛ tsp
cumin, ground, 1½ tsp
Italian Seasoning (page 234), ½ tsp
oregano leaves, 1½ tsp

PANTRY ITEMS

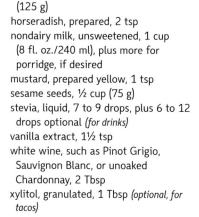

almond flour, blanched,
⅓ cup (40 g)
almond meal, ¼ cup (28 g)
apple cider vinegar, ¼ cup
(60 ml)
balsamic vinegar (preferably NUCO
balsamic-style coconut vinegar), 2 Tbsp
Brazil nuts, raw, 4
chia seeds, 1 Tbsp
coconut milk, full-fat, 2 Tbsp
coffee, ground, ½ cup plus 1 Tbsp (45 g),
or tea of choice, 2 Tbsp loose tea or
6 bags
collagen peptides, ¼ cup plus 3 Tbsp
(70 g)
Dijon mustard, 2¼ tsp
erythritol, confectioners'-style, 1 Tbsp
flax seeds, whole, 1 Tbsp plus 1½ tsp
gelatin, unflavored, ¼ cup (40 g)
green tea, 1 Tbsp loose tea or 4 bags
hemp seeds, hulled, ¾ cup plus 1 Tbsp
(125 g)
horseradish, prepared, 2 tsp
nondairy milk, unsweetened, 1 cup
(8 fl. oz./240 ml), plus more for
porridge, if desired
mustard, prepared yellow, 1 tsp
sesame seeds, ½ cup (75 g)
stevia, liquid, 7 to 9 drops, plus 6 to 12
drops optional *(for drinks)*
vanilla extract, 1½ tsp
white wine, such as Pinot Grigio,
Sauvignon Blanc, or unoaked
Chardonnay, 2 Tbsp
xylitol, granulated, 1 Tbsp *(optional, for
tacos)*

	MEAL 1	MEAL 2	MEAL 3	SNACKS	DAY MACROS/TOTALS	
DAY 8	ROCKET FUEL LATTE ·P428·	SHREDDED BEEF TACOS ½ ·P314·	*Leftover* Verde Caesar Salad with Crispy Capers **AND** BALSAMIC TURKEY THIGHS[1] ½ ❄ ·P338· **AND** ZOODLES ·P376· *tossed in 2 Tbsp. mayonnaise*		*fat* **79%**	*chol.* **224**
					carbs **3%**	*sodium* **1549**
					protein **18%**	*carbs* **11.8**
					calories **1663**	*fiber* **4.8**
					total fat **146**	*net carbs* **7**
					sat. fat **52.9**	*protein* **76.3**
DAY 9	FATTY GREEN TEA ·P419·	*Leftover* Shredded Beef Tacos **AND** ZOODLES ·P376· *drizzled with* GARLIC-INFUSED OIL ·P230·	MICHAEL'S PEPPERONI MEATZZA[2] ❄ ·P312·	*Leftover* Bacon Fudge	*fat* **78%**	*chol.* **335**
					carbs **4%**	*sodium* **1445**
					protein **18%**	*carbs* **18.2**
					calories **1644**	*fiber* **5.5**
					total fat **142**	*net carbs* **12.7**
					sat. fat **53.2**	*protein* **74.3**
DAY 10	GRAIN-FREE HEMP SEED PORRIDGE ·P244·	*Leftover* Shredded Beef Tacos	*Leftover* Bacon Lovers' Quiche **AND** ZOODLES *tossed in 2 Tbsp. mayonnaise* ·P376·		*fat* **74%**	*chol.* **364**
					carbs **7%**	*sodium* **1344**
					protein **19%**	*carbs* **31.5**
					calories **1738**	*fiber* **19.4**
					total fat **143**	*net carbs* **12.1**
					sat. fat **34.1**	*protein* **82.3**
DAY 11	*Leftover* Grain-Free Hemp Seed Porridge *with 1 Tbsp. coconut oil and 2 Tbsp. collagen stirred in*	CAJUN PORK BELLY CHOPPED SALAD ½ ·P286·	*Leftover* Bacon Lovers' Quiche **AND** ZOODLES *tossed in 2 Tbsp. mayonnaise* ·P376·		*fat* **82%**	*chol.* **321**
					carbs **6%**	*sodium* **1066**
					protein **12%**	*carbs* **34.5**
					calories **2482**	*fiber* **21.4**
					total fat **228**	*net carbs* **13.1**
					sat. fat **73.1**	*protein* **76.2**
DAY 12	FATTY GREEN TEA ·P419·	*Leftover* Michael's Pepperoni Meatzza	BEEF STROGANOFF[3] ½ ❄ ·P300·	*Leftover* Bacon Crackers *dipped in 2 Tbsp. mayonnaise*	*fat* **76%**	*chol.* **369**
					carbs **4%**	*sodium* **1738**
					protein **20%**	*carbs* **15.5**
					calories **1688**	*fiber* **3.6**
					total fat **143**	*net carbs* **11.9**
					sat. fat **59.8**	*protein* **85**
DAY 13	*Leftover* Flaxseed Cinnamon Bun Muffins **AND** ROCKET FUEL LATTE *with 2 Tbsp. additional collagen* ·P428·	*Leftover* Cajun Pork Belly Chopped Salad		*Leftover* Bacon Fudge	*fat* **88%**	*chol.* **221**
					carbs **4%**	*sodium* **688**
					protein **9%**	*carbs* **19**
					calories **2031**	*fiber* **11.8**
					total fat **198**	*net carbs* **7.2**
					sat. fat **87.7**	*protein* **43.2**
DAY 14	ROCKET FUEL LATTE ·P428·	*Leftover* Michael's Pepperoni Meatzza	*Leftover* Balsamic Turkey Thighs **AND** BACON-WRAPPED ASPARAGUS WITH HORSERADISH SAUCE ½ ·P262·		*fat* **77%**	*chol.* **176**
					carbs **2%**	*sodium* **1772**
					protein **21%**	*carbs* **7.9**
					calories **1342**	*fiber* **3.5**
					total fat **115**	*net carbs* **4.4**
					sat. fat **41.6**	*protein* **69.9**

½ HALF BATCH

❄ FREEZE

UPPERCASE RECIPES are to be made fresh.

[1] Freeze 1 serving of Shredded Beef Tacos to enjoy after the plan.

[2] Freeze 1 serving of Balsamic Turkey Thighs for week 3 and 1 serving for week 4.

[3] Freeze 2 servings of Meatzza for week 3 and 1 serving for week 4.

[4] Freeze 2 servings of Beef Stroganoff for week 4 and 1 serving for use after the plan.

SHOPPING LIST FOR WEEK 3

FRESH PRODUCE
avocados, Hass, 2 large
cauliflower, 1 medium head
celery, 2 large stalks
chives, 1½ tsp sliced
cilantro leaves, ½ oz.
   (15 g), plus more for
   garnish *(optional, for Sloppy Jolenes)*
dill, ¾ tsp finely chopped
endive, 1
garlic, 3 small cloves
ginger root, 6-inch (15-cm) piece
lemons, 2 large
onion, red, 1 small
onion, white, 1 small
onions, green, 4
parsley, 1 small bunch
tomato, 1 small

MEAT AND BROTH
broth, any type, 2 cups
   (16 fl. oz./475 ml)
   *(If making homemade broth, see page 152 for
   ingredients.)*
chicken bone broth, ½ cup
   (4 fl. oz./120 ml)
chicken thigh, boneless, 1
chicken thigh skins, 6 (about 4½ oz./
   125 g)
ground beef, 20% to 30% fat, ½ lb
   (225 g)
sausages, 4 (about 8 oz./225 g)

FATS AND OILS
avocado oil, refined, ⅓ cup
   (2⅔ fl. oz./80 ml)
cacao butter, 3 Tbsp
coconut oil, 1¼ cups plus
   3 Tbsp (345 ml)
lard, ⅓ cup (69 g)
mayonnaise, made with avocado oil,
   ½ cup (105 g) *(If making homemade mayo,
   see page 220 for ingredients.)*

DRIED HERBS AND SPICES
Cajun Seasoning (page 232), 2 Tbsp
cardamom, ground, 1¾ tsp
cayenne pepper, 1 pinch
cinnamon, ground, ¼ tsp
cumin seeds, ½ tsp
Curry Powder (page 235), 1 tsp
ginger powder, 2 tsp
paprika, 2¼ tsp
parsley, 1 tsp
Seasoning Salt (page 235), 2¾ tsp

PANTRY ITEMS
apple cider vinegar, 1 Tbsp
   plus 1 tsp
chili, dried, 1 whole
coconut milk, full-fat, ½ cup plus 2 Tbsp
   (5 fl. oz./150 ml)
coffee, ground, ½ cup plus 1 Tbsp (45 g),
   or tea of choice, 2 Tbsp loose tea or
   6 bags
collagen peptides, ¼ cup plus 3 Tbsp
   (70 g)
erythritol, confectioners'-style, 2 Tbsp
gelatin, unflavored, ¼ cup (40 g)
green tea, 2 Tbsp loose tea or 8 bags
hemp seeds, hulled, 3 Tbsp
macadamia nut halves, raw, 1 oz. (28 g)
orange extract, ½ tsp
stevia, liquid, ¼ tsp, plus 6 to 12 drops
   optional *(for drinks)*
tomato sauce, sugar-free, ¾ cup plus
   1½ Tbsp (6¾ fl. oz./135 g)
vanilla extract or powder, 1¼ tsp
walnut pieces, raw, 2⅔ oz. (75 g)

	MEAL 1	MEAL 2	MEAL 3	SNACKS	DAY MACROS/TOTALS	
DAY 15	**FATTY GREEN TEA** P419	*Leftover* **Bacon Lovers' Quiche** AND *Leftover* **Bacon-Wrapped Asparagus with Horseradish Sauce**	**EARLY-DAY JAMBALAYA** *drizzled with* Garlic-Infused Oil P242	**ROCKET FUEL BONE BROTH** P426	*fat* 77% · *carbs* 6% · *protein* 17% · *calories* 1671 · *total fat* 143 · *sat. fat* 49.4	*chol.* 295 · *sodium* 2061 · *carbs* 25.3 · *fiber* 10.3 · *net carbs* 14.4 · *protein* 70.3
DAY 16	*(fasted morning)*	*Leftover* **Early-Day Jambalaya** *drizzled with* **RANCH DRESSING** ¼ P226	*Leftover* **Bacon Lovers' Quiche** AND **AVOCADO FRIES WITH DIPPING SAUCE** P378	*Leftover* **Rocket Fuel Bone Broth**	*fat* 79% · *carbs* 7% · *protein* 14% · *calories* 1597 · *total fat* 140 · *sat. fat* 38.1	*chol.* 277 · *sodium* 2157 · *carbs* 27.4 · *fiber* 17 · *net carbs* 10.4 · *protein* 57.1
DAY 17	**ROCKET FUEL LATTE** P428	*Leftover* **Early-Day Jambalaya** *drizzled with* Garlic-Infused Oil	*Leftover* **Michael's Pepperoni Meatzza** *covered in* 2 Tbsp. mayonnaise		*fat* 81% · *carbs* 3% · *protein* 16% · *calories* 1569 · *total fat* 142 · *sat. fat* 53.4	*chol.* 309 · *sodium* 1679 · *carbs* 13 · *fiber* 5.9 · *net carbs* 7.1 · *protein* 60.7
DAY 18	**FATTY GREEN TEA** P419	*Leftover* **Bacon Lovers' Quiche** *drizzled with* **Ranch Dressing**	*Leftover* **Balsamic Turkey Thighs** AND *Leftover* **Avocado Fries with Dipping Sauce**		*fat* 75% · *carbs* 7% · *protein* 18% · *calories* 1385 · *total fat* 116 · *sat. fat* 27.7	*chol.* 153 · *sodium* 1550 · *carbs* 23.1 · *fiber* 14.2 · *net carbs* 8.9 · *protein* 63.5
DAY 19	*Leftover* **Flaxseed Cinnamon Bun Muffins** AND **ROCKET FUEL LATTE** *with 2 Tbsp. additional collagen* P428	**BOMBAY SLOPPY JOLENES**[1] ½ 🌀 P302	**CHICKEN CRISPS**[2] *dipped in* **Ranch Dressing** ½ 🌀 P248	*Leftover* **Avocado Fries with Dipping Sauce**	*fat* 80% · *carbs* 7% · *protein* 13% · *calories* 1467 · *total fat* 130 · *sat. fat* 51	*chol.* 154 · *sodium* 2058 · *carbs* 27.2 · *fiber* 18.8 · *net carbs* 8.4 · *protein* 47.9
DAY 20	*Leftover* **Early-Day Jambalaya** *drizzled with* Garlic-Infused Oil	**ROCKET FUEL LATTE** P428	*Leftover* **Michael's Pepperoni Meatzza** AND *Leftover* **Avocado Fries with Dipping Sauce**		*fat* 81% · *carbs* 5% · *protein* 14% · *calories* 1724 · *total fat* 154 · *sat. fat* 55.7	*chol.* 253 · *sodium* 1921 · *carbs* 21.3 · *fiber* 14.4 · *net carbs* 6.9 · *protein* 62.3
DAY 21	**KETO MILKSHAKE** P423	*Leftover* **Bacon Lovers' Quiche**	*Leftover* **Bombay Sloppy Jolenes** *drizzled with* **Ranch Dressing**	**CARDAMOM ORANGE BARK**[3] 🌀 P395	*fat* 82% · *carbs* 5% · *protein* 13% · *calories* 2072 · *total fat* 188 · *sat. fat* 105	*chol.* 408 · *sodium* 1808 · *carbs* 28 · *fiber* 12.8 · *net carbs* 15.2 · *protein* 66.3

½ HALF BATCH
¼ QUARTER BATCH
🌀 FREEZE

UPPERCASE RECIPES are to be made fresh.

[1]Freeze 2 servings of Sloppy Jolenes for use in week 4. The fresh ingredients for these 2 servings have been added to the shopping list for week 4.
[2]Freeze 5 servings of Chicken Crisps for use in week 4.
[3]Freeze 4 servings of Cardamom Orange Bark for use in week 4.

SHOPPING LIST FOR WEEK 4

FRESH PRODUCE
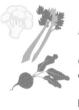
avocados, Hass, 1½ large
berries, couple of handfuls
  (optional, for granola)
cabbage, red, ¼ small head
celery, 1 large stalk
cilantro, 3 oz. (80 g)
cucumber, 1
endive, 1
garlic, 2 small cloves
ginger root, ½-inch (1.25-cm) piece
lemons, 6
lime, 1 wedge
okra, 8 oz. (225 g)
onion, red, 1 small *(optional, for
  Curried Okra Salad)*
onion, white, 1 small
onions, green, 3
parsley, fresh, 6 or 7 sprigs
rutabaga, 1 small
spinach, 12 oz. (340 g)
strawberries, 6
tomato, 1 small
zucchini, 2 medium

MEAT, EGGS, AND BROTH
bacon, 9 strips
broth, any type, 2 cups (16 fl. oz./475 ml)
  *(If making homemade broth, see page 152 for
  ingredients.)*
egg, 1 large
flank steak, 13 oz. (370 g)
sausages, precooked, 2 (about 4 oz./
  115 g)

FATS AND OILS

avocado oil, refined, ½ cup
  (120 ml)
coconut cream, 1 (13½-oz./400-ml) can
coconut oil, 1 cup (240 ml), plus more for
  the pan
lard, 2 Tbsp

DRIED HERBS AND SPICES

cayenne pepper, 1 pinch
chili powder, ¾ tsp
cinnamon, ground, 3 Tbsp
cloves, ground, ⅛ tsp
Curry Powder (page 235),
  1 tsp
garlic powder, ¼ tsp
mustard, ground, ¼ tsp
onion powder, ½ tsp

PANTRY ITEMS
apple cider vinegar, 1½ Tbsp
capers, 1 Tbsp
cashews, raw, 3 oz. (85 g)
chia seeds, 1½ oz. (40 g)
chocolate chips, stevia-sweetened,
  couple of handfuls *(optional, for granola)*
coconut, unsweetened shredded, 2 cups
  (200 g)
coconut milk, full-fat, ⅓ cup (2¾ fl. oz./
  80 ml), plus more for granola
collagen peptides, ½ cup (80 g)
Dijon mustard, 1½ tsp
erythritol, confectioners'-style, 2 Tbsp,
  plus 1 Tbsp optional *(for Coconut Whipped
  Cream)*
gelatin, unflavored, ¼ cup (40 g)
hemp seeds, hulled, 5½ oz. (155 g)
nutritional yeast, 2 Tbsp
pecans, raw, 1¼ oz. (35 g)
red wine vinegar, 2 Tbsp
sesame seeds, 5½ oz. (155 g)
stevia, liquid, ¼ tsp plus 4 drops
tea of choice, 3 bags
vanilla extract, 2 tsp, plus 1 tsp optional
  (for Coconut Whipped Cream)

	MEAL 1	MEAL 2	MEAL 3	SNACKS	DAY MACROS/TOTALS	
DAY 22	**ROCKET FUEL BONE BROTH** P426	*Leftover* **Michael's Pepperoni Meatzza**	*Leftover* **Beef Stroganoff** *drizzled with* **Garlic-Infused Oil**	*Leftover* **Chicken Crisps**	fat 77% carbs 3% protein 20% calories 1536 total fat 131 sat. fat 50.6	chol. 306 sodium 2312 carbs 11.3 fiber 2.9 net carbs 8.4 protein 78.4
DAY 23	*Leftover* **Rocket Fuel Bone Broth** *with 2 Tbsp. collagen blended in* *Leftover* **Cardamom Orange Bark**	*Leftover* **Bacon Lovers' Quiche** AND **CURRIED OKRA SALAD** ½ P296	**ICED TEA LEMONADE GUMMIES** P406 AND *Leftover* **Chicken Crisps**		fat 79% carbs 6% protein 15% calories 1578 total fat 138 sat. fat 63.3	chol. 184 sodium 1967 carbs 23.1 fiber 10.6 net carbs 12.5 protein 60.2
DAY 24	**SAUSAGE AND GREENS HASH BOWL** *drizzled with* **Garlic-Infused Oil** P243 AND *Leftover* **Chicken Crisps**	*Leftover* **Beef Stroganoff** AND 1 small cucumber, sliced		*Leftover* **Iced Tea Lemonade Gummies** AND *Leftover* **Cardamom Orange Bark**	fat 79% carbs 5% protein 16% calories 1777 total fat 155 sat. fat 71	chol. 215 sodium 1831 carbs 24.3 fiber 9 net carbs 15.3 protein 70.6
DAY 25	(fasted morning)	*Leftover* **Sausage and Greens Hash Bowl** AND 4 strips bacon	*Leftover* **Bombay Sloppy Jolenes** AND *Leftover* **Curried Okra Salad**	*Leftover* **Iced Tea Lemonade Gummies**	fat 79% carbs 7% protein 14% calories 1687 total fat 148 sat. fat 56.1	chol. 189 sodium 2116 carbs 31 fiber 13.4 net carbs 16.5 protein 56.9
DAY 26	**NO-NUTS GRANOLA WITH CLUSTERS** P246 *topped with* **COCONUT WHIPPED CREAM** P414	**BERRY AVOCADO SALAD** ½ P294 AND *Leftover* **Balsamic Turkey Thighs**		1 large stalk celery AND **BACON SPINACH DIP** ½ P255 AND *Leftover* **Cardamom Orange Bark**	fat 78% carbs 9% protein 13% calories 1568 total fat 136 sat. fat 63	chol. 23 sodium 868 carbs 33.4 fiber 18.8 net carbs 14.6 protein 52.1
DAY 27	*Leftover* **No-Nuts Granola with Clusters** *topped with leftover* **Coconut Whipped Cream**	**SPINACH SALAD WITH FLANK STEAK** ½ P292	*Leftover* **Berry Avocado Salad** AND *Leftover* **Chicken Crisps** AND *Leftover* **Bacon Spinach Dip**	*Leftover* **Cardamom Orange Bark**	fat 78% carbs 8% protein 14% calories 1886 total fat 163 sat. fat 73.2	chol. 109 sodium 1228 carbs 37.8 fiber 21.2 net carbs 16.6 protein 67.3
DAY 28	*Leftover* **Cardamom Orange Bark**	*Leftover* **Bombay Sloppy Jolenes**	*Leftover* **Spinach Salad with Flank Steak**	*Leftover* **Chicken Crisps** AND *Leftover* **Bacon Spinach Dip**	fat 76% carbs 6% protein 18% calories 1465 total fat 125 sat. fat 48.3	chol. 143 sodium 1730 carbs 21.5 fiber 7.8 net carbs 13.7 protein 64.8

½ HALF BATCH

UPPERCASE RECIPES are to be made fresh.

EXTRA LEFTOVERS NOT USED IN THE PLAN: 5 servings Bacon Spinach Dip, 2 servings Bacon-Wrapped Asparagus with Horseradish Sauce, 1 serving Beef Stroganoff, 5 servings Coconut Whipped Cream, 1 serving Garlic-Infused Oil, 1 serving Iced Tea Lemonade Gummies, 10 servings No-Nuts Granola with Clusters, 1 serving Shredded Beef Tacos, 1 serving Spinach Salad with Flank Steak

This plan is for the Pumped Keto Fat Fueled Profile (find out more on page 47). This profile can be followed indefinitely. If you decide to switch from Pumped Keto to another Fat Fueled Profile that includes carb-ups, follow this plan until you're fat-adapted (read about the signs of becoming adapted on pages 63 to 65) before switching to the Full Keto or Adapted Fat Burner meal plan.

Not enough food for you? The simplest way to add bulk to the meals without having to worry about it affecting your macros is to increase the fat and protein in your Rocket Fuel Lattes, enjoy jerky with a handful of nuts or seeds, or double up on serving sizes, doubling recipes as needed.

Too much protein for you? Switch to the Classic Keto meal plan (page 176).

SHOPPING LIST FOR WEEK 1

FRESH PRODUCE
carrot, 1 medium
celery, 2 medium stalks
chives, 2 Tbsp sliced
fennel bulb, 1 large
   (about 10½ oz./300 g)
garlic, 11 small cloves
ginger root, 2½-inch (6.35-cm) piece
grape tomatoes, 1½ cups (210 g)
herbs of choice, such as thyme and/or
   rosemary, 1 Tbsp chopped
lemons, 3
onions, green, 3 bunches
onions, white, 2 small
parsley, 1 large bunch
radishes, 2 bunches
rosemary, 2 sprigs
zucchini, green or yellow, 2
   medium

MEAT, EGGS, AND BROTH
bacon, 8 strips (about 8½ oz./240 g)
bone broth, any type, 2 cups (16 fl.
   oz./475 ml) *(If making homemade broth, see
   page 152 for ingredients.)*
calamari rings, uncooked, 12 oz. (340 g)
chicken bone broth, 7 cups (56 fl. oz./
   1.7 L), or more as needed *(for ribs)*
chicken breasts, bone-in, skin-on, 4
   (about 2 lbs/910 g)
chicken thighs, boneless, skinless, 1 lb
   (455 g)
eggs, 2 large
ground beef, 10% fat, ½ lb (225 g)
ground beef, 20% to 30% fat, 1 lb
   (455 g)
pork chops, boneless center-cut, 6
   (5½ oz./155 g each)
pork ribs, country-style, 1⅔ lbs (750 g)

FATS AND OILS
avocado oil, refined, 1 cup
   (240 ml)
cacao butter, ½ cup (120 g)
coconut oil, ¾ cup plus 2 Tbsp plus 1 tsp
   (215 ml)
extra-virgin olive oil, 1 cup plus 2 Tbsp
   plus 1½ tsp (280 ml)
lard, 3 Tbsp
MCT oil, ¾ cup (180 g)

DRIED HERBS AND SPICES
basil, ½ tsp
cayenne pepper, 1 pinch
cinnamon, ground, ¼ tsp
cloves, ground, ¼ tsp
garlic powder, ¾ tsp
Greek Seasoning (page 232), 1 Tbsp
onion powder, 2 tsp
oregano leaves, 1 tsp
parsley, dried, 1 tsp
red pepper flakes, ¼ tsp
rosemary leaves, ½ tsp
sage, ground, 1 tsp
smoked sea salt, ½ tsp
thyme leaves, ½ tsp

PANTRY ITEMS
almond butter, unsweetened,
   2 Tbsp
apple cider vinegar, 1½ tsp
baking powder, ¾ tsp
coconut aminos, 1 Tbsp
coconut flour, ¾ cup (75 g)
coconut milk, full-fat, ¼ cup (2 fl. oz./
   60 ml)
coffee, ground, ¼ cup plus 2 Tbsp
   (32 g), or tea of choice, 4 tsp loose tea
   or 4 bags
collagen peptides, ½ cup plus 2 Tbsp
   (100 g)
gelatin, unflavored, 3 Tbsp plus 1½ tsp
green tea, 1 Tbsp loose tea or 4 bags
hemp seeds, hulled, ½ cup (75 g)
kalamata olives, pitted, 2 (13½-oz./
   400-ml) cans plus ½ cup (60 g)
mustard, prepared yellow, 1 Tbsp
nutritional yeast, ⅓ cup (22 g)
pork dust, 3 oz. (85 g)
red wine vinegar, 1 Tbsp
stevia, liquid, ¼ tsp, plus ¼ to ½ tsp
   optional *(for RFL)*
vanilla extract, 2 tsp

Finely ground gray sea salt and ground black pepper will be needed for many of the recipes. Purchase once and use throughout the plan.

	MEAL 1	MEAL 2	MEAL 3	SNACKS	DAY MACROS/TOTALS	
DAY 1	**ROCKET FUEL LATTE** P428 AND **JERKY COOKIES**[1] *(eat 2 servings)* ½ P271	**BACON-WRAPPED MINI MEATLOAVES**[2] P298 AND **HERB-CRUSTED PORK CHOPS**[3] P326	**BAKED OLIVE CHICKEN**[4] *(eat 2 servings)* P336		*fat* 62% / *carbs* 5% / *protein* 33% / *calories* 1742 / *total fat* 119 / *sat. fat* 46.1	*chol.* 422 / *sodium* 3109 / *carbs* 20.5 / *fiber* 7.3 / *net carbs* 12.2 / *protein* 146
DAY 2	**ROCKET FUEL BONE BROTH** P426	**CALAMARI SALAD** *(eat 2 servings)* P288	*Leftover* **Herb-Crusted Pork Chops**		*fat* 59% / *carbs* 3% / *protein* 38% / *calories* 1758 / *total fat* 116 / *sat. fat* 27.8	*chol.* 1717 / *sodium* 3747 / *carbs* 10.5 / *fiber* 3.2 / *net carbs* 7.3 / *protein* 168
DAY 3	*Leftover* **Rocket Fuel Bone Broth**	*Leftover* **Baked Olive Chicken** *(eat 2 servings)*	*Leftover* **Calamari Salad**		*fat* 57% / *carbs* 7% / *protein* 36% / *calories* 1706 / *total fat* 108 / *sat. fat* 24.5	*chol.* 1049 / *sodium* 3642 / *carbs* 32.4 / *fiber* 10.2 / *net carbs* 22.2 / *protein* 152
DAY 4	**FATTY GREEN TEA** *(drink 2 servings)* P419	*Leftover* **Calamari Salad**	*Leftover* **Bacon-Wrapped Mini Meatloaves** *(eat 2 servings)*		*fat* 61% / *carbs* 6% / *protein* 34% / *calories* 1629 / *total fat* 111 / *sat. fat* 46.6	*chol.* 931 / *sodium* 3260 / *carbs* 23.1 / *fiber* 7 / *net carbs* 16.1 / *protein* 134
DAY 5	**ROCKET FUEL LATTE** P428	**CHICKEN NOODLE SOUP**[5] P276	*Leftover* **Baked Olive Chicken** *(eat 2 servings)*	*Leftover* **Jerky Cookies**	*fat* 58% / *carbs* 8% / *protein* 33% / *calories* 1683 / *total fat* 109 / *sat. fat* 41.4	*chol.* 396 / *sodium* 2972 / *carbs* 34.6 / *fiber* 11.9 / *net carbs* 22.2 / *protein* 140
DAY 6	*Leftover* **Chicken Noodle Soup**	*Leftover* **Bacon-Wrapped Mini Meatloaves** AND **HERBED RADISHES** P384	**SALT AND PEPPER RIBS**[6] *(eat 2 servings)* ½ P330	*Leftover* **Fatty Green Tea**	*fat* 64% / *carbs* 5% / *protein* 31% / *calories* 1903 / *total fat* 135 / *sat. fat* 35.1	*chol.* 214 / *sodium* 3420 / *carbs* 23.5 / *fiber* 5.6 / *net carbs* 17.9 / *protein* 149
DAY 7	*(fasted morning)*	*Leftover* **Herb-Crusted Pork Chops**	*Leftover* **Chicken Noodle Soup**	**CLASSIC BUTTER BISCUITS**[7] with 2 Tbsp. almond butter ½ P368 AND 2 Tbsp. collagen mixed into your favorite tea AND *Leftover* **Jerky Cookies**	*fat* 62% / *carbs* 6% / *protein* 32% / *calories* 1391 / *total fat* 96.2 / *sat. fat* 37.7	*chol.* 299 / *sodium* 1808 / *carbs* 21 / *fiber* 10.8 / *net carbs* 9.7 / *protein* 114

½ HALF BATCH

❄ FREEZE

UPPERCASE RECIPES are to be made fresh.

[1] Freeze 1 serving of Jerky Cookies for day 7, 1 serving for week 2, and 3 servings for week 4.

[2] Freeze 1 serving of meatloaf for day 6, 1 serving for week 2, and 2 servings for week 3.

[3] Freeze 1 serving of pork chops for day 7, 1 serving for week 2, and 1 serving for week 3.

[4] Freeze 2 servings of Baked Olive Chicken for week 2 and 1 serving for week 3.

[5] Freeze 1 serving of Chicken Noodle Soup for week 2.

[6] Reserve half of the ribs for day 8.

[7] Freeze 5 biscuits for use in weeks 3 and 4.

PATH 2
PUMPED KETO

WEEK 2

SHOPPING LIST FOR WEEK 2

FRESH PRODUCE

apple, 1
asparagus, 1 lb (455 g)
cauliflower, 1 medium
  head and 1 large head
chives, 1 Tbsp sliced
dill, 1½ tsp finely chopped
garlic, 6 small cloves
ginger root, 2½-inch (6.35-cm) piece
lemons, 8, plus 1 optional *(for Hamburger
  Dinner)* and ½ optional *(for liver)*
onion, white, 1 small
oregano, 1 bunch
parsley, 1 small bunch
thyme, 1 bunch

MEAT, EGGS, AND BROTH

bacon, 9 strips
beef bone broth, ½ cup (4 fl. oz./120 ml)
  *(If making homemade broth, see page 152 for
  ingredients.)*
bone broth, any type, 2 cups (16 fl. oz./
  475 ml)
chicken, 1 whole (3½ lbs/1.6 kg), with
  giblets
chicken livers, ½ lb (225 g)
eggs, 2 large
ground beef, 20% to 30% fat, 1 lb
  (455 g)
turkey thighs, bone-in, skin-on, 2½ lbs
  (1.2 kg)

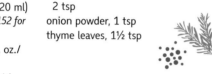

FATS AND OILS

avocado oil, refined, ¼ cup
  plus 3 Tbsp (105 ml)
cacao butter, ½ cup (120 g)
coconut oil, 2 Tbsp
duck fat, 3 Tbsp
mayonnaise, made with avocado oil,
  ½ cup (105 g) *(If making homemade mayo,
  see page 220 for ingredients.)*
MCT oil, ¾ cup (180 ml)

DRIED HERBS AND SPICES

cayenne pepper, 1 pinch
cinnamon, ground, ¼ tsp
garlic powder, ¼ tsp
Greek Seasoning (page 232), 1 Tbsp plus
  1½ tsp
Italian Seasoning (page 234), 1 Tbsp plus
  2 tsp
onion powder, 1 tsp
thyme leaves, 1½ tsp

PANTRY ITEMS

apple cider vinegar, 1 Tbsp
balsamic vinegar, ¼ cup (60 ml)
coconut milk, full-fat, ¼ cup (2 fl. oz./
  60 ml)
coffee, ground, ¼ cup plus 2 Tbsp (32 g),
  or tea of choice, 4 bags or 4 tsp loose
  tea
collagen peptides, 1 cup (160 g)
Dijon mustard, 1 Tbsp
erythritol, confectioners'-style, 2 Tbsp
gelatin, unflavored, ½ cup (80 g)
green tea, 1 Tbsp loose tea or 4 bags
hemp seeds, hulled, ½ cup (75 g)
mustard, prepared yellow, 2 tsp
nondairy milk, unsweetened, 2 cups
  (16 fl. oz./475 ml)
nutritional yeast, ½ cup plus 1 Tbsp plus
  1 tsp (40 g)
pork dust, 2 oz. (60 g) plus ¼ cup plus
  2 Tbsp (25 g)
stevia, liquid, 6 to 8 drops, plus ¼ to ½
  tsp optional *(for RFL)*
tapioca starch, 1 tsp
tea of choice, 3 bags
vanilla extract or powder, 2 tsp

	MEAL 1	MEAL 2	MEAL 3	SNACKS	DAY MACROS/TOTALS	
DAY 8	**FATTY GREEN TEA** with 2 Tbsp. collagen **P419**	*Leftover* **Salt and Pepper Ribs** *(eat 2 servings)* **AND** *Leftover* **Herbed Radishes**		*Leftover* **Jerky Cookies** **AND** **RANCH DRESSING** ½ **P226**	fat 66% / carbs 4% / protein 30% / calories 1347 / total fat 99.4 / sat. fat 23.1	chol. 46 / sodium 1964 / carbs 13.4 / fiber 1.3 / net carbs 11.6 / protein 99.8
DAY 9	**ROCKET FUEL BONE BROTH** **P426**	**THE ONLY WAY I'LL EAT LIVER** drizzled with **Ranch Dressing** *(eat 2 servings)* ½ **P274**	*Leftover* **Herb-Crusted Pork Chops** *(eat 2 servings)*	*Leftover* **Fatty Green Tea**	fat 67% / carbs 2% / protein 31% / calories 1675 / total fat 125 / sat. fat 34.8	chol. 383 / sodium 2754 / carbs 4.6 / fiber 0 / net carbs 4.6 / protein 132
DAY 10	*Leftover* **Rocket Fuel Bone Broth** with 2 Tbsp. collagen blended in	*Leftover* **The Only Way I'll Eat Liver** *(eat 2 servings)*	**BACON MAC 'N' CHEESE** *(eat 2 servings)* **P320**	2 Tbsp. collagen mixed into your favorite tea	fat 59% / carbs 8% / protein 34% / calories 1717 / total fat 112 / sat. fat 37.9	chol. 326 / sodium 3762 / carbs 32.5 / fiber 13.2 / net carbs 19.3 / protein 145
DAY 11	**ROCKET FUEL LATTE** with 2 Tbsp. additional collagen **P428**	*Leftover* **The Only Way I'll Eat Liver** drizzled with **Ranch Dressing**	*Leftover* **Chicken Noodle Soup** with 2 Tbsp. collagen **AND** **BALSAMIC TURKEY THIGHS**[1] ✱ **P338**		fat 66% / carbs 3% / protein 31% / calories 1468 / total fat 108 / sat. fat 40.7	chol. 141 / sodium 2271 / carbs 9.3 / fiber 3.3 / net carbs 6 / protein 115
DAY 12	*(fasted morning)*	*Leftover* **Bacon Mac 'n' Cheese** *(eat 2 servings)*	*Leftover* **The Only Way I'll Eat Liver** *(eat 2 servings)* drizzled with **Ranch Dressing**	**ICED TEA LEMONADE GUMMIES**[2] **P406**	fat 58% / carbs 8% / protein 34% / calories 1527 / total fat 98.1 / sat. fat 30.7	chol. 307 / sodium 3307 / carbs 32.7 / fiber 13.2 / net carbs 19.5 / protein 128
DAY 13	**ROCKET FUEL LATTE** **P428** **AND** *Leftover* **Iced Tea Lemonade Gummies**	*Leftover* **Baked Olive Chicken** *(eat 2 servings)* drizzled with **Ranch Dressing**		*Leftover* **Iced Tea Lemonade Gummies**	fat 60% / carbs 8% / protein 32% / calories 1468 / total fat 97.7 / sat. fat 36.8	chol. 265 / sodium 2218 / carbs 30.3 / fiber 9.6 / net carbs 20.7 / protein 117
DAY 14	**ONE-POT HAMBURGER DINNER**[3] drizzled with **Ranch Dressing** ✱ **P310**	**GREEK CHICKEN WITH GRAVY AND ASPARAGUS**[4] *(eat 2 servings)* ✱ **P346**	*Leftover* **Bacon-Wrapped Mini Meatloaves** drizzled with **Ranch Dressing**		fat 65% / carbs 4% / protein 31% / calories 2112 / total fat 152 / sat. fat 46.2	chol. 656 / sodium 2587 / carbs 22.4 / fiber 10 / net carbs 12.4 / protein 164

½ HALF BATCH

✱ FREEZE

UPPERCASE RECIPES are to be made fresh.

[1] Freeze 6 servings of Balsamic Turkey Thighs for week 3 and 1 serving for week 4.

[2] Reserve 1 serving of Iced Tea Lemonade Gummies for day 16.

[3] Reserve 1 serving of One-Pot Hamburger Dinner for day 17. Freeze 1 serving for week 3 and 1 serving for week 4.

[4] Freeze 4 servings of Greek Chicken for week 3.

SHOPPING LIST FOR WEEK 3

FRESH PRODUCE
cilantro, 1 handful
garlic, 3 small cloves
ginger root, 1½-inch (3.75-
   cm) piece
onion, yellow, 1 small
onions, green, 2

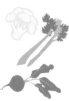

FATS AND OILS

cacao butter, ½ cup (120 g)
coconut oil, ⅓ cup (80 ml)
MCT oil, ¾ cup (180 ml)

PANTRY ITEMS

almond flour, blanched, 3 Tbsp
coconut milk, full-fat, ⅓ cup
   (2¾ fl. oz./80 ml)
coffee, ground, ¼ cup plus
   2 Tbsp (32 g), or tea of choice, 4 tsp
   loose tea or 4 bags
collagen peptides, 1¼ cups (200 g)
hemp seeds, hulled, ½ cup (75 g)
stevia, liquid, ¼ to ½ tsp *(optional, for RFL)*
tea of choice, 2 tsp loose tea or 2 bags
tomatoes, diced, 1 (14½-oz./400-g/
   428-ml) can
vanilla extract, 2 tsp

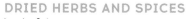

MEAT AND BROTH
bone broth, any type, 2 cups (16 fl. oz./
   475 ml) *(If making homemade broth, see
   page 152 for ingredients.)*
chicken bone broth, 1 cup (240 ml)
chicken thighs, boneless, skinless,
   1⅓ lbs (600 g)

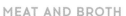

DRIED HERBS AND SPICES
bay leaf, 1
cardamom, ground, ⅛ tsp
cayenne pepper, 1 pinch
cinnamon, ground, ¼ tsp
cloves, ground, ¼ tsp
coriander, ground, ½ tsp
cumin, ground, 1 tsp
garam masala, 1 Tbsp

	MEAL 1	MEAL 2	MEAL 3	SNACKS	DAY MACROS/TOTALS	
DAY 15	*Leftover* **Greek Chicken with Gravy and Asparagus**	*Leftover* **Baked Olive Chicken**	**BUTTER CHICKEN¹** ⊕ P340 AND *Leftover* **Classic Butter Biscuits**		fat 63% / carbs 7% / protein 30% / calories 1759 / total fat 122 / sat. fat 58.2	chol. 487 / sodium 2063 / carbs 32.3 / fiber 12.9 / net carbs 19.4 / protein 132
DAY 16	*Leftover* **Butter Chicken** AND *Leftover* **Classic Butter Biscuits**	*Leftover* **Herb-Crusted Pork Chops**	*Leftover* **Greek Chicken with Gravy and Asparagus**	*Leftover* **Iced Tea Lemonade Gummies**	fat 63% / carbs 4% / protein 33% / calories 1815 / total fat 127 / sat. fat 60.6	chol. 520 / sodium 1851 / carbs 20.4 / fiber 8.6 / net carbs 11.8 / protein 148
DAY 17	*Leftover* **One-Pot Hamburger Dinner**	*Leftover* **Greek Chicken with Gravy and Asparagus** AND *Leftover* **Classic Butter Biscuits**	*Leftover* **Bacon-Wrapped Mini Meatloaves** *(eat 2 servings)*		fat 64% / carbs 6% / protein 30% / calories 1959 / total fat 139 / sat. fat 58.4	chol. 498 / sodium 3264 / carbs 29.6 / fiber 14.6 / net carbs 15 / protein 147
DAY 18	**ROCKET FUEL LATTE** *with 2 Tbsp. additional collagen* P428	*Leftover* **Balsamic Turkey Thighs**	*Leftover* **Greek Chicken with Gravy and Asparagus**	*2 Tbsp. collagen mixed into your favorite tea*	fat 67% / carbs 2% / protein 31% / calories 1324 / total fat 99 / sat. fat 37.7	chol. 231 / sodium 1039 / carbs 5 / fiber 2.9 / net carbs 2.1 / protein 103
DAY 19	**ROCKET FUEL BONE BROTH** *with 2 Tbsp. additional collagen* P426	*Leftover* **Balsamic Turkey Thighs** *(eat 2 servings)* AND *Leftover* **Classic Butter Biscuits**	*Leftover* **Bacon-Wrapped Mini Meatloaves** AND *2 Tbsp. collagen mixed into your favorite tea*		fat 69% / carbs 3% / protein 28% / calories 1652 / total fat 126 / sat. fat 41.8	chol. 107 / sodium 2683 / carbs 14.3 / fiber 6.5 / net carbs 7.8 / protein 115
DAY 20	*Leftover* **Rocket Fuel Bone Broth** AND *Leftover* **One-Pot Hamburger Dinner**	*Leftover* **Butter Chicken**	*Leftover* **Balsamic Turkey Thighs**		fat 65% / carbs 5% / protein 30% / calories 1419 / total fat 103 / sat. fat 39.5	chol. 251 / sodium 2564 / carbs 17.9 / fiber 6.4 / net carbs 11.5 / protein 105
DAY 21	**ROCKET FUEL LATTE** *with 2 Tbsp. additional collagen* P428	*Leftover* **Balsamic Turkey Thighs** *(eat 2 servings)*	*Leftover* **Butter Chicken**	*2 Tbsp. collagen mixed into your favorite tea*	fat 68% / carbs 2% / protein 30% / calories 1527 / total fat 115 / sat. fat 47.2	chol. 126 / sodium 1998 / carbs 9 / fiber 3.2 / net carbs 5.8 / protein 115

⊕ FREEZE   ¹Freeze 2 servings of Butter Chicken, separately, for days 20 and 21.

UPPERCASE RECIPES are to be made fresh.

SHOPPING LIST FOR WEEK 4

FRESH PRODUCE

bell pepper, green, 1 small
bell pepper, yellow, 1 small
carrot, 1 medium
celery, 2 medium stalks
cilantro, 2 Tbsp finely
    chopped, plus more for garnish
dill, 2 packed Tbsp, plus more for garnish
English cucumbers, 2
fennel bulb, 1 large (about 10½ oz./
    300 g)
garlic, 12 small cloves
ginger root, 2-inch (5-cm) piece
grape tomatoes, 1½ cups (210 g)
kale, 2 cups (95 g) chopped
lemons, 3
lime, 1
mint, 1 Tbsp finely chopped
onions, green, 2 bunches
onions, white, 2 small
parsley, 1 small bunch
radishes, ⅓ cup (55 g) diced
rosemary, 2 sprigs
tomatoes, 2 small
zucchini, green or yellow,
    2 medium

MEAT, EGGS, AND BROTH

calamari rings, uncooked, 12 oz. (340 g)
chicken bone broth, 6 cups (48 fl. oz./
    1.4 L) *(If making homemade broth, see page
    152 for ingredients.)*
chicken breasts, bone-in, skin-on, 4
    (about 2 lbs/910 g)
chicken thighs, boneless, skinless, 1 lb
    (455 g)
crab leg meat, cooked, 1 cup (230 g)
eggs, 3 large
smoked salmon, 8 oz. (225 g)

FATS AND OILS

avocado oil, refined, ¾ cup
    plus 1 Tbsp (195 ml)
cacao butter, ½ cup (120 g)
coconut oil, ⅓ cup plus 2 Tbsp (110 ml)
extra-virgin olive oil, 3 Tbsp
MCT oil, ½ cup (120 ml), or coconut oil,
    ½ cup (105 g)

DRIED HERBS AND SPICES

basil, ½ tsp
cinnamon, ground, ¼ tsp
Greek Seasoning (page 232), 1 Tbsp
oregano leaves, ½ tsp
Seasoning Salt (page
    235), 1 Tbsp *(optional, for
    tortillas)*

PANTRY ITEMS

apple cider vinegar, 1 Tbsp plus
    1½ tsp
coconut milk, full-fat, ⅓ cup
    (2¾ fl. oz./80 ml)
coffee, ground, ¼ cup plus 2 Tbsp
    (32 g), or tea of choice, 4 tsp loose tea
    or 4 bags
collagen peptides, ½ cup (80 g)
gelatin, unflavored, 2 Tbsp
green tea, 1 Tbsp loose tea or 4 bags
hemp seeds, hulled, ½ cup (75 g)
kalamata olives, pitted, 2 (13½-oz./
    400-ml) cans plus ½ cup (60 g)
pork dust, 1⅓ cups (85 g)
red wine vinegar, 1 Tbsp
sesame seeds, ¼ cup (40 g)
Sriracha sauce, 2 Tbsp
stevia, liquid, 6 to 8 drops, plus ¼ to
    ½ tsp optional *(for RFL)*
vanilla extract, 2 tsp

	MEAL 1	MEAL 2	MEAL 3	SNACKS	DAY MACROS/TOTALS	
DAY 22	*Leftover* **One-Pot Hamburger Dinner** AND *Leftover* **Classic Butter Biscuits**	*Leftover* **Balsamic Turkey Thighs** AND *Leftover* **Jerky Cookies**	**BAKED OLIVE CHICKEN** P336		fat 60% / carbs 8% / protein 32% / calories 1472 / total fat 97.8 / sat. fat 35.3	chol. 254 / sodium 2611 / carbs 30.2 / fiber 13 / net carbs 16.7 / protein 118
DAY 23	**CHICKEN NOODLE SOUP** P276	**CRAB TACOS** *(eat 2 servings)* P354	*Leftover* **Baked Olive Chicken** *(eat 2 servings)*		fat 54% / carbs 9% / protein 37% / calories 1891 / total fat 113 / sat. fat 24.7	chol. 631 / sodium 4150 / carbs 44.1 / fiber 13.1 / net carbs 31 / protein 174
DAY 24	*Leftover* **Baked Olive Chicken** *(eat 2 servings)* AND **KALE PÂTÉ** ½ P259	**SHAVED CUCUMBER AND SMOKED SALMON SALAD** *(eat 2 servings)* ½ P297	*Leftover* **Crab Tacos** *(eat 2 servings)*		fat 56% / carbs 11% / protein 33% / calories 2024 / total fat 126 / sat. fat 29.1	chol. 544 / sodium 6162 / carbs 56.5 / fiber 17.7 / net carbs 38.8 / protein 166
DAY 25	**ROCKET FUEL LATTE** P428	*Leftover* **Chicken Noodle Soup** *(eat 2 servings)*	**CALAMARI SALAD** P288		fat 61% / carbs 5% / protein 34% / calories 1588 / total fat 108 / sat. fat 44.1	chol. 991 / sodium 2974 / carbs 18.3 / fiber 7.2 / net carbs 11.1 / protein 136
DAY 26	**FATTY GREEN TEA** P419	*Leftover* **Chicken Noodle Soup**	*Leftover* **Baked Olive Chicken** *(eat 2 servings)* AND *Leftover* **Kale Pâté**		fat 58% / carbs 10% / protein 32% / calories 1711 / total fat 110 / sat. fat 30.8	chol. 373 / sodium 2967 / carbs 43.2 / fiber 13.3 / net carbs 29.9 / protein 137
DAY 27	*Leftover* **Fatty Green Tea**	*Leftover* **Calamari Salad** *(eat 2 servings)*	*Leftover* **Jerky Cookies** AND *Leftover* **Kale Pâté**		fat 59% / carbs 5% / protein 36% / calories 1475 / total fat 97.3 / sat. fat 26.3	chol. 1553 / sodium 2991 / carbs 19.2 / fiber 5.6 / net carbs 13.1 / protein 131
DAY 28	**ROCKET FUEL LATTE** P428	**SHAVED CUCUMBER AND SMOKED SALMON SALAD** *(eat 2 servings)* ½ P297	*Leftover* **Calamari Salad** AND *Leftover* **Jerky Cookies** *(eat 2 servings)* AND *Leftover* **Kale Pâté**		fat 63% / carbs 7% / protein 30% / calories 1444 / total fat 101 / sat. fat 42.8	chol. 837 / sodium 4482 / carbs 25.2 / fiber 9.5 / net carbs 14.7 / protein 108

½ HALF BATCH

UPPERCASE RECIPES are to be made fresh.

EXTRA LEFTOVERS NOT USED IN THE PLAN:
1 serving Bacon-Wrapped Mini Meatloaves, 1 serving Baked Olive Chicken, 4 Bendy Tortillas

PATH 3
FULL KETO

WEEK 1

This plan is for the Full Keto Fat Fueled Profile (find out more on page 48). Follow this plan after you've become fat-adapted (see pages 63 to 65 for more on how to tell whether you are fat-adapted) by following either the Classic Keto or the Pumped Keto meal plan. This plan is similar to the Adapted Fat Burner meal plan to allow for switching between the two profiles as you find the profile that suits you best.

You'll start this plan with a carb-up (assuming that you've become fat-adapted by following plan 1 or 2) and then practice a carb-up every 6 or 7 days.

Not enough food for you? The simplest way to add bulk to the meals without having to worry about it affecting your macros is to increase the fat in your Rocket Fuel Lattes, whip up a fat bomb (see the chart beginning on page 432) and enjoy it after a meal, or double up on serving sizes, doubling the recipes as needed. If you need more carbs following a carb-up, visit healthfulpursuit.com/carbup to download the complimentary PDF "Carb-Up Recipes," simply adding additional carbs to your meal or post-meal dessert.

Instructions for evening carb-ups are below the plan for each week.

SHOPPING LIST FOR WEEK 1

FRESH PRODUCE

avocados, Hass, 3 large
bell pepper, green, ¼
cabbage, green, ½ large head
cauliflower, 1 medium head
cilantro, 1 bunch
collards, 2 bunches (about 18 oz./510 g)
cucumber, 1
garlic, 5 small cloves
ginger root, 1-inch (2.5-cm) piece
limes, 2
mint leaves, 1 packed Tbsp
onion, red, 1 small
onion, white, 1 small
parsley, 1 bunch
pineapple, 1 small
shallots, 3 medium
spinach, 1 packed cup (70 g)
sweet potatoes, 2 medium
thyme, 4 sprigs
turnips, 3 medium

MEAT, EGGS, AND BROTH

bacon, 14 strips
chicken bone broth, 5 cups plus
  1 Tbsp plus 1 tsp (41 fl. oz./1.2 L)
  (If making homemade broth, see page 152 for ingredients.)
chicken wings, 1 lb (455 g)
egg, 1 large
ground beef, 20% to 30% fat, ½ lb (225 g)
ground chicken, ½ lb (225 g)
ground lamb, 1 lb (455 g)
ground pork, ½ plus ⅓ lb (375 g)
pork rib roast, boneless, 2 lbs (910 g)
pork stewing pieces, 1 lb (455 g)
pork stir-fry pieces, ½ lb (277 g)

FATS AND OILS

avocado oil, refined, 1 cup
  plus 3 Tbsp (285 ml)
cacao butter, ¾ cup (180 ml)
coconut cream, 2 Tbsp
coconut oil, ½ cup (120 ml)
lard, ⅔ cup (140 g)
MCT oil, ¼ cup (60 ml)
sesame oil, toasted, 1 Tbsp
tallow, 1 Tbsp

DRIED HERBS AND SPICES

Bahārāt Seasoning (page 233), 1 Tbsp
chai spice (page 392), 1 Tbsp plus 1 tsp
chili powder, 2¼ tsp
chipotle powder, ½ plus ⅛ tsp
cinnamon, ground, ¼ tsp
cumin, ground, ¾ tsp
garlic powder, ½ tsp
Italian Seasoning (page 234), 1 Tbsp
  plus 2 tsp
onion powder, ¼ tsp
oregano leaves, 2¼ tsp
paprika, 1 tsp
Shichimi Seasoning (page 234), 1 Tbsp
smoked paprika, ¼ tsp
tarragon leaves, 1 Tbsp

PANTRY ITEMS

almond butter, unsweetened smooth,
  ½ cup plus 2 Tbsp (175 g)
almonds, 3 Tbsp
apple cider vinegar, ¼ cup plus 2 Tbsp
  (90 ml)
baking powder, ¾ tsp
cassava flour, ¼ cup (30 g)
chilis, dried, 2 to 4
cocoa powder, 2 Tbsp
coconut aminos, ¼ cup plus 1 Tbsp (75 ml)

coconut flour, ¾ cup (75 g)
coconut milk, full-fat, ¾ cup
  (6 fl. oz./180 ml)
coconut palm sugar, 1 Tbsp
coffee, ground, ¼ cup plus
  2 Tbsp (32 g), or tea of choice,
  4 tsp loose tea or 4 bags
collagen peptides, ¼ cup plus 2 Tbsp
  (60 g)
erythritol, confectioners'-style, 1 Tbsp
  plus 1½ tsp
gelatin, unflavored, 3 Tbsp plus 1½ tsp
green tea, 1½ tsp loose tea or 2 bags
hemp seeds, hulled, 2 Tbsp
lemon extract, 1 tsp
macadamia nuts, 12
magnesium powder, lemon-flavored,
  2 tsp *(optional, for Lemon Drops)*
mustard, prepared yellow, 1 Tbsp
nondairy milk, unsweetened, 2 Tbsp
pork dust, 2 oz. (57 g)
rice, white, 2 cups (1120 g)
rooibos tea, 2½ tsp loose tea or 3 bags
sesame seeds *(optional, for garnishing
  collards)*
stevia, liquid, 10 drops, plus ¼ tsp
  optional *(for drinks)*
tapioca starch, 1 tsp
tomatoes, crushed, 1¼ cups (300 ml)
tomatoes, whole, ½ (14½-oz/408-g/
  428-ml) can
vanilla extract, 1½ tsp
white wine, such as Pinot Grigio,
  Sauvignon Blanc, or unoaked
  Chardonnay, ¼ cup (2 fl. oz./60 ml)

*Finely ground gray sea salt and ground
black pepper will be needed for many
of the recipes. Purchase once and use
throughout the plan.*

	MEAL 1	MEAL 2	MEAL 3	SNACKS	DAY MACROS/TOTALS	
DAY 1	(fasted morning)	**CHIPOTLE-SPICED MEATBALL SUBS** (eat 2 servings) ½ P322	**LAMB KEBABS[1]** with white rice ❄ ⊕ P318 AND Mug Cake[2] ⊕		fat 47% / carbs 35% / protein 18% / calories 1482 / total fat 77.4 / sat. fat 29.7	chol. 358 / sodium 1464 / carbs 128 / fiber 13.7 / net carbs 114 / protein 68.5
DAY 2	**ROCKET FUEL LATTE** with 2 Tbsp. additional collagen P428	**STUFFED PORK ROAST[3]** ❄ P334 AND **CAULIFLOWER RICE** P364 AND **SHICHIMI COLLARDS** P379	**ALMOND CHAI TRUFFLES[4]** ❄ P392		fat 74% / carbs 6% / protein 20% / calories 1389 / total fat 114 / sat. fat 49.3	chol. 111 / sodium 1867 / carbs 22.5 / fiber 11.4 / net carbs 11.1 / protein 68.8
DAY 3	**MOJITO SMOOTHIE** P425 AND **LEMON DROPS[5]** ❄ P407	Leftover Chipotle-Spiced Meatball Subs (eat 3 servings)	**BACON SOUP[6]** ❄ P280		fat 72% / carbs 8% / protein 20% / calories 1898 / total fat 151 / sat. fat 68.9	chol. 270 / sodium 2267 / carbs 39.7 / fiber 12.9 / net carbs 26.8 / protein 94.9
DAY 4	Leftover Mojito Smoothie	Leftover Stuffed Pork Roast with Herb Gravy AND Leftover Cauliflower Rice	**SALT AND PEPPER CHICKEN WINGS[7]** P270 AND Leftover Shichimi Collards (eat 2 servings)		fat 75% / carbs 8% / protein 17% / calories 1672 / total fat 138 / sat. fat 42.8	chol. 192 / sodium 2594 / carbs 33.9 / fiber 16.9 / net carbs 17 / protein 72.8
DAY 5	**CLASSIC BUTTER BISCUITS[8]** ½ ❄ P368 AND **ROCKET FUEL LATTE** with 2 Tbsp. additional collagen P428	Leftover Chipotle-Spiced Meatball Subs (eat 2 servings) AND Leftover Shichimi Collards		Leftover Lemon Drops	fat 76% / carbs 9% / protein 15% / calories 1589 / total fat 134 / sat. fat 79.1	chol. 104 / sodium 1609 / carbs 34.5 / fiber 15.6 / net carbs 18.9 / protein 60.2
DAY 6	**ACV ICED TEA** P418	Leftover Salt and Pepper Chicken Wings AND Leftover Cauliflower Rice	**CHILI-STUFFED AVOCADOS[9]** (eat 2 servings) ½ P304	Leftover Almond Chai Truffles (eat 2 servings)	fat 77% / carbs 8% / protein 15% / calories 1725 / total fat 146 / sat. fat 45.9	chol. 205 / sodium 961 / carbs 36.1 / fiber 21.9 / net carbs 14.4 / protein 65.7
DAY 7	4 strips bacon AND Leftover Cauliflower Rice AND Leftover Salt and Pepper Chicken Wings	**KUNG PAO PORK[10]** with roasted sweet potatoes ❄ ⊕ P328 AND Pineapple Cream Bowl[11] ⊕			fat 61% / carbs 23% / protein 16% / calories 1718 / total fat 117 / sat. fat 35.7	chol. 220 / sodium 1144 / carbs 97.3 / fiber 16.3 / net carbs 79.9 / protein 69.2

½ HALF BATCH
⊕ CARB-UP
❄ FREEZE

UPPERCASE RECIPES are to be made fresh.

[1] Follow the carb-up instructions for the Lamb Kebabs recipe. Serve with 2 cups (1120 g) white rice, cooked. Adjusted recipe provides 4 carb-up servings. Freeze 1 serving for week 2 and 1 serving for week 4.

[2] Follow steps for preparation under Cassava/Microwave in the free "Carb-Up Recipes" PDF available at healthfulpursuit.com/carbup. Makes 1 serving.

[3] Freeze 1 serving of Stuffed Pork Roast with Herb Gravy for week 2, 3 servings for week 3, and 2 servings for week 4.

[4] Freeze 6 servings of truffles for use in weeks 3 and 4.

[5] Freeze 2 servings of Lemon Drops for week 2.

[6] Freeze 1 serving of soup for week 2, 3 servings for week 3, and 1 serving for week 4.

[7] Reserve 1 serving of chicken wings for week 2.

[8] Freeze 5 biscuits for use in weeks 2, 3, and 4.

[9] Reserve 2 servings of chili for use in week 2 along with fresh ingredients.

[10] Follow the carb-up instructions for the Kung Pao Pork recipe. Serve with roasted sweet potatoes (2 medium), as outlined in the free "Carb-Up Recipes" PDF available at healthfulpursuit.com/carbup. Adjusted recipe provides 2 carb-up servings. Freeze 1 serving for week 3.

[11] Prepare 2 cups (330 g) cubed pineapple. Enjoy with 2 Tbsp coconut cream. Makes 1 serving.

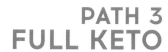

SHOPPING LIST FOR WEEK 2

FRESH PRODUCE

apple, 1
avocado, Hass, ½ large
cauliflower, 1 large head
chives, 2 Tbsp sliced
cilantro, 1 bunch
dill, 2 Tbsp
garlic, 4 small cloves
ginger root, 3-inch (7.5-cm) piece
herbs of choice, fresh, such as thyme
    and/or rosemary, 1 Tbsp chopped
lemons, 3
lime, 1, plus 1 optional *(for Cajun Pork Belly*
    Salad)
mint, 2 Tbsp chopped
onions, green, 2
parsley, 1 bunch
radishes, 3 bunches
rosemary, 1 sprig
sage, 1 sprig
thyme, 1 sprig
turmeric root, 6-in (15-cm) piece
turnips, 2 large
zucchini, 1 large

MEAT, EGGS, AND BROTH

bacon, 7 strips
eggs, 7 large, plus 1 optional
    (for Keto Milkshake)
lard, 3 Tbsp
MCT oil, ¼ cup plus 2 Tbsp
    (90 ml)
pork belly, side of, ½ lb (225 g)
salmon, 2 (7½-oz./213-g) cans
sirloin steak (aka strip steak or beef strip
    loin steak), boneless, about 1 inch
    (2.5 cm) thick, 13 oz. (370 g)

FATS AND OILS

avocado oil, refined, 3 Tbsp
    plus 1½ tsp
coconut cream, ¾ cup (180 g)
coconut oil, 3 Tbsp
extra-virgin olive oil, ¼ cup plus 3 Tbsp
    (105 ml)
tallow, ¼ cup plus 2 Tbsp (78 g)

DRIED HERBS AND SPICES

Cajun Seasoning (page 232), ¾ Tbsp
cinnamon, ground, 1 tsp
cumin, ground, ¼ tsp
garlic powder, ½ tsp
Italian Seasoning, 1 Tbsp
nutmeg, ground, ½ tsp
onion powder, ½ tsp
paprika, 1 pinch
parsley, 1 pinch
thyme leaves, 1 tsp

PANTRY ITEMS

cacao powder, 2 Tbsp
coconut milk, full-fat, 2⅓ cups
    (18½ fl. oz./550 ml)
collagen peptides, ¼ cup plus 2 Tbsp
    (60 g)
gelatin, unflavored, 3 Tbsp
green tea, 1 Tbsp plus 2 tsp loose tea or
    6 bags
mustard, prepared yellow, 1 tsp
nondairy milk, unsweetened, 4 cups
    (32 fl. oz./940 ml)
nutritional yeast, 2 Tbsp plus 2 tsp
pork dust, 1 oz. (30 g)
stevia, liquid, ¼ to ½ tsp
tahini, 2 Tbsp
vanilla extract, 1 tsp

	MEAL 1	MEAL 2	MEAL 3	SNACKS	DAY MACROS/TOTALS	
DAY 8	2 eggs cooked in 1 Tbsp. tallow **AND** 4 strips bacon **AND** **FAT-BURNING GOLDEN MILKSHAKE** P416	*Leftover* **Salt and Pepper Chicken Wings** **AND** **CREAMY MASHED TURNIPS** ½ P382	*Leftover* **Chili-Stuffed Avocados**		fat 80% / carbs 6% / protein 14% / calories 1782 / total fat 158 / sat. fat 74.5	chol. 534 / sodium 1665 / carbs 27.5 / fiber 10.3 / net carbs 16.2 / protein 61.2
DAY 9	**FATTY GREEN TEA** P419	*Leftover* **Stuffed Pork Roast with Herb Gravy** **AND** *Leftover* **Creamy Mashed Turnips**	*Leftover* **Chili-Stuffed Avocados** **AND** **HERBED RADISHES** *(eat 2 servings)* P384	*Leftover* **Almond Chai Truffles**	fat 71% / carbs 10% / protein 19% / calories 1740 / total fat 138 / sat. fat 55.3	chol. 185 / sodium 1673 / carbs 41.3 / fiber 13.2 / net carbs 28.2 / protein 84
DAY 10	*Leftover* **Fatty Green Tea**	**SALMON CAKES WITH DILL CREAM SAUCE**[1] ❄ P360	**STEAK WITH TALLOW HERB BUTTER**[2] ❄ P306 **AND** *Leftover* **Creamy Mashed Turnips**	**NO-BEANS HUMMUS** ½ P256 **AND** **ITALIAN ZUCCHINI ROUNDS**[3] ½ ❄ P250 **AND** *Leftover* **Lemon Drops**	fat 78% / carbs 7% / protein 15% / calories 1609 / total fat 140 / sat. fat 69.2	chol. 215 / sodium 1713 / carbs 26.1 / fiber 7.2 / net carbs 18.9 / protein 61.6
DAY 11	**FAT-BURNING GOLDEN MILKSHAKE** P416	*Leftover* **Salmon Cakes with Dill Cream Sauce** **AND** *Leftover* **Italian Zucchini Rounds** **AND** *Leftover* **No-Beans Hummus**	*Leftover* **Steak with Tallow Herb Butter** **AND** *Leftover* **Creamy Mashed Turnips** **AND** *Leftover* **No-Beans Hummus**		fat 79% / carbs 8% / protein 13% / calories 1678 / total fat 147 / sat. fat 72.1	chol. 215 / sodium 2088 / carbs 33.2 / fiber 10 / net carbs 23.2 / protein 55.2
DAY 12	*(fasted morning)*	*Leftover* **Salmon Cakes with Dill Cream Sauce** **AND** *Leftover* **Creamy Mashed Turnips**	*Leftover* **Bacon Soup** **AND** *Leftover* **Italian Zucchini Rounds** **AND** *Leftover* **No-Beans Hummus**		fat 72% / carbs 8% / protein 20% / calories 1432 / total fat 114 / sat. fat 40.9	chol. 254 / sodium 2974 / carbs 30.5 / fiber 7.6 / net carbs 22.9 / protein 70.4
DAY 13	*Leftover* **Classic Butter Biscuits** **AND** 2 eggs cooked in 1 Tbsp. tallow	**CAJUN PORK BELLY CHOPPED SALAD**[4] ½ P286		*Leftover* **Lemon Drops**	fat 90% / carbs 3% / protein 7% / calories 1811 / total fat 180 / sat. fat 87	chol. 458 / sodium 479 / carbs 15.2 / fiber 7.3 / net carbs 7.9 / protein 32.9
DAY 14	**KETO MILKSHAKE** with 2 Tbsp. additional collagen P423	**BACON MAC 'N' CHEESE**[5] ½ P320	*Leftover* **Lamb Kebabs** with white rice ➕ **AND** **Cooked Apple**[6] ➕		fat 57% / carbs 27% / protein 16% / calories 2314 / total fat 146 / sat. fat 87.2	chol. 428 / sodium 1901 / carbs 156 / fiber 24.6 / net carbs 131 / protein 95.1

½ HALF BATCH
➕ CARB-UP
❄ FREEZE

UPPERCASE RECIPES are to be made fresh.

[1] Freeze 1 serving of Salmon Cakes for week 3. In the shopping lists, the fresh ingredients for the sauce have been reduced this week and transferred to week 3 to be prepared as a quarter batch.

[2] Freeze 1 serving of steak for week 2 and 1 serving for week 3.

[3] Freeze 2 servings of Italian Zucchni Rounds for week 3.

[4] Reserve half of the Cajun Pork Belly Salad for week 3.

[5] Reserve 1 serving of Bacon Mac 'n' Cheese for day 15.

[6] Using 1 apple, follow the steps for preparation in the free "Carb-Up Recipes" PDF available at healthfulpursuit.com/carbup under Apple > Microwave or Roast. Makes 1 serving.

PATH 3
FULL KETO

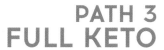

SHOPPING LIST FOR WEEK 3

FRESH PRODUCE

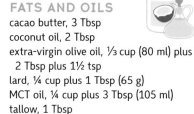

Brussels sprouts, trimmed and halved, 2½ cups (300 g)
cauliflower, 1 small head
chives, 2 Tbsp sliced
dill, 2 tsp
garlic, 1 small clove
ginger root, ½ tsp grated
herbs of choice, such as thyme and/or rosemary, 1 Tbsp chopped
lemons, 2
parsley, 1 bunch
radishes, 2 bunches
thyme, 2 sprigs

MEAT, EGGS, AND BROTH

bacon, 3 strips
bone broth, any type, 2 cups (16 fl. oz./ 475 ml) *(If making homemade broth, see page 152 for ingredients.)*
chicken bone broth, 1 cup (8 fl. oz./ 240 ml), or more as needed *(for ribs)*
eggs, 4 large
pork ribs, country-style, 1⅔ lbs (750 g)

FATS AND OILS

cacao butter, 3 Tbsp
coconut oil, 2 Tbsp
extra-virgin olive oil, ⅓ cup (80 ml) plus 2 Tbsp plus 1½ tsp
lard, ¼ cup plus 1 Tbsp (65 g)
MCT oil, ¼ cup plus 3 Tbsp (105 ml)
tallow, 1 Tbsp

DRIED HERBS AND SPICES

cayenne pepper, 1 pinch
cinnamon, ground, ¼ tsp
cloves, ground, ⅛ tsp
garlic powder, ½ tsp
onion powder, 1¾ tsp

PANTRY ITEMS

apple cider vinegar, 2 Tbsp
baking powder, ¼ tsp
cassava flour, ¼ cup (30 g)
cocoa powder, 2 Tbsp
coconut milk, full-fat, ¼ cup (2 fl. oz./60 ml)
coconut palm sugar, 1 Tbsp
coffee, ground, ½ cup plus 1 Tbsp (56 g), or tea of choice, 2 Tbsp loose tea or 6 bags
collagen peptides, 3 Tbsp
Dijon mustard, ¼ tsp
gelatin, unflavored, 1 Tbsp
hemp seeds, hulled, 3 Tbsp
mustard, prepared yellow, 1 tsp
nondairy milk, unsweetened, 1 cup plus 2 Tbsp (9 fl. oz./270 ml)
nutritional yeast, ¼ cup plus 4 tsp (22 g)
pork dust, 1 oz. (30 g)
rooibos tea, 2½ tsp loose tea or 3 bags
stevia, liquid, 11 drops, plus 6 to 12 optional drops *(for RFL)*
sun-dried tomatoes, 1½ oz. (40 g)
vanilla extract, ¾ tsp
walnut pieces, raw, ¼ cup plus 2 Tbsp (40 g)

196   Chapter 12: MEAL PLANS AND SHOPPING LISTS

	MEAL 1	MEAL 2	MEAL 3	SNACKS	DAY MACROS/TOTALS	
DAY 15	*(fasted morning)*	**ROCKET FUEL BONE BROTH** `P426` `AND` *Leftover* **Bacon Mac 'n' Cheese**	*Leftover* **Stuffed Pork Roast with Herb Gravy** `AND` *Leftover* **Classic Butter Biscuits**		*fat* **68%** / *carbs* **7%** / *protein* **25%** / *calories* **1413** / *total fat* **107** / *sat. fat* **48.6**	*chol.* **247** / *sodium* **2374** / *carbs* **24.8** / *fiber* **11.1** / *net carbs* **13.7** / *protein* **87.5**
DAY 16	*Leftover* **Rocket Fuel Bone Broth**	*Leftover* **Cajun Pork Belly Chopped Salad**	*Leftover* **Stuffed Pork Roast with Herb Gravy** `AND` *Leftover* **Italian Zucchini Rounds**		*fat* **83%** / *carbs* **3%** / *protein* **14%** / *calories* **1899** / *total fat* **176** / *sat. fat* **55**	*chol.* **236** / *sodium* **2213** / *carbs* **12.2** / *fiber* **3.7** / *net carbs* **8.5** / *protein* **66.9**
DAY 17	*2 eggs cooked in 1 Tbsp. tallow* `AND` *Leftover* **Classic Butter Biscuits** `AND` **ROCKET FUEL LATTE** `P428`	*Leftover* **Bacon Soup**	*Leftover* **Salmon Cakes with Dill Cream Sauce** `AND` *Leftover* **Italian Zucchini Rounds**		*fat* **77%** / *carbs* **5%** / *protein* **18%** / *calories* **2024** / *total fat* **173** / *sat. fat* **90.7**	*chol.* **595** / *sodium* **2972** / *carbs* **26.6** / *fiber* **9.1** / *net carbs* **17.5** / *protein* **90.6**
DAY 18	**ROCKET FUEL LATTE** `P428` `AND` *Leftover* **Almond Chai Truffles**	**SALT AND PEPPER RIBS**[1] ½ ❋ `P330`	**BACON MAC 'N' CHEESE** ½ `P320`		*fat* **70%** / *carbs* **6%** / *protein* **24%** / *calories* **1349** / *total fat* **105** / *sat. fat* **40.9**	*chol.* **128** / *sodium* **1933** / *carbs* **20** / *fiber* **10** / *net carbs* **10** / *protein* **80.1**
DAY 19	**ACV ICED TEA** `P418`	*Leftover* **Bacon Mac 'n' Cheese**	*Leftover* **Steak with Tallow Herb Butter** `AND` **HERBED RADISHES** *(eat 2 servings)* `P384`	*Leftover* **Almond Chai Truffles** *(eat 2 servings)*	*fat* **72%** / *carbs* **9%** / *protein* **19%** / *calories* **1585** / *total fat* **127** / *sat. fat* **49.4**	*chol.* **239** / *sodium* **1514** / *carbs* **36.9** / *fiber* **12.6** / *net carbs* **24.3** / *protein* **74.1**
DAY 20	*(fasted morning)*	*Leftover* **Bacon Soup** `AND` *Leftover* **Almond Chai Truffles**	*Leftover* **Stuffed Pork Roast with Herb Gravy** `AND` **ROASTED BRUSSELS SPROUTS**[2] ½ ❋ `P388`		*fat* **69%** / *carbs* **7%** / *protein* **24%** / *calories* **1464** / *total fat* **112** / *sat. fat* **37**	*chol.* **215** / *sodium* **2443** / *carbs* **24.6** / *fiber* **7.8** / *net carbs* **16.8** / *protein* **89**
DAY 21	**ROCKET FUEL LATTE** `P428`	*Leftover* **Bacon Soup** `AND` *Leftover* **Roasted Brussels Sprouts**	*Leftover* **Kung Pao Pork** *with roasted sweet potatoes* ➕ `AND` *Mug Cake*[3] ➕		*fat* **62%** / *carbs* **20%** / *protein* **18%** / *calories* **2109** / *total fat* **144** / *sat. fat* **65**	*chol.* **349** / *sodium* **2337** / *carbs* **108** / *fiber* **21.3** / *net carbs* **86.6** / *protein* **94.3**

½ HALF BATCH
➕ CARB-UP
❋ FREEZE

UPPERCASE RECIPES are to be made fresh.

[1] Freeze 3 servings of ribs for week 4.
[2] Reserve 1 serving of Brussels sprouts for week 4.
[3] Follow the steps for preparation in the free "Carb-Up Recipes" PDF available at healthfulpursuit.com/carbup under Cassava > Microwave. Makes 1 serving.

WEEK 4

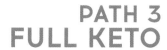

PATH 3
FULL KETO

SHOPPING LIST FOR WEEK 4

FRESH PRODUCE

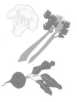

avocado, Hass, 1 large

cabbage, green, 1 medium head

carrots, 1 medium

cauliflower, 1 small head

celery, 3 large stalks

cucumbers, 2 small

garlic, 3 small cloves

ginger root, ½ tsp grated

kale, 2 cups (85 g) chopped

limes, 2

mint leaves, 1 packed Tbsp

onion, white, 1 small

onions, green, 4

spinach, 1 packed cup (70 g)

MEAT, EGGS, AND BROTH

bacon, 6 strips

bone broth, any type, 2 cups (16 fl. oz./ 475 ml) *(If making homemade broth, see page 152 for ingredients.)*

chicken bone broth, 2 cups (16 fl. oz./ 475 ml)

chicken thighs, boneless, skinless, 1 lb (455 g)

egg, 1 large, plus 1 optional *(for milkshake)*

FATS AND OILS

avocado oil, refined, ¼ cup plus 2 Tbsp (90 ml)

cacao butter, 2 Tbsp

coconut oil, ½ cup (120 ml)

MCT oil, ½ cup plus 2 Tbsp (150 ml)

DRIED HERBS AND SPICES

cayenne pepper, 1 pinch

cinnamon, ground, ¼ tsp

garlic powder, ½ tsp

onion powder, 1 tsp

PANTRY ITEMS

apple cider vinegar, 2 Tbsp plus 1½ tsp

cacao powder, 2 Tbsp

coconut flour, ¼ cup plus 2 Tbsp (40 g)

coconut milk, full-fat, 2 cups (16 fl. oz./ 480 ml)

coffee, ground, ¼ cup plus 2 Tbsp (32 g), or tea of choice, 4 tsp loose tea or 4 bags

collagen peptides, ½ cup (80 g)

green tea, 1½ tsp loose tea or 2 bags

hemp seeds, hulled, 2 Tbsp

macadamia nuts, 12

rice, white, 2 cups (1120 g)

rooibos tea, 2½ tsp loose tea or 3 bags

sesame seeds, ¼ cup (40 g)

stevia, liquid, ¼ tsp, plus 8 to 14 optional drops *(for drinks)*

vanilla extract, 1½ tsp

	MEAL 1	MEAL 2	MEAL 3	SNACKS	DAY MACROS/TOTALS	
DAY 22	*(fasted morning)*	*Leftover* **Salt and Pepper Ribs** **AND** **ROASTED BRUSSELS SPROUTS** ¼ P388	**CHICKEN POT PIE CRUMBLE**[1] ❄ P344 **AND** **KALE PÂTÉ** ½ P259 **AND** *1 large stalk celery*	**ROCKET FUEL BONE BROTH** P426	fat 73% · chol. 167 carbs 7% · sodium 2132 protein 20% · carbs 29.6 calories 1622 · fiber 11.8 total fat 131 · net carbs 17.8 sat. fat 44.1 · protein 80.9	
DAY 23	**MOJITO SMOOTHIE** P425	*Leftover* **Chicken Pot Pie Crumble** **AND** **PORKY CABBAGE** P385	*Leftover* **Salt and Pepper Ribs** **AND** *Leftover* **Kale Pâté** **AND** *1 large stalk celery*		fat 73% · chol. 167 carbs 8% · sodium 2045 protein 19% · carbs 31.9 calories 1611 · fiber 14.3 total fat 131 · net carbs 17.6 sat. fat 52.2 · protein 75.8	
DAY 24	*Leftover* **Mojito Smoothie**	*Leftover* **Stuffed Pork Roast with Herb Gravy** **AND** *Leftover* **Porky Cabbage**	*Leftover* **Classic Butter Biscuits** **AND** *Leftover* **Kale Pâté** **AND** *Leftover* **Rocket Fuel Bone Broth** *with 2 Tbsp. collagen blended in*		fat 76% · chol. 149 carbs 7% · sodium 2338 protein 17% · carbs 29.4 calories 1762 · fiber 13 total fat 150 · net carbs 16.4 sat. fat 65.4 · protein 74	
DAY 25	*(fasted morning)*	*Leftover* **Stuffed Pork Roast with Herb Gravy** **AND** *Leftover* **Kale Pâté** **AND** *1 small cucumber, sliced*	*Leftover* **Chicken Pot Pie Crumble**	**KETO MILKSHAKE** P423	fat 75% · chol. 442 carbs 6% · sodium 1775 protein 19% · carbs 28.3 calories 2043 · fiber 11 total fat 171 · net carbs 17.3 sat. fat 101 · protein 97.7	
DAY 26	**ROCKET FUEL LATTE** P428	*Leftover* **Salt and Pepper Ribs** **AND** *Leftover* **Porky Cabbage**	*Leftover* **Chicken Pot Pie Crumble** **AND** *1 small cucumber, sliced*		fat 71% · chol. 167 carbs 7% · sodium 1857 protein 22% · carbs 23 calories 1420 · fiber 9.1 total fat 112 · net carbs 13.9 sat. fat 57.3 · protein 79.4	
DAY 27	**ACV ICED TEA** P418	*Leftover* **Bacon Soup** **AND** *Leftover* **Classic Butter Biscuits**	*Leftover* **Steak with Tallow Herb Butter** **AND** *Leftover* **Porky Cabbage**	*Leftover* **Almond Chai Truffles**	fat 73% · chol. 219 carbs 8% · sodium 2307 protein 19% · carbs 30.1 calories 1555 · fiber 10.8 total fat 126 · net carbs 19.3 sat. fat 62.2 · protein 75.3	
DAY 28	**ROCKET FUEL LATTE** P428 **AND** *Leftover* **Almond Chai Truffles**	*Leftover* **Lamb Kebabs** *with white rice (eat 2 servings)*	➕		fat 52% · chol. 180 carbs 33% · sodium 1318 protein 15% · carbs 143 calories 1713 · fiber 6.4 total fat 98.8 · net carbs 136 sat. fat 46.3 · protein 63	

½ HALF BATCH

¼ QUARTER BATCH

➕ CARB-UP

❄ FREEZE

UPPERCASE RECIPES are to be made fresh.

[1] Freeze 1 serving for day 26.

EXTRA LEFTOVERS NOT USED IN THE PLAN: 1 serving Chili-Stuffed Avocados, 1 serving Chipotle-Spiced Meatball Subs, 1 serving Roasted Brussels Sprouts

PATH 3
ADAPTED FAT BURNER

Follow this plan after you've become fat-adapted by following either the Classic Keto (plan 1) or the Pumped Keto (plan 2) meal plan (find out more on page 47). You'll start with a carb-up (assuming that you've become fat-adapted by following plan 1 or 2) and then practice a carb-up twice a week.

This plan is similar to the Full Keto meal plan to allow for switching between the two profiles as you find the profile that suits you best.

Not enough food for you? The simplest way to add bulk to the daytime meals without having to worry about it affecting your macros is to increase the fat in your Rocket Fuel Latte (RFL), whip up a fat bomb (see the chart beginning on page 432) and enjoy after a meal, or double up on recipes. If more carbs are needed following your carb-up, visit healthfulpursuit.com/carbup to download the complimentary PDF "Carb-Up Recipes," simply adding additional carbs to your meal or post-meal dessert.

Instructions for evening carb-ups are below the plan for each week.

SHOPPING LIST FOR WEEK 1

FRESH PRODUCE
apple, red, 1
avocados, Hass, 3 large
bell pepper, green, 1
blackberries, 1 cup (145 g)
cabbage, green, 1 large head
cauliflower, 1 medium head
celery, 1 medium stalk
cilantro, 1 bunch *(optional, for subs)*
collards, 1 bunch
garlic, 1 small clove
lemon, 1
lime, 1
mint leaves, 1 packed Tbsp
onion, red, 1 small
onion, white, 1 small
parsley, 2 bunches
pineapple, 1 small
raspberries, 1 cup (125 g)
rosemary, 1 sprig
sage, 1 sprig
shallots, 3 medium
spinach, 1 packed cup (70 g)
strawberries, 1 cup (150 g)
thyme, 1 bunch
tomatoes, hothouse, 2
turnips, 3 medium

MEAT, EGGS, AND BROTH
bacon, 14 strips
chicken bone broth, 5 cups plus 2 Tbsp (41 fl. oz./1.2 L) *(If making homemade broth, see page 152 for ingredients.)*
chicken breasts, skinless, 1 cup plus 3 Tbsp (150 g) diced
chicken wings, 1 lb (455 g)
egg, 1 large
ground beef, 20% to 30% fat, ½ lb (225 g)
ground chicken, ½ lb (225 g)
ground lamb, 1 lb (455 g)
ground pork, 13¼ oz. (375 g)
pork rib roast, boneless, 2 lbs (910 g)
pork stewing pieces, 1 lb (455 g)
sirloin steak (aka strip steak or beef strip loin steak), boneless, 6½ oz. (185 g), about 1 inch (2.5 cm) thick

FATS AND OILS
avocado oil, refined, 1 cup plus 1 Tbsp (255 ml)
cacao butter, ¾ cup (180 g)
coconut cream, 2 Tbsp
coconut oil, ¾ cup plus 2 Tbsp (210 ml)
lard, ⅔ cup (140 g)
mayonnaise, made with avocado oil, 2 Tbsp *(If making homemade mayo, see page 220 for ingredients.)*
MCT oil, ¼ cup (60 ml)
tallow, 3 Tbsp (40 g)

DRIED HERBS AND SPICES
Bahārāt Seasoning (page 233), 1 Tbsp
chai spice (page 392), 1 Tbsp plus 1 tsp
chili powder, 2¼ tsp
chipotle powder, ½ plus ⅛ tsp
cinnamon, ground, ¼ tsp
cumin, ground, ¾ tsp
garlic powder, ¾ tsp
Italian Seasoning (page 234), 1 Tbsp plus 2 tsp
onion powder, ¼ tsp
oregano leaves, 2¼ tsp
paprika, 1 tsp
Shichimi Seasoning (page 234), 1½ tsp
smoked paprika, ¼ tsp
tarragon leaves, 1 Tbsp

PANTRY ITEMS
almond butter, unsweetened smooth, ½ cup (140 g)
almonds, 3 Tbsp
apple cider vinegar, 3 Tbsp plus 2 tsp
baking powder, ¾ tsp
cassava flour, ¼ cup (30 g)
cocoa powder, 2 Tbsp
coconut aminos, 1 Tbsp
coconut flour, ¾ cup (75 g)
coconut milk, full-fat, ¾ cup (6 fl. oz./180 ml)
coconut palm sugar, 1 Tbsp
coffee, ground, 3 Tbsp, or tea of choice, 2 tsp loose tea or 2 bags
collagen peptides, ¼ cup plus 2 Tbsp (60 g)
erythritol, confectioners'-style, 1½ Tbsp
gelatin, unflavored, 3 Tbsp plus 1½ tsp
green tea, 1 Tbsp loose tea or 4 bags
hemp seeds, hulled, 2 Tbsp
lemon extract, 1 tsp
macadamia nuts, 12
magnesium powder, lemon-flavored, 2 tsp
mustard, prepared yellow, 1 Tbsp
nondairy milk, unsweetened, 2 Tbsp
pork dust, 2 oz. (57 g)
raisins, ¼ cup (57 g)
rice, white, 2 cups (1120 g)
rooibos tea, 1½ tsp loose tea or 2 bags
sesame seeds *(optional, for Shichimi Collards)*
stevia, liquid, 9 drops, plus ¼ tsp optional *(for drinks)*
tapioca starch, 1 tsp
tomatoes, crushed, 1¼ cups (300 ml)
tomatoes, whole, ½ (14½-oz./408-g) can
vanilla extract, 1½ tsp
white wine, such as Pinot Grigio, Sauvignon Blanc, or unoaked Chardonnay, ¼ cup (2 fl. oz./60 ml)

Finely ground gray sea salt and ground black pepper will be needed for many of the recipes. Purchase once and use throughout the plan.

	MEAL 1	MEAL 2	MEAL 3	SNACKS	DAY MACROS/TOTALS	
DAY 1	*(fasted morning)*	**CHIPOTLE-SPICED MEATBALL SUBS** *(eat 2 servings)*[1] ½ ❄ P322	**LAMB KEBABS** *with white rice*[2] ❄ ➕ P318 AND *Mug Cake*[3] ➕		fat 47% / carbs 34% / protein 18% / calories 1482 / total fat 77.4 / sat. fat 29.7	chol. 358 / sodium 1464 / carbs 128 / fiber 13.7 / net carbs 114 / protein 68.5
DAY 2	**MOJITO SMOOTHIE** *with 2 Tbsp. collagen* P425	**STUFFED PORK ROAST**[4] ❄ P334 AND **CAULIFLOWER RICE** ½ P364 AND **SHICHIMI COLLARDS** ½ P379	**STEAK WITH TALLOW HERB BUTTER**[5] ½ ❄ P306	**ALMOND CHAI TRUFFLES**[6] ❄ P392	fat 73% / carbs 7% / protein 20% / calories 1664 / total fat 135 / sat. fat 52.3	chol. 186 / sodium 1863 / carbs 28.1 / fiber 14.4 / net carbs 13.7 / protein 83.4
DAY 3	*Leftover* **Mojito Smoothie** AND **LEMON DROPS**[7] ❄ P407	*Leftover* **Chipotle-Spiced Meatball Subs** *(3 servings)*	**BACON SOUP**[8] ❄ P280		fat 72% / carbs 8% / protein 20% / calories 1898 / total fat 151 / sat. fat 68.9	chol. 270 / sodium 2267 / carbs 39.7 / fiber 12.9 / net carbs 26.8 / protein 94.9
DAY 4	**ROCKET FUEL LATTE** P428	*Leftover* **Stuffed Pork Roast with Herb Gravy** AND *Leftover* **Cauliflower Rice**	**WALDORF-STUFFED TOMATOES**[9] ½ ➕ P351 AND *Pineapple Cream Bowl*[10] ➕		fat 59% / carbs 22% / protein 19% / calories 1593 / total fat 104 / sat. fat 49.4	chol. 172 / sodium 1421 / carbs 88.2 / fiber 11.8 / net carbs 76.4 / protein 76.5
DAY 5	**CLASSIC BUTTER BISCUITS**[11] ½ ❄ P368 AND **ROCKET FUEL LATTE** *with 2 Tbsp. additional collagen* P428	*Leftover* **Chipotle-Spiced Meatball Subs** *(eat 2 servings)* AND *Leftover* **Shichimi Collards**		*Leftover* **Lemon Drops**	fat 76% / carbs 9% / protein 15% / calories 1589 / total fat 134 / sat. fat 79.1	chol. 104 / sodium 1609 / carbs 34.5 / fiber 15.6 / net carbs 18.9 / protein 60.2
DAY 6	**ACV ICED TEA** P418	**SALT AND PEPPER CHICKEN WINGS**[12] P270 AND **CAULIFLOWER RICE** ½ P364	**CHILI-STUFFED AVOCADOS**[13] *(eat 2 servings)* ½ P304	*Leftover* **Almond Chai Truffles** *(eat 2 servings)*	fat 77% / carbs 8% / protein 15% / calories 1725 / total fat 146 / sat. fat 45.9	chol. 205 / sodium 961 / carbs 36.1 / fiber 21.9 / net carbs 14.4 / protein 65.7
DAY 7	*(fasted morning)*	*Leftover* **Salt and Pepper Chicken Wings** AND *Leftover* **Cauliflower Rice** AND *4 strips bacon*	*Leftover* **Waldorf-Stuffed Tomatoes** ➕ AND *Bowl of berries*[14] ➕		fat 61% / carbs 23% / protein 16% / calories 1445 / total fat 99.6 / sat. fat 27.6	chol. 216 / sodium 1283 / carbs 82.1 / fiber 24 / net carbs 58.1 / protein 60.2

½ HALF BATCH
➕ CARB-UP
❄ FREEZE

UPPERCASE RECIPES are to be made fresh.

[1] Freeze 1 serving for day 5. Fresh ingredients can remain in the fridge.
[2] Follow the carb-up instructions for the Lamb Kebabs recipe. Serve with 2 cups (1120 g) white rice, cooked (½ cup [280 g] per serving). Adjusted recipe provides 4 servings. Freeze 1 serving for week 2 and 1 serving for use after the plan.
[3] Follow the steps for preparing the Mug Cake in the free "Carb-Up Recipes" PDF available at healthfulpursuit.com/carbup under Cassava>Microwave. Makes 1 serving.
[4] Freeze 2 servings of Stuffed Pork Roast with Herb Gravy for week 2, 2 servings for week 3, and 2 servings for week 4.
[5] Freeze 1 serving of steak with tallow butter for week 3.
[6] Freeze 7 servings of truffles for use in weeks 2, 3, and 4.

[7] Freeze 1 serving of Lemon Drops for week 2 and 1 serving for week 3.
[8] Freeze 2 servings of Bacon Soup for week 2, 2 servings for week 3, and 1 serving for week 4.
[9] Follow the carb-up instructions for the Waldorf-Stuffed Tomatoes recipe.
[10] Enjoy 2 cups (330 g) cubed pineapple with 2 Tbsp coconut cream. Makes 1 serving.
[11] Freeze 5 biscuits for use in weeks 2, 3, and 4.
[12] Reserve 2 servings of chicken wings for day 8.
[13] Reserve 2 servings of Chili-Stuffed Avocados for week 2. Fresh ingredients can be stored in the fridge for later use.
[14] Place 1 cup (145 g) blackberries, 1 cup (125 g) raspberries, and 1 cup (150 g) strawberries in a bowl and enjoy. Makes 1 serving.

PATH 3
ADAPTED FAT BURNER

SHOPPING LIST FOR WEEK 2

FRESH PRODUCE
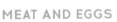
cauliflower, 1 medium head
cilantro, 1 bunch
cucumber, 1 small
dill, 3 Tbsp chopped
garlic, 8 small cloves
ginger root, 4-in (10-cm) piece
lemons, 3
limes, 2
mint, 2 Tbsp chopped
onions, green, 2
pineapple, 1 small
radishes, 1 bunch
sweet potatoes, 2 medium
turmeric root, 9-in (23-cm) piece
turnips, 2 large
zucchini, 1 large

MEAT AND EGGS
eggs, 6 large
pork belly, side of, ½ lb (225 g)
pork stir-fry pieces, ½ lb (225 g)
salmon, 2 (7½-oz./213-g) cans

FATS AND OILS
avocado oil, refined, 3 Tbsp
  plus 1½ tsp (52 ml)
coconut cream, 1 cup plus
  2 Tbsp (270 ml)
coconut oil, 2 Tbsp
extra-virgin olive oil, ¼ cup plus 3 Tbsp
  (125 ml)
MCT oil, ¼ cup plus 2 Tbsp (90 ml)
sesame oil, toasted, 1 Tbsp
tallow, 2 Tbsp

DRIED HERBS AND SPICES
Cajun Seasoning (page 232), 2¼ tsp
cinnamon, ground, 1 tsp
cumin, ground, ¼ tsp
Italian Seasoning (page 234), 1 Tbsp
paprika, 1 pinch
parsley, 1 pinch
thyme leaves, 1 tsp

PANTRY ITEMS
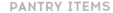
almond butter, unsweetened
  smooth, 2 Tbsp
apple cider vinegar, 2 Tbsp
chilis, dried, 2 to 4
coconut aminos, 3 Tbsp
coconut milk, full-fat, ⅓ cup (2¾ fl. oz./
  80 ml)
collagen peptides, 2 Tbsp
gelatin, unflavored, 2 Tbsp
green tea, 1 Tbsp loose tea or 4 bags
nondairy milk, unsweetened, 4½ cups
  (34 fl. oz./1 L)
stevia, liquid, ¼ to ½ tsp
tahini, 2 Tbsp
vanilla extract, ¾ tsp

	MEAL 1	MEAL 2	MEAL 3	SNACKS	DAY MACROS/TOTALS	
DAY 8	2 eggs cooked in 1 Tbsp. tallow **AND** **FAT-BURNING GOLDEN MILKSHAKE** P416	Leftover **Salt and Pepper Chicken Wings** (eat 2 servings) **AND** **CREAMY MASHED TURNIPS** ½ P382	Leftover **Chili-Stuffed Avocados**		fat 78% / carbs 6% / protein 16% / calories 1791 / total fat 156 / sat. fat 69.8	chol. 557 / sodium 1392 / carbs 26.7 / fiber 10.3 / net carbs 16.5 / protein 69.8
DAY 9	**FATTY GREEN TEA** P419	Leftover **Stuffed Pork Roast with Herb Gravy** **AND** Leftover **Creamy Mashed Turnips** (eat 2 servings)	Leftover **Chili-Stuffed Avocados**	Leftover **Almond Chai Truffles**	fat 68% / carbs 11% / protein 21% / calories 1387 / total fat 105 / sat. fat 43.5	chol. 149 / sodium 1588 / carbs 36.3 / fiber 13.9 / net carbs 22.5 / protein 73.7
DAY 10	Leftover **Fatty Green Tea**	**SALMON CAKES** P360 **AND** **NO-BEANS HUMMUS** ½ P256 **AND** **ITALIAN ZUCCHINI ROUNDS** ½ P250	**KUNG PAO PORK** with roasted sweet potatoes[1] ➕ P328 **AND** Pineapple Cream Bowl[2] ➕		fat 59% / carbs 24% / protein 17% / calories 1761 / total fat 115 / sat. fat 43.7	chol. 205 / sodium 1443 / carbs 107 / fiber 18.5 / net carbs 88 / protein 74.4
DAY 11	**FAT-BURNING GOLDEN MILKSHAKE** P416	Leftover **Salmon Cakes** with Dill Cream Sauce	Leftover **Stuffed Pork Roast with Herb Gravy** **AND** Leftover **Italian Zucchini Rounds** **AND** Leftover **No-Beans Hummus** (eat 2 servings)		fat 77% / carbs 6% / protein 17% / calories 1715 / total fat 147 / sat. fat 66.1	chol. 235 / sodium 2458 / carbs 25.6 / fiber 8.1 / net carbs 17.5 / protein 73.1
DAY 12	(fasted morning)	Leftover **Salmon Cakes** with Dill Cream Sauce **AND** Leftover **Creamy Mashed Turnips** (eat 2 servings)	Leftover **Bacon Soup** **AND** Leftover **Italian Zucchini Rounds** **AND** Leftover **No-Beans Hummus**		fat 71% / carbs 10% / protein 19% / calories 1525 / total fat 120 / sat. fat 44.3	chol. 254 / sodium 3235 / carbs 38.7 / fiber 9.5 / net carbs 29.2 / protein 71.7
DAY 13	2 eggs cooked in 1 Tbsp. tallow **AND** Leftover **Classic Butter Biscuits**	**CAJUN PORK BELLY CHOPPED SALAD**[3] ½ P286		Leftover **Lemon Drops**	fat 89% / carbs 3% / protein 8% / calories 1811 / total fat 180 / sat. fat 87	chol. 458 / sodium 479 / carbs 15.2 / fiber 7.3 / net carbs 7.9 / protein 32.9
DAY 14	**FAT-BURNING GOLDEN MILKSHAKE** with 2 Tbsp. collagen blended in P416	Leftover **Bacon Soup**	Leftover **Lamb Kebabs** with white rice ➕		fat 58% / carbs 22% / protein 20% / calories 1547 / total fat 100 / sat. fat 59	chol. 204 / sodium 2215 / carbs 85.5 / fiber 4 / net carbs 81.5 / protein 75.8

½ HALF BATCH
➕ CARB-UP

UPPERCASE RECIPES are to be made fresh.

[1] Follow the carb-up instructions for the Kung Pao Pork recipe. Serve with roasted sweet potatoes (2 medium), as outlined in the free "Carb-Up Recipes" PDF available at healthfulpursuit.com/carbup. Adjusted recipe provides 2 servings.
[2] For the Pineapple Cream Bowl, prepare 2 cups (330 g) cubed pineapple. Enjoy with 2 Tbsp coconut cream. Makes 1 serving.
[3] Reserve 1 serving of Cajun Pork Belly Chopped Salad for day 16. Fresh ingredients can be stored in the fridge for later use.

SHOPPING LIST FOR WEEK 3

FRESH PRODUCE

apple, 1
Brussels sprouts, 2½ cups (300 g) trimmed and halved
carrot, 1 medium
cauliflower, 1 large head
celery, 2 medium stalks
garlic, 1 small clove
ginger root, ½ tsp grated
lemon, 1
onions, green, 1 bunch
parsley, 1 bunch
thyme, 2 sprigs
yams, 2 medium

MEAT, EGGS, AND BROTH

bacon, 6 strips (about 6 oz./170 g)
bone broth, any type, 2 cups (16 fl. oz./ 475 ml) *(If making homemade broth, see page 152 for ingredients.)*
chicken bone broth, 7 cups (56 fl. oz./ 1.7 L), or more as needed
chicken breasts, boneless, skinless, 1 lb (455 g)
eggs, 5 large
pork ribs, country-style, 1⅔ lbs (750 g)

FATS AND OILS

cacao butter, ¼ cup (60 g)
coconut oil, ½ cup (120 ml)
extra-virgin olive oil, ½ cup (120 ml)
lard, 2 Tbsp
MCT oil, ¼ cup (60 ml)
tallow, 1 Tbsp

DRIED HERBS AND SPICES

basil, ½ tsp
cayenne pepper, 1 pinch
cinnamon, ground, 1 tsp
cloves, ground, ⅛ tsp
garlic powder, ¾ tsp
nutmeg, ground, ½ tsp
onion powder, 2⅛ tsp
oregano leaves, ½ tsp

PANTRY ITEMS

apple cider vinegar, 1 Tbsp
baking powder, ¼ tsp
cassava flour, ¼ cup (30 g)
cocoa powder, 2 Tbsp
coconut palm sugar, 1 Tbsp
coffee, ground, ¼ cup plus 2 Tbsp (32 g), or tea of choice, 4 tsp loose tea or 4 bags
collagen peptides, ¼ cup (40 g)
Dijon mustard, ¼ tsp
gelatin, unflavored, 2 Tbsp
hemp seeds, hulled, ¼ cup (38 g)
mustard, prepared yellow, 2 tsp
nondairy milk, unsweetened, 2 cups plus 2 Tbsp (17 fl. oz./505 ml)
nutritional yeast, ¾ cup (50 g)
pork dust, 2 oz. (60 g)
stevia, liquid, 2 to 3 drops, plus ⅛ to ¼ tsp optional *(for RFL)*
sun-dried tomatoes, 1½ oz. (42 g)
vanilla extract, 1 tsp
walnut pieces, raw, ¼ cup plus 2 Tbsp (42 g)

	MEAL 1	MEAL 2	MEAL 3	SNACKS	DAY MACROS/TOTALS	
DAY 15	*(fasted morning)* **AND** **ROCKET FUEL BONE BROTH** `P426`	**BACON MAC 'N' CHEESE** ½ `P320`	*Leftover* **Stuffed Pork Roast with Herb Gravy** **AND** *Leftover* **Italian Zucchini Rounds** **AND** *Leftover* **Classic Butter Biscuits**		*fat* 70% / *carbs* 7% / *protein* 23% / *calories* 1560 / *total fat* 122 / *sat. fat* 50.7	*chol.* 247 / *sodium* 3124 / *carbs* 27.7 / *fiber* 12 / *net carbs* 15.7 / *protein* 88.5
DAY 16	*Leftover* **Rocket Fuel Bone Broth**	*Leftover* **Cajun Pork Belly Chopped Salad**	**STEAK WITH TALLOW HERB BUTTER** `P306`	*Cooked Apples*[1] ⊕	*fat* 75% / *carbs* 15% / *protein* 10% / *calories* 1982 / *total fat* 166 / *sat. fat* 63.9	*chol.* 216 / *sodium* 837 / *carbs* 73.2 / *fiber* 15.3 / *net carbs* 57.9 / *protein* 48.1
DAY 17	**ROCKET FUEL LATTE** `P428` **AND** *2 eggs cooked in 1 Tbsp. tallow* **AND** *Leftover* **Classic Butter Biscuits**	*Leftover* **Bacon Mac 'n' Cheese** **AND** *Leftover* **Italian Zucchini Rounds**	*Leftover* **Salmon Cakes with Dill Cream Sauce**		*fat* 75% / *carbs* 7% / *protein* 18% / *calories* 1893 / *total fat* 158 / *sat. fat* 82.6	*chol.* 609 / *sodium* 2516 / *carbs* 31.5 / *fiber* 14.6 / *net carbs* 16.9 / *protein* 85.4
DAY 18	**ROCKET FUEL LATTE** `P428`	**SALT AND PEPPER RIBS**[2] ½ ❄ `P330` **AND** **ROASTED BRUSSELS SPROUTS**[3] ½ `P388`	**BACON MAC 'N' CHEESE** ½ `P320`	*Leftover* **Almond Chai Truffles**	*fat* 71% / *carbs* 7% / *protein* 21% / *calories* 1612 / *total fat* 128 / *sat. fat* 45.4	*chol.* 134 / *sodium* 2137 / *carbs* 29.9 / *fiber* 14.3 / *net carbs* 15.6 / *protein* 85.9
DAY 19	**ROCKET FUEL LATTE** `P428` **AND** *Leftover* **Almond Chai Truffles** *(eat 2 servings)*	*Leftover* **Bacon Mac 'n' Cheese**	**CHICKEN NOODLE SOUP** *with yam noodles*[4] ❄ ⊕ `P276`		*fat* 61% / *carbs* 16% / *protein* 23% / *calories* 1606 / *total fat* 108 / *sat. fat* 51.3	*chol.* 217 / *sodium* 1940 / *carbs* 63.1 / *fiber* 19.3 / *net carbs* 43.8 / *protein* 94.5
DAY 20	*(fasted morning)*	*Leftover* **Bacon Soup**	*Leftover* **Stuffed Pork Roast with Herb Gravy** **AND** *Leftover* **Roasted Brussels Sprouts**	*Leftover* **Almond Chai Truffles** **AND** *Leftover* **Lemon Drops**	*fat* 73% / *carbs* 6% / *protein* 21% / *calories* 1722 / *total fat* 141 / *sat. fat* 59.2	*chol.* 215 / *sodium* 2443 / *carbs* 24.8 / *fiber* 7.8 / *net carbs* 17 / *protein* 89
DAY 21	**ROCKET FUEL LATTE** `P428`	*Leftover* **Bacon Soup** **AND** *Leftover* **Roasted Brussels Sprouts**	*Leftover* **Kung Pao Pork** *with roasted sweet potatoes* ⊕ **AND** *Mug Cake*[5] ⊕		*fat* 62% / *carbs* 20% / *protein* 18% / *calories* 2109 / *total fat* 144 / *sat. fat* 65	*chol.* 349 / *sodium* 2337 / *carbs* 108 / *fiber* 21.3 / *net carbs* 86.6 / *protein* 94.3

½ HALF BATCH
⊕ CARB-UP
❄ FREEZE

UPPERCASE RECIPES are to be made fresh.

[1]Using 1 apple, follow the steps for preparation in the free "Carb-Up Recipes" PDF available at healthfulpursuit.com/carbup under Apple > Microwave or Roast. Makes 1 serving.

[2]Freeze 3 servings of ribs for week 4.

[3]Reserve 1 serving of Brussels sprouts for day 22.

[4]Follow the carb-up instructions for the Chicken Noodle Soup recipe, adding 2 medium spiral-sliced yams to the soup.

[5]Follow the steps for preparation in the free "Carb-Up Recipes" PDF available at healthfulpursuit.com/carbup under Cassava>Microwave. Makes 1 serving.

SHOPPING LIST FOR WEEK 4

FRESH PRODUCE

apple, 1
avocado, Hass, 1 large
cabbage, green, 1 medium
  head
carrot, 1 medium
cauliflower, 1 small head
celery, 3 large stalks
cucumber, 1 small
garlic, 3 small cloves
ginger root, ½ tsp grated
kale, 2 cups (95 g) chopped
limes, 2
mint leaves, 1 packed Tbsp
onions, green, 4
onion, white, 1 small
spinach, 1 packed cup (70 g)

MEAT, EGGS, AND BROTH

bacon, 6 strips
bone broth, any type, 2 cups (16 fl. oz./
  475 ml) (If making homemade, see page 152
  for ingredients.)
chicken bone broth, 2 cups (16 fl. oz./
  475 ml)
chicken thighs, boneless, skinless, 1 lb
  (455 g)
egg, 1 large

FATS AND OILS

avocado oil, refined, ¼ cup
  plus 1 Tbsp (75 ml)
bacon grease, ¼ cup (35 g)
cacao butter, ¼ cup (60 g)
coconut oil, ¾ cup plus 1 tsp (182 ml)
MCT oil, ¼ cup (60 ml)

DRIED HERBS AND SPICES

cayenne pepper, 1 pinch
cinnamon, ground, ¾ tsp
garlic powder, ½ tsp
nutmeg, ground, ½ tsp
onion powder, 1 tsp

PANTRY ITEMS

apple cider vinegar, 1 Tbsp plus
  1½ tsp
cacao powder, 2 Tbsp (10 g)
coconut flour, ¼ cup plus 2 Tbsp (40 g)
coffee, ground, ¼ cup plus 2 Tbsp
  (32 g), or tea of choice, 4 tsp loose tea
  or 4 bags
collagen peptides, 2 Tbsp
erythritol, confectioners'-style, 1 Tbsp
  plus 1½ tsp
green tea, 1½ tsp loose tea or 2 bags
hemp seeds, hulled, 2 Tbsp
macadamia nuts, 12
sesame seeds, ¼ cup (40 g)
stevia, liquid, 8 to 14 drops (optional, for
  sweetening drinks)
vanilla extract, 1½ tsp

	MEAL 1	MEAL 2	MEAL 3	SNACKS	DAY MACROS/TOTALS	
DAY 22	*(fasted morning)* AND **ROCKET FUEL BONE BROTH** P426	*Leftover* **Salt and Pepper Ribs** AND *Leftover* **Roasted Brussels Sprouts**	**CHICKEN POT PIE CRUMBLE** P344 AND **KALE PÂTÉ** ½ P259 AND *1 large stalk celery*		fat 73% / carbs 7% / protein 20% / calories 1622 / total fat 131 / sat. fat 44.1	chol. 167 / sodium 2132 / carbs 29.6 / fiber 11.8 / net carbs 17.8 / protein 80.9
DAY 23	**MOJITO SMOOTHIE** P425	*Leftover* **Chicken Pot Pie Crumble**	*Leftover* **Salt and Pepper Ribs** AND *Leftover* **Kale Pâté** AND *1 large stalk celery*		fat 73% / carbs 7% / protein 20% / calories 1396 / total fat 114 / sat. fat 46.4	chol. 137 / sodium 1493 / carbs 24.3 / fiber 11.5 / net carbs 12.8 / protein 68.9
DAY 24	*Leftover* **Mojito Smoothie** AND *Leftover* **Classic Butter Biscuits**	*Leftover* **Stuffed Pork Roast with Herb Gravy** AND **PORKY CABBAGE** P385	*Leftover* **Chicken Noodle Soup** *with yam noodles* ⊕		fat 62% / carbs 15% / protein 23% / calories 1660 / total fat 113 / sat. fat 55.6	chol. 214 / sodium 2261 / carbs 62.1 / fiber 18.2 / net carbs 43.9 / protein 97.6
DAY 25	*Leftover* **Rocket Fuel Bone Broth**	*Leftover* **Stuffed Pork Roast with Herb Gravy** AND *Leftover* **Kale Pâté** AND *Cucumber (1 small)*	*Leftover* **Chicken Pot Pie Crumble**	**BACON FUDGE** ½ P394	fat 77% / carbs 5% / protein 18% / calories 1839 / total fat 156 / sat. fat 69.9	chol. 283 / sodium 2038 / carbs 24.5 / fiber 8.5 / net carbs 16 / protein 83.3
DAY 26	*Leftover* **Rocket Fuel Latte** AND *Leftover* **Bacon Fudge**	*Leftover* **Salt and Pepper Ribs** AND *Leftover* **Porky Cabbage**	*Leftover* **Chicken Pot Pie Crumble** AND *1 small cucumber, sliced*		fat 77% / carbs 5% / protein 18% / calories 1832 / total fat 156 / sat. fat 79.2	chol. 194 / sodium 1974 / carbs 25.5 / fiber 10.6 / net carbs 14.9 / protein 80.9
DAY 27	**ROCKET FUEL BONE BROTH** P426	*Leftover* **Classic Butter Biscuits** AND *Leftover* **Kale Pâté** AND *Leftover* **Bacon Soup**		*Leftover* **Almond Chai Truffles**	fat 77% / carbs 7% / protein 16% / calories 1534 / total fat 131 / sat. fat 58.4	chol. 138 / sodium 2358 / carbs 28.2 / fiber 9.7 / net carbs 18.5 / protein 59.3
DAY 28	**ROCKET FUEL LATTE** P428 AND *Leftover* **Almond Chai Truffles**	*Leftover* **Porky Cabbage** *(eat 2 servings)*	*Leftover* **Chicken Noodle Soup** *with yam noodles* ⊕ AND *Cooked Apples*[1] ⊕		fat 55% / carbs 28% / protein 17% / calories 1760 / total fat 108 / sat. fat 55.3	chol. 149 / sodium 2060 / carbs 124 / fiber 28.4 / net carbs 95.9 / protein 71.4

½ HALF BATCH
⊕ CARB-UP

UPPERCASE RECIPES are to be made fresh.

[1] Using 1 apple, follow the steps for preparation in the free "Carb-Up Recipes" PDF available at healthfulpursuit.com/carbup under Apple>Microwave or Roast. Makes 1 serving.

EXTRA LEFTOVERS NOT USED IN THE PLAN: 1 serving Chicken Noodle Soup with yam noodles, 1 serving Lamb Kebabs with white rice, 1 serving Rocket Fuel Bone Broth

This plan is for the Daily Fat Burner Fat Fueled Profile (find out more on page 49).

Not enough food for you? The simplest way to add bulk to the meals without having to worry about it affecting your macros is to increase the fat in your Rocket Fuel Latte (RFL), whip up a fat bomb (see the chart beginning on page 432) and enjoy after a meal, or double up on serving sizes. If you need more carbs following your carb-up, visit healthfulpursuit.com/carbup to download the complimentary PDF "Carb-Up Recipes," simply adding additional carbs to your meal or post-meal dessert.

Instructions for evening carb-ups are below the plan for each week.

SHOPPING LIST FOR WEEK 1

FRESH PRODUCE

apples, 3
bell pepper, red, 1 small
butter lettuce, 1 small head
cantaloupe, 1 small
cauliflower, 1 medium head
celery, 3 medium stalks
chives, 1 Tbsp sliced
dill, 1½ tsp finely chopped
English cucumber, 1 small
fennel bulb, ½ large
garlic, 11 small cloves
ginger root, ½-inch (1.25-cm) piece
kabocha squash, 1 small
lemons, 2, plus 1 optional *(for Hamburger Dinner)*
lime, 1 small
onion, white, 1 small
onions, green, 1 bunch
parsley, 2 bunches
pineapple, 1 small
radishes, 4
romaine lettuce, 8 leaves
rosemary, 1 sprig
spinach, 2 cups (140 g)
tomatoes, hothouse, 4 (about 1 lb/455 g)
turmeric root, 3-inch (7.5-cm) piece

MEAT, EGGS, AND BROTH

bone broth, 1½ cups (350 ml)
  (If making homemade broth, see page 152 for ingredients.)
beef brisket or chuck roast, 1½ lbs (680 g)
chicken breasts, boneless, skinless, 5 (about 2½ lbs/1.1 kg)
chicken thighs, boneless, skinless, ¾ lb (340 g)

eggs, 7 large
ground beef, 20% to 30% fat, 1 lb (455 g)
pork shoulder blade chops (aka shoulder chops, blade steaks, or pork shoulder steaks), bone-in, about ½ inch (1.25 cm) thick, 1¼ lbs (600 g)
sardines, 2 (4.375-oz/125-g) cans

FATS AND OILS

avocado oil, refined, ¼ cup plus 2 Tbsp plus 1½ tsp (100 ml)
cacao butter, 1 cup (240 g)
coconut oil, 1 cup plus 1 Tbsp plus 1 tsp (260 ml)
mayonnaise, made with avocado oil, 1¼ cups (265 g) *(If making homemade mayo, see page 220 for ingredients.)*
MCT oil, ¼ cup plus 2 Tbsp (90 ml)

DRIED HERBS AND SPICES

Cajun Seasoning (page 232), 2 tsp
cardamom, ground, 1¾ tsp
cinnamon, ground, 2 Tbsp plus 1½ tsp
cloves, ground, ⅛ tsp
cumin, ground, 1½ tsp
ginger powder, 2 tsp
Greek Seasoning (page 232), 1½ tsp
Italian Seasoning (page 234), 1 Tbsp plus 1 tsp
oregano leaves, 1½ tsp
thyme leaves, ½ tsp

PANTRY ITEMS

almond flour, blanched, ½ cup (55 g)
apple cider vinegar, 1½ tsp
baking powder, 1 Tbsp
coconut milk, full-fat, ½ cup plus 1 Tbsp plus 1 tsp (4¾ fl. oz./140 ml)
coconut, unsweetened shredded, ½ cup (50 g)
coffee, ground, ¾ cup (64 g), or tea of choice, 8 tsp loose tea or 8 bags
collagen peptides, ¼ cup plus 2 Tbsp (60 g)
erythritol, confectioners'-style, ⅓ cup plus 2 Tbsp (68 g)
flax seeds, roughly ground, 2 cups (256 g)
gelatin, unflavored, 1 Tbsp
hemp seeds, hulled, ¼ cup (38 g)
kalamata olives, pitted, 1 (13½-oz./400-ml) can
nondairy milk, unsweetened, 1½ cups (12 fl. oz./350 ml)
nutritional yeast, ¼ cup (17 g)
orange extract, ½ tsp
raisins, ½ cup (115 g)
stevia, liquid, 3 to 5 drops, plus ⅛ to ¼ tsp optional *(for RFL)*
vanilla extract, 3¾ tsp
walnut pieces, raw, ⅔ cup (75 g)
white wine, such as Pinot Grigio, Sauvignon Blanc, or unoaked Chardonnay, 2 Tbsp plus 1 tsp
xylitol, granulated, 1 Tbsp *(optional, for tacos)*

Finely ground gray sea salt and ground black pepper will be needed for many of the recipes. Purchase once and use throughout the plan.

	MEAL 1	MEAL 2	MEAL 3	SNACKS	DAY MACROS/TOTALS	
DAY 1	FLAXSEED CINNAMON BUN MUFFINS[1] ½ ⊛ P239 AND ROCKET FUEL LATTE P428	SPINACH SALAD WITH BREADED CHICKEN STRIPS ½ P284	BAKED OLIVE CHICKEN[2] *with fruit bowl* ½ ⊛ ⊕ P336		fat 64%, carbs 14%, protein 22%, calories 1769, total fat 126, sat. fat 57.3	chol. 255, sodium 1847, carbs 60.1, fiber 22.5, net carbs 37.6, protein 99.5
DAY 2	ROCKET FUEL LATTE P428	ONE-POT HAMBURGER DINNER[3] ⊛ P310	WALDORF-STUFFED TOMATOES[4] ⊕ P351	CARDAMOM ORANGE BARK[5] *(at bedtime)* ½ ⊛ P395	fat 68%, carbs 13%, protein 19%, calories 1398, total fat 105, sat. fat 60.3	chol. 162, sodium 1429, carbs 46.5, fiber 8.6, net carbs 37.9, protein 66.4
DAY 3	*Leftover* Spinach Salad with Breaded Chicken Strips	SHREDDED BEEF TACOS[6] ½ ⊛ P314	*Leftover* Baked Olive Chicken *with fruit bowl* ⊕		fat 59%, carbs 13%, protein 28%, calories 1685, total fat 111, sat. fat 33.3	chol. 338, sodium 2080, carbs 54, fiber 15.8, net carbs 38.2, protein 117
DAY 4	*Leftover* Flaxseed Cinnamon Bun Muffins AND ROCKET FUEL LATTE *with 2 Tbsp. additional collagen* P428	*Leftover* Shredded Beef Tacos	SARDINE FRITTER WRAPS[7] *with grilled kabocha squash* ⊛ ⊕ P362		fat 69%, carbs 9%, protein 22%, calories 1632, total fat 125, sat. fat 44.6	chol. 486, sodium 1783, carbs 37.3, fiber 13.2, net carbs 24.1, protein 89.1
DAY 5	FAT-BURNING GOLDEN MILKSHAKE *with 2 Tbsp. additional collagen* P416	SHOULDER CHOPS WITH LEMON-THYME GRAVY[8] ½ ⊛ P332	*Leftover* Waldorf-Stuffed Tomatoes ⊕		fat 65%, carbs 14%, protein 21%, calories 1260, total fat 91.6, sat. fat 52.9	chol. 179, sodium 1178, carbs 43.9, fiber 3.8, net carbs 40.1, protein 65.1
DAY 6	*Leftover* Flaxseed Cinnamon Bun Muffins	*Leftover* One-Pot Hamburger Dinner *drizzled with* GARLIC-INFUSED OIL[9] P230	*Leftover* Waldorf-Stuffed Tomatoes ⊕ AND Apple and Cinnamon[10] ⊕		fat 51%, carbs 28%, protein 21%, calories 1181, total fat 66.2, sat. fat 19.5	chol. 239, sodium 1304, carbs 83.2, fiber 18.8, net carbs 64.4, protein 63.2
DAY 7	*Leftover* Flaxseed Cinnamon Bun Muffins AND ROCKET FUEL LATTE P428	*Leftover* Shredded Beef Tacos	*Leftover* Waldorf-Stuffed Tomatoes ⊕ AND Apple and Cinnamon[10] ⊕		fat 60%, carbs 21%, protein 19%, calories 1485, total fat 98.9, sat. fat 41.8	chol. 298, sodium 1140, carbs 79.3, fiber 16.4, net carbs 62.9, protein 69.6

½ HALF BATCH
⊕ CARB-UP
⊛ FREEZE

UPPERCASE RECIPES are to be made fresh.

[1] Freeze 1 muffin for week 2 and 1 muffin for week 3.

[2] Follow the carb-up instructions for the Baked Olive Chicken recipe. Adjusted recipe provides 3 servings. Freeze 1 serving for week 2. Enjoy 2/3 cup (107 g) cubed cantaloupe and 2/3 cup (110 g) cubed pineapple with each serving. Fresh ingredients for the third serving of fruit have been added to the shopping list for week 2.

[3] Freeze 2 servings of One-Pot Hamburger Dinner for week 2.

[4] Follow the carb-up instructions for the Waldorf-Stuffed Tomatoes recipe. Adjusted recipe provides 4 servings.

[5] Freeze 2 servings of Cardamom Orange Bark for week 2 and 3 servings for week 4.

[6] Freeze 1 serving of tacos for week 2. Fresh ingredients have been added to the shopping list for week 2.

[7] Follow the carb-up instructions for the Sardine Fritter Wraps recipe. Serve with grilled kabocha squash (1 small/600 g), as outlined in the free "Carb-Up Recipes" PDF available at healthfulpursuit.com/carbup. Adjusted recipe provides 3 servings. Freeze 2 servings for week 2.

[8] Freeze 1 serving of Shoulder Chops for week 3 and 1 serving for week 4.

[9] Reserve 2 servings of Garlic-Infused Oil for week 2, 1 serving for week 3, and 1 serving for week 4. Five additional servings are not used in the plan.

[10] Slice an apple and sprinkle with ¼ tsp ground cinnamon. Makes 1 serving; prepare twice this week (once for day 6 and once for day 7).

PATH 3
DAILY FAT BURNER

SHOPPING LIST FOR WEEK 2

FRESH PRODUCE
apple, 1
asparagus, 1 lb (455 g)
berries, any type *(optional, for porridge)*
blackberries, 1 cup (142 g)
butter lettuce, 1 small head
cabbage, red, 1 medium head
cantaloupe, 1 small
cauliflower, 1 small head
celery, 3 medium stalks
chives, 1½ tsp sliced
cilantro, 1 bunch (about 2 oz./56 g)
cucumber, 1
dill, ¾ tsp finely chopped
garlic, 9 small cloves
ginger root, 3-inch (7.5-cm) piece
kale, 4 cups (190 g) chopped
lemons, 2
limes, 2
mint, 2 Tbsp chopped
onions, green, 2 bunches
onion, red, 1 small
onion, white, 1 small
oregano, 1 bunch
parsley, 1 bunch
pineapple, 1 small
plantains, green, 4 medium
radishes, 1 bunch, plus 2
sweet potatoes, 2 medium
thyme, 6 sprigs
tomato, 1 small
zucchini, ½ large

MEAT, EGGS, AND BROTH
chicken, 1 whole (3½ lbs/ 1.6 kg), with giblets
chicken bone broth, ¾ cup (6 fl. oz./180 ml) *(If making homemade broth, see page 152 for ingredients.)*
chicken thighs, skinless, 1 cup (180 g) cubed cooked
eggs, 2 large
ground beef, 20% to 30% fat, 1 lb (455 g)
pepperoni, sliced, ¾ cup (105 g)
pork belly, side of, ½ lb (225 g)
pork stir-fry pieces, ½ lb (225 g)
salmon steaks, 4 (6 oz./170 g each)
sausages, 4 (about 8 oz./225 g)

FATS AND OILS
avocado oil, refined, 1 cup plus 1 Tbsp (255 ml)
cacao butter, 3 Tbsp
coconut oil, ¼ cup plus 1 Tbsp (75 ml)
duck fat, 1 Tbsp plus 1½ tsp
lard, ⅓ cup (69 g)
mayonnaise, made with avocado oil, ¼ cup (70 g) *(If making homemade mayo, see page 220 for ingredients.)*
MCT oil, 3 Tbsp
sesame oil, toasted, 1 Tbsp

DRIED HERBS AND SPICES
Cajun Seasoning (page 232), 2 Tbsp plus 2¼ tsp
cinnamon, ground, 1 tsp
Greek Seasoning (page 232), 1 Tbsp plus 1½ tsp
Italian Seasoning (page 234), 1 Tbsp

PANTRY ITEMS
almond butter, unsweetened smooth, 2 Tbsp
almond flour, blanched, ⅓ cup (36 g)
almond meal, ¼ cup (28 g)
apple cider vinegar, ¼ cup plus 2 Tbsp plus ¾ tsp (95 ml)
balsamic vinegar, 1 Tbsp
Brazil nuts, raw, 4
cashews, raw, ¼ cup (40 g)
chia seeds, 1 Tbsp
chilis, dried, 2 to 4
coconut aminos, 3 Tbsp
coconut milk, full-fat, 2 Tbsp
coffee, ground, ½ cup plus 1 Tbsp (56 g), or tea of choice, 2 Tbsp loose tea or 6 bags
collagen peptides, ¼ cup plus 1 Tbsp (50 g)
erythritol, confectioners'-style, 1 Tbsp
flax seeds, 2 Tbsp roughly ground
gelatin, unflavored, 2 Tbsp
green tea, 1 Tbsp loose tea or 4 bags
hemp seeds, hulled, 1 cup plus 1 Tbsp (160 g)
nondairy milk, unsweetened, 1 cup (8 fl. oz./240 ml), plus more for serving with porridge, if desired
red wine, such as Pinot Noir, Merlot, or Cabernet Sauvignon, ⅓ cup (80 ml)
sesame seeds, ½ cup (75 g)
stevia, liquid, 9 to 11 drops, plus 6 to 12 drops optional *(for RFL)*
tapioca starch, ½ tsp
vanilla extract, 1½ tsp

	MEAL 1	MEAL 2	MEAL 3	SNACKS	DAY MACROS/TOTALS	
DAY 8	**ROCKET FUEL LATTE** P428 **AND** *Leftover* **Cardamom Orange Bark**	*Leftover* **One-Pot Hamburger Dinner**	*Leftover* **Sardine Fritter Wraps** *with grilled kabocha squash* ⊕		fat 72% / carbs 9% / protein 19% / calories 1640 / total fat 132 / sat. fat 63.1	chol. 350 / sodium 2020 / carbs 35.8 / fiber 11.1 / net carbs 24.7 / protein 77.5
DAY 9	**EARLY-DAY JAMBALAYA[1]** ❄ P242	*Leftover* **One-Pot Hamburger Dinner** *drizzled with* **Garlic-Infused Oil**	*Leftover* **Sardine Fritter Wraps** *with grilled kabocha squash* ⊕		fat 67% / carbs 10% / protein 23% / calories 1551 / total fat 115 / sat. fat 29	chol. 450 / sodium 2420 / carbs 40 / fiber 12.6 / net carbs 27.4 / protein 89.3
DAY 10	**GRAIN-FREE HEMP SEED PORRIDGE** P244	*Leftover* **Shredded Beef Tacos**	*Leftover* **Baked Olive Chicken** *with fruit bowl[2]* ⊕		fat 61% / carbs 14% / protein 25% / calories 1639 / total fat 110 / sat. fat 27.5	chol. 185 / sodium 1685 / carbs 58.1 / fiber 22 / net carbs 36.1 / protein 104
DAY 11	*Leftover* **Flaxseed Cinnamon Bun Muffins** **AND** **ROCKET FUEL LATTE** *with 2 Tbsp. additional collagen* P428	**CAJUN PORK BELLY CHOPPED SALAD** ½ P286	**CRISPY SALMON STEAKS WITH SWEET CABBAGE[3]** *and blackberries* ❄ ⊕ P356		fat 75% / carbs 8% / protein 17% / calories 2090 / total fat 173 / sat. fat 68.5	chol. 294 / sodium 1238 / carbs 41.5 / fiber 22.4 / net carbs 19.1 / protein 90.7
DAY 12	**FATTY GREEN TEA** P419	**MICHAEL'S PEPPERONI MEATZZA** P312	**KUNG PAO PORK** *with roasted sweet potatoes[4]* ⊕ P328	*Leftover* **Cardamom Orange Bark** *(at bedtime)*	fat 66% / carbs 15% / protein 19% / calories 1515 / total fat 111 / sat. fat 51	chol. 213 / sodium 983 / carbs 55.4 / fiber 11 / net carbs 44.4 / protein 73.3
DAY 13	*Leftover* **Grain-Free Hemp Seed Porridge** *with 1 Tbsp. coconut oil*	*Leftover* **Cajun Pork Belly Chopped Salad**	**GREEK CHICKEN WITH GRAVY AND ASPARAGUS** *with boiled plantains[5]* ½ ❄ ⊕ P346		fat 77% / carbs 11% / protein 12% / calories 2246 / total fat 192 / sat. fat 58.4	chol. 229 / sodium 416 / carbs 61.4 / fiber 18.8 / net carbs 42.6 / protein 67.9
DAY 14	**ROCKET FUEL LATTE** P428	*Leftover* **Michael's Pepperoni Meatzza** *drizzled with* **RANCH DRESSING[6]** ¼ P226	*Leftover* **Kung Pao Pork** *with roasted sweet potatoes* ⊕		fat 67% / carbs 14% / protein 19% / calories 1441 / total fat 107 / sat. fat 42.4	chol. 218 / sodium 1223 / carbs 50.1 / fiber 10.3 / net carbs 39.8 / protein 69.4

½ HALF BATCH
¼ QUARTER BATCH
⊕ CARB-UP
❄ FREEZE

UPPERCASE RECIPES are to be made fresh.

[1] Freeze 3 servings of Jambalaya for week 3.
[2] Serve with ⅔ cup (107 g) cubed cantaloupe and ⅔ cup (110 g) pineapple chunks.
[3] Follow the carb-up instructions for the Crispy Salmon Steaks recipe. Adjusted recipe provides 3 servings. Freeze 2 servings for week 3.
[4] Follow the carb-up instructions in the Kung Pao Pork recipe. Serve with roasted sweet potatoes (2 medium), as outlined in the free "Carb-Up Recipes" PDF available at healthfulpursuit.com/carbup. Adjusted recipe provides 2 servings.
[5] Follow the carb-up instructions in the Greek Chicken recipe. Serve with boiled green plantains (4 medium), as outlined in the free "Carb-Up Recipes" PDF available at healthfulpursuit.com/carbup. Adjusted recipe provides 6 servings. Freeze 3 servings for week 3 and 2 servings for week 4.
[6] Reserve 3 servings of Ranch Dressing for use in week 3.

SHOPPING LIST FOR WEEK 3

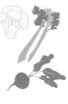

FRESH PRODUCE

asparagus, ½ bunch (about 6½ oz./185 g)
blackberries, 2 cups (283 g)
chives *(for garnishing quiche)*
ginger root, 4-inch (10-cm) piece
lemons, 3
parsley, 1 Tbsp finely chopped

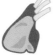

FATS AND OILS

cacao butter, ½ cup (120 g)
lard, 1 Tbsp, plus more for the pans
mayonnaise, made with avocado oil, 2 Tbsp plus 2 tsp *(If making homemade mayo, see page 220 for ingredients.)*
MCT oil, ½ cup (120 ml)

PANTRY ITEMS

almond flour, blanched, 1 cup (110 g)
coconut milk, full-fat, ⅔ cup (5⅓ fl. oz./158 ml)
coffee, ground, ¼ cup plus 2 Tbsp (32 g), or tea of choice, 4 tsp loose tea or 4 bags
collagen peptides, ½ cup plus 2 Tbsp (100 g)
Dijon mustard, ¾ tsp
gelatin, unflavored, ¼ cup (40 g)
green tea, 2 Tbsp loose tea or 8 bags
hemp seeds, hulled, ½ cup (75 g)
horseradish, prepared, 2 tsp
nutritional yeast, 3 Tbsp
rice, white, 2 cups (1120 g)
stevia, liquid, ¼ tsp, plus ¼ to ½ tsp optional
vanilla extract, 2 tsp

MEAT AND EGGS

bacon, 8 strips regular (not thick-cut)
eggs, 3 medium
ground lamb, 1 lb (455 g)

DRIED HERBS AND SPICES

Bahārāt Seasoning (page 233), 1 Tbsp
cinnamon, ground, ¼ tsp
nutmeg, ground, 1 pinch

	MEAL 1	MEAL 2	MEAL 3	SNACKS	DAY MACROS/TOTALS	
DAY 15	**FATTY GREEN TEA** P419	**BACON LOVERS' QUICHE**[1] ❄ ½ P240 AND **BACON-WRAPPED ASPARAGUS WITH HORSERADISH SAUCE**[2] ½ P262	*Leftover* **Crispy Salmon Steaks with Sweet Cabbage** *and blackberries* ➕		fat 60% / carbs 13% / protein 27% / calories 1285 / total fat 85.3 / sat. fat 26.8	chol. 271 / sodium 1625 / carbs 41.2 / fiber 18.9 / net carbs 22.3 / protein 88.1
DAY 16	*Leftover* **Fatty Green Tea**	*Leftover* **Early-Day Jambalaya** *with* **Ranch Dressing**	*Leftover* **Greek Chicken with Gravy and Asparagus** *and boiled plantains* ➕ AND *Apple and Cinnamon*[3] ➕		fat 56% / carbs 26% / protein 18% / calories 1297 / total fat 80.5 / sat. fat 33	chol. 217 / sodium 866 / carbs 83.7 / fiber 13.4 / net carbs 70.3 / protein 59.7
DAY 17	**ROCKET FUEL LATTE** P428	*Leftover* **Early-Day Jambalaya** *with* **Ranch Dressing**	*Leftover* **Greek Chicken with Gravy and Asparagus** *and boiled plantains* ➕		fat 68% / carbs 15% / protein 17% / calories 1319 / total fat 99.5 / sat. fat 45.9	chol. 217 / sodium 1051 / carbs 48.8 / fiber 8 / net carbs 40.8 / protein 57.1
DAY 18	**FATTY GREEN TEA** P419	*Leftover* **Bacon Lovers' Quiche** *with* **Ranch Dressing**	**LAMB KEBABS**[4] *with white rice* ❄ ➕ P318		fat 56% / carbs 26% / protein 18% / calories 1286 / total fat 79.7 / sat. fat 28.2	chol. 238 / sodium 1310 / carbs 83.2 / fiber 7.2 / net carbs 76 / protein 59
DAY 19	*Leftover* **Flaxseed Cinnamon Bun Muffins** AND **ROCKET FUEL LATTE** *with 2 Tbsp. additional collagen* P428	*Leftover* **Shoulder Chops with Lemon-Thyme Gravy**	*Leftover* **Greek Chicken with Gravy and Asparagus** *and boiled plantains* ➕		fat 64% / carbs 14% / protein 22% / calories 1500 / total fat 107 / sat. fat 51.2	chol. 307 / sodium 1132 / carbs 51.8 / fiber 11 / net carbs 40.8 / protein 83.6
DAY 20	*Leftover* **Early-Day Jambalaya** *drizzled with* **Garlic-Infused Oil**	*Leftover* **Michael's Pepperoni Meatzza** AND *Leftover* **Bacon-Wrapped Asparagus with Horseradish Sauce**	*Leftover* **Crispy Salmon Steaks with Sweet Cabbage** *and blackberries* ➕		fat 66% / carbs 9% / protein 25% / calories 1725 / total fat 127 / sat. fat 33.7	chol. 376 / sodium 2399 / carbs 39.3 / fiber 18.1 / net carbs 21.2 / protein 106
DAY 21	*(fasted morning)*	*Leftover* **Bacon Lovers' Quiche** AND *Leftover* **Bacon-Wrapped Asparagus with Horseradish Sauce**	*Leftover* **Lamb Kebabs** *with white rice* ➕		fat 56% / carbs 26% / protein 18% / calories 1217 / total fat 75.4 / sat. fat 19.2	chol. 261 / sodium 1508 / carbs 80.5 / fiber 7.6 / net carbs 72.9 / protein 54

½ HALF BATCH
➕ CARB-UP
❄ FREEZE

UPPERCASE RECIPES are to be made fresh.

[1]Freeze 1 quiche for use on days 21 and 23.
[2]Reserve 1 serving of Bacon-Wrapped Asparagus with Horseradish Sauce for week 4.
[3]Slice an apple and sprinkle with ¼ tsp ground cinnamon. Makes 1 serving.
[4]Follow the carb-up instructions in the Lamb Kebabs recipe. Serve with 2 cups (1120 g) white rice, cooked. Adjusted recipe provides 4 servings. Freeze 2 servings for week 4.

dfb

WEEK 4

PATH 3
DAILY FAT BURNER

SHOPPING LIST FOR WEEK 4

FRESH PRODUCE

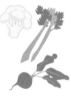

apple, 1
avocados, Hass, 2 large
berries, any type *(optional, for granola)*
cabbage, red, 1 cup (85 g) sliced
carrot, 1 medium
celery, 2 medium stalks
cilantro leaves, 1½ packed tsp
garlic, 3 small cloves
ginger root, ½-inch (1.25-cm) piece
lemon, 1
lime, 1
onion, white, 1 small
onions, green, 2 bunches
parsley, 1 bunch
rutabaga, 1 small
spinach, 6 cups (420 g)
strawberries, 6
yams, 2 medium
zucchini, 1 smalll

FATS AND OILS

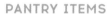

avocado oil, refined, 1 Tbsp plus 1½ tsp
coconut cream, 1 (13½-oz./400-ml) can
coconut oil, ¾ cup (180 ml)
extra-virgin olive oil, ¼ cup plus 1 Tbsp (75 ml)
lard, 2 Tbsp
MCT oil, ¼ cup (60 ml)

DRIED HERBS AND SPICES

basil, ½ tsp
cayenne pepper, 1 pinch
chili powder, ¾ tsp
cinnamon, ground, 3 Tbsp plus ¼ tsp
cloves, ground, ⅛ tsp
oregano leaves, ½ tsp

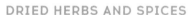

PANTRY ITEMS

capers, 1 Tbsp
chia seeds, ¼ cup (38 g)
coconut, unsweetened shredded, 2 cups (200 g)
coconut milk, full-fat *(amount as desired, for serving with granola)*
collagen peptides, ½ cup (80 g)
Dijon mustard, 1½ tsp
erythritol, confectioners'-style, 1 Tbsp *(optional, for Coconut Whipped Cream)*
hemp seeds, hulled, 1 cup (150 g)
pecans, raw, ¼ cup (35 g) roughly chopped
red wine vinegar, 2 Tbsp
sesame seeds, 1 cup (150 g)
stevia, liquid, ¼ tsp plus 5 drops
vanilla extract, 2 tsp, plus 1 tsp optional *(for Coconut Whipped Cream)*

MEAT, EGGS, AND BROTH

bacon, 6 strips
bone broth, any type, 2 cups (16 fl. oz./ 475 ml) *(If making homemade broth, see page 152 for ingredients.)*
chicken bone broth, 6 cups (48 fl. oz./ 1.4 L)
chicken breasts, boneless, skinless, 1 lb (455 g)
egg, 1 large
flank steak, 13 oz. (375 g)
sausages, precooked, 2 (about 4 oz./ 115 g)

	MEAL 1	MEAL 2	MEAL 3	SNACKS	DAY MACROS/TOTALS	
DAY 22	**ROCKET FUEL BONE BROTH** P426	*Leftover* Michael's Pepperoni Meatzza — AND — *Leftover* Bacon-Wrapped Asparagus with Horseradish Sauce	*Leftover* Greek Chicken with Gravy and Asparagus *and boiled plantains* ⊕		fat 66% / carbs 14% / protein 20% / calories 1358 / total fat 98.9 / sat. fat 30.8	chol. 312 / sodium 1661 / carbs 47.7 / fiber 6 / net carbs 41.7 / protein 69.1
DAY 23	*Leftover* Rocket Fuel Bone Broth	*Leftover* Bacon Lovers' Quiche — AND — **BERRY AVOCADO SALAD** ½ P294	**CHICKEN NOODLE SOUP** *made with yam noodles*[1] ⊛ ⊕ P276	*Leftover* Cardamom Orange Bark *(at bedtime)*	fat 66% / carbs 15% / protein 19% / calories 1705 / total fat 124 / sat. fat 47.8	chol. 256 / sodium 1973 / carbs 65.4 / fiber 22.8 / net carbs 42.6 / protein 81.3
DAY 24	**SAUSAGE AND GREENS HASH BOWL** *drizzled with* Garlic-Infused Oil P243 — AND — *Leftover* Cardamom Orange Bark	**SPINACH SALAD WITH FLANK STEAK** ½ P292	*Leftover* Greek Chicken with Gravy and Asparagus *and boiled plantains* ⊕		fat 71% / carbs 12% / protein 17% / calories 2003 / total fat 159 / sat. fat 56	chol. 262 / sodium 1169 / carbs 60 / fiber 13.9 / net carbs 46.1 / protein 83.2
DAY 25	*(fasted morning)*	*Leftover* Sausage and Greens Hash Bowl — AND — *4 strips bacon*	*Leftover* Lamb Kebabs *with white rice* ⊕		fat 64% / carbs 22% / protein 14% / calories 1500 / total fat 107 / sat. fat 34.4	chol. 229 / sodium 1817 / carbs 81.6 / fiber 7.5 / net carbs 73 / protein 52.7
DAY 26	**NO-NUTS GRANOLA WITH CLUSTERS** P246 *with* **COCONUT WHIPPED CREAM** P414	*Leftover* Spinach Salad with Flank Steak	*Leftover* Lamb Kebabs *with white rice* ⊕	*Leftover* Berry Avocado Salad	fat 62% / carbs 21% / protein 17% / calories 1916 / total fat 132 / sat. fat 49.3	chol. 175 / sodium 1053 / carbs 99.8 / fiber 21.1 / net carbs 78.7 / protein 82.8
DAY 27	*Leftover* No-Nuts Granola with Clusters *with* leftover Coconut Whipped Cream	*Leftover* Spinach Salad with Flank Steak	*Leftover* Chicken Noodle Soup ⊕		fat 59% / carbs 15% / protein 26% / calories 1503 / total fat 97.8 / sat. fat 41.5	chol. 174 / sodium 1168 / carbs 57.8 / fiber 16.6 / net carbs 41.2 / protein 97.9
DAY 28	*Leftover* Cardamom Orange Bark	*Leftover* Shoulder Chops with Lemon-Thyme Gravy	*Leftover* Chicken Noodle Soup ⊕ — AND — *Apple and Cinnamon*[2] ⊕		fat 56% / carbs 21% / protein 23% / calories 1411 / total fat 87.5 / sat. fat 42.5	chol. 207 / sodium 1454 / carbs 75.9 / fiber 13.6 / net carbs 62.3 / protein 80

½ HALF BATCH
⊕ CARB-UP

UPPERCASE RECIPES are to be made fresh.

[1] Follow the carb-up instructions in the Chicken Noodle Soup recipe, using 2 medium yams that have been spiral-sliced and added to the soup. Adjusted recipe provides 4 servings. Freeze 1 serving for day 28.

[2] Slice an apple and sprinkle with ¼ tsp ground cinnamon. Makes 1 serving.

EXTRA LEFTOVERS NOT USED IN THE PLAN: 1 serving Chicken Noodle Soup with yam noodles, 5 servings Coconut Whipped Cream, 3 servings Garlic-Infused Oil, 2 servings Michael's Pepperoni Meatzza, 10 servings No-Nuts Granola with Clusters

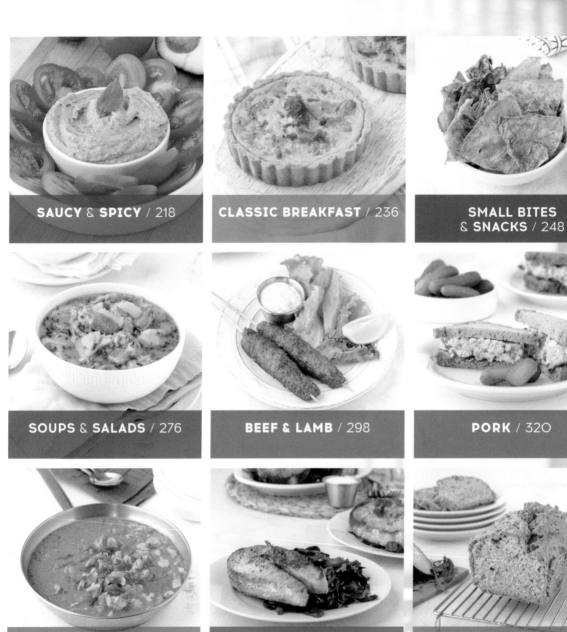
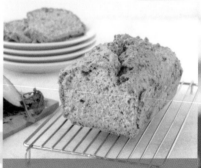
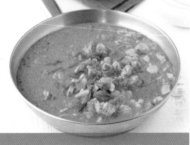
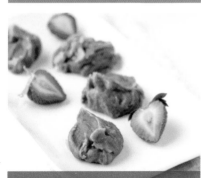
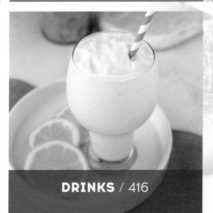

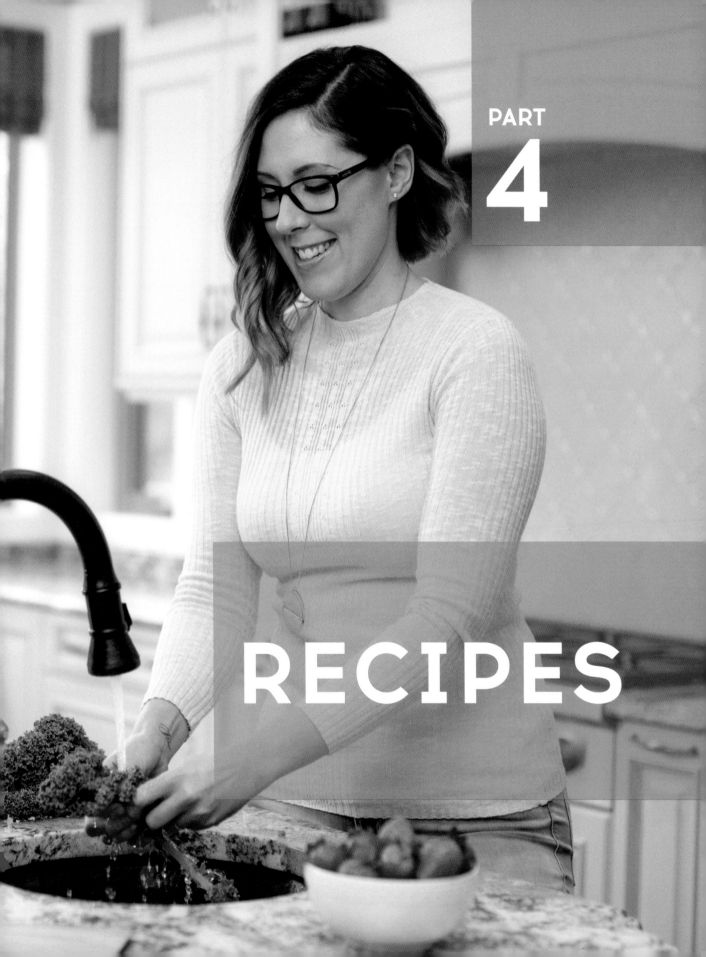

PART
4

RECIPES

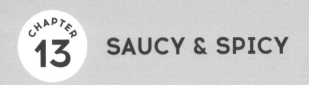

CHEESE SAUCE

   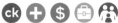

PREP TIME: **5 minutes, plus 1 hour to soak sesame seeds** · COOK TIME: **10 minutes** · MAKES: **1 cup (240 ml) (8 servings)**

EGG-FREE · NIGHTSHADE-FREE · NUT-FREE · OPTIONS: COCONUT-FREE · LOW-FODMAP · VEGAN

If you haven't discovered the wonders of nutritional yeast, you must try it, despite its unappetizing name. It's cheesy, not yeasty! And if you're doing keto without dairy, nutritional yeast can be a fabulous way to add "cheese" without actual cheese. For this sauce, I didn't want any coconut flavor to seep in, so I used refined coconut oil to ensure that all you taste is cheese.

¾ cup (180 ml) chicken bone broth (see page 152)

⅓ cup (22 g) nutritional yeast

¼ cup (38 g) sesame seeds, soaked for 1 hour, then drained and rinsed

¼ cup (60 ml) melted refined coconut oil

1 tablespoon plus 1 teaspoon fresh lemon juice

1½ teaspoons ground mustard

¾ teaspoon onion powder

¼ teaspoon garlic powder

¼ teaspoon finely ground gray sea salt

1. Place the broth, nutritional yeast, sesame seeds, coconut oil, and lemon juice in a high-powered blender or food processor fitted with the "S" blade. Blend on high for 30 seconds, or until smooth.

2. Transfer the mixture to a small saucepan and bring to a boil over medium heat, whisking occasionally.

3. Reduce the heat to medium-low, add the spices and salt, and whisk to combine. Continue to lightly simmer the sauce, whisking constantly, for 5 minutes, or until thickened.

STORE IT: *Keep in an airtight container in the fridge for up to 1 week.*

REHEAT IT: *Place in a saucepan, cover, and reheat on low, whisking occasionally, until the desired temperature is reached.*

SERVE IT WITH: *Toss with Zoodles or Doodles (page 376) and your favorite protein. This sauce also tastes great on Bacon-Wrapped Asparagus (page 262) in place of the Horseradish Sauce or on Roasted Cajun Broccoli (page 266).*

MAKE IT COCONUT-FREE: *Replace the coconut oil with ghee (if tolerated), refined avocado oil, tallow, or lard.*

MAKE IT LOW-FODMAP: *Replace 2 tablespoons of the coconut oil with Garlic-Infused Oil (page 230) made with refined avocado oil or extra-virgin olive oil and omit the onion and garlic powder.*

MAKE IT VEGAN: *Use vegetable stock in place of the chicken bone broth.*

MAKE IT A CARB-UP: *Replace half of the coconut oil with water. Serve alongside the carb of your choice (find ideas on page 117, or visit healthfulpursuit.com/carbup to download the complimentary PDF "Carb-Up Recipes"). It's delicious with cassava, delicata squash, or parsnips.*

NUTRIENT INFORMATION (PER 2-TABLESPOON SERVING):

calories: 107 | calories from fat: 84 | total fat: 9.4g | saturated fat: 2.6g | cholesterol: 0mg

sodium: 98mg | carbs: 2.6g | dietary fiber: 1.2g | net carbs: 1.4g | sugars: 0g | protein: 2.9g

RATIOS:

fat:	carbs:	protein:
79%	10%	11%

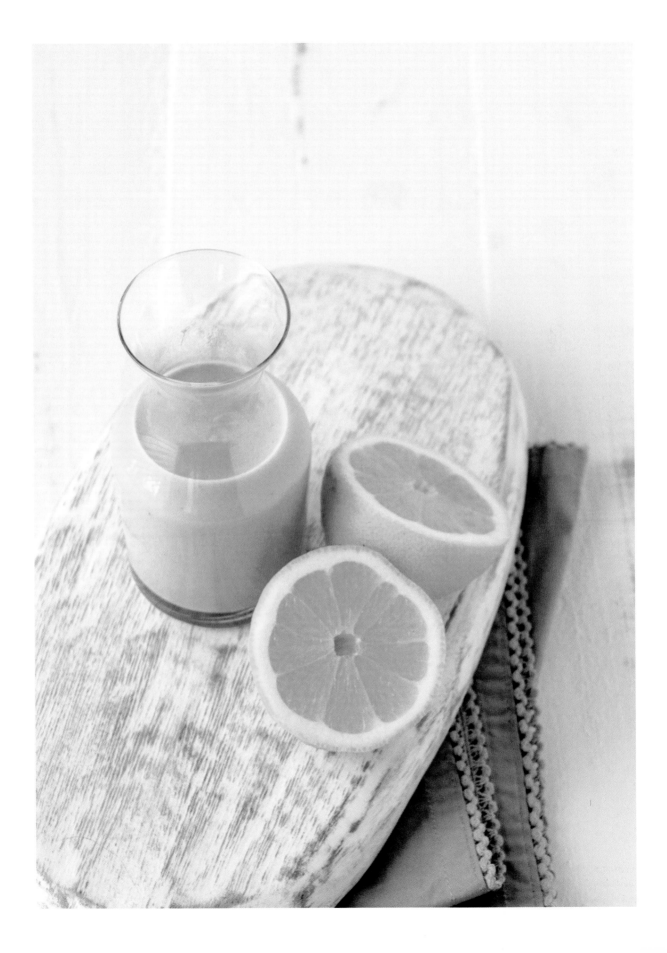

MAYONNAISE

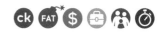

PREP TIME: **5 minutes**   MAKES: **1¼ cups (260 g) (10 servings)**

COCONUT-FREE • LOW-FODMAP • NIGHTSHADE-FREE • NUT-FREE • VEGETARIAN   OPTIONS: EGG-FREE • VEGAN

No keto diet is complete without mayo. It's my go-to sauce for basically everything. No time to make salad dressing? Add mayo to it. Need more fat on a steak? Add mayo to it. Need a dipping sauce for your favorite jerky? Mayo, for real. And for those who are sensitive to eggs, I've got you covered with an egg-free variation.

1 large egg

2 large egg yolks

1 tablespoon fresh lemon juice

1 tablespoon plus 1 teaspoon white wine vinegar or 1 tablespoon apple cider vinegar

1 teaspoon Dijon mustard

¼ teaspoon finely ground gray sea salt

⅛ teaspoon ground black pepper

1 cup (240 ml) light-tasting oil such as refined avocado oil, refined olive oil, or unrefined canola oil

If using a countertop blender, put all the ingredients, except the oil, in the blender. Mix just enough to combine. With the blender running on medium speed, slowly drizzle in the oil, taking at least 2 minutes to add all the oil. After all the oil has been added, continue to blend until the mixture is the consistency of mayonnaise.

If using an immersion blender, put all the ingredients, including the oil, in the blending jar or beaker. (If your immersion blender didn't come with a jar, use a wide-mouthed quart-sized jar or similar-sized container.) Insert the blender into the jar, turn it to high speed, and keep it at the base of the jar for 25 seconds. Then move the blender up and down in the jar until the ingredients are well incorporated.

TIP: *For homemade mayo, an immersion blender or high-powered blender is best. Otherwise, it's better to buy a keto-friendly mayo.*

STORE IT: *Keep in an airtight container in the fridge for up to 1 week.*

VARIATION: EGG-FREE MAYONNAISE. *While not completely keto diet–approved because it uses the liquid from a can of chickpeas (called aquafaba), this is a fabulous mayo alternative for those who are sensitive to eggs. In a blender, combine 6 tablespoons of chickpea liquid, 2 tablespoons of lemon juice, 1 tablespoon plus 1 teaspoon of Dijon mustard, 1 tablespoon of apple cider vinegar, ½ teaspoon of ground black pepper, and ½ teaspoon of finely ground gray sea salt. Turn on the blender to medium speed and slowly drizzle in 1½ cups (350 ml) of a light-tasting oil, such as refined avocado oil, light refined oil, or unrefined canola oil, while the blender is running, taking at least 2 minutes to add all the oil. After all the oil has been added, continue to run the blender until the mixture is the consistency of mayonnaise. Or, if using an immersion blender, follow the instructions in Step 2 above. Makes 1¾ cups (365 g), or 14 servings.*

MAKE IT EGG-FREE/VEGAN: *Prepare the egg-free variation.*

NUTRIENT INFORMATION (PER 2-TABLESPOON SERVING OF EGG-BASED MAYO):

calories: 200 | calories from fat: 192 | total fat: 21.6g | saturated fat: 3.4g | cholesterol: 61g

sodium: 62mg | carbs: 0.3g | dietary fiber: 0g | net carbs: 0.3g | sugars: 0g | protein: 1.2g

RATIOS:

fat:	carbs:	protein:
97%	1%	2%

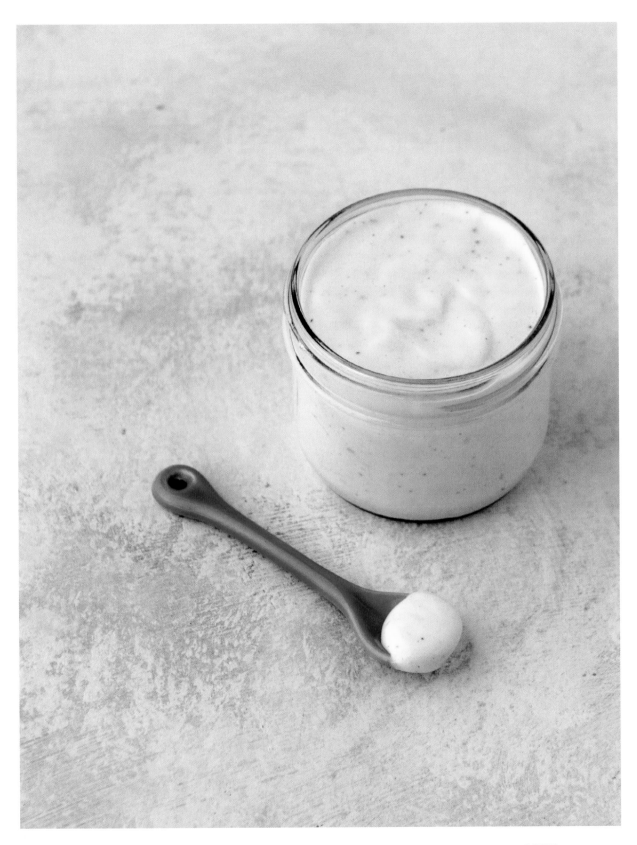

NUTRIENT INFORMATION (PER 2-TABLESPOON SERVING OF EGG-FREE MAYO):
calories: 190 | calories from fat: 190 | total fat: 21.9g | saturated fat: 3.1g | cholesterol: 0mg
sodium: 82mg | carbs: 0.4g | dietary fiber: 0g | net carbs: 0.4g | sugars: 0g | protein: 0.3g

RATIOS:
fat: carbs: protein:
99% 1% 0%

BASIL AVOCADO SPREAD

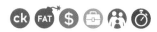

PREP TIME: **5 minutes**   MAKES: **1¹/₃ cups (410 g) (10 servings)**

COCONUT-FREE • EGG-FREE • NIGHTSHADE-FREE • NUT-FREE • VEGAN

I love slathering this spread on fresh vegetables! It's my go-to condiment when my meals are in need of a fat boost and I don't feel like using mayonnaise.

2 small Hass avocados, peeled and pitted (about 8½ ounces/210 g flesh)

½ cup (32 g) fresh basil leaves

¼ cup (60 ml) white balsamic vinegar

¼ cup (60 ml) MCT oil

¼ cup (38 g) hulled hemp seeds

2 teaspoons onion powder

½ teaspoon finely ground gray sea salt

¾ teaspoon ground black pepper

Place all the ingredients in a blender or the bowl of a food processor. Pulse or blend on medium speed until smooth.

STORE IT: *Keep in an airtight container in the fridge for up to 3 days.*

SERVE IT WITH: *Serve with sliced fresh vegetables and cold cuts, or use as a sauce for Zoodles or Doodles (page 376).*

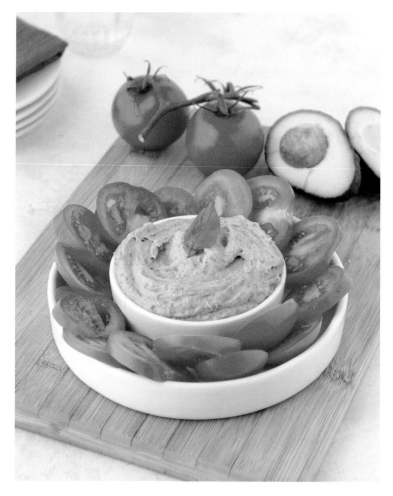

NUTRIENT INFORMATION (PER 2-TABLESPOON SERVING):

calories: 122 | calories from fat: 103 | total fat: 11.5g | saturated fat: 6.7g | cholesterol: 0mg

sodium: 96mg | carbs: 2.8g | dietary fiber: 1.9g | net carbs: 0.9g | sugars: 0g | protein: 1.9g

RATIOS:

fat:	carbs:	protein:
85%	9%	6%

KICKIN' KETCHUP

COCONUT-FREE • EGG-FREE • NUT-FREE • VEGAN   OPTION: LOW-FODMAP

I use this ketchup all the time in my cooking. You'd be amazed at the flavor it provides—it's a one-stop-shop flavor booster in a bottle! If you're planning on cooking with this ketchup, make it with refined avocado oil. Refined avocado oil is more heat-stable than olive oil, making it a better choice if you plan to use the ketchup as more than a condiment at the table.

3 ounces (85 g) sun-dried tomatoes

⅔ cup (160 ml) extra-virgin olive oil or refined avocado oil

2 tablespoons apple cider vinegar

2 teaspoons onion powder

½ teaspoon garlic powder

½ teaspoon finely ground gray sea salt

½ teaspoon ground black pepper

¼ teaspoon ground cloves

5 drops liquid stevia

STORE IT: *Keep in an airtight container in the refrigerator for up to 5 days.*

MAKE IT LOW-FODMAP: *Omit the onion and garlic powder and replace 2 tablespoons of the oil with Garlic-Infused Oil (page 230).*

1. Place the sun-dried tomatoes in a heat-safe bowl and cover with boiling water. Allow to soak for 10 minutes.

2. Meanwhile, place the remaining ingredients in a blender or food processor.

3. After the tomatoes have soaked for 10 minutes, strain ⅓ cup (80 ml) of the soaking liquid into the blender, then drain the tomatoes. Transfer the drained tomatoes to the blender.

4. Blend the mixture until smooth, 1 to 2 minutes.

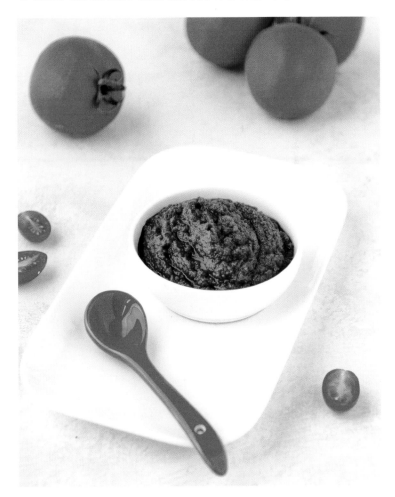

NUTRIENT INFORMATION (PER 1-TABLESPOON SERVING):

calories: 62 | calories from fat: 51 | total fat: 5.7g | saturated fat: 0.8g | cholesterol: 0mg

sodium: 113mg | carbs: 2.2g | dietary fiber: 0g | net carbs: 2.2g | sugars: 1.4g | protein: 0.5g

RATIOS:

fat:	carbs:	protein:
83%	**14%**	**3%**

CLASSIC CAESAR DRESSING

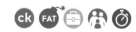

PREP TIME: **5 minutes**   MAKES: **1 cup (240 ml) (8 servings)**

NIGHTSHADE-FREE · NUT-FREE   OPTIONS: COCONUT-FREE · EGG-FREE · LOW-FODMAP · VEGAN

Who needs dairy in a Caesar salad when you have a dressing recipe like this one? Answer: no one. I promise, you'll be impressed with the flavor of this dressing and even more thrilled when you top your salad with hulled hemp seeds and coat it in this delicious dressing. Hulled hemp seeds lend a texture that's amazingly like the Parmesan cheese found in a classic Caesar salad—so you won't miss the dairy! If this is your first time making Caesar dressing, you may have a bit of a hard time finding anchovies at the store. This is because they're hiding. They aren't always in the canned fish aisle, as you may suspect. Check the seafood section where they keep the lobsters and other fresh fish. The anchovies will likely be in that area.

½ cup (120 ml) MCT oil

¼ cup (53 g) mayonnaise, homemade (page 220) or store-bought

1¾ ounces (50 g) anchovy fillets (about 8)

3 tablespoons fresh lemon juice

1 tablespoon plus 1 teaspoon Dijon mustard

2 small cloves garlic, minced if not using a high-powered blender

¼ teaspoon ground black pepper

Pinch of finely ground gray sea salt

Place all the ingredients in a blender and blend until smooth.

STORE IT: *Keep in an airtight container in the fridge for up to 3 days.*

PREP AHEAD: *Always have a batch of mayonnaise on hand.*

MAKE IT COCONUT-FREE: *Replace the MCT oil with extra-virgin olive oil, unrefined canola oil, or refined avocado oil.*

MAKE IT EGG-FREE: *Use egg-free mayonnaise.*

MAKE IT LOW-FODMAP: *For both the original recipe and the vegan variation, replace 2 tablespoons of the MCT oil or extra-virgin olive oil with Garlic-Infused Oil (page 230). If you are severely sensitive to FODMAPs, you may react to the amount of avocado used in this dressing. Be cautious.*

MAKE IT VEGAN: *Prepare the Vegan Caesar Dressing variation below.*

VARIATION: VEGAN CAESAR DRESSING. *Place the flesh of 1 large ripe Hass avocado, peeled and pitted (about 6 ounces/170 g of flesh), 3 tablespoons of lemon juice, 2 tablespoons of extra-virgin olive oil, 3 cloves of minced garlic, 1 tablespoon of caper brine, 1 tablespoon of capers, 2 teaspoons of Dijon mustard, and a pinch each of finely ground gray sea salt and ground black pepper in a food processor or blender. Blend until smooth. If it needs some thinning, add more olive oil. Transfer to a bowl and stir in ¼ cup (37 g) of hulled hemp seeds for the "Parmesan." Makes 1¼ cups (300 ml), or 10 servings.*

NUTRIENT INFORMATION (PER 2-TABLESPOON SERVING OF CLASSIC VERSION):

calories: 187 | calories from fat: 161 | total fat: 19.8g | saturated fat: 14.8g | cholesterol: 3mg

sodium: 96mg | carbs: 0.6g | dietary fiber: 0g | net carbs: 0.6g | sugars: 0g | protein: 1.6g

RATIOS:

fat:	carbs:	protein:
96%	1%	3%

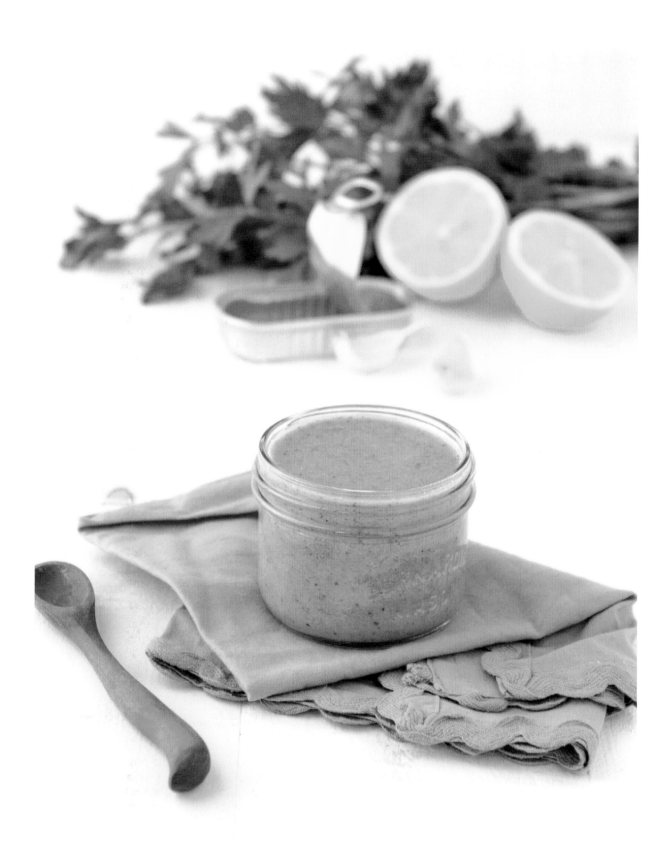

NUTRIENT INFORMATION (PER 2-TABLESPOON SERVING OF VEGAN VERSION):

calories: 107 | calories from fat: 95 | total fat: 10.6g | saturated fat: 1.9g | cholesterol: 0mg

sodium: 73mg | carbs: 3.6g | dietary fiber: 2.2g | net carbs: 1.4g | sugars: 0g | protein: 1g

RATIOS:

fat:	carbs:	protein:
84%	12%	4%

RANCH DRESSING

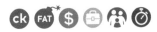

PREP TIME: **5 minutes**   MAKES: **2 cups (475 ml) (16 servings)**

NIGHTSHADE-FREE · NUT-FREE · VEGETARIAN   OPTIONS: **EGG-FREE · LOW-FODMAP · VEGAN**

Creamy and delicious, this dressing does triple duty: in addition to being yummy on a salad, it's great as a dip for baked chicken tenders (page 284) and also works as a meat or vegetable marinade—just add to an oven-safe casserole dish with chicken thighs or breasts or pork cutlets and bake until cooked through.

1 cup (210 g) mayonnaise, homemade (page 220) or store-bought

½ cup (120 ml) full-fat coconut milk

2 small cloves garlic, minced if not using a high-powered blender

1 tablespoon fresh lemon juice

1 tablespoon apple cider vinegar

1 tablespoon chopped white onions

¼ teaspoon finely ground gray sea salt

⅛ teaspoon ground black pepper

2 tablespoons sliced fresh chives

3 tablespoons finely chopped fresh parsley

1 tablespoon finely chopped fresh dill

1. Place the mayonnaise, coconut milk, garlic, lemon juice, vinegar, onions, salt, and pepper in a blender. Blend on high until smooth, about 1 minute.

2. Add the chives, parsley, and dill and pulse only once, just to combine.

STORE IT: *Keep in an airtight container in the fridge for up to 5 days.*

MAKE IT EGG-FREE/VEGAN: *Use egg-free mayonnaise.*

MAKE IT LOW-FODMAP: *Omit the garlic or replace it with 1 tablespoon of Garlic-Infused Oil (page 230) made with olive oil. Increase the amount of chives to ¼ cup (18 g).*

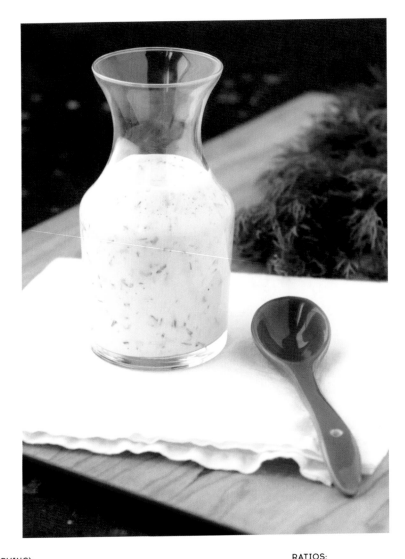

NUTRIENT INFORMATION (PER 2-TABLESPOON SERVING):

calories: 107 | calories from fat: 104 | total fat: 11.5g | saturated fat: 2.9g | cholesterol: 5mg

sodium: 104mg | carbs: 0.7g | dietary fiber: 0g | net carbs: 0.7g | sugars: 0g | protein: 0.2g

RATIOS:

fat:	carbs:	protein:
96%	3%	1%

RED WINE VINAIGRETTE

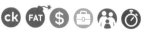

COCONUT-FREE • EGG-FREE • NIGHTSHADE-FREE • NUT-FREE • VEGAN   OPTION: LOW-FODMAP

Whether I'm using it to flavor (and give a keto boost to) a batch of pan-steamed vegetables or tossing a salad with it, this is one of my go-to homemade dressings.

½ cup (120 ml) extra-virgin olive oil

¼ cup (60 ml) red wine vinegar

1 tablespoon Dijon mustard

1 small clove garlic, minced if not using a high-powered blender

½ teaspoon ground black pepper

¼ teaspoon finely ground gray sea salt

4 drops liquid stevia

Place all the ingredients in a blender and blend on high speed until smooth.

STORE IT: *Keep in an airtight container in the fridge for up to 1 week.*

MAKE IT LOW-FODMAP: *Replace the Dijon mustard with 1 teaspoon of ground mustard seed. Omit the garlic clove and replace 1 tablespoon of the olive oil with Garlic-Infused Oil (page 230) made with olive oil or refined avocado oil.*

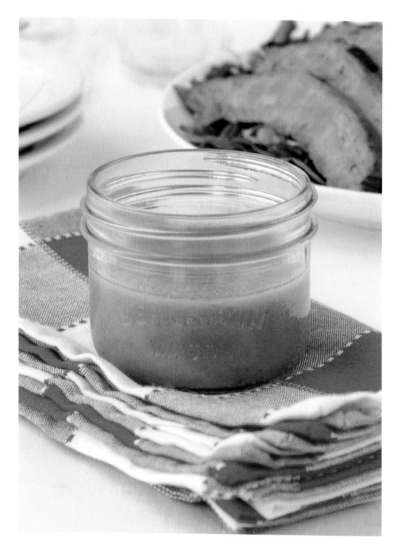

NUTRIENT INFORMATION (PER 1-TABLESPOON SERVING):

calories: 78 | calories from fat: 75 | total fat: 8.5g | saturated fat: 1.2g | cholesterol: 0mg

sodium: 54mg | carbs: 0.3g | dietary fiber: 0g | net carbs: 0.3g | sugars: 0g | protein: 0.1g

RATIOS:

fat: carbs: protein:

98%   **2%**   **0%**

INFUSED OIL

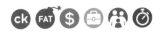

PREP TIME: **5 minutes**   COOK TIME: **5 minutes**   MAKES: **½ cup (120 ml) (8 servings)**

COCONUT-FREE • EGG-FREE • LOW-FODMAP • NIGHTSHADE-FREE • NUT-FREE • VEGAN

Infused oils are at the center of my keto diet. I use them to flavor dishes when I'm too pressed for time to get creative, when I want to add a garlic flavor to a recipe but don't want to deal with the tummy pains that follow, or when I want to up the fat content of my meal. A tablespoon of infused oil adds about 14 grams of fat to a meal, just like a tablespoon of regular oil.

I highly recommend having a couple of these oils on hand at all times. Although the process of infusing oils may sound tedious, it's not tedious at all. In just 10 minutes, you can transform a couple of ingredients into something you can use over and over again to save you time in the kitchen and pack flavor into your recipes.

Which type of oil you use is entirely up to you. I like refined avocado oil or coconut oil for infused oils that I plan on heating and extra-virgin olive oil for infused oils that I plan on adding to salads. If I want to use the infused oil both heated and cold, I go with refined avocado oil.

The key to infusing oil is to heat the ingredients only until bubbly, but not allow them to cook beyond that point. If the mixture continues to

bubble, you risk burning it and ruining your oil. After removing the oil from the heat, transfer it to a heatproof jar or bowl to cool for 1 hour. The longer you allow the ingredients to steep, the stronger the flavor of the infused oil will be. Once the oil is cool, strain it through a fine-mesh sieve. (*Note:* The only flavoring ingredients that absolutely must be strained before the oil is bottled are soft herbs, which, if left in the oil, will go bad.)

Infused oil keeps best when protected from light. Store it in glass bottles, preferably dark glass, and keep it in the pantry or another dark place. It will keep for months if stored correctly, depending on the shelf life of the individual oil (see pages 138 and 139). Remember to label your bottles with a piece of masking tape and permanent marker. (*Note:* If you're storing your oil in a jar with a lid, place the label on the lid rather than on the side of the jar to prevent smudges from dripping oil.)

If you have concerns about your oil going rancid, the chart on pages 138 and 139 also provides details on oil stability, which will help you choose the best type of oil for your needs.

GUIDE TO INFUSING INGREDIENTS—BY TYPE

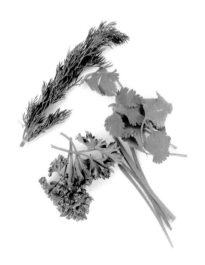

SOFT HERBS, FRESH

EXAMPLES: *basil, cilantro, parsley, dill*

Though not herbs, green onions and chives work well here.

RATIO: *a handful of herbs (about ⅔ ounce/20 g) to ½ cup (120 ml) oil*

Place the herb (stems and leaves) in a blender with the oil of your choice and pulse until broken down. Transfer the mixture to a small saucepan and heat on medium heat until bubbles form, about 5 minutes.

WOODY HERBS, FRESH

EXAMPLES: *rosemary, thyme, tarragon, mint, oregano, sage, lemongrass*

Though not an herb, fresh ginger root works well here.

RATIO: *a handful of herbs (about ⅔ ounce/20 g) to ½ cup (120 ml) oil*

Place the herb sprigs in a small saucepan with the oil of your choice. Heat on medium heat until bubbles form, about 5 minutes.

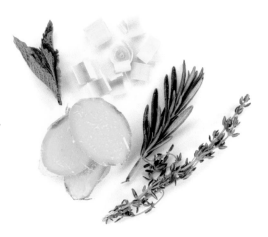

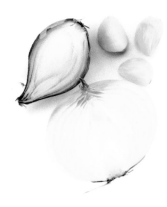

ROASTED AROMATICS

EXAMPLES: *garlic, onions, shallots*

RATIO: *½ ounce (15 g) aromatics to ½ cup (120 ml) oil*

Roasting is optional for aromatics but adds a deeper flavor. If you choose not to roast the aromatics, simply place the raw ingredients in the saucepan with the oil.

Roast the peeled aromatic in a preheated 350°F (177°C) oven for 15 to 25 minutes, until lightly golden and fragrant. Transfer to a small saucepan with the oil of your choice. Heat on medium heat until bubbles form, about 5 minutes.

CITRUS

EXAMPLES: *lemon, lime, orange, grapefruit*

RATIO: *1 teaspoon citrus zest to ½ cup (120 ml) oil*

Place the citrus zest in a small saucepan with the oil of your choice. Heat on medium heat until bubbles form, about 5 minutes.

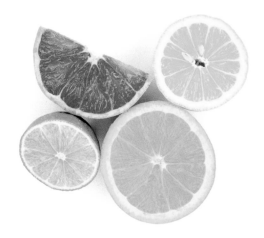

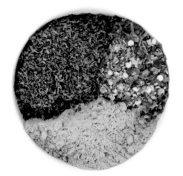

DRIED SPICES AND/OR HERBS

EXAMPLES: *crushed red pepper, cumin seeds, dried oregano leaves, any spice mixture from pages 232 to 235*

RATIO: *1 teaspoon dried spices/herbs to ½ cup (120 ml) oil*

Place the spices/herbs in a small saucepan with the oil of your choice. Heat on medium heat until bubbles form, about 5 minutes.

MY FAVORITE INFUSED OIL BLENDS

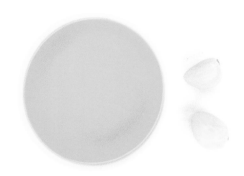

GARLIC-INFUSED OIL
(AROMATIC)

Peel 4 cloves of garlic and place on an unlined rimmed baking sheet. Roast in a preheated 350°F (177°C) oven for 15 to 20 minutes, until lightly golden and fragrant. Place ½ cup (120 ml) refined avocado oil in a saucepan along with the roasted garlic cloves. Heat on medium heat until bubbles form, about 5 minutes.

ONION-INFUSED OIL
(AROMATIC)

Quarter a small onion (red, yellow, white—your choice) and place on an unlined rimmed baking sheet. Roast in a preheated 350°F (177°C) oven for 20 to 25 minutes, until lightly golden and fragrant. Place ½ cup (120 ml) refined avocado oil in a saucepan along with the roasted onion. Heat on medium heat until bubbles form, about 5 minutes.

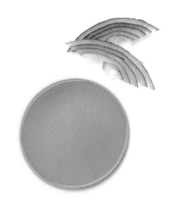

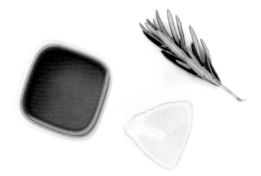

ROSEMARY LEMON–INFUSED
OIL (WOODY HERB + CITRUS)

Place ½ cup (120 ml) refined avocado oil, the leaves from ½ sprig rosemary, and the zest from ½ lemon in a small saucepan. Heat on medium heat until bubbles form, about 5 minutes.

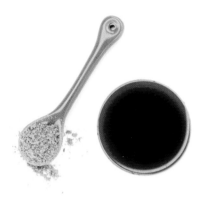

MEDITERRANEAN-INFUSED OIL (DRIED SPICES)

Place ½ cup (120 ml) extra-virgin olive oil and 1 teaspoon Mediterranean seasoning (page 233) in a small saucepan. Heat on medium heat until bubbles form, about 5 minutes.

CILANTRO, GINGER, SHALLOT, AND GARLIC-INFUSED OIL
(SOFT HERB + AROMATICS)

Place 2 peeled garlic cloves and 2 halved and peeled shallots on an unlined rimmed baking sheet and roast in a preheated 350°F (177°C) oven for 20 to 25 minutes. Meanwhile, place ½ cup (120 ml) melted coconut oil and ¼ cup (15 g) cilantro leaves in a blender and pulse until broken down. Transfer the mixture to a saucepan. Chop a 1-inch (2.5-cm) piece of fresh ginger and add it to the saucepan along with the roasted garlic cloves and shallots. Heat on medium heat until bubbles form, about 5 minutes.

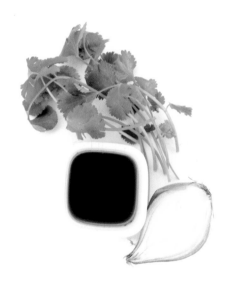

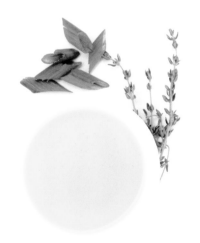

GREEN ONION AND THYME OIL
(SOFT HERB + WOODY HERB)

Place ½ cup (120 ml) refined avocado oil and ⅓ cup (27 g) chopped green onions in a blender and pulse until broken down. Transfer the mixture to a saucepan. Add 1 fresh thyme sprig. Heat on medium heat until bubbles form, about 5 minutes.

HOMEMADE SPICE MIXTURES

PREP TIME: **5 minutes**   COOK TIME: **– (not including toasting of spices for some blends)**

COCONUT-FREE • EGG-FREE • NUT-FREE • VEGAN

You probably noticed a lot of mentions of "your favorite fresh or dried spice mixtures" in the One-Pan Meal Strategies on pages 161 and 162. And maybe you were like, okay…chili powder. If you feel creatively limited in your use of spices, you're not alone.

If it were up to me, I'd put basil on everything. But sometimes it's nice to step out of your comfort zone and do something fun with the flavors in your everyday meals. The easiest way to mix it up is with homemade spice mixtures. I prep a bunch of these every couple of months so I have lots of different flavors on hand for quick spice action. A dash here, a sprinkle there, and boom! These mixtures massively change the flavor of a meal.

GREEK SEASONING

MAKES: ½ cup (75 g) • NIGHTSHADE-FREE • OPTION: LOW-FODMAP

Use in stuffed peppers or salad dressing, or mix with dairy-free yogurt or full-fat coconut milk for a tasty vegetable dip.

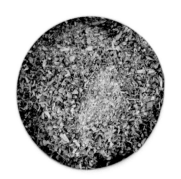

- 1 tablespoon plus 1 teaspoon finely ground gray sea salt
- 1 tablespoon plus 1 teaspoon garlic powder
- 1 tablespoon plus 1 teaspoon dried basil
- 1 tablespoon plus 1 teaspoon dried oregano leaves
- 2 teaspoons dried parsley
- 2 teaspoons dried ground rosemary
- 2 teaspoons dried ground marjoram
- 2 teaspoons dried thyme leaves
- 1 teaspoon ground black pepper
- ½ teaspoon ground cinnamon
- ½ teaspoon ground nutmeg

MAKE IT LOW-FODMAP: *Omit the garlic powder.*

Place all the ingredients in a ½-cup (120-ml) glass jar with an airtight lid. Cover and shake. Store in the pantry for up to 3 months.

CAJUN SEASONING

MAKES: ½ cup (82 g)

Use as a rub for chicken or turkey or as a topping on shrimp, or mix into a sausage scramble.

- 2 tablespoons plus 2 teaspoons paprika
- 1½ tablespoons finely ground gray sea salt
- 1½ tablespoons garlic powder
- 1 tablespoon onion powder
- 1 tablespoon dried oregano leaves
- 1 teaspoon ground black pepper
- 1 teaspoon dried thyme leaves
- ½ teaspoon cayenne pepper
- ½ teaspoon red pepper flakes

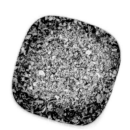

Place the ingredients in a ½-cup (120-ml) glass jar with an airtight lid. Cover and shake. Store in the pantry for up to 3 months.

MEDITERRANEAN SEASONING

MAKES: ½ cup (50 g) • LOW-FODMAP • NIGHTSHADE-FREE

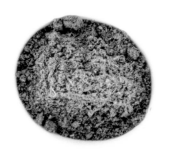

Use in chicken tacos, salad dressings, or kebabs.

3 tablespoons dried rosemary leaves

2 tablespoons ground cumin

2 tablespoons ground coriander

1 tablespoon dried oregano leaves

2 teaspoons ground cinnamon

½ teaspoon finely ground gray sea salt

Place the spices and salt in a ½-cup (120-ml) glass jar with an airtight lid. Cover and shake. Store in the pantry for up to 3 months.

BAHĀRĀT SEASONING

MAKES: ⅔ cup (72 g) • LOW-FODMAP

Bahārāt means "spice" in Arabic. It is used as an all-purpose seasoning in Middle Eastern cooking with a couple of variations to the recipe depending on country. Some combinations include mint, saffron, dried rose petals, or turmeric powder, which you could add to this base recipe if you're feeling a little crazy!

Bahārāt can be used in cooked eggplant, lamb burgers, chicken, meat, riced cauliflower, or grilled fish.

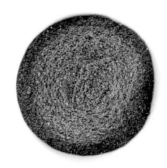

2 tablespoons paprika

2 tablespoons ground black pepper

1½ tablespoons ground cumin

1 tablespoon ground cinnamon

1 tablespoon ground cloves

1 tablespoon ground coriander

2 teaspoons ground nutmeg

1 teaspoon ground allspice

½ teaspoon ground cardamom

Place the spices in a ½-cup (120-ml) glass jar with an airtight lid. Cover and shake. Store in the pantry for up to 6 months.

SHICHIMI SEASONING

MAKES: ½ cup (110 g)

Shichimi togarashi is called seven spice; *shichi* means "seven" in Japanese. And while seven ingredients is the norm for the classic mixture, I can't help but add a bit of ginger to the mix when I make a batch! Because this seasoning particularly shines in fatty dishes, it is a pantry staple in a keto kitchen.

You should be able to find these ingredients in the ethnic aisle of a big chain grocery store. Use this seasoning mixture in a variety of ways: add to mayo as a dip, use as a meat rub, or sprinkle on bacon.

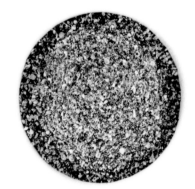

2 tablespoons dried orange peel

3 to 4 whole dried red chili peppers (depending on your tolerance for heat)

1 tablespoon plus 1 teaspoon wakame flakes

1 tablespoon plus 1 teaspoon sesame seeds

1 tablespoon plus 1 teaspoon poppy seeds

1 tablespoon plus 1 teaspoon garlic powder

1 tablespoon plus 1 teaspoon ginger powder

1 tablespoon plus 1 teaspoon ground black pepper

1. Place the spices in a coffee grinder and grind until powdered.

2. Place the spice blend in a ½-cup (120-ml) glass jar with an airtight lid. Store in the pantry for up to 6 months.

ITALIAN SEASONING

MAKES: ½ cup (30 g) • LOW-FODMAP • NIGHTSHADE-FREE

Use Italian seasoning to spice up chicken or turkey or dishes that contain tomatoes, eggplant, garlic, onions, or zucchini.

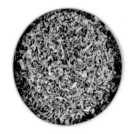

3 tablespoons dried basil

3 tablespoons dried oregano leaves

2 tablespoons dried parsley

1 tablespoon dried rosemary leaves

1 tablespoon dried thyme leaves

1½ teaspoons dried ground sage

¾ teaspoon ground black pepper

Place the ingredients in a ½-cup (120-ml) glass jar with an airtight lid. Cover and shake. Store in the pantry for up to 3 months.

CURRY POWDER

MAKES: ½ cup (40 g) • LOW-FODMAP • OPTION: NIGHTSHADE-FREE

Use curry powder in a variety of ways, including on roasted vegetables, fried sausages, or cauliflower rice (page 364).

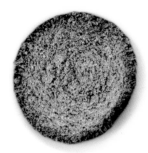

¼ cup coriander seeds or 2 tablespoons ground coriander

2 teaspoons cumin seeds

1 teaspoon yellow mustard seeds

1 (6-in/15-cm) piece cinnamon bark

20 whole cloves

2 to 4 whole dried red chili peppers (depending on your tolerance for heat)

2 teaspoons ground cardamom

2 teaspoons turmeric powder

1. If using whole coriander seeds, place them along with the cumin and mustard seeds in a small cast-iron frying pan over medium heat. Toast for 2 to 3 minutes, until golden, shaking the pan continuously to prevent the seeds from burning.

2. Drop the toasted seeds into a coffee or spice grinder and add the cinnamon bark, cloves, and dried chilis. Grind until powdered.

3. Transfer the mixture to a ½-cup (120-ml) glass jar with an airtight lid along with the cardamom, turmeric, and ground coriander (if you didn't use whole coriander seeds in Step 1). Cover and shake. Store in the pantry for up to 6 months.

MAKE IT NIGHTSHADE-FREE:
Omit the dried chili peppers.

SEASONING SALT

MAKES: ½ cup (80 g) • OPTION: NIGHTSHADE-FREE

Use as a dry rub for meat, or sprinkle over eggs or roasted jicama.

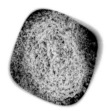

3 tablespoons ground coriander

2 tablespoons onion powder

2 tablespoons finely ground gray sea salt

2 teaspoons ground mustard

2 teaspoons paprika

1¼ teaspoons turmeric powder

¾ teaspoon ground celery seed

¾ teaspoon dried parsley

½ teaspoon ground black pepper

Place the ingredients in a ½-cup (120-ml) glass jar with an airtight lid. Cover and shake. Store in the pantry for up to 3 months.

MAKE IT NIGHTSHADE-FREE:
Omit the paprika.

CHAPTER 14

CLASSIC BREAKFAST

PANCAKES

PREP TIME: **10 minutes**   COOK TIME: **40 minutes**   MAKES: **4 pancakes (2 servings)**

LOW-FODMAP • NIGHTSHADE-FREE   OPTION: **NUT-FREE**

This is a HealthfulPursuit.com classic, and one of the first keto recipes that I created and shared on my blog. While it's a fabulous recipe and I continue to make it to this day, the initial reaction to it wasn't all that fabulous. Before I shared this recipe, ingredients like pork rinds never, ever made it to the blog because until I went keto, *Healthful Pursuit* was primarily a vegan blog! You can imagine the backlash this recipe received when I posted it. Yikes. Over time, as I've grown into the keto space, this recipe has become one of my most popular. I chose to revisit it for this book and have adjusted a couple of the instructions to make the end result easier to achieve. I hope you love it! Be sure to use your nonstick pan; it's essential to success on this one.

PANCAKES:

2.8 ounces (80 g) unseasoned pork rinds

2 teaspoons ground cinnamon, plus more for garnish (optional)

½ teaspoon baking powder

4 large eggs

½ cup (120 ml) full-fat coconut milk

¼ scant teaspoon liquid stevia

2 tablespoons coconut oil, divided, for the pan

SAUCE:

2 tablespoons coconut oil

2 tablespoons unsweetened smooth almond butter

1. Place the pork rinds in a spice grinder or blender. Grind to a very fine but clumping powder (it will clump together when pinched because of the fat content in the pork rinds).

2. Transfer the ground pork rinds to a small bowl and add the cinnamon and baking powder. Stir to combine.

3. In a larger bowl, whisk together the eggs, coconut milk, and stevia. Add the pork rind mixture and stir to incorporate.

4. In an 8-inch (20-cm) nonstick frying pan, melt ½ tablespoon of coconut oil over medium-low heat.

5. Preheat your oven to the lowest temperature possible.

6. Pour a quarter of the batter into the hot oiled pan and spread the batter evenly into a circle with the back of a spoon or by rotating the pan. Do not allow the batter to migrate too far up the sides of the pan, or it will burn. Cook the pancake for 4 to 5 minutes, until bubbles form all over. Flip carefully and cook for another 4 to 5 minutes.

7. Transfer the completed pancake to a clean oven-safe plate and place in the preheated oven.

8. Add another ½ tablespoon of coconut oil to the pan. The batter may have thickened while sitting. If so, add water, a splash at a time, and mix until the batter returns to its original consistency, being careful not to add too much water.

9. Pour another quarter of the batter into the pan, form it into a circle, and cook, following Step 6. Repeat with the remaining coconut oil and batter.

10. While the last pancake is cooking, prepare the sauce: Melt the 2 tablespoons of coconut oil and put it in a small bowl along with the almond butter. Stir to combine.

MAKE IT NUT-FREE: *Use coconut butter in place of the almond butter.*

11. When the pancakes are ready, divide between 2 plates and drizzle with the almond butter sauce. Sprinkle with additional cinnamon, if desired.

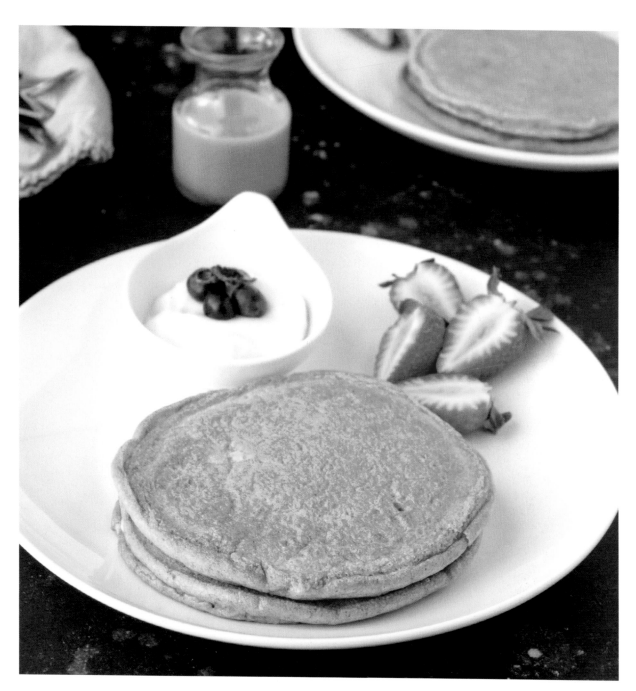

NUTRIENT INFORMATION (PER 2 PANCAKES):

calories: 885 | calories from fat: 641 | total fat: 71.3g | saturated fat: 44g | cholesterol: 342mg

sodium: 920mg | carbs: 8.1g | dietary fiber: 3.2g | net carbs: 4.9g | sugars: 2.2g | protein: 52.8g

RATIOS:

fat:	carbs:	protein:
72%	**4%**	**24%**

ALLSPICE MUFFINS

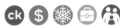

PREP TIME: 15 minutes, plus 30 minutes to cool COOK TIME: 25 minutes MAKES: 12 muffins (12 servings)

NIGHTSHADE-FREE • VEGETARIAN

I'm not much of a sweets-for-breakfast gal, but you may be, so I've included this recipe especially for you! If I were a sweets-for-breakfast gal, I would enjoy these muffins with an epic Rocket Fuel Latte (page 428), and I might slather a little butter-infused coconut oil on the muffin to fatten it up even more.

Raw nuts are fine to use, but for health reasons, it's better to soak and roast them before using them in this recipe (see page 157).

DRY INGREDIENTS:

1½ cups (165 g) blanched almond flour

½ cup (64 g) roughly ground flax seeds

½ cup (80 g) confectioners'-style erythritol

2 teaspoons baking powder

1 tablespoon plus 1 teaspoon ground allspice

½ teaspoon finely ground gray sea salt

WET INGREDIENTS:

6 large eggs

½ cup (120 ml) melted (but not hot) coconut oil

½ cup (120 ml) full-fat coconut milk

Grated zest of 1 lemon

1 teaspoon vanilla extract

TOPPING:

¼ cup (28 g) raw walnut pieces

1. Preheat the oven to 350°F (177°C) and line a muffin pan with 12 paper liners, or have on hand a 12-cavity silicone muffin pan.

2. Place the dry ingredients in a medium-sized bowl and mix until fully blended.

3. In a large bowl, whisk the eggs, coconut oil, coconut milk, lemon zest, and vanilla. Once combined, add the dry mixture to the wet. Stir with a spatula just until incorporated.

4. Pour the batter into the prepared muffin cups, filling each about three-quarters full. Sprinkle the tops with the walnuts.

5. Bake for 22 to 25 minutes, until the tops are golden and a toothpick inserted in the middle comes out clean.

6. Allow the muffins to cool in the pan for 30 minutes before removing and serving.

STORE IT: *Keep in an airtight container on the counter for up to 3 days, in the fridge for up to 1 week, or in the freezer for up to 1 month.*

REHEAT IT: *Place on a plate and microwave until the desired temperature is reached. Or place in a covered casserole dish and reheat in a preheated 300°F (150°C) oven for 5 minutes, or until warmed through.*

THAW IT: *Allow to thaw completely on the counter. Once defrosted, enjoy cold or use the reheating instructions above.*

SERVE IT WITH: *To make this a complete meal, serve with a Rocket Fuel Latte (page 428). These muffins taste great slathered with Coconut Whipped Cream (page 414).*

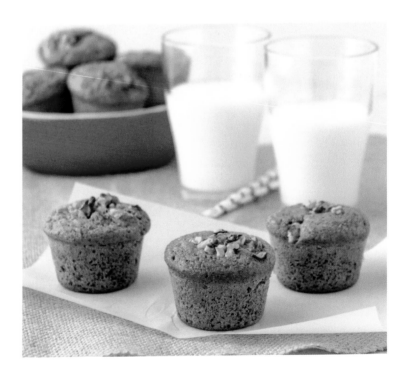

NUTRIENT INFORMATION (PER MUFFIN):

calories: 273 | calories from fat: 217 | total fat: 24.1g | saturated fat: 11.3g | cholesterol: 93mg

sodium: 120mg | carbs: 5.8g | dietary fiber: 3.5g | net carbs: 2.3g | sugars: 1.1g | protein: 8.1g

RATIOS:

fat:	carbs:	protein:
80%	8%	12%

FLAXSEED CINNAMON BUN MUFFINS

PREP TIME: 10 minutes, plus 20 minutes to cool   COOK TIME: 15 minutes   MAKES: 12 muffins (12 servings)

NIGHTSHADE-FREE • NUT-FREE • VEGETARIAN   OPTION: COCONUT-FREE

Enjoy the flavor of cinnamon buns without the carbs with these flourless grain-free, sugar-free muffins made entirely from flax seeds. You'll be amazed at the texture.

2 cups (256 g) roughly ground flax seeds

⅓ cup (53 g) confectioners'-style erythritol, ¼ cup (58 g) granulated xylitol, or ¾ teaspoon liquid stevia

2 tablespoons ground cinnamon

1 tablespoon baking powder

½ teaspoon finely ground gray sea salt

5 large eggs

½ cup (120 ml) water, at room temperature

⅓ cup (80 ml) melted (but not hot) coconut oil or refined avocado oil

2 teaspoons vanilla extract

STORE IT: *Keep in the fridge for up to 4 days or in the freezer for up to 3 months.*

PREP AHEAD: *Measure out the dry ingredients—ground flax seeds, xylitol (if using), cinnamon, baking powder, and salt— and store in a baggie in the pantry for up to 1 month. When you're ready to make a batch of muffins, place the dry mixture in a bowl. Preheat the oven and prepare the pan as described in Step 1, then continue with Step 3.*

SERVE IT WITH: *To make this a complete meal, slather a muffin with coconut oil and sprinkle it with gray sea salt.*

MAKE IT COCONUT-FREE: *Replace the coconut oil with refined avocado oil, melted ghee (if tolerated), or macadamia nut oil.*

1. Preheat the oven to 350°F and line a 12-count muffin pan with paper liners.

2. In a large bowl, whisk the flax seeds with the erythritol or xylitol (if using one of these sweetener options), cinnamon, baking powder, and salt until fully combined.

3. Place the eggs, water, oil, vanilla, and stevia (if using this sweetener option) in a blender. Blend on high speed for 30 seconds, until foamy.

4. Transfer the liquid mixture to the bowl with the flaxseed mixture. Stir with a spatula just until incorporated. The batter will be very fluffy. Allow to sit for 3 minutes.

5. Spoon the batter into prepared muffin pan, filling each cavity 90 percent of the way up. Bake for 13 to 15 minutes, until a toothpick inserted in the middle comes out clean.

6. Immediately take the muffins out of the pan and place them on a cooling rack. Allow to cool for at least 20 minutes before you grab one for yourself.

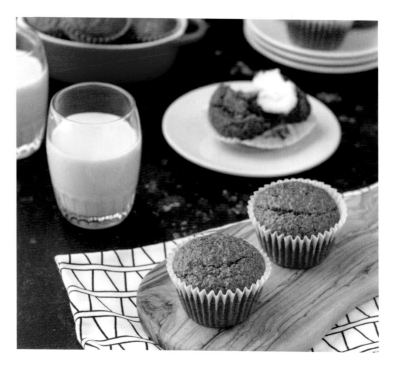

NUTRIENT INFORMATION (PER MUFFIN, MADE WITH ERYTHRITOL OR STEVIA):
calories: 199 | calories from fat: 137 | total fat: 15.2g | saturated fat: 6.5g | cholesterol: 77mg
sodium: 116mg | carbs: 8.8g | dietary fiber: 6.5g | net carbs: 2.3g | sugars: 0g | protein: 6.8g

RATIOS:
fat:	carbs:	protein:
68%	18%	14%

BACON LOVERS' QUICHE

PREP TIME: 20 minutes, plus 30 minutes to cool   COOK TIME: 45 minutes   MAKES: four 4-inch (10-cm) mini quiches (8 servings)

NIGHTSHADE-FREE   OPTION: VEGETARIAN

There's good quiche—crispy crust, fully cooked yet tender interior, lightly seasoned, and packed with flavor. And there's not-so-good quiche—soggy crust, runny or overdone and rubbery insides, and bland, tasting like nothing but eggs. This is the good quiche you write home about. Heck, this is the quiche you bring home *with* you. Make some for the fam-jam, or keep it all for yourself. I promise you won't be disappointed because…bacon! And the crust really is phenomenal.

If you'd like to make one large quiche, go for it! You'll need a 9-inch (23-cm) tart pan. Increase the par-baking time for the crust by 2 to 4 minutes and the baking time for the quiche by 5 to 8 minutes.

CRUST:

2 cups (220 g) blanched almond flour

1 large egg

2 tablespoons melted lard, plus more for the pans

⅛ teaspoon finely ground gray sea salt

FILLING:

6 strips bacon (about 6 ounces/170 g)

1⅓ cups (315 ml) full-fat coconut milk

4 large eggs

¼ cup plus 2 tablespoons (25 g) nutritional yeast

¼ teaspoon finely ground gray sea salt

¼ teaspoon ground black pepper

⅛ teaspoon ground nutmeg

FOR GARNISH (OPTIONAL):

Cooked chopped bacon (reserved from above)

Sliced fresh chives

1. Preheat the oven to 350°F (177°C) and lightly grease four 4-inch (10-cm) tart pans with lard.

2. Make the crusts: In a large bowl, combine the almond flour, egg, lard, and salt. Mix with a fork until completely incorporated.

3. Divide the dough into 4 pieces and place each piece in a prepared tart pan. Press the dough into the pans, pushing it evenly up the sides. It should be about ⅛ inch (3 mm) thick.

4. Place the tart pans on a rimmed baking sheet and par-bake for 13 to 15 minutes, until the crusts are lightly golden.

5. Meanwhile, prepare the filling: Cook the bacon in a frying pan over medium heat until crispy, then roughly chop or crumble it; reserve the bacon grease. Put the coconut milk, eggs, nutritional yeast, salt, pepper, and nutmeg in a bowl. Add the bacon pieces (setting a small amount aside for garnish if you wish) and still-warm reserved bacon grease and whisk to combine.

6. Remove the par-baked crusts from the oven and reduce the temperature to 325°F (163°C). Leaving the crusts on the baking sheet, fill them all the way to the brim with the egg filling.

7. Return the quiches to the oven and bake for 30 minutes, or until the tops are lightly golden. Allow to cool for 30 minutes before serving. Garnish each quiche with the reserved bacon pieces and/or sliced chives, if desired.

STORE IT: *Keep in an airtight container in the fridge for up to 3 days or in the freezer for up to 1 month.*

REHEAT IT: *Place on a plate and microwave until the desired temperature is reached. Or place on a rimmed baking sheet and reheat in a preheated 300°F (150°C) oven for 10 minutes, or until warmed through.*

THAW IT: *Allow to thaw completely in the fridge. Once defrosted, enjoy cold or use the reheating instructions above.*

PREP AHEAD: *Prepare the bacon bits up to a month ahead and store in the freezer in an airtight container. When ready to use, simply add to the recipe. In Step 5, use 3 tablespoons plus 1 teaspoon of melted bacon grease.*

SERVE IT WITH: *To make this a complete meal, serve on a bed of arugula drizzled with olive oil and apple cider vinegar. This quiche tastes great paired with Roasted Brussels Sprouts with Walnut "Cheese" (page 388).*

MAKE IT VEGETARIAN: *Replace the lard with coconut oil. Replace the bacon with 6 cremini mushrooms, sliced and sautéed in 2 tablespoons of coconut oil for 5 to 7 minutes.*

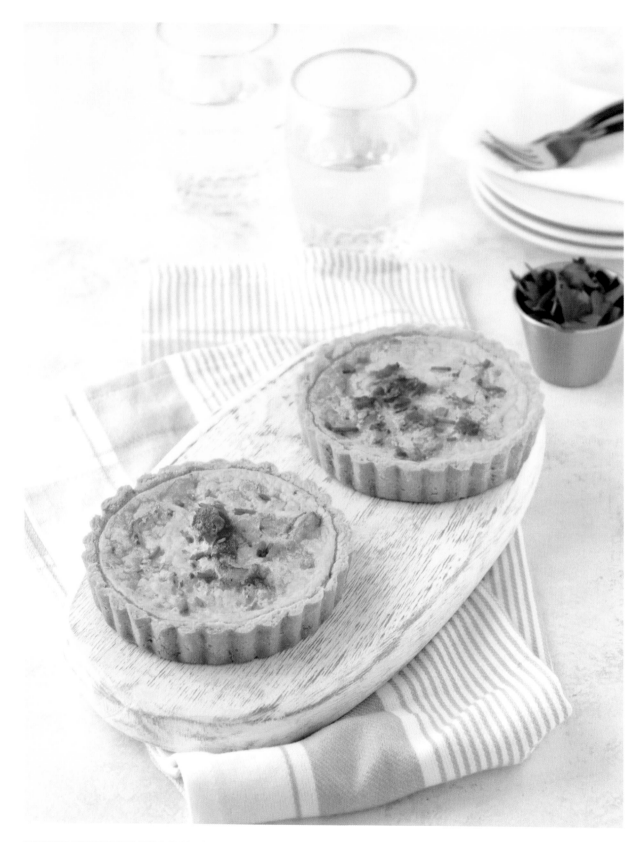

NUTRIENT INFORMATION (PER ½ QUICHE):

calories: 404 | calories from fat: 276 | total fat: 30.7g | saturated fat: 6.2g | cholesterol: 143mg
sodium: 646mg | carbs: 9g | dietary fiber: 5g | net carbs: 4g | sugars: 1.2g | protein: 22.9g

RATIOS:

fat:	carbs:	protein:
68%	9%	23%

EARLY-DAY JAMBALAYA

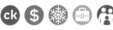

PREP TIME: **25 minutes**   COOK TIME: **25 minutes**   SERVES: **4**

COCONUT-FREE • EGG-FREE • LOW-FODMAP • NUT-FREE   OPTION: NIGHTSHADE-FREE

Have a bit of leftover chicken that you don't know what to do with? Look no further than this egg-free breakfast recipe; it will stick to your ribs until dinner, no joke. If you're a volume eater and need the volume to spark fullness, try serving this jambalaya on a bed of spinach or arugula. Though there is quite a bit of prep work involved in making this hearty breakfast, it comes together quickly when several of the components are made ahead (see below).

⅓ cup (69 g) lard

4 sausages (about 8 ounces/225 g), cooked and chopped

1 cup (180 g) cubed cooked skinless chicken thighs

1¼ cups (210 g) diced celery

½ packed cup chopped green onions

2 tablespoons Cajun Seasoning (page 232)

2½ cups (400 g) riced cauliflower florets (see page 163)

½ cup (120 ml) chicken bone broth (see page 152)

¼ cup (50 g) diced tomatoes

Handful of chopped fresh parsley (optional)

1. Melt the lard in a large frying pan over medium heat, then add the chopped sausages, cubed chicken thighs, celery, green onions, and Cajun seasoning. Cook for 10 minutes, or until the celery has softened.

2. Add the cauliflower and bone broth. Cover and cook for 5 minutes, or until the cauliflower is fork-tender.

3. Stir in the diced tomatoes and increase the heat to high. Cook, uncovered, for 5 to 7 minutes, until most of the liquid has evaporated.

4. Remove from the heat, toss in a handful of chopped fresh parsley, if desired, and divide among 4 small serving bowls.

STORE IT: *Keep in an airtight container in the fridge for up to 3 days or in the freezer for up to 1 month.*

REHEAT IT: *Microwave, covered, until the desired temperature is reached or reheat in a frying pan, covered, on medium.*

THAW IT: *Allow to thaw completely in the fridge. Once defrosted, use the reheating instructions above (it's better to pan-fry).*

PREP AHEAD: *Use the leftover protein of your choice in place of the cooked chicken thighs (leftover meat from the Balsamic Turkey Thighs on page 338 works well). Cook the sausages ahead, purchase fully cooked sausage, or replace the sausage with 6 to 8 Paleovalley Fermented Beef Sticks, which are sold fully cooked. Rice the cauliflower the evening before. Have the broth and Cajun seasoning made ahead of time.*

MAKE IT NIGHTSHADE-FREE: *Replace the Cajun seasoning with Greek seasoning (page 232) and omit the tomatoes.*

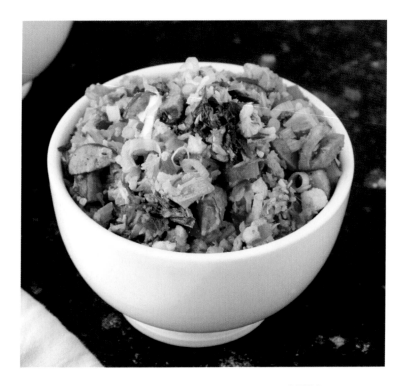

NUTRIENT INFORMATION (PER SERVING):

calories: 458 | calories from fat: 338 | total fat: 37.6g | saturated fat: 13.2g | cholesterol: 100mg

sodium: 643mg | carbs: 7.6g | dietary fiber: 3.5g | net carbs: 4.1g | sugars: 3.4g | protein: 22.4g

RATIOS:

fat:	carbs:	protein:
74%	**7%**	**19%**

SAUSAGE AND GREENS HASH BOWL

PREP TIME: **25 minutes**　COOK TIME: **25 minutes**　SERVES: **2**

COCONUT-FREE • EGG-FREE • NIGHTSHADE-FREE • NUT-FREE　OPTION: LOW-FODMAP

This is the base of just about every breakfast I eat, varying the meats and vegetables based on what I have on hand. The sausage can be replaced with just about any leftover meat, from brisket to ground pork to chicken thighs and beyond. The rutabaga could be swapped for cauliflower, zucchini, asparagus, or bok choy. And the spinach could be endive, arugula, or chard. You get the picture. Switch it up and make it work for you on a day-to-day basis. If you tolerate eggs, this dish is tasty topped with a couple of poached eggs.

HASH:

⅔ cup (100 g) peeled and ½-inch-cubed rutabaga

2 tablespoons lard

2 precooked sausages (about 4 ounces/ 115 g), cut into ½-inch cubes

¼ cup (20 g) chopped green onions, green parts only

FOR THE BOWLS:

2 cups (140 g) fresh spinach

½ large Hass avocado, sliced

2 strips bacon, cooked and cut into bite-sized pieces

1 teaspoon finely chopped fresh parsley

STORE IT: *Keep the hash and ingredients for the bowls in separate airtight containers in the fridge for up to 3 days.*

REHEAT IT: *Microwave the hash, covered, until the desired temperature is reached or reheat in a frying pan, covered, on medium.*

MAKE IT LOW-FODMAP: *Use only one-quarter of an avocado and add a handful of raw macadamia nuts or hulled hemp seeds.*

1. Steam the rutabaga for 8 to 10 minutes, until fork-tender.

2. Melt the lard in a medium-sized frying pan over medium heat. Add the steamed rutabaga and cook for 7 to 10 minutes, until the rutabaga begins to brown.

3. Add the sausages and green onions and cook for 3 to 5 minutes, until the sausages begin to brown.

4. Meanwhile, assemble the bowls: Divide the spinach equally between 2 medium-sized serving bowls. When the hash is ready, divide it equally between the bowls, laying it on top of the bed of spinach. Place equal amounts of the sliced avocado, bacon pieces, and parsley on top.

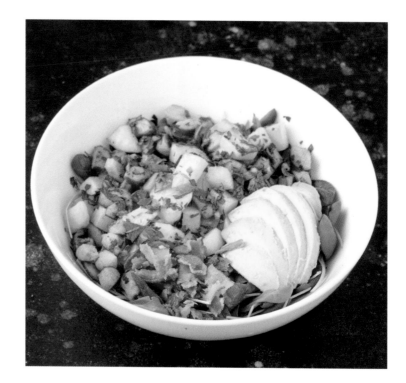

NUTRIENT INFORMATION (PER SERVING):

calories: 560 | calories from fat: 447 | total fat: 49.7g | saturated fat: 16g | cholesterol: 81mg

sodium: 699mg | carbs: 11.6g | dietary fiber: 6g | net carbs: 5.6g | sugars: 3.6g | protein: 16.6g

RATIOS:

fat:	carbs:	protein:
79%	8%	13%

GRAIN-FREE HEMP SEED PORRIDGE

PREP TIME: **2 minutes**   COOK TIME: **3 minutes**   MAKES: **1½ cups (2 servings)**

EGG-FREE • NIGHTSHADE-FREE • VEGAN   OPTIONS: COCONUT-FREE • LOW-FODMAP • NUT-FREE

This grain-free keto porridge is made with only nuts and seeds and then topped with more nuts. Brazil nuts are my choice for the topping: they provide a day's worth of thyroid-supporting selenium in each hearty bowl. With more than 24 grams of fiber in every serving, this porridge is a hearty meal that's gluten-free, dairy-free, vegan, low-carb, and Paleo. The coarser texture of almond meal works best for this recipe, though fine-textured blanched almond flour can also be used. Raw nuts are fine, but for health reasons, it's better to soak and roast them before using them in this recipe (see page 157).

PORRIDGE:

1 cup (240 ml) nondairy milk

½ cup (75 g) hulled hemp seeds

2 tablespoons roughly ground flax seeds

2 tablespoons coconut oil

1 tablespoon chia seeds

1 tablespoon confectioners'-style erythritol or granulated xylitol or 5 drops liquid stevia

¾ teaspoon vanilla extract

¾ teaspoon ground cinnamon

¼ cup (28 g) almond meal or blanched almond flour (see note, above)

TOPPINGS:

4 raw Brazil nuts or small handful of nuts of choice, roughly chopped

2 tablespoons hulled hemp seeds

Fresh berries (optional)

Additional nondairy milk, for serving (optional)

1. Put all the ingredients for the porridge, except the almond meal, in a small saucepan. Stir to combine, then bring to a gentle boil over medium heat.

2. Once bubbling lightly, stir, then cover and cook for 1 to 2 minutes.

3. Remove from the heat, stir in the almond meal, and divide between 2 serving bowls. Divide the toppings evenly between the bowls and eat immediately with a splash of nondairy milk, if desired.

STORE IT: *Keep in an airtight container in the fridge for up to 3 days.*

REHEAT IT: *Place in a small saucepan and reheat on medium-low until warmed through. If the mixture has thickened up in the fridge, add a splash of nondairy milk while reheating.*

PREP AHEAD: *Put all the dry ingredients—hemp seeds, flax seeds, chia seeds, xylitol (if using), ground cinnamon, and almond meal—in a baggie. When ready to eat, empty the contents of the baggie into a saucepan and add the wet ingredients: nondairy milk, coconut oil, stevia (if using), and vanilla.*

PRESSURE-COOK IT: *Place all the ingredients, except the toppings, in a pressure cooker. Secure the lid and cook on low pressure for 1 minute. Allow the pressure to release, then remove the lid.*

MAKE IT COCONUT-FREE: *Replace the coconut oil with cacao butter, macadamia nut oil, or ghee (if tolerated).*

MAKE IT LOW-FODMAP: *Avoid using cashew or pistachio milk. Replace the flax seeds with 1 tablespoon of ground chia seeds. Use stevia rather than erythritol or xylitol. Replace the almond meal with ground hulled sunflower seeds or ground hulled pumpkin seeds.*

MAKE IT NUT-FREE: *Replace the almond meal with ground hulled sunflower seeds or ground hulled pumpkin seeds. Raw seeds are fine to use, but for health reasons, it's better to soak and roast them before grinding (see page 157). Omit the nut topping.*

NUTRIENT INFORMATION (PER SERVING, MADE WITH ERYTHRITOL OR STEVIA):

calories: 660 | calories from fat: 502 | total fat: 55.7g | saturated fat: 17.1g | cholesterol: 0mg

sodium: 95mg | carbs: 15.2g | dietary fiber: 12.5g | net carbs: 2.7g | sugars: 1.1g | protein: 24.5g

RATIOS:

fat:	carbs:	protein:
76%	9%	15%

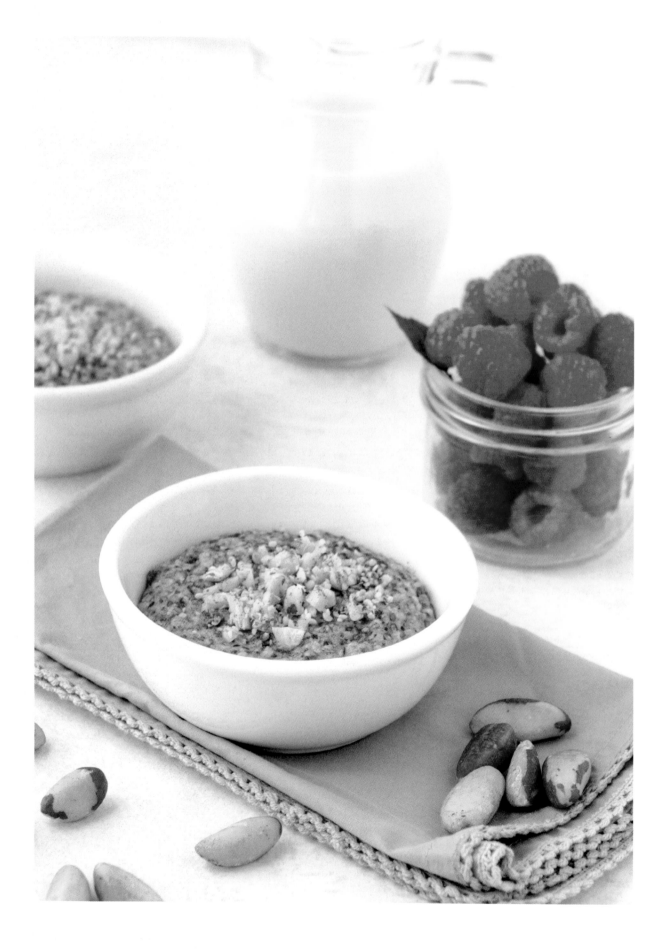

NO-NUTS GRANOLA WITH CLUSTERS

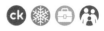

PREP TIME: 20 minutes   COOK TIME: 50 minutes   MAKES: 6 cups (720 g) (12 servings)

LOW-FODMAP • NIGHTSHADE-FREE • NUT-FREE   OPTION: COCONUT-FREE

Granola clusters remind me of my childhood. By the time my siblings and I reached the age of eight, our parents expected us to be able to pack our own lunches, and that's what we did. Often, mine consisted of bologna and ketchup sandwiches, carrot sticks, and four granola bars. Yes, four. Not the chewy granola bars, but the crunchy ones. When I'd get to school, I'd crush the packages between my hands before opening them so that I could snack on the granola clusters. Ah, memories.

While these clusters don't come with a set of bologna sandwiches, I'd like to think that they're tastier than an eight-year-old's smashed store-bought granola bars.

Shredded coconut makes up the bulk of the ingredients in this recipe. If you're sensitive to FODMAPs, you may find that the recommended serving size is too much for you. If so, cut the portion in half, to ¼ cup (25 g), and sprinkle it over the top of another food instead of making it the star of the show. If you don't tolerate coconut at all, follow the coconut-free option below.

½ cup (120 ml) melted coconut oil, plus more for the pan

½ cup (80 g) collagen peptides

1 large egg

3 tablespoons ground cinnamon

2 teaspoons vanilla extract

¼ teaspoon liquid stevia

¼ teaspoon finely ground gray sea salt

2 cups (200 g) shredded unsweetened coconut

1 cup (150 g) sesame seeds

1 cup (150 g) hulled hemp seeds

¼ cup (38 g) chia seeds

SERVING SUGGESTIONS:

Full-fat coconut milk

Fresh berries or stevia-sweetened chocolate chips

STORE IT: *Keep in an airtight container on the counter for up to a week or in the freezer for up to 2 months. Remove from the freezer and use immediately.*

MAKE IT COCONUT-FREE: *Replace the shredded coconut with additional hemp and/or sesame seeds and the coconut oil with cacao butter, macadamia nut oil, or ghee (if tolerated).*

1. Preheat the oven to 300°F (150°C) and grease a 13 by 9-inch (33 by 23-cm) baking pan with a dab of coconut oil.

2. Place the melted coconut oil, collagen, egg, cinnamon, vanilla, stevia, and salt in a medium-sized bowl and whisk until combined. The consistency will be a bit odd, but don't worry, keep going!

3. In a separate large bowl, combine the shredded coconut, sesame seeds, hemp seeds, and chia seeds. Pour the liquid mixture into the bowl with the seed mixture and stir with a spatula until all the seeds are coated.

4. Transfer the mixture to the prepared pan and press it down firmly with your hands. Really pressing it in there is what creates those yummy clusters.

5. Bake for 30 minutes, or until the top and corners begin to turn golden.

6. Break the granola into large pieces with a metal spatula, keeping as many clusters intact as possible. Flip the pieces over and return the pan to the oven for another 15 to 20 minutes, until the pieces are golden.

7. Allow the clusters to cool in the pan for 1 hour before using.

8. When ready to serve, place ½ cup (60 g) of granola in a bowl and pour coconut milk over the top. Fresh berries or chocolate chips are a nice touch. Enjoy!

NUTRIENT INFORMATION (PER ½-CUP/60-G SERVING):

calories: 384 | calories from fat: 288 | total fat: 32g | saturated fat: 19g | cholesterol: 16mg

sodium: 104mg | carbs: 9.7g | dietary fiber: 6.3g | net carbs: 3.4g | sugars: 1.4g | protein: 14.4g

RATIOS:

fat:	carbs:	protein:
75%	10%	15%

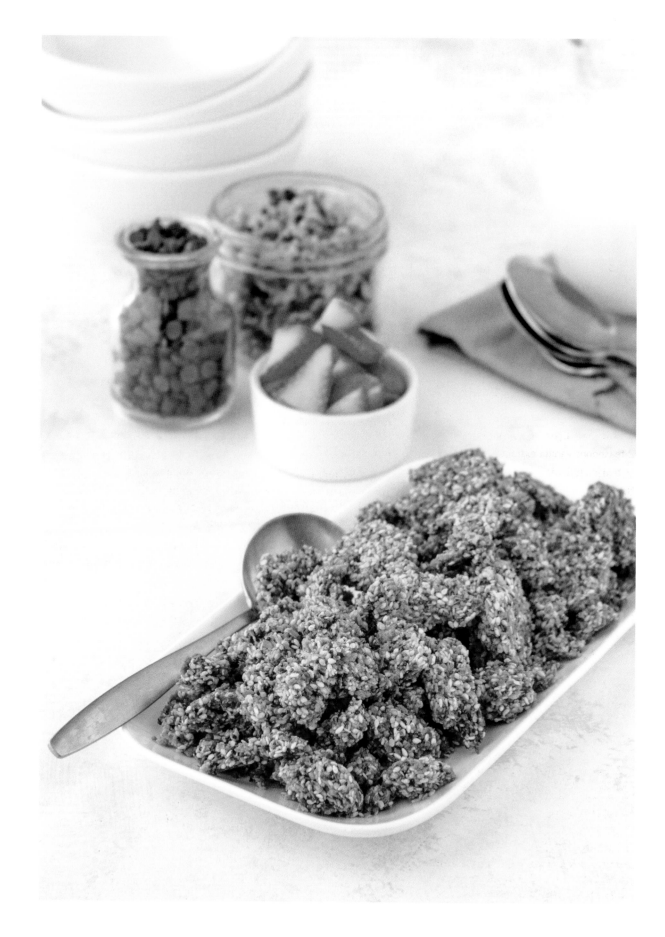

CHICKEN CRISPS

   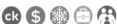

PREP TIME: **2 minutes**   COOK TIME: **20 minutes**   MAKES: **12 crisps (12 servings)**

COCONUT-FREE • EGG-FREE   OPTIONS: LOW-FODMAP • NIGHTSHADE-FREE

When I buy chicken thighs, I remove and reserve the skins for this recipe, then bake the skinless thighs, eat the meat, and use the bones for bone broth. All the pieces get used and enjoyed! In fact, a lot of fat will collect in the baking sheet while the skins are baking. After completing this recipe, you could transfer the fat to a frying pan and use it to make your next meal.

I prefer chicken thigh skins over chicken breast skins for this recipe because of their size. Enjoy these babies as a snack, plain or with a dip, like a simple mayonnaise (page 220).

12 chicken thigh skins (about 9 ounces/ 250 g)

1 tablespoon Seasoning Salt (page 235)

1. Preheat the oven to 325°F (163°C). Line a rimmed baking sheet with parchment paper, then cut a second piece of parchment to the same size and set it aside, along with a slightly smaller second baking sheet. (You want the second baking sheet slightly smaller than the first one so that it can be nestled inside it.)

2. Place the chicken skins in a large bowl and sprinkle with the Seasoning Salt. Toss with your hands until the skins are evenly coated.

3. Spread the skins evenly on the larger baking sheet, placing them as close together as you can.

4. Lay the second piece of parchment over the skins and set the smaller baking sheet on top. This will help keep the skins flat during baking.

5. Bake the skins for 15 to 20 minutes, flipping them over halfway through. Once crisp, remove from the oven and allow to cool for 5 minutes before enjoying.

STORE IT: *Wrap in parchment paper and keep in an airtight container in the fridge for up to 5 days or in the freezer for up to 1 month. Remove from the freezer and enjoy immediately.*

PREP AHEAD: *Store reserved chicken skins in the freezer for up to 3 months; defrost in the fridge before using them to make crisps.*

SERVE IT WITH: *These crisps taste great with Bacon Spinach Dip (page 255) or mayonnaise.*

MAKE IT LOW-FODMAP: *Replace the Seasoning Salt with one of the low-FODMAP spice mixtures on pages 232 to 235. If using a spice mix that doesn't contain salt, add ¼ teaspoon of salt to it.*

MAKE IT NIGHTSHADE-FREE: *Replace the Seasoning Salt with one of the nightshade-free spice mixtures on pages 232 to 235. If using a spice mix that doesn't contain salt, add ¼ teaspoon of salt to it.*

NUTRIENT INFORMATION (PER CRISP):

calories: 93 | calories from fat: 76 | total fat: 8.5g | saturated fat: 2.4g | cholesterol: 17mg

sodium: 595mg | carbs: 0g | dietary fiber: 0g | net carbs: 0g | sugars: 0g | protein: 4.2g

RATIOS:

fat:	carbs:	protein:
82%	0%	18%

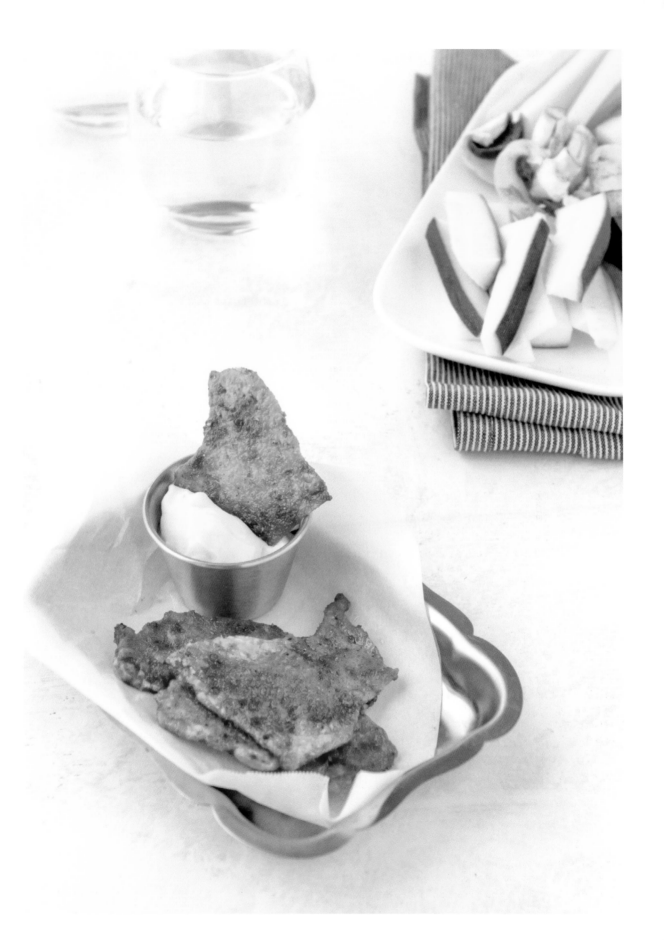

ITALIAN ZUCCHINI ROUNDS

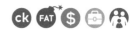

PREP TIME: **10 minutes**   COOK TIME: **80 minutes**   MAKES: **about 70 rounds (10 servings)**

COCONUT-FREE • EGG-FREE • LOW-FODMAP • NIGHTSHADE-FREE • NUT-FREE • VEGAN

This is my favorite way to enjoy zucchini. And the eggplant variation is even better because it's fattier! These rounds are a great way to add fat to a salad or burger. Have patience with the low-and-slow baking method: it's worth it! I'm always up for shortcuts, but in this case, the lower oven temperature works best. I tested these at a higher temperature to cut down the baking time, and the flavor wasn't as bold.

1 large zucchini (about 1⅓ pounds/ 600 g), sliced into extremely thin rounds

½ cup (120 ml) extra-virgin olive oil

2 tablespoons Italian Seasoning (page 234)

¼ teaspoon finely ground gray sea salt

1. Preheat the oven to 250°F (120°C) and line 2 baking sheets with parchment paper or silicone baking mats.

2. Place all the ingredients in a large bowl and toss with your hands until every round is coated in the seasoning mixture. Transfer the rounds to the baking sheets, placing them as close together as possible.

3. Bake the rounds for 80 minutes, flipping them over halfway through, until lightly browned, completely dry in the center, and still flexible enough to bend but not break. Some of the chips may be ready at the 60-minute mark, depending on how thin the slices are. Remove the chips that are done to a cooling rack.

4. If some of the chips still aren't done after 80 minutes, transfer them to a bare rimmed baking sheet and return to the oven. Lower the oven temperature to 170°F (77°C) and dry the rounds for 30 to 45 minutes, until dried through but still bendy.

STORE IT: *Keep in an airtight container in the fridge for up to 3 days.*

VARIATION: SPICED EGGPLANT CHIPS. *Use a large eggplant (about 19 ounces/510 g) in place of the zucchini. Slice the eggplant into thin rounds and place them, along with ¾ cup (180 ml) of olive oil and 1 tablespoon of Seasoning Salt (page 235), in a bowl and toss to coat. Bake the coated rounds for 70 minutes, flipping them over halfway through and beginning to remove the browned chips at about the 50-minute mark.* Makes about 30 chips.

NUTRIENT INFORMATION (PER 10 ZUCCHINI ROUNDS):

calories: 147 | calories from fat: 131 | total fat: 14.6g | saturated fat: 2.1g | cholesterol: 0mg

sodium: 750mg | carbs: 2.9g | dietary fiber: 0.9g | net carbs: 2g | sugars: 1.5g | protein: 1g

RATIOS:

fat:	carbs:	protein:
89%	8%	3%

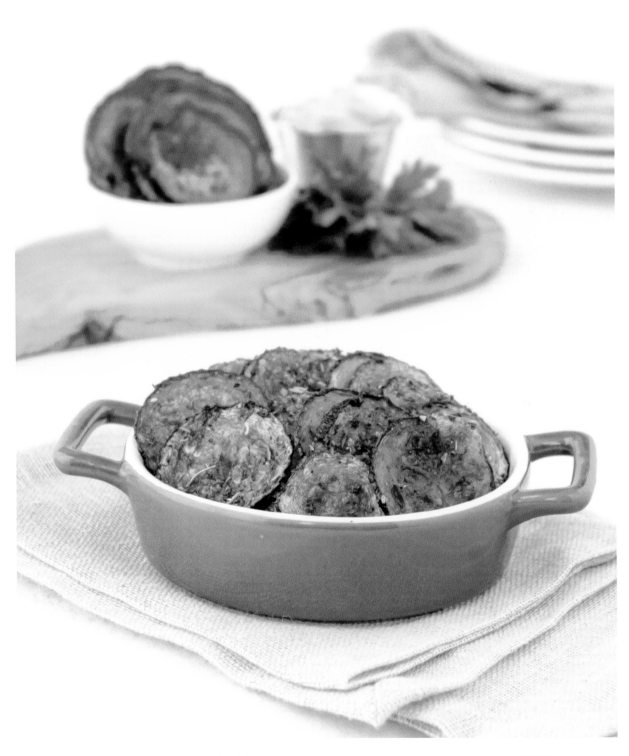

NUTRIENT INFORMATION (PER 3 EGGPLANT ROUNDS):

calories: 143 | calories from fat: 137 | total fat: 15.2g | saturated fat: 2.2g | cholesterol: 0mg

sodium: 745mg | carbs: 3.1g | dietary fiber: 1.9g | net carbs: 1.2g | sugars: 1.6g | protein: 0.5g

RATIOS:

fat:	carbs:	protein:
91%	8%	1%

ZESTY NACHO CABBAGE CHIPS

PREP TIME: **30 minutes**   COOK TIME: **4 hours**   SERVES: **8**

COCONUT-FREE · EGG-FREE · NUT-FREE · VEGAN   OPTIONS: **LOW-FODMAP · NIGHTSHADE-FREE**

I really enjoy these chips. Kevin, my husband, says that they're less like "chips" and more like "spicy leaves." But if I had called this recipe "Nacho Spicy Leaves," every man, woman, and child would avoid making it, and all the time I spent making this recipe would have been wasted. I say, if they're great with guacamole, awesome with salsa, and pretty darn delicious with a bowl of ranch dressing (page 226), then they're chips in my book. And hey, this *is* my book! When preparing the cabbage leaves for this recipe, you should have about 64 chips when all is said and done.

2 medium heads green cabbage

SAUCE:

¼ cup (60 ml) refined avocado oil or extra-virgin olive oil

½ cup (75 g) raw hulled sunflower seeds, soaked for 8 hours, then drained and rinsed

½ white onion, roughly chopped

2 small carrots (about 2 ounces/55 g), roughly chopped

2 tablespoons tahini

2 tablespoons apple cider vinegar

3 small cloves garlic

2 teaspoons fresh lemon juice

2 teaspoons chipotle powder

3 drops liquid stevia

STORE IT: *Keep in an airtight container on the counter for up to 5 days.*

SERVE IT WITH: *These chips taste great with Mind-Blowing Burgers (page 308).*

MAKE IT LOW-FODMAP: *Replace the white onion with ½ cup (40 g) of sliced green onions. Omit the garlic. Omit the chipotle powder or replace it with your favorite seasoning, or one from pages 232 to 235. If using a spice mix that doesn't contain salt, you'll need to add salt to taste.*

MAKE IT NIGHTSHADE-FREE: *Omit the chipotle powder or replace it with your favorite seasoning, or one from pages 232 to 235. If using a spice mix that doesn't contain salt, you'll need to add salt to taste.*

1. Preheat the oven to 170°F (77°C) and line 3 rimmed baking sheets with parchment paper or silicone baking mats.

2. Place one of the cabbages on a cutting board and cut it in half crosswise. Lay one half flat side down and cut it into quarters. Begin peeling off the leaves, being careful not to rip them. When it gets too difficult to access flatter, easy-to-remove leaves, continue with the next quarter. Place the usable leaves in a large bowl and the excess that you can't work with in a sealable container for use in another recipe. Repeat this process with the other half, then with the second head of cabbage. When done, you should have 1⅓ pounds (600 g) of leaves.

3. Prepare the sauce: Place the ingredients for the sauce in a high-powered blender or food processor and blend or pulse on high for 1 minute, or until smooth.

4. Pour the sauce over the cabbage leaves and massage it into the leaves with your hands, coating each leaf in sauce.

5. Transfer the coated leaves to the prepared baking sheets, laying them in a single layer, close together.

6. Place the baking sheets in the oven, layering them on top of one another if needed, crisscrossing them so the bottom of one sheet isn't touching the tops of the cabbage chips in the tray below it, but the edge of the bottom tray is holding up the second tray over the top of it.

7. Bake for 2 hours before checking on the chips. If any are crisp, transfer them to a cooling rack, then continue to cook for an additional 2 hours, checking for completed chips every 30 minutes.

8. Allow the chips to cool for 5 to 10 minutes before enjoying.

NUTRIENT INFORMATION (PER 8 CHIPS):
calories: 120 | calories from fat: 70 | total fat: 7.8g | saturated fat: 0.9g | cholesterol: 0mg
sodium: 26mg | carbs: 8.6g | dietary fiber: 3.5g | net carbs: 5.1g | sugars: 3.6g | protein: 3.9g

RATIOS:
fat: carbs: protein:
59%   **28%**   **13%**

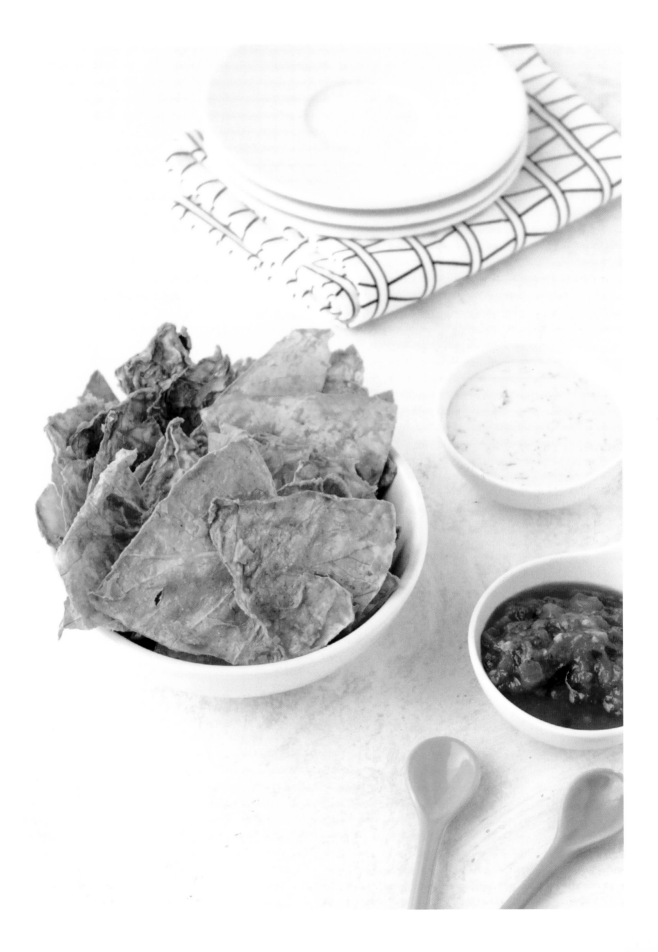

BACON CRACKERS

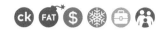

PREP TIME: **10 minutes**   COOK TIME: **20 minutes**   MAKES: **60 crackers (6 servings)**

COCONUT-FREE • EGG-FREE • LOW-FODMAP • NIGHTSHADE-FREE • NUT-FREE

These bacon crackers are the perfect keto accompaniment to a variety of high-fat sauces, many of which you'll find in the Saucy chapter of this book. They're great for lunches, picnics, or traveling long distances—I took them on a plane from Calgary to Germany with no problems.

Accept that strips of bacon aren't cut perfectly, so your crackers won't be, either. If you can get your paws on a pack of hearty, thick-cut bacon, it makes awesome crackers. If you're using thicker-cut bacon, the baking time will be closer to the 20-minute mark. You'll have a lot of bacon grease left over after making these crackers. Save it for making Bacon Fudge (page 394)!

13 strips bacon (about 13 ounces/370 g), preferably thick-cut

> **STORE IT:** *Keep in an airtight container in the fridge for up to 5 days or in the freezer for up to 1 month. Remove from the freezer and use immediately.*

> **SERVE IT WITH:** *These crackers taste great with MCT Guacamole (page 260) or No-Beans Hummus (page 256).*

1. Preheat the oven to 400°F (205°C) and line a rimmed baking sheet with parchment paper or a silicone baking mat.

2. Cut the strips of bacon into roughly 2-inch (5-cm) squares, about 6 per strip. Place the squares on the prepared baking sheet, leaving a small gap between crackers.

3. Bake the crackers until crisp, about 15 minutes if using regular bacon or 20 minutes if using thick-cut bacon.

4. Allow the crackers to cool on the baking sheet for 10 minutes. Transfer to a serving plate and enjoy.

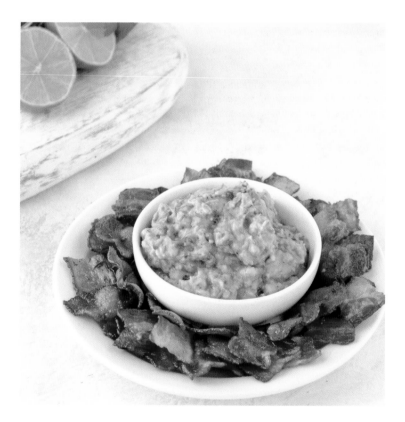

NUTRIENT INFORMATION (PER 10 CRACKERS):

calories: 258 | calories from fat: 223 | total fat: 24.8g | saturated fat: 8.3g | cholesterol: 43mg

sodium: 414mg | carbs: 0.8g | dietary fiber: 0g | net carbs: 0.8g | sugars: 0g | protein: 7.9g

RATIOS:

fat:	carbs:	protein:
87%	1%	12%

BACON SPINACH DIP

PREP TIME: **10 minutes, plus 4 hours to soak cashews**   COOK TIME: **8 minutes**   MAKES: **2 cups (475 ml) (16 servings)**

EGG-FREE • NIGHTSHADE-FREE   OPTIONS: **COCONUT-FREE • VEGAN**

Creamy, spreadable, and downright delicious! I use this dip on just about everything. Don't let the "dip" title box you in; you could use this as a topping on a bowl of cauliflower rice (page 364), dollop it onto a plate of greens, or use it as a spread on your next steak! It's really good spread over the shoulder chops on page 332 if you don't want to make the thyme gravy.

6 strips bacon (about 6 ounces/170 g)

1 cup (160 g) raw cashews, soaked for 4 hours, then drained and rinsed

⅔ cup (160 ml) full-fat coconut milk

¼ cup (17 g) nutritional yeast

3 tablespoons apple cider vinegar

1 teaspoon finely ground gray sea salt

1 teaspoon onion powder

½ teaspoon garlic powder

½ teaspoon ground mustard

¼ teaspoon ground black pepper

1 cup (70 g) spinach, chopped

1. Place the bacon in a large frying pan over medium heat and cook until crisp. Remove from the pan and, when cool enough to handle, crumble and set aside. Transfer the bacon grease in the frying pan to a food processor or blender. (Don't clean the pan; you will use it again shortly.)

2. To the food processor or blender, add the soaked cashews, coconut milk, nutritional yeast, vinegar, salt, and spices. Blend until smooth.

3. Meanwhile, sauté the spinach in the frying pan over medium-low heat just until wilted, about 30 seconds.

4. Add the crumbled bacon and sautéed spinach to the food processor or blender. Pulse just until mixed.

5. Transfer to a serving bowl and dig in!

STORE IT: *Keep in an airtight container in the fridge for up to 3 days.*

PREP AHEAD: *Prepare the bacon bits up to a month ahead of time and store them in the freezer in an airtight container. When ready to use, simply add the bacon bits as directed in Step 4, and use 3 tablespoons plus 1 teaspoon of bacon grease in Step 1.*

SERVE IT WITH: *To make this a complete meal, serve it alongside steamed vegetables. This dip tastes great paired with Buffalo Chicken Tots (page 264).*

MAKE IT COCONUT-FREE: *Replace the coconut milk with ½ cup (120 ml) of your favorite nondairy milk.*

MAKE IT VEGAN: *Omit the bacon, add 3 tablespoons of refined avocado oil or olive oil, and replace the gray sea salt with finely ground smoked sea salt.*

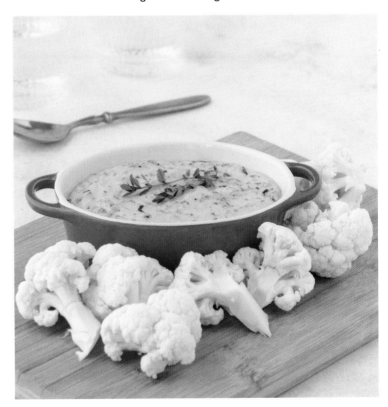

NUTRIENT INFORMATION (PER 2-TABLESPOON SERVING):

calories: 132 | calories from fat: 100 | total fat: 11.1g | saturated fat: 4.2g | cholesterol: 7mg

sodium: 84mg | carbs: 4.5g | dietary fiber: 0.6g | net carbs: 3.9g | sugars: 0.8g | protein: 3.6g

RATIOS:

fat:	carbs:	protein:
75%	**13%**	**12%**

NO-BEANS HUMMUS

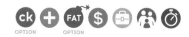

PREP TIME: **5 minutes**   MAKES: **2 cups (660 g) (8 servings)**

COCONUT-FREE • EGG-FREE • NUT-FREE • VEGAN   OPTIONS: **LOW-FODMAP • NIGHTSHADE-FREE**

Hummus lovers, unite! Here are three of my favorite ways to make keto-friendly hummus when I'm craving the good stuff. I used to tolerate beans so well, but in recent years they've started to aggravate my stomach. Perhaps I met my life's quota of beans when I was vegan for as long as I was. In any case, you won't be swooning over bowls of conventional hummus when you have this recipe in your back pocket. It makes a great pack-along snack for your lunch kit paired with celery sticks and extra olive oil, or you can make a batch and share with your friends the next time you're invited to a potluck.

My favorite way to scoop the hummus is with NUCO coconut wraps cut into squares, as pictured. So good!

1 medium head cauliflower, cored and separated into florets (about 15½ ounces/445 g florets)

¼ cup (65 g) tahini

6 tablespoons (90 ml) extra-virgin olive oil, divided

¼ cup (60 ml) fresh lemon juice

2 small cloves garlic, minced

¾ teaspoon finely ground gray sea salt

½ teaspoon ground cumin

Pinch of paprika, for garnish

Pinch of dried parsley, for garnish

1. Place the cauliflower florets, tahini, 4 tablespoons (60 ml) of the olive oil, lemon juice, garlic, salt, and cumin in a food processor or blender. Pulse until somewhat smooth, or until it reaches the desired hummus-like consistency.

2. Transfer the mixture to a serving bowl. Drizzle with the remaining olive oil and sprinkle with the paprika and parsley.

STORE IT: *Keep in an airtight container in the fridge for up to 4 days.*

SERVE IT WITH: *To make this a complete meal, spread it over a collard leaf, fill with your favorite sandwich fillings, and enjoy. This hummus tastes great with Chicken Crisps (page 248).*

VARIATION: ROASTED GARLIC NO-BEANS HUMMUS. *Replace the minced garlic with 6 cloves of roasted garlic.*

VARIATION: MACADAMIA NUT HUMMUS. *Make a low-FODMAP hummus by soaking 1 cup (160 g) of raw macadamia nuts in water for 24 hours, then drain and rinse. Place in a food processor along with 3 tablespoons of Garlic-Infused Oil (page 230), 3 tablespoons of lemon juice, 3 tablespoons of roasted sesame seeds, ¼ teaspoon of ground cumin, and ¼ teaspoon of finely ground gray sea salt. Pulse until somewhat smooth, or until the desired hummus-like consistency is reached. Transfer the hummus to a serving bowl, drizzle with 2 tablespoons of extra-virgin olive oil, and sprinkle with a pinch each of paprika and dried parsley flakes. Makes 1¼ cups (320 g), or 5 servings.*

MAKE IT HIT CLASSIC KETO RATIOS OR MAKE IT A FAT BOMB: *Prepare the macadamia nut variation.*

MAKE IT LOW-FODMAP: *Make the macadamia nut variation.*

MAKE IT NIGHTSHADE-FREE: *Omit the paprika.*

MAKE IT A CARB-UP: *Replace half of the olive oil with water. Serve alongside the carb of your choice (find ideas on page 117, or visit healthfulpursuit.com/carbup to download the complimentary PDF "Carb-Up Recipes"). It's fabulous with roasted sweet potatoes, green plantain chips, or raw jicama slices.*

NUTRIENT INFORMATION (PER ¼-CUP/82-G SERVING, FOR CAULIFLOWER-BASED VERSIONS):

calories: 162 | calories from fat: 132 | total fat: 14.7g | saturated fat: 2.1g | cholesterol: 0mg

sodium: 203mg | carbs: 5g | dietary fiber: 2.1g | net carbs: 2.9g | sugars: 1.5g | protein: 2.5g

RATIOS:

fat:	carbs:	protein:
82%	**12%**	**6%**

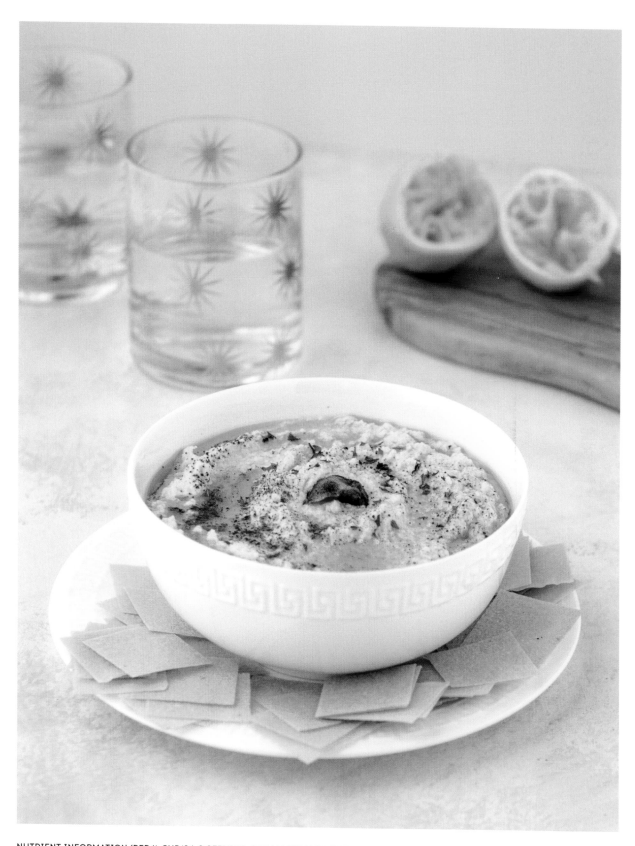

NUTRIENT INFORMATION (PER ¼-CUP/64-G SERVING, FOR MACADAMIA NUT–BASED HUMMUS):
calories: 335 | calories from fat: 319 | total fat: 35.4g | saturated fat: 5.5g | cholesterol: 0mg
sodium: 98mg | carbs: 5.9g | dietary fiber: 3.5g | net carbs: 2.4g | sugars: 1.7g | protein: 3.6g

RATIOS:
fat: carbs: protein:
89% 7%   4%

PIZZA PÂTÉ

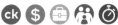

PREP TIME: 10 minutes, plus 12 hour to soak almonds   MAKES: 2½ cups (575 g) (20 servings)

EGG-FREE   OPTIONS: COCONUT-FREE • NUT-FREE

If liver isn't your jam but you love the idea of a fat-rich, protein-based spread for crackers, raw veggies, or the side of your dinner plate, look no further than this pizza pâté! It has all the flavors of pizza without the crust. When purchasing tomato sauce for this recipe, look for a sugar-free variety (usually available in cans as opposed to jars). Because of the coconut oil, the pâté will be quite hard straight from the fridge. Set it out on the counter for 10 to 15 minutes before serving.

1 cup (190 g) chopped pepperoni

¾ cup (120 g) raw almonds, soaked for 12 hours, then drained and rinsed

½ cup (120 ml) melted coconut oil

⅓ cup (80 ml) tomato sauce (see above)

¼ cup (17 g) nutritional yeast

2 teaspoons apple cider vinegar

2 teaspoons onion powder

1 teaspoon garlic powder

¼ teaspoon finely ground gray sea salt

1 tablespoon finely chopped fresh basil

1. Place all the ingredients except the basil in a high-powered blender or food processor. Blend or pulse until smooth, about 1 minute.

2. Add the basil and pulse until just mixed in.

STORE IT: *Keep in an airtight container in the fridge for up to 5 days.*

PREP AHEAD: *Soak, drain, and rinse the almonds and freeze for up to 1 month before using in this recipe.*

SERVE IT WITH: *To make this a complete meal, serve it with your favorite low-carb crackers or spread on pieces of fresh fennel bulb. It tastes great spread over a piece of Egg-Free Flaxseed Focaccia (page 373).*

MAKE IT COCONUT-FREE: *Replace the coconut oil with unrefined canola oil, extra-virgin olive oil, or refined avocado oil.*

MAKE IT NUT-FREE: *Replace the almonds with raw, hulled sunflower seeds soaked for at least 8 hours, then drained and rinsed.*

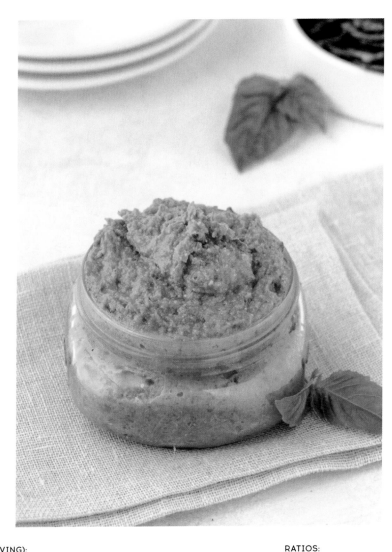

NUTRIENT INFORMATION (PER 2-TABLESPOON SERVING):
calories: 144 | calories from fat: 115 | total fat: 12.8g | saturated fat: 6.3g | cholesterol: 10mg
sodium: 209mg | carbs: 2.8g | dietary fiber: 1.4g | net carbs: 1.4g | sugars: 0.5g | protein: 4.5g

RATIOS:
fat:	carbs:	protein:
80%	8%	12%

KALE PÂTÉ

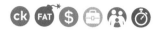

PREP TIME: **10 minutes**   MAKES: **2 cups (450 g) (8 servings)**

COCONUT-FREE · EGG-FREE · LOW-FODMAP · NIGHTSHADE-FREE · NUT-FREE · VEGAN

A couple of summers ago, I spent nearly two weeks visiting one of my close girlfriends, who is as in love with creating tasty, easy recipes as I am. We picked oodles of kale from her garden and created this dish. I can't take credit for it in the slightest; it was all her. Thanks for the recipe, Sprout. Love you bunches!

2 tablespoons refined avocado oil, for the pan

4 cups (190 g) chopped kale

½ cup (75 g) sesame seeds

½ cup (120 ml) refined avocado oil or extra-virgin olive oil

8 green onions, green parts only, roughly chopped

3 tablespoons apple cider vinegar

1¼ teaspoons finely ground gray sea salt

STORE IT: *Keep in an airtight container in the fridge for up to 1 week.*

SERVE IT WITH: *To make this a complete meal, slather it over cooked vegetables, toss it into a batch of Zoodles or Doodles (page 376), or serve it over roasted brisket. It tastes great with Italian Zucchini Rounds (page 250).*

1. Place 2 tablespoons of avocado oil and the chopped kale in a large frying pan over medium heat. Cover and cook until the kale is slightly crispy, stirring occasionally, 3 to 6 minutes.

2. Meanwhile, place the remaining ingredients in a blender or food processor. When the kale is done, add it to the blender or food processor. Blend on high speed until smooth, about 1 minute.

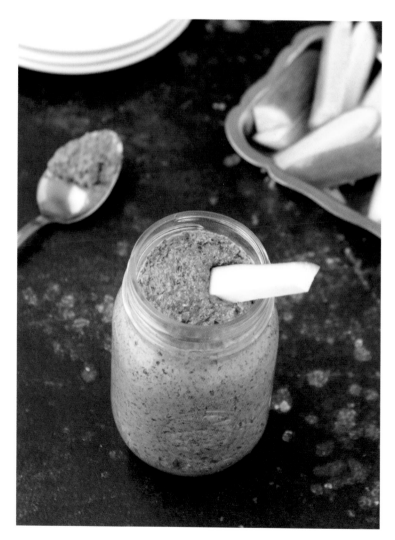

NUTRIENT INFORMATION (PER ¼-CUP/56-G SERVING):

calories: 228 | calories from fat: 195 | total fat: 21.7g | saturated fat: 2.9g | cholesterol: 0mg

sodium: 306mg | carbs: 5.5g | dietary fiber: 1.7g | net carbs: 3.8g | sugars: 0g | protein: 2.6g

RATIOS:

fat:	carbs:	protein:
86%	10%	4%

MCT GUACAMOLE

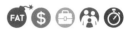

EGG-FREE • NIGHTSHADE-FREE • NUT-FREE • VEGAN   OPTION: COCONUT-FREE

I created this recipe years ago, late at night, while we were hosting a game night. We'd made our way through all the snacks we'd prepared, but many of us were still snacky and, believe it or not, we didn't have much food left in the house. But we did have avocados…and pork rinds. With a little ingenuity, I created a simple guacamole that didn't use the classic onion, tomato, and pepper mixture. Since that day, I've never made any other guac. This one does the trick. The original version didn't have lime zest and juice or fresh chives and cilantro; I've added them to the recipe over time. If you don't have those ingredients on hand, don't worry! It'll still turn out wonderful.

1 large Hass avocado, peeled and pitted (about 6 ounces/170 g of flesh) (optional: reserve the pit for leftovers)

¼ cup plus 2 tablespoons (90 ml) MCT oil

1 tablespoon plus 1 teaspoon apple cider vinegar

Grated zest of 1 lime

Juice of 1 lime

1 tablespoon plus 1 teaspoon dried oregano leaves

½ teaspoon finely ground gray sea salt

½ teaspoon ground black pepper

2 tablespoons fresh cilantro leaves, finely chopped

2 teaspoons sliced fresh chives

1. Place the avocado flesh, oil, vinegar, lime zest, lime juice, dried oregano, salt, and pepper in a large bowl. Mash with a potato masher or the back of a fork to the desired consistency.

2. Stir in the cilantro and chives and you're ready to party!

STORE IT: *Transfer the guacamole to an airtight container and place the reserved pit in the guacamole to keep it fresh. Store in the fridge for up to 3 days.*

SERVE IT WITH: *To make this a complete meal, serve it with a bowl of Chicken Crisps (page 248) or your favorite pork rinds, spread it on roasted chicken, or add a dollop to a bowl of cooked ground beef. As a snack, this tastes great paired with Zesty Nacho Cabbage Chips (page 252).*

MAKE IT COCONUT-FREE: *Replace the MCT oil with refined avocado oil.*

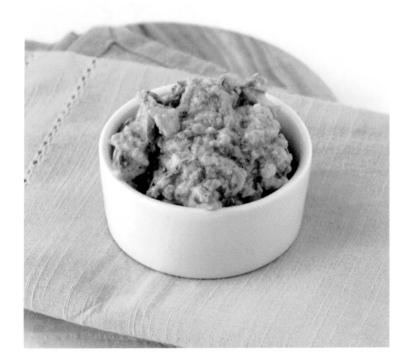

NUTRIENT INFORMATION (PER 3-TABLESPOON SERVING):
calories: 213 | calories from fat: 181 | total fat: 20.2g | saturated fat: 13.6g | cholesterol: 0mg
sodium: 133mg | carbs: 5.9g | dietary fiber: 5.3g | net carbs: 0.6g | sugars: 0g | protein: 1.8g

RATIOS:
fat: carbs: protein:
86%   11%   3%

BAHĀRĀT BALLS

PREP TIME: **50 minutes**   MAKES: **14 balls (14 servings)**

EGG-FREE • LOW-FODMAP • NUT-FREE • VEGAN   OPTIONS: **COCONUT-FREE • NIGHTSHADE-FREE**

When I surveyed the Healthful Pursuit community on what recipes they wanted to see in this book, "savory fat bombs" won, hands down. I love fat bombs, but I'm more of a sweet fat bomb person, so I was a bit apprehensive when I sat down to plan the savory fat bombs that you'll find in *The Keto Diet*. But wow, I must say…these are pretty darn good! If you're not a Bahārāt seasoning person, no worries; you can use any of the other seasoning mixes in this book (pages 232 to 235) or your favorite store-bought variety.

1½ cups (223 g) hulled hemp seeds, divided

1⅓ cups (200 g) roasted sesame seeds

½ cup (120 ml) melted coconut oil

1 tablespoon Bahārāt Seasoning (page 233)

1 tablespoon fresh lemon juice

1 small clove garlic, coarsely chopped if not using a high-powered blender

½ teaspoon finely ground gray sea salt

STORE IT: *Keep in an airtight container in the fridge for up to 1 week or in the freezer for up to 1 month.*

THAW IT: *Allow to thaw on the counter for 10 to 15 minutes.*

PREP AHEAD: *Roast the sesame seeds using the instructions on page 157 and store in the freezer for quick additions to recipes.*

SERVE IT WITH: *To make this a complete meal, crumble and serve it over your favorite salad.*

MAKE IT COCONUT-FREE: *Use ghee instead of coconut oil, if tolerated.*

MAKE IT NIGHTSHADE-FREE: *Replace the Bahārāt seasoning with one of the nightshade-free spice mixtures on pages 232 to 235.*

1. Line a baking sheet with parchment paper or a silicone baking mat.

2. Place ¼ cup (37 g) of the hemp seeds, the roasted sesame seeds, coconut oil, seasoning, lemon juice, garlic, and salt in a blender. Blend on high speed for 30 seconds, or until almost smooth with a bit of chunkiness left.

3. Transfer the mixture to a large bowl. Add the remaining 1¼ cups (185 g) of hemp seeds and stir with a spatula to combine.

4. Scoop up a heaping tablespoon of the mixture, roll it into a ball between your palms, and place on the prepared baking sheet. Repeat with the remaining mixture.

5. Transfer the sheet to the fridge and let the balls set for 1½ hours, or place them in the freezer to set for 25 minutes. Once set, they're ready to enjoy.

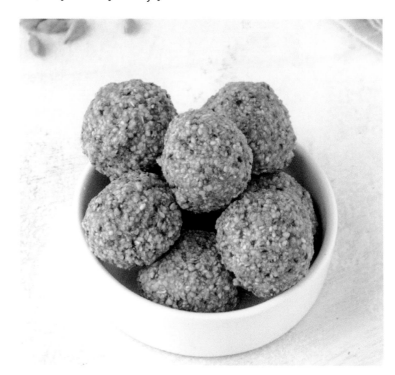

NUTRIENT INFORMATION (PER BALL):

calories: 249 | calories from fat: 197 | total fat: 21.9g | saturated fat: 8.5g | cholesterol: 0mg

sodium: 68mg | carbs: 5g | dietary fiber: 3.3g | net carbs: 1.7g | sugars: 0g | protein: 7.9g

RATIOS:

fat: 79% carbs: 8% protein: 13%

BACON-WRAPPED ASPARAGUS WITH HORSERADISH SAUCE

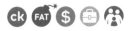

PREP TIME: **20 minutes**   COOK TIME: **15 minutes**   SERVES: **8**

COCONUT-FREE · NIGHTSHADE-FREE · NUT-FREE   OPTION: EGG-FREE

Bacon makes everything better! Especially asparagus. After making a batch of these bacon-wrapped asparagus, I find myself snacking on cold pieces from the fridge when hunger strikes. They make a great snack! This recipe works best with regular bacon as opposed to the thick, hearty stuff; thick-cut bacon will never cook through and the asparagus tips will burn.

10 strips regular (not thick-cut) bacon (about 10 ounces/285 g)

1 bunch asparagus (about 13 ounces/ 370 g), tough ends removed

HORSERADISH SAUCE:

⅓ cup (70 g) mayonnaise, homemade (page 220) or store-bought

1 tablespoon plus 1 teaspoon prepared horseradish

1½ teaspoons Dijon mustard

1 teaspoon fresh lemon juice

FOR GARNISH:

1 tablespoon finely chopped fresh parsley

1. Preheat the oven to 400°F (205°C) and line a rimmed baking sheet with parchment paper or a silicone baking mat.

2. Cut the bacon lengthwise into 2 or 3 strips, depending on the width of the bacon (you want each strip to be about ½ inch/ 1.25 cm wide).

3. Take an asparagus spear in one hand and, beginning at the base, wrap a bacon strip around the spear. When you're approximately 1 inch (2.5 cm) from the tip, place the bacon-wrapped asparagus on the baking sheet and repeat with the remaining spears. You can nestle the wrapped asparagus quite close to one another on the sheet.

4. Bake for 12 to 15 minutes, until the bacon is crisp and the tips of the asparagus are beginning to brown.

5. Meanwhile, place the ingredients for the sauce in a small bowl. Whisk to combine.

6. Allow the asparagus to cool on the pan for 5 minutes before transferring to a serving plate. Serve with the sauce on the side and sprinkle everything with parsley.

STORE IT: *Keep in an airtight container in the fridge for up to 3 days.*

REHEAT IT: *Place on a plate and microwave until the desired temperature is reached. Or place in a covered casserole dish and reheat in a 300°F (150°C) oven for 10 minutes, or until warmed through. Or reheat in a frying pan, covered, on medium.*

SERVE IT WITH: *To make this a complete meal, serve it alongside the salad of your choice. This dish tastes great paired with Creamy Mashed Turnips (page 382) or Marinated Bok Choy Salad (page 295).*

MAKE IT EGG-FREE: *Use egg-free mayonnaise.*

NUTRIENT INFORMATION (PER 2 TO 3 SPEARS WITH ¾ TEASPOON SAUCE):
calories: 224 | calories from fat: 191 | total fat: 21.2g | saturated fat: 5.9g | cholesterol: 28mg
sodium: 307mg | carbs: 2.6g | dietary fiber: 1.1g | net carbs: 1.5g | sugars: 1.1g | protein: 5.7g

RATIOS:		
fat:	carbs:	protein:
85%	5%	10%

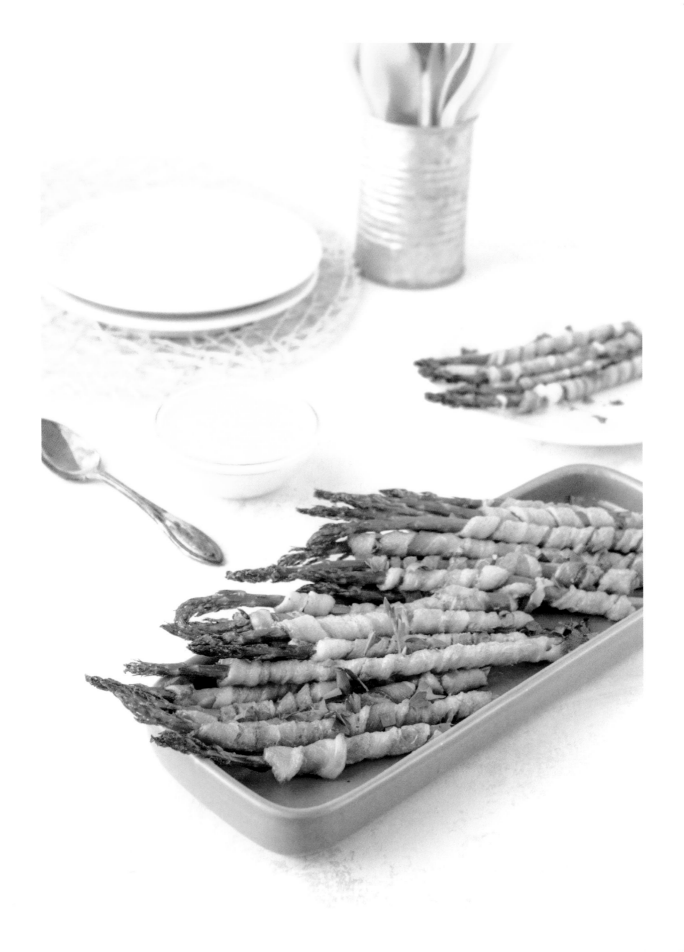

BUFFALO CHICKEN TOTS

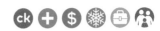

PREP TIME: **15 minutes**   COOK TIME: **30 minutes**   MAKES: **24 to 36 pieces (6 servings)**

NUT-FREE   OPTIONS: **COCONUT-FREE · EGG-FREE**

If you love spice, this is so totally your recipe! You could go with bone-in, skin-on chicken thighs as I do and remove the skin and bones yourself. The benefits of going this route are that you save money, the bones can be used for a batch of chicken bone broth (see page 152), and the skins can be frozen for up to 3 months before being used for a batch of Chicken Crisps (page 248). If you're unsure of how to remove the bones from a chicken thigh, Serious Eats is a good resource.

1 pound (455 g) boneless, skinless chicken thighs

⅓ cup (54 g) Cajun Seasoning (page 232)

½ cup (120 ml) refined avocado oil or melted chicken fat, for the pan

BUFFALO SAUCE:

2 tablespoons Sriracha sauce or hot sauce

1 tablespoon melted butter-infused coconut oil

1 tablespoon fresh lemon juice

½ teaspoon garlic powder

FOR SERVING:

½ cup (120 ml) Ranch Dressing (page 226)

Celery sticks (optional)

1. Preheat the oven to 400°F (205°C) and line a rimmed baking sheet with parchment paper or a silicone baking mat.

2. Cut the chicken thighs into roughly 1-inch (2.5-cm) squares and set aside.

3. Place the Cajun seasoning in a bowl. Add a couple of pieces of chicken and toss to coat lightly, then transfer to a plate. Repeat with the remaining chicken.

4. Pour the avocado oil into a large frying pan and heat on medium-high for 2 minutes, or until it begins to crackle lightly.

5. Transfer the chicken pieces to the frying pan, leaving a small gap between pieces. Once the pan is full, cook for 2 to 3 minutes before flipping the chicken pieces over and cooking for another 2 to 3 minutes. The chicken should be crisp on the outside. Transfer to a clean plate and repeat with the remaining pieces.

6. Meanwhile, place the ingredients for the Buffalo sauce in a medium-sized bowl and whisk to combine. When all the chicken is done, transfer it to the bowl with the sauce and toss to coat.

7. Spread the coated chicken tots on the prepared baking sheet and bake for 20 minutes, or until the sauce on the edges of the chicken begins to blacken.

8. Serve the chicken tots with ranch dressing and celery sticks, if desired.

STORE IT: *Keep in an airtight container in the fridge for up to 3 days or in the freezer for up to 1 month.*

REHEAT IT: *Place on a plate and microwave until the desired temperature is reached. Or place in a covered casserole dish and reheat in a 300°F (150°C) oven for 5 minutes, or until warmed through. Or reheat in a frying pan with a drizzle of refined avocado oil, covered, on medium-low.*

THAW IT: *Allow to thaw completely in the fridge. Once defrosted, use the reheating instructions above, or enjoy cold.*

MAKE IT COCONUT-FREE: *Replace the coconut oil with refined olive oil or ghee (if tolerated) and omit the ranch dressing.*

MAKE IT EGG-FREE: *Make the egg-free ranch dressing variation.*

MAKE IT A CARB-UP: *Replace the ranch dressing with the carb of your choice (find ideas on page 117, or visit healthfulpursuit.com/carbup to download the complimentary PDF "Carb-Up Recipes"). These tots are amazing with raw pineapple, roasted mango, or grilled acorn squash.*

NUTRIENT INFORMATION (PER 4 TO 6 PIECES WITH 1⅓ TABLESPOONS RANCH DRESSING):
calories: 371 | calories from fat: 312 | total fat: 34.6g | saturated fat: 8.2g | cholesterol: 64mg
sodium: 305mg | carbs: 1.6g | dietary fiber: 0g | net carbs: 1.6g | sugars: 0g | protein: 13.2g

RATIOS:
fat:	carbs:	protein:
84%	2%	14%

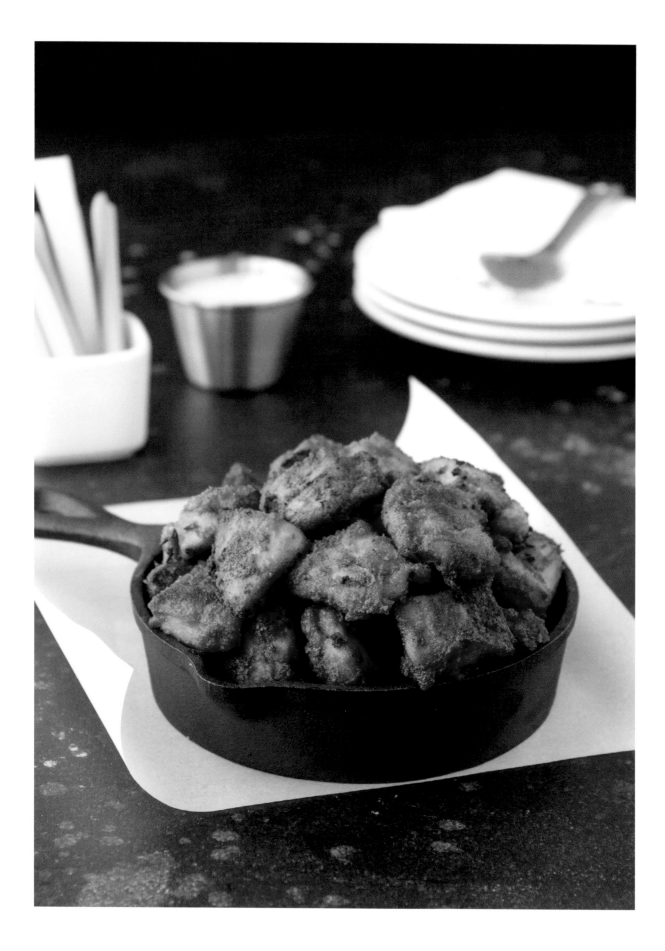

ROASTED CAJUN BROCCOLI

PREP TIME: **15 minutes**   COOK TIME: **27 minutes**   SERVES: **8**

VEGETARIAN   OPTIONS: **COCONUT-FREE** • **LOW-FODMAP** • **NIGHTSHADE-FREE** • **VEGAN**

Technically, any more than ½ cup (36 g) of broccoli is too much FODMAP for those who are sensitive. So if you are sensitive to FODMAPs but want to try this recipe, keep it to 1 floret per serving, as there are almonds in this dish as well.

I kept the florets large, about 8 for the whole recipe, because it's fun. If you're serving this dish to a group as finger food, make about 16 smaller florets and check the broccoli for doneness at around the 18- to 20-minute mark.

EGG WASH:

¼ cup (60 ml) refined avocado oil or melted coconut oil

2 large eggs

DRY COATING:

½ cup (55 g) blanched almond flour

3 tablespoons Cajun Seasoning (page 232)

1 large head broccoli, broken into 8 large florets (about 10½ ounces/300 g florets)

1 batch Cheese Sauce (page 218), for serving

1. Preheat the oven to 375°F (190°C) and line a rimmed baking sheet with parchment paper or a silicone baking mat.

2. Place the avocado oil and eggs in a medium-sized bowl. Whisk to combine.

3. In a separate bowl, combine the almond flour and Cajun seasoning.

4. Dip one floret at a time into the egg mixture and make sure that it's well coated. Pull the floret out of the egg mixture and give it a shake to remove the excess.

5. Take the floret in your other hand and use that hand to coat it in the almond flour mixture. Once thoroughly coated, shake off the excess and place on the prepared baking sheet. Repeat this process, keeping each hand assigned to its own bowl so you don't get a floury mess in the egg bowl or vice versa.

6. Bake the coated florets for 25 to 27 minutes, until the tops are beginning to brown. Allow to cool for 5 minutes before transfering to a serving dish alongside a bowl of cheese sauce.

STORE IT: *Keep in an airtight container in the fridge for up to 3 days.*

REHEAT IT: *Place on a plate and microwave until the desired temperature is reached. Or place in a covered casserole dish and reheat in a 300°F (150°C) oven for 10 minutes, or until warmed through. Or place in a frying pan with 2 to 3 tablespoons of oil and fry on medium-low.*

MAKE IT COCONUT-FREE: *Use avocado oil and make the coconut-free version of the Cheese Sauce.*

MAKE LOW-FODMAP: *Replace the Cajun seasoning with one of the low-FODMAP spice mixtures on pages 232 to 235. If using a spice mix that doesn't contain salt, you'll need to add ¾ teaspoon to the flour coating.*

MAKE IT NIGHTSHADE-FREE: *Replace the Cajun seasoning with one of the nightshade-free spice mixtures on pages 232 to 235. If using a spice mix that doesn't contain salt, you'll need to add ¾ teaspoon to the flour coating.*

MAKE IT VEGAN: *Follow the Make It Vegan instructions in the cheese sauce recipe.*

NUTRIENT INFORMATION (PER 1 LARGE BROCCOLI FLORET WITH 2 TABLESPOONS SAUCE):
calories: 216 | calories from fat: 161 | total fat: 17.9g | saturated fat: 7.4g | cholesterol: 47mg
sodium: 186mg | carbs: 6.5g | dietary fiber: 2.9g | net carbs: 3.6g | sugars: 1.2g | protein: 7.2g

RATIOS:

fat:	carbs:	protein:
75%	12%	13%

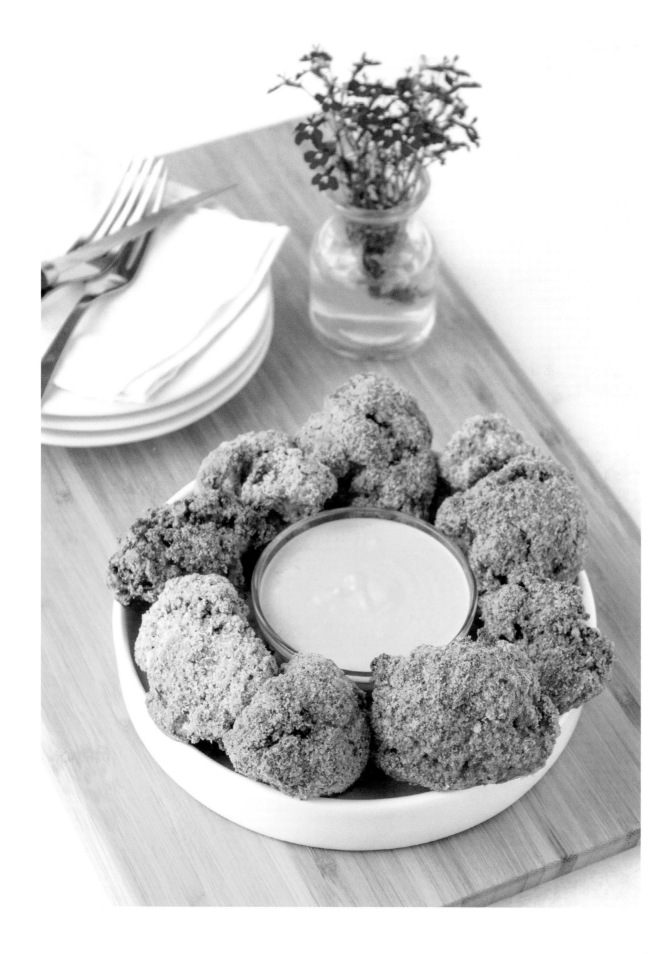

NORI ROLLS WITH ALMOND DIPPING SAUCE

PREP TIME: **30 minutes**   COOK TIME: **5 minutes**   SERVES: **8**

EGG-FREE · VEGETARIAN   OPTIONS: **COCONUT-FREE · NIGHTSHADE-FREE · NUT-FREE · VEGAN**

I learned how to make sushi from my longtime friend Crystal, whom I met in holistic nutrition school almost a decade ago. She'd come over to my one-bedroom basement suite, which I shared with three other people, and we'd make sushi rolls filled with quinoa, nuts, and various exciting Asian vegetables.

If the sushi wrapping technique seems scary, jump on YouTube to watch a how-to video. A couple of minutes after watching the videos and trying it yourself, you will have mastered the art!

NORI ROLLS:

8 nori sheets

2 large Hass avocados, skinned, cored, and sliced (about 12 ounces/340 g flesh)

½ English cucumber, sliced thin

3 tablespoons roasted sesame seeds

½ packed cup (35 g) fresh cilantro leaves, roughly chopped

ALMOND DIPPING SAUCE:

1 teaspoon toasted sesame oil

2 small cloves garlic, minced

½ cup (140 g) unsweetened smooth almond butter

⅓ cup (80 ml) MCT oil

1 tablespoon fresh lime juice

1 tablespoon fish sauce

2 teaspoons coconut aminos

1 teaspoon Sriracha sauce

2 drops liquid stevia

1 tablespoon apple cider vinegar

1. Place a nori sheet on a sushi mat and, using your finger dabbed in water, lightly dampen the bottom three-quarters of the sheet. Stack the nori roll ingredients along the bottom of the sheet, 1 inch (2.5 cm) from the end, placing one-eighth of the avocado, then one-eighth of the cucumber, followed by a sprinkle of sesame seeds and chopped cilantro.

2. Pick up the edge of the sushi mat and roll it into itself, over the fillings, being careful not to push the ingredients up the nori sheet. Continue to roll until you get to the last one-quarter section that isn't damp yet. Dampen that area, then roll onto it, pressing down to seal. Rotate the roll in the mat for a couple of seconds to secure the sheet. Remove the roll from the sushi mat and place on a clean plate. If you find that the roll is a bit dry, dampen it all over with additional water.

3. Repeat with the remaining nori roll ingredients. Once complete, use a sharp knife to cut each roll into 6 pieces. Set on a clean plate.

4. Prepare the almond sauce: Place the sesame oil and minced garlic in a small saucepan. Heat on low just until fragrant, about 2 minutes.

5. Add the almond butter, MCT oil, lime juice, fish sauce, aminos, Sriracha, and stevia. Cook, whisking occasionally, until the mixture is smooth and only lightly simmering.

6. Stir in the vinegar and let the sauce sit for 2 minutes before using. Drizzle the sauce over the rolls and serve extra on the side for dipping.

STORE IT: Store the sauce and rolls in separate airtight containers in the fridge, wrapping the rolls in plastic wrap to keep them as fresh as possible. The sauce will keep for up to 5 days, and the rolls up to 3 days. To keep the avocado from browning, store the leftover pits with the rolls. Uncut rolls will keep better than cut rolls.

PREP AHEAD: Prepare the sauce up to 2 days before making the rolls.

MAKE IT COCONUT-FREE: Use refined avocado oil in place of the MCT oil. Replace the coconut aminos with a wheat-free soy sauce, if you tolerate soy.

MAKE IT NIGHTSHADE-FREE: Omit the Sriracha sauce.

MAKE IT NUT-FREE: Use sunflower seed butter in place of the almond butter.

MAKE IT VEGAN: Omit the fish sauce.

MAKE IT A CARB-UP: Replace the MCT oil with water, omit one of the avocados, and fill the nori rolls with the carb of your choice (find ideas on page 117, or visit healthfulpursuit.com/carbup to download the complimentary PDF "Carb-Up Recipes").

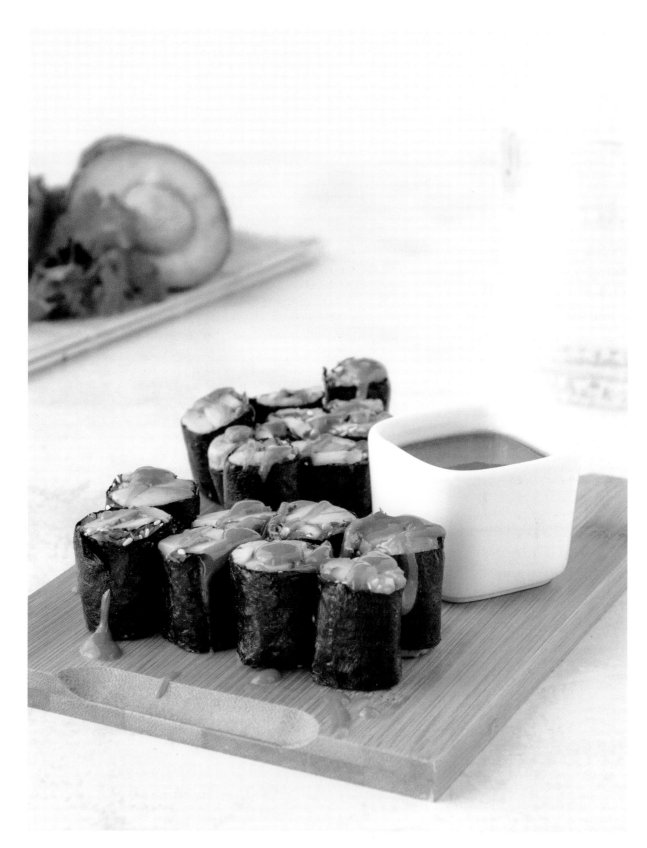

NUTRIENT INFORMATION (PER 1 ROLL WITH 2 TABLESPOONS SAUCE):

calories: 321 | calories from fat: 260 | total fat: 28.9g | saturated fat: 12.4g | cholesterol: 0mg

sodium: 188mg | carbs: 9g | dietary fiber: 6.4g | net carbs: 2.6g | sugars: 1.2g | protein: 6.2g

RATIOS:

fat:	carbs:	protein:
81%	11%	8%

SALT AND PEPPER CHICKEN WINGS

PREP TIME: **5 minutes**   COOK TIME: **35 minutes**   SERVES: **4**

COCONUT-FREE · EGG-FREE · LOW-FODMAP · NIGHTSHADE-FREE · NUT-FREE

There's nothing I love more than a plate of chicken wings. Often I'll make a batch and split them between lunch and dinner with a large bowl of green salad—simple and easy!

1 pound (455 g) chicken wings

¼ cup (60 ml) refined avocado oil

¼ teaspoon finely ground gray sea salt

1 teaspoon ground black pepper, divided

STORE IT: *Keep in an airtight container in the fridge for up to 3 days.*

REHEAT IT: *Place on a plate and microwave until the desired temperature is reached. Or place in a covered casserole dish and reheat in a preheated 300°F (150°C) oven for 5 minutes, or until warmed through. Or reheat in a frying pan with a drizzle of refined avocado oil, covered, on medium-low.*

1. Preheat the oven to 400°F (205°C).

2. Place the wings, oil, salt, and ¼ teaspoon of the pepper in a medium-sized bowl. Toss to coat the wings.

3. Transfer the coated wings to a cast-iron pan, unlined rimmed baking sheet, or 1½-quart (1.4-L) casserole dish. Sprinkle with the remaining pepper.

4. Bake for 30 minutes, or until lightly golden. If using a baking sheet, rotate the pan halfway through cooking.

5. Turn the oven broiler to low (if your oven doesn't have a low broil setting, simply "broil" is fine) and crisp the wings for 3 minutes. Allow to cool on the pan for 5 minutes before enjoying.

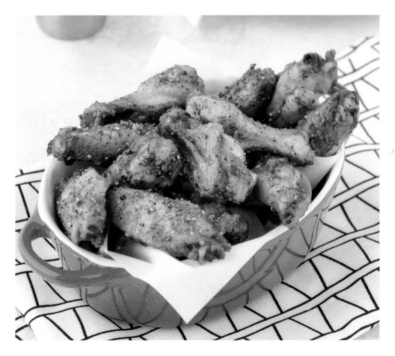

NUTRIENT INFORMATION (PER SERVING):

calories: 360 | calories from fat: 282 | total fat: 31.3g | saturated fat: 6.6g | cholesterol: 81mg

sodium: 290mg | carbs: 0.3g | dietary fiber: 0g | net carbs: 0.3g | sugars: 0g | protein: 19.3g

RATIOS:

fat:	carbs:	protein:
79%	0%	21%

JERKY COOKIES

PREP TIME: **15 minutes**   COOK TIME: **6 hours**   MAKES: **18 cookies (18 servings)**

EGG-FREE • NUT-FREE   OPTIONS: **COCONUT-FREE • LOW-FODMAP • NIGHTSHADE-FREE**

Kevin, my husband, eats so much jerky. If it were up to him, he'd have a full bag with him at all times. As you can imagine, his love of jerky crushes our grocery budget. I decided to start making jerky for him, but making it from expensive cuts of meat didn't save us much money. Then I discovered that jerky could be made with ground meat! You can imagine my excitement. These jerky cookies have all the flavor of jerky without the high cost!

1 pound (455 g) ground beef (10% fat)

2 tablespoons coconut aminos

1 teaspoon smoked sea salt

1 teaspoon ground black pepper

½ teaspoon garlic powder

½ teaspoon red pepper flakes

STORE IT: *Keep in an airtight container in the fridge for up to 5 days or in the freezer for up to 1 month.*

THAW IT: *Allow to thaw on the counter for 1 hour before enjoying.*

SERVE IT WITH: *These cookies taste great with Kale Pâté (page 259), Bacon Spinach Dip (page 255), or mayonnaise.*

MAKE IT COCONUT-FREE: *Replace the coconut aminos with a wheat-free soy sauce, if you tolerate soy.*

MAKE IT LOW-FODMAP: *Replace the coconut aminos, salt, black pepper, garlic, and red pepper flakes with 1 tablespoon of one of the low-FODMAP spice mixtures on pages 232 to 235. If using a spice mix that doesn't contain salt, you'll need to add 1 teaspoon of salt to it. If using a spice mix that doesn't contain black pepper, you'll need to add 1 teaspoon of pepper.*

MAKE IT NIGHTSHADE-FREE: *Omit the red pepper flakes.*

1. Place 2 oven racks as close to the middle of the oven as possible. Preheat the oven to 170°F (77°C) and line 2 baking sheets with parchment paper or a silicone baking mat.

2. Place all the ingredients in a medium-sized bowl and combine with your hands until well mixed.

3. Scooping a heaping tablespoon of the meat mixture into your palm, roll it into a ball, and then flatten it into a 2-inch (5-cm) round. Transfer to a prepared baking sheet and repeat with the remaining mixture.

4. Bake the cookies for 6 hours, flipping them over halfway through cooking. From time to time, rotate the pans from one oven rack to the other to ensure even baking. The cookies are done when they are chewy like jerky.

5. Transfer the cookies to a cooling rack and allow to cool for 30 minutes.

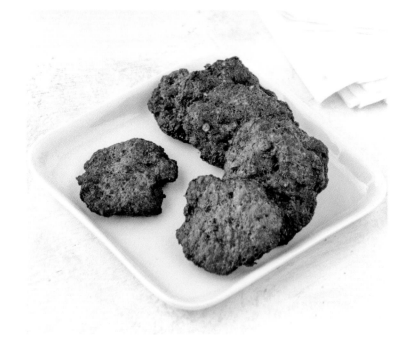

NUTRIENT INFORMATION (PER COOKIE):

calories: 47 | calories from fat: 14 | total fat: 1.6g | saturated fat: 0.6g | cholesterol: 23mg

sodium: 124mg | carbs: 0.5g | dietary fiber: 0g | net carbs: 0.5g | sugars: 0g | protein: 7.7g

RATIOS:

fat:	carbs:	protein:
31%	4%	65%

THANKSGIVING BALLS

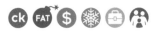

PREP TIME: **20 minutes**   COOK TIME: **35 minutes**   MAKES: **14 balls (14 servings)**

COCONUT-FREE · EGG-FREE · NIGHTSHADE-FREE

These meatballs remind me of the Paleo-friendly stuffing recipe that I shared on HealthfulPursuit.com a couple of years ago. What I love about that recipe, and this one as well, is how easy it is to prepare. Need to shave off even more time? I've included a variation that's even quicker to make. Make a couple of batches of these meatballs, store them in the freezer, and add them to just about any meal as a protein source—salads, scrambles, bowls with all sorts of goodies—or enjoy them on their own.

The sausage you use will impact the flavor of the dish. I opted for a light apple chicken sausage that has only 1 gram of carbs per sausage. I recommend staying away from heavily spiced sausages if you want to retain the Thanksgiving flavor. Original-flavor fermented beef sticks from Paleovalley would work wonders in this recipe and save you time since they are fully cooked.

¼ cup (52 g) duck fat

4½ ounces (125 g) chicken sausages, chopped

½ cup (85 g) chopped celery

3 white mushrooms (about 2¼ ounces/ 65 g), chopped

2 small cloves garlic, minced

2 teaspoons dried thyme leaves

½ teaspoon dried ground sage

½ teaspoon finely ground gray sea salt

¼ teaspoon ground black pepper

¾ cup (85 g) raw walnut pieces, soaked for 12 hours, then drained and rinsed

¼ packed cup (16 g) fresh parsley leaves, finely chopped

1. Preheat the oven to 350°F (177°C) and line a rimmed baking sheet with parchment paper or a silicone baking mat.

2. Place the duck fat, sausages, celery, mushrooms, and garlic in a frying pan over medium heat. Cook for 7 to 10 minutes, until the celery is fork-tender and the sausages reach an internal temperature of 165°F (74°C).

3. Add the thyme, sage, salt, and pepper and continue to cook for 1 to 2 minutes, until fragrant. Remove from the heat and transfer the contents of the pan to a blender or food processor.

4. Add the walnuts and pulse until the ingredients are broken down but still have some texture.

5. Transfer 3 tablespoons of the mixture to a bowl, then blend the rest until smooth.

6. Transfer the blended-smooth ingredients to the bowl and stir in the parsley.

7. Scoop up a heaping tablespoon of the mixture, roll it into a ball, and place it on the prepared baking sheet. Repeat with the remaining mixture.

8. Bake the meatballs for 22 to 25 minutes, until browned and lightly cracked on the tops. Allow to cool on the baking sheet for 30 minutes before serving.

STORE IT: *Keep in an airtight container in the fridge for up to 2 days or in the freezer for up to 1 month.*

REHEAT IT: *Place on a plate and microwave until the desired temperature is reached. Or place in a covered casserole dish and reheat in a preheated 300°F (150°C) oven for 5 minutes, or until warmed through.*

THAW IT: *Allow to thaw completely in the fridge. Once defrosted, enjoy cold or use the reheating instructions above.*

VARIATION: QUICKER THANKSGIVING BALLS. *If you don't care too much about presentation, the balls are ready for consumption following Step 7. Instead of baking them, place the baking sheet in the fridge to firm up the balls for an hour or two, then enjoy.*

SERVE IT WITH: *To make this a complete meal, use the balls as the protein source for your favorite salad, or break them up and add them to a morning scramble.*

NUTRIENT INFORMATION (PER BALL):

calories: 82 | calories from fat: 70 | total fat: 7.7g | saturated fat: 1.7g | cholesterol: 5mg

sodium: 88mg | carbs: 1.4g | dietary fiber: 0.7g | net carbs: 0.7g | sugars: 0g | protein: 1.7g

RATIOS:

fat:	carbs:	protein:
85%	7%	8%

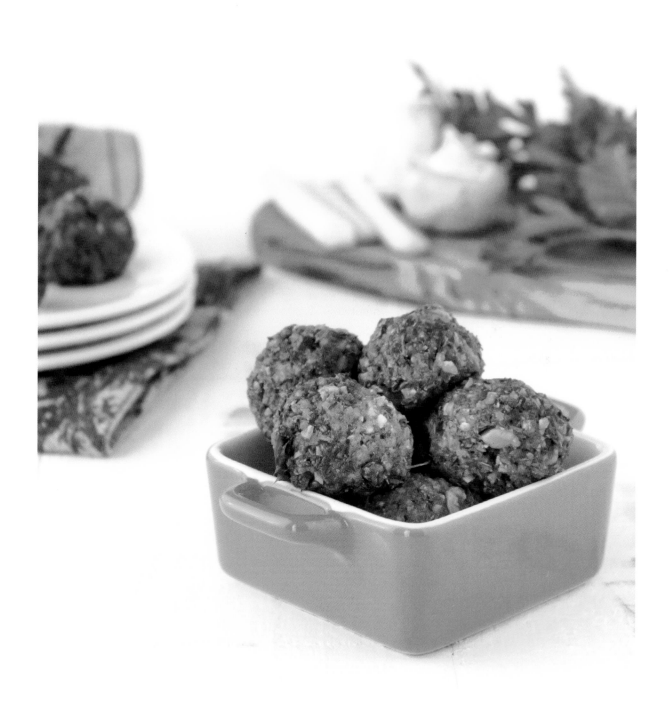

THE ONLY WAY I'LL EAT LIVER

PREP TIME: **15 minutes, plus time to soak overnight**   COOK TIME: **20 minutes**   SERVES: **6**

COCONUT-FREE · EGG-FREE · LOW-FODMAP · NIGHTSHADE-FREE · NUT-FREE

Please, for the love of liver, do not skip the vinegar soak in this recipe. Soaking these babies in vinegar takes the edge off, making the flavor a lot smoother. It's best to cover the pan with a mesh cover so that the livers don't hit you in the face. I'm not kidding. While they cook, they like to jump! If you're easing your way into eating liver, note that chicken livers are milder than beef liver. Eat the cooked livers with a side of mayonnaise, or use them as the protein on a salad. Leftovers can be heated up or enjoyed cold.

1 pound (455 g) chicken livers, rinsed and cut into bite-sized pieces

1 tablespoon apple cider vinegar

6 ounces (170 g) bacon (about 6 strips), cut into small pieces

SEASONED "BREADING":

¾ cup (50 g) pork dust or ground pork rinds

1 tablespoon dried thyme leaves

¾ teaspoon finely ground gray sea salt

1 teaspoon ground black pepper

1 lemon, cut into wedges, for serving (optional)

STORE IT: *Keep in an airtight container in the fridge for up to 3 days.*

REHEAT IT: *Place on a plate and microwave until the desired temperature is reached. Or place in a covered casserole dish and reheat in a preheated 300°F (150°C) oven for 5 minutes, or until warmed through. Or reheat in a frying pan with a drizzle of refined avocado oil, covered, on medium-low.*

PREP AHEAD: *Prepare the bacon bits as much as a month ahead of time. Store in an airtight container in the freezer. When ready to use, simply add to the recipe. If preparing this way, place 3 tablespoons of refined avocado oil in the frying pan in Step 6 to replace the bacon grease.*

1. Place the chicken liver pieces in a large glass or stainless-steel bowl. Cover with water and add the vinegar. Stir with a spoon until the vinegar is thoroughly mixed into the water. Cover and place in the fridge overnight.

2. When ready to complete the recipe, cook the bacon pieces in a large frying pan over medium heat until crisp, 8 to 10 minutes.

3. While the bacon is cooking, combine the ingredients for the breading in a medium-sized bowl.

4. Drain and rinse the soaked livers. Transfer half of the livers to the bowl with the breading mixture and toss in the breading until coated.

5. Remove the cooked bacon pieces to a plate, leaving the grease in the pan.

6. Transfer the coated livers to the frying pan with the bacon grease and reduce the heat to medium-low. Cook for 10 to 12 minutes, until no longer pink or only slightly pink on the inside, flipping them over halfway through.

7. Transfer the cooked livers to a serving plate. Bread and cook the remaining liver pieces as described in Steps 4 and 6.

8. When the second batch is complete, move to a serving plate, garnish with the reserved bacon bits, and dig in!

NUTRIENT INFORMATION (PER ⅓-CUP/115-G SERVING):
calories: 246 | calories from fat: 145 | total fat: 16.1g | saturated fat: 5.1g | cholesterol: 23mg
sodium: 624mg | carbs: 0.9g | dietary fiber: 0g | net carbs: 0.9g | sugars: 0g | protein: 24.4g

RATIOS:

fat:	carbs:	protein:
59%	1%	40%

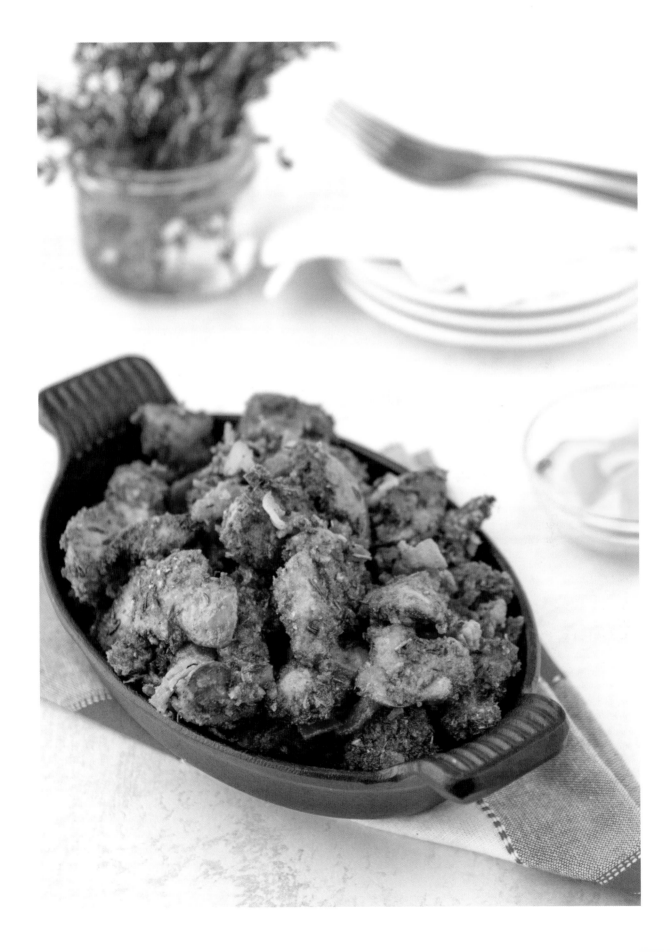

CHICKEN NOODLE SOUP

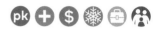

PREP TIME: **10 minutes**   COOK TIME: **35 minutes**   SERVES: **4**

EGG-FREE · NIGHTSHADE-FREE · NUT-FREE   OPTIONS: COCONUT-FREE · LOW-FODMAP

Homemade bone broth takes this soup to new heights, but if you don't have any on hand, store-bought will do the trick. Instead of using raw chicken thighs to make this soup, I often use leftover cooked chicken from a roasted bird; it adds great flavor, is a time-saver, and is a great way to use up leftovers. If you end up using leftover, cooked chicken pieces, go for about 10½ ounces (300 g) of cooked meat. While this is a "chicken" noodle soup recipe, the soup is really great with pork, too! If using raw pork versus leftover cooked pork, sliced tenderloin is a good choice. If using cooked pork, any cut will do.

⅓ cup (70 g) coconut oil or duck fat

1 pound (455 g) boneless, skinless chicken thighs, sliced

1 cup (170 g) diced celery

1 cup (80 g) chopped green onions, green parts only

½ cup (80 g) diced carrots

6 cups (1.4 L) chicken bone broth (see page 152)

2 teaspoons finely ground gray sea salt

½ teaspoon dried basil

½ teaspoon dried oregano leaves

⅛ teaspoon ground black pepper

2 cups (200 g) Zoodles or Doodles (page 376)

1. Heat the oil in a large saucepan over medium-high heat, then add the sliced chicken. Brown the chicken on both sides, about 10 minutes total.

2. Add the celery, onions, and carrots to the pan and continue to cook for 5 minutes.

3. Add the broth, salt, basil, oregano, and pepper. Cover and bring to a boil. Once boiling, reduce the heat to medium-low and cook for 20 minutes. In the last 2 minutes of cooking, add the Zoodles.

4. Remove from the heat and divide the soup among 4 medium-sized serving bowls.

STORE IT: *Keep in an airtight container in the fridge for up to 4 days or in the freezer for up to 1 month.*

REHEAT IT: *Microwave until the desired temperature is reached, or place in a saucepan and reheat, covered, on medium-low.*

THAW IT: *Allow to thaw completely in the fridge. Once defrosted, use the reheating instructions above.*

PRESSURE-COOK IT: *Complete Step 1 using the sauté function on your pressure cooker. Add the remaining ingredients, except the noodles, seal the lid, and set on high pressure for 8 minutes. Allow the pressure to release, then remove the lid, add the noodles and cover for 2 minutes before serving.*

SERVE IT WITH: *This soup tastes great with Classic Butter Biscuits (page 368).*

MAKE IT COCONUT-FREE: *Use duck fat instead of coconut oil.*

MAKE IT LOW-FODMAP: *Reduce the amount of celery to ½ cup (85 g).*

MAKE IT A CARB-UP: *Replace the chicken thighs with boneless, skinless chicken breasts, reduce the amount of oil to 1 tablespoon, and replace the Zoodles or Doodles with spiral-sliced parsnips, yams, or sweet potatoes (see page 154 for spiral-slicing instructions), adding them 10 minutes before the end of the cooking time.*

NUTRIENT INFORMATION (PER 2-CUP/475-ML SERVING):
calories: 371 | calories from fat: 200 | total fat: 22.2g | saturated fat: 6.9g | cholesterol: 113mg

sodium: 752mg | carbs: 6.5g | dietary fiber: 2.3g | net carbs: 4.2g | sugars: 2.9g | protein: 36.4g

RATIOS:

fat:	carbs:	protein:
54%	7%	39%

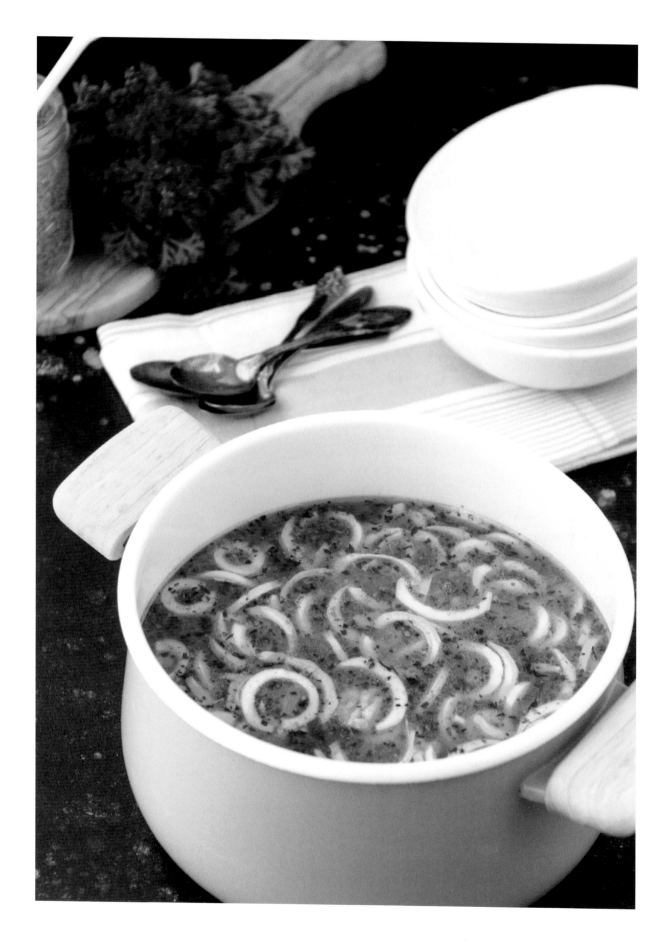

SHRIMP CHOWDER

PREP TIME: **10 minutes**   COOK TIME: **40 minutes**   SERVES: **6**

EGG-FREE • NUT-FREE   OPTIONS: COCONUT-FREE • LOW-FODMAP • NIGHTSHADE-FREE

This recipe totally happened by accident. Originally, I'd planned to bake fish in a mushroom cream sauce, but the grocery store had run out of trout, so I was stuck with shrimp. Then, when I went to make the cream sauce, I realized I was out of egg yolks (which is what I was planning on thickening the sauce with). In the end, though, I'm happy that nothing went as planned, because the result couldn't have been better if I'd planned it from the very start! If you're a chowder person like I am, you're going to love this!

¼ cup (60 ml) refined avocado oil or melted ghee (if tolerated)

1⅔ cups (140 g) diced mushrooms

⅓ cup (55 g) diced yellow onions

10½ ounces (300 g) small raw shrimp, shelled and deveined

1 can (13½-ounce/400-ml) full-fat coconut milk

⅓ cup (80 ml) chicken bone broth (see page 152)

2 tablespoons apple cider vinegar

1 teaspoon onion powder

1 teaspoon paprika

1 bay leaf

¾ teaspoon finely ground gray sea salt

½ teaspoon dried oregano leaves

¼ teaspoon ground black pepper

12 radishes (about 6 ounces/170 g), cubed

1 medium zucchini (about 7 ounces/ 200 g), cubed

1. Heat the avocado oil in a large saucepan on medium for a couple of minutes, then add the mushrooms and onions. Sauté for 8 to 10 minutes, until the onions are translucent and mushrooms are beginning to brown.

2. Add the remaining ingredients, except the radishes and zucchini. Cover and bring to a boil, then reduce the heat to low and simmer for 20 minutes.

3. After 20 minutes, add the radishes and zucchini. Continue to cook for 10 minutes, until the vegetables are fork-tender.

4. Remove the bay leaf, divide among 6 small soup bowls, and enjoy.

STORE IT: *Keep in an airtight container in the fridge for up to 3 days or in the freezer for up to 1 month.*

REHEAT IT: *Microwave or place in a saucepan, cover, and heat on medium until the desired temperature is reached.*

THAW IT: *Allow to thaw completely in the fridge. Once defrosted, use the reheating instructions above.*

PRESSURE-COOK IT: *Complete Step 1 using the sauté feature of your pressure cooker. Add the rest of the ingredients, including the radishes and zucchini. Secure the lid and set to high pressure for 8 minutes. Allow the pressure to release, then remove the lid and serve, following Step 4.*

SERVE IT WITH: *This chowder tastes great served over Zoodles or Doodles (page 376) or with Classic Flaxseed Focaccia (page 373).*

MAKE IT COCONUT-FREE: *Use a nondairy milk of your choice.*

MAKE IT LOW-FODMAP: *Omit the diced onions and onion powder. Replace 2 tablespoons of the avocado oil with Onion-Infused Oil (page 230), and replace the diced yellow onions with ¼ cup chopped green onions, green parts only.*

MAKE IT NIGHTSHADE-FREE: *Omit the paprika.*

NUTRIENT INFORMATION (PER 1-CUP/240-ML SERVING):
calories: 301 | calories from fat: 213 | total fat: 23.7g | saturated fat: 13.9g | cholesterol: 105mg

sodium: 410mg | carbs: 7.4g | dietary fiber: 1.5g | net carbs: 5.9g | sugars: 3.2g | protein: 14.5g

RATIOS:
fat: carbs: protein:
71%   10%   19%

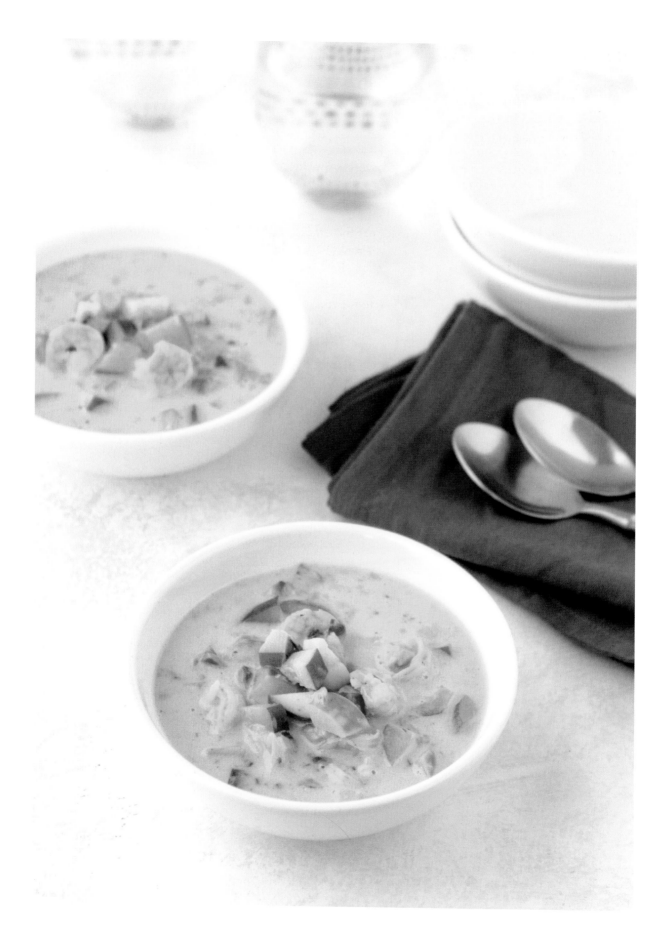

BACON SOUP

PREP TIME: **10 minutes**   COOK TIME: **1 hour, 20 minutes**   SERVES: **6**

EGG-FREE • NIGHTSHADE-FREE • NUT-FREE   OPTIONS: COCONUT-FREE • LOW-FODMAP

If you really want to get crazy with this soup, you could replace the pork stewing pieces with your favorite low-carb sausage and serve it alongside a big bowl of sauerkraut, maybe even with a drizzle of mustard on top. Along with the stovetop method, I've included a set-it-and-forget slow cooker method and a hurry-up-and-get-it-done pressure cooker method.

⅓ cup (69 g) lard

1 pound (455 g) pork stewing pieces

¾ cup (110 g) sliced shallots

10 strips bacon (about 10 ounces/285 g), cut into about ½-inch (1.25-cm) pieces

1¾ cups (415 ml) chicken bone broth (see page 152)

3 medium turnips (about 12½ ounces/ 355 g), cubed

¼ cup (60 ml) white wine, such as Pinot Grigio, Sauvignon Blanc, or unoaked Chardonnay

1 tablespoon prepared yellow mustard

4 sprigs fresh thyme

½ cup (120 ml) full-fat coconut milk

2 tablespoons apple cider vinegar

2 tablespoons unflavored gelatin

1 tablespoon dried tarragon leaves

1. Melt the lard in a large saucepan over medium heat. Once the lard has melted, add the pork pieces and cook for 8 minutes, or until lightly browned on the outside.

2. Add the sliced shallots and bacon pieces. Sauté for an additional 5 minutes or until the shallots become fragrant.

3. Add the bone broth, turnips, wine, mustard, and thyme sprigs. Cover and bring to a boil, then reduce the heat to medium-low and cook until the meat and turnips are fork-tender, about 1 hour.

4. Remove the thyme sprigs and add the coconut milk, vinegar, gelatin, and tarragon. Increase the heat to medium and boil, covered, for another 10 minutes.

5. Divide the soup among 6 small bowls and serve.

STORE IT: *Keep in an airtight container in the fridge for up to 3 days or in the freezer for up to 1 month.*

REHEAT IT: *Microwave until the desired temperature is reached. Or place in a covered casserole dish and reheat in a 300°F (150°C) oven for 10 to 15 minutes, until warmed through. Or reheat in a saucepan, covered, on medium-low for 5 minutes.*

THAW IT: *Allow to thaw completely in the fridge. Once defrosted, use the reheating instructions above.*

PRESSURE-COOK IT: *Complete Steps 1 and 2 using the sauté function on your pressure cooker. Add the bone broth, turnips, wine, mustard, and thyme sprigs, then seal the pressure cooker and set it to high pressure for 30 minutes. Allow the pressure to release, then remove the lid. Remove the thyme sprigs and set the pressure cooker to sauté. Cover and boil for 10 minutes, then serve.*

SLOW-COOK IT: *Complete Steps 1 and 2, then transfer the sautéed meat and shallots to a slow cooker. Add the bone broth, turnips, wine, mustard, and thyme sprigs. Cover and cook on high for 4 hours or low for 6 hours. Remove the thyme sprigs and add the coconut milk, vinegar, gelatin, and tarragon. Cook, covered, for an additional 30 minutes on high.*

MAKE IT COCONUT-FREE: *Replace the coconut milk with another nondairy milk. Unsweetened almond milk would be good.*

MAKE IT LOW-FODMAP: *Replace the shallots with sliced green onions, green parts only.*

NUTRIENT INFORMATION (PER ¾-CUP/180-ML SERVING):

calories: 571 | calories from fat: 372 | total fat: 41.4g | saturated fat: 16.9g | cholesterol: 114mg

sodium: 1429mg | carbs: 9.7g | dietary fiber: 1.1g | net carbs: 8.6g | sugars: 2.8g | protein: 39.8g

RATIOS:

fat:	carbs:	protein:
65%	7%	28%

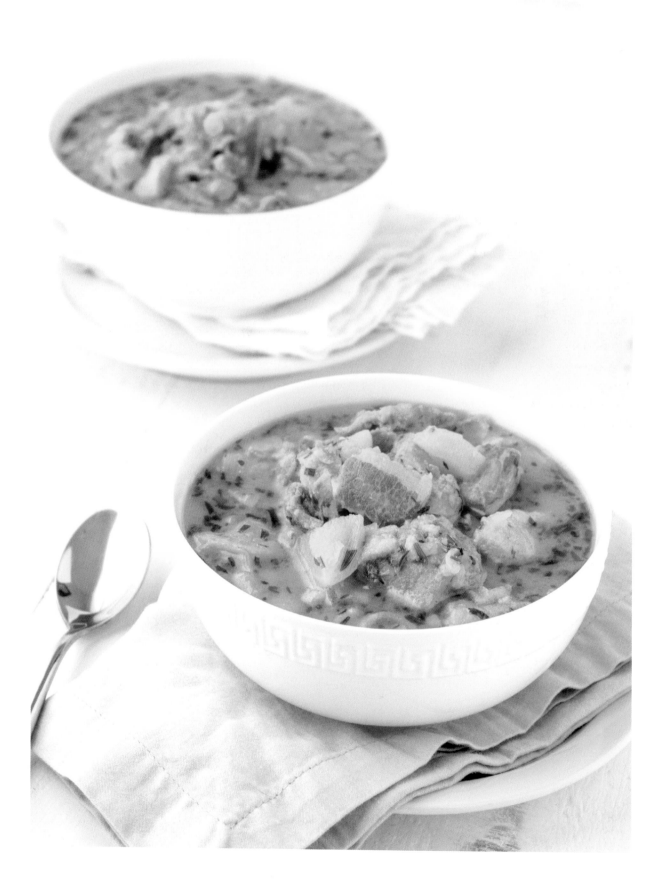

VEGAN CREAM OF BROCCOLI SOUP

PREP TIME: **20 minutes**   COOK TIME: **15 minutes**   SERVES: **6**

EGG-FREE • NIGHTSHADE-FREE • NUT-FREE • VEGAN   OPTION: COCONUT-FREE

This soup is a year-round dairy-free delight that even masquerades as a sauce. When chilled, it's a perfect summertime meal, tossed with Doodles and topped with cooked strips of chicken thighs. If it's wintertime and the thought of cold noodles has you shaking from the inside out, the soup is delicious served hot! Try it with a side of Egg-Free Flax Focaccia (page 373).

Butter-infused olive oil is extra-virgin olive oil that's been infused with herbs to create the flavor of butter, without the dairy. There's butter-flavored coconut oil as well. My favorite is from Ellyndale Foods, a division of NOW Foods. You can find both products at many health food stores. If it's too tricky of an ingredient and you can tolerate ghee or butter, use one of them!

2 cups (475 ml) vegetable stock

1 (13½-ounce/400-ml) can full-fat coconut milk

1 small head cauliflower (about 14 ounces/400 g), cored and cut into large florets

6 green onions, green parts only, roughly chopped

2 medium celery sticks, chopped

1 teaspoon finely ground gray sea salt

1 large head broccoli, cored and cut into large florets (about 11½ ounces/325 g florets)

⅓ cup (80 ml) butter-infused olive oil or melted butter-infused coconut oil

¼ teaspoon ground black pepper

¼ teaspoon ground white pepper (optional)

FOR GARNISH (OPTIONAL):

1 green onion, sliced on the diagonal

1. Place the vegetable stock, coconut milk, cauliflower florets, green onions, chopped celery, and salt in a large saucepan. Cover and bring to a boil. Cook for 15 minutes, or until the florets are soft when poked with a knife.

2. Meanwhile, steam the broccoli until it's fork-tender.

3. Transfer the cauliflower mixture to a blender along with the infused olive oil, black pepper, and white pepper, if using. Blend on high for 1 minute, or until smooth.

4. Add the steamed broccoli and pulse 3 or 4 times, just to break up the broccoli (allow some bite-sized pieces to remain).

5. Divide among 6 small soup bowls, garnish with sliced green onions, if desired, and serve.

STORE IT: *Keep in an airtight container in the fridge for up to 4 days or in the freezer for up to 1 month.*

REHEAT IT: *Microwave, covered, until the desired temperature is reached or reheat in a saucepan, covered, on medium.*

THAW IT: *Allow to thaw completely in the fridge. Once defrosted, use the reheating instructions above.*

SERVE IT WITH: *To make this a complete meal, serve over Doodles (page 376) and top with hulled hemp seeds, your favorite nut/seed mixture, or (if you're eating meat) cooked ground or sliced chicken or pork. This soup tastes great with Egg-Free Flax Focaccia (page 373).*

MAKE IT COCONUT-FREE: *Use your favorite nondairy milk in place of the coconut milk, and use olive oil instead of coconut oil.*

NUTRIENT INFORMATION (PER ¾ CUP PLUS 2 TABLESPOONS/210-ML SERVING):

calories: 279 | calories from fat: 210 | total fat: 23.3g | saturated fat: 12.4g | cholesterol: 0mg

sodium: 518mg | carbs: 10.3g | dietary fiber: 3.6g | net carbs: 6.7g | sugars: 4g | protein: 6.9g

RATIOS:

fat:	carbs:	protein:
75%	15%	10%

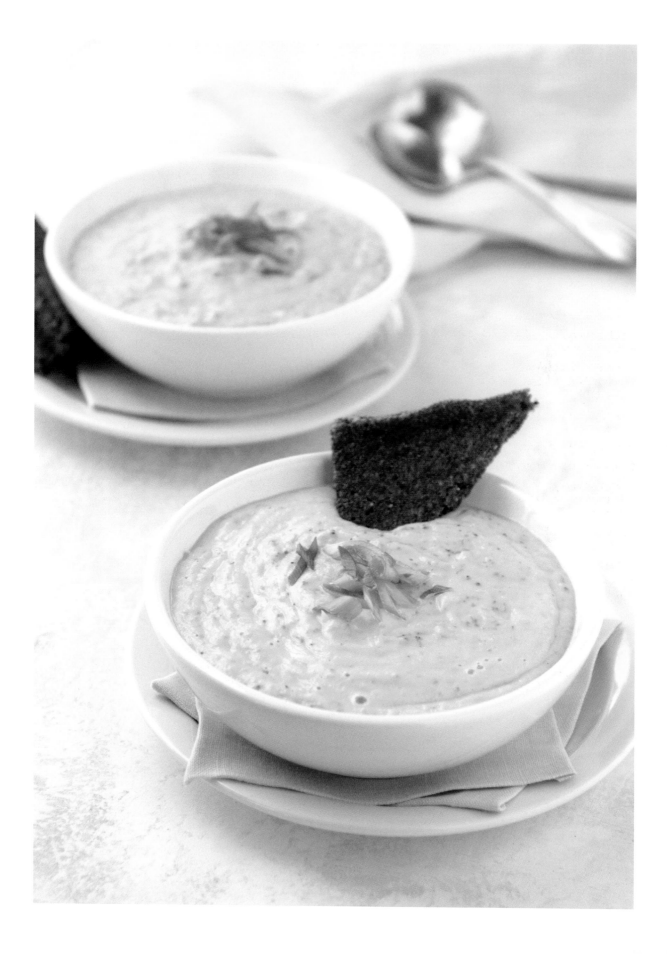

SPINACH SALAD WITH BREADED CHICKEN STRIPS

PREP TIME: **15 minutes**   COOK TIME: **25 minutes**   SERVES: **4**

NUT-FREE   OPTIONS: COCONUT-FREE · EGG-FREE · LOW-FODMAP · NIGHTSHADE-FREE

If you're looking for perfectly crispy chicken tenders, set the oven to broil just after baking and broil the tenders on low for 1 minute or so. Just watch them! Shredded coconut burns quickly.

3 tablespoons refined avocado oil, for the pan

CHICKEN:

1 cup (100 g) unsweetened shredded coconut

1 tablespoon plus 1 teaspoon Cajun Seasoning (page 232)

1½ pounds (680 g) boneless, skinless chicken thighs

SALAD:

4 cups (280 g) fresh spinach

½ cup (85 g) roughly chopped celery

½ cup (40 g) sliced green onions

1 cup (240 ml) Ranch Dressing (page 226)

1. Preheat the oven to 375°F (190°C) and heavily grease a rimmed baking sheet with the avocado oil.

2. Place the coconut in a blender or food processor and pulse until coarsely ground, but not to a powder.

3. Combine the coconut and Cajun seasoning in a medium-sized bowl. Toss to combine.

4. Place a chicken thigh between 2 pieces of plastic wrap. Using a mallet or the flat surface of a heavy object, such as a small cast-iron frying pan or mug, pound the chicken until it's ¼ inch (6 mm) thick. Transfer to the bowl of seasoned coconut and roll it around until well coated. Place the breaded thigh on the prepared baking sheet and repeat with the remaining chicken. Once all the chicken is breaded, bake for 25 minutes. (*Note:* For extra-crispy chicken, follow the instructions in the note above.)

5. Meanwhile, divide the spinach among 4 large dinner plates. Top with the celery and green onions. Divide the dressing among 4 small ramekins and set to the side of the salads.

6. Slice the chicken and divide among the salads.

STORE IT: *Keep the salad ingredients and cooked chicken in separate airtight containers in the fridge for up to 3 days.*

REHEAT IT: *Microwave the chicken until the desired temperature is reached. Or place the chicken in a covered casserole dish and reheat in a preheated 300°F (150°C) oven for 10 to 15 minutes, until warmed through.*

MAKE IT COCONUT-FREE: *Replace the coconut with 1 cup (150 g) of hulled sunflower seeds.*

MAKE IT EGG-FREE: *Use the egg-free variation of the ranch dressing.*

MAKE IT LOW-FODMAP: *Replace the Cajun seasoning with an equal amount of one of the low-FODMAP spice mixtures on pages 232 to 235. If using a spice mix that doesn't contain salt, you'll need to add 1½ teaspoons of finely ground gray sea salt to this recipe. Replace the celery with an equal amount of cucumbers, and use only the green parts of the green onions. Use the low-FODMAP variation of the ranch dressing.*

MAKE IT NIGHTSHADE-FREE: *Replace the Cajun seasoning with an equal amount of one of the nightshade-free spice mixtures on pages 232 to 235. If using a spice mix that doesn't contain salt, you'll need to add 1½ teaspoons of finely ground gray sea salt to this recipe.*

NUTRIENT INFORMATION (PER SERVING):
calories: 706 | calories from fat: 511 | total fat: 56.8g | saturated fat: 22.9g | cholesterol: 153mg
sodium: 490mg | carbs: 11.1g | dietary fiber: 6.3g | net carbs: 4.8g | sugars: 2.9g | protein: 37.7g

RATIOS:

fat:	carbs:	protein:
73%	6%	21%

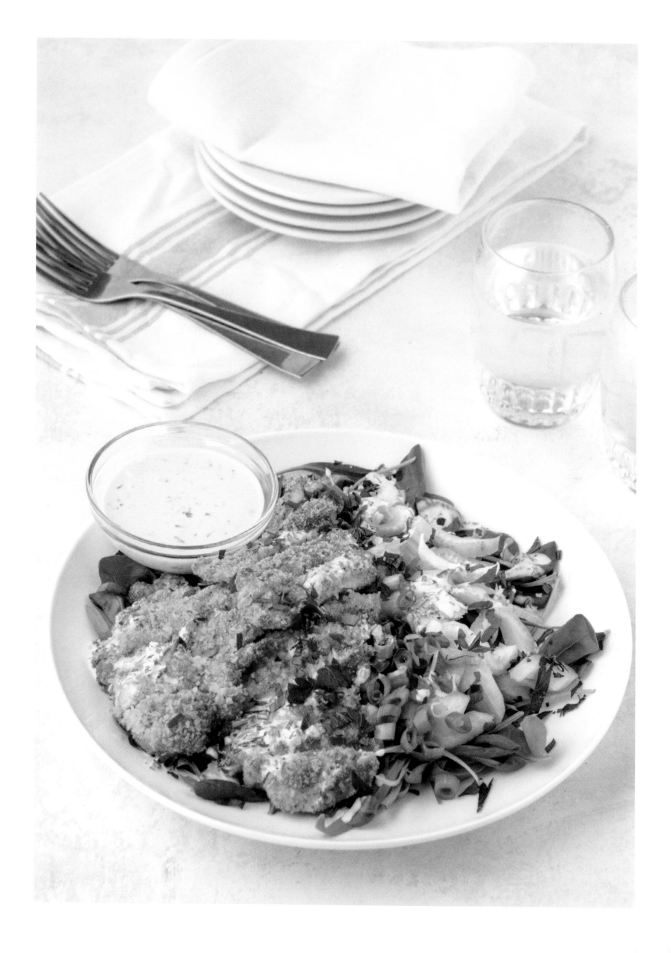

CAJUN PORK BELLY CHOPPED SALAD

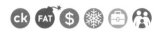

PREP TIME: **15 minutes + overnight**   COOK TIME: **1 hour 45 minutes**   SERVES: **4**

COCONUT-FREE · EGG-FREE · NUT-FREE   OPTIONS: LOW-FODMAP · NIGHTSHADE-FREE

I'm a sucker for crispy pork skin, and this recipe has the crispiest layer you'll find in just about any dish. The top is one large cracklin, the inside is juicy, and the whole darn thing is full of Cajun flavor. Topped with a cooling salad, there's nothing I'd change about this recipe. Nothing.

1 pound (455 g) side pork belly

1 tablespoon refined avocado oil

1½ tablespoons Cajun Seasoning (page 232)

SALAD:

2 cups (240 g) sliced radishes

3 green onions, sliced

1 bunch fresh cilantro (about 1¾ ounces/ 50 g), chopped

¼ cup (15 g) chopped fresh mint

1 large zucchini (about 10½ ounces/ 300 g), diced

¼ cup (60 ml) refined avocado oil or extra-virgin olive oil

Juice of 2 limes

¼ teaspoon finely ground gray sea salt

2 drops liquid stevia

FOR SERVING (OPTIONAL):

Lime wedges

1. Remove the pork belly from its packaging and place it fat side up on a cutting board. Using a sharp knife, score the top with diagonal lines about ½ inch (1.25 cm) apart. Drizzle the entire pork belly with the avocado oil, and top with the Cajun seasoning. Rub thoroughly. Wrap in plastic wrap and set in the fridge for at least 2 hours and up to 24 hours.

2. When ready to cook the pork belly, preheat the oven to 500°F (260°C) and place the pork belly, fat side up, in a cast-iron or other broiler-safe pan. Cook for 15 minutes, until browned. Reduce the oven temperature to 325°F (163°C) and continue cooking for 1½ hours, or until the top and sides are dark brown and the internal temperature reaches 165°F (74°C). Remove the pork belly from the oven and set it on a cutting board; allow to rest for 5 minutes.

3. Meanwhile, prepare the salad: Place all the ingredients in a large bowl. Toss to combine, then spread out the salad on a large serving platter.

4. Using a sharp knife, slice the pork belly, then arrange the slices on top of the salad. Serve with lime wedges on the side, if desired.

STORE IT: *Keep in an airtight container in the fridge for up to 4 days or freeze the meat only for up to 1 month.*

REHEAT IT: *Microwave the meat until the desired temperature is reached; place the meat in a covered casserole dish and reheat in a 300°F (150°C) oven for 10 to 15 minutes, until warmed through; or reheat in a frying pan, covered, on medium-low.*

THAW IT: *Allow the frozen meat to thaw completely in the fridge. Once defrosted, use the reheating instructions above.*

MAKE IT LOW-FODMAP: *Replace the Cajun seasoning with an equal amount of one of the low-FODMAP spice mixtures on pages 232 to 235. If using a spice mix that doesn't have salt, you'll need to add ½ teaspoon finely ground gray sea salt to this recipe. For the green onions, use the green parts only.*

MAKE IT NIGHTSHADE-FREE: *Replace the Cajun seasoning with an equal amount of one of the nightshade-free spice mixtures on pages 232 to 235. If using a spice mix that doesn't have salt, you'll need to add ½ teaspoon of finely ground gray sea salt to this recipe.*

NUTRIENT INFORMATION (PER SERVING):
calories: 1045 | calories from fat: 948 | total fat: 105.4g | saturated fat: 34.4g | cholesterol: 117mg
sodium: 209mg | carbs: 6.7g | dietary fiber: 2.8g | net carbs: 3.9g | sugars: 2.9g | protein: 17.4g

RATIOS:
fat: carbs: protein:
91%   2%   7%

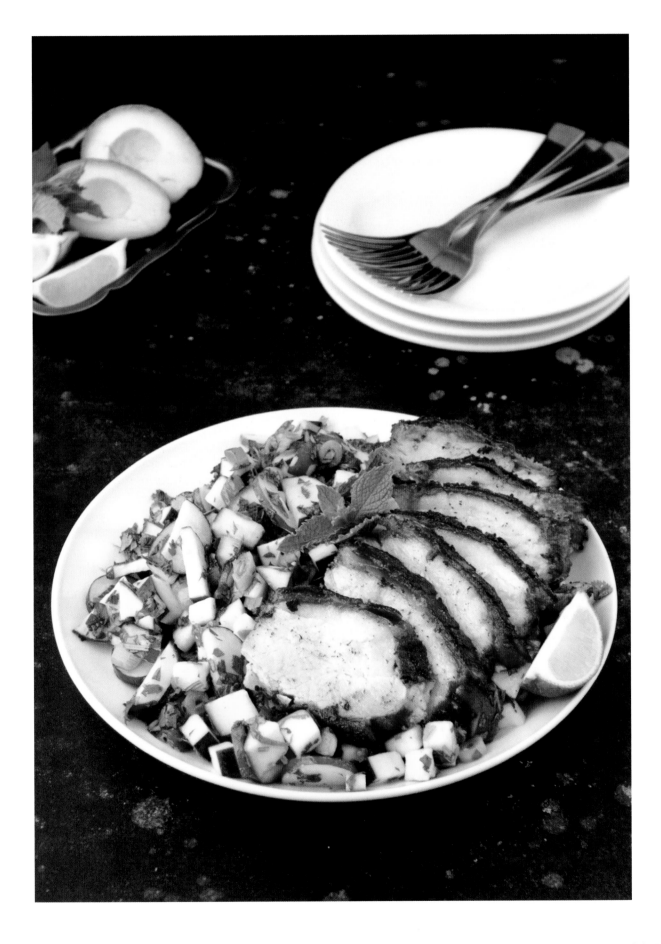

CALAMARI SALAD

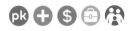

PREP TIME: **10 minutes**   COOK TIME: **7 minutes**   SERVES: **4**

COCONUT-FREE • EGG-FREE • NUT-FREE   OPTIONS: LOW-FODMAP • NIGHTSHADE-FREE

Wah! This salad is so good. I could eat it every day . . . and I don't even like squid! If you can do dairy, I bet feta cheese would be unreal on this. The whole time I was eating it (I made it four times just to be sure I had it right), I was cursing my dairy allergy to the moon and back. Feta cheese or not, this salad is good . . . and quick!

12 ounces (340 g) uncooked calamari rings, defrosted

1½ cups (210 g) grape tomatoes, halved

½ cup (60 g) pitted kalamata olives, halved

½ packed cup (35 g) chopped fresh parsley

¼ cup (20 g) sliced green onions

DRESSING:

½ cup (120 ml) extra-virgin olive oil or refined avocado oil

1 tablespoon red wine vinegar

Grated zest of ½ lemon

Juice of ½ lemon

2 small cloves garlic, minced

¼ teaspoon finely ground gray sea salt

¼ teaspoon ground black pepper

1. Place the calamari in a steamer and steam for 7 minutes. Transfer to the freezer to cool for a couple of minutes.

2. Meanwhile, make the dressing: Place the ingredients for the dressing in a small bowl. Whisk to combine and set aside.

3. Once the calamari has cooled, place it in a large bowl along with the grape tomatoes, olives, parsley, and green onions. Add the dressing and toss to coat.

4. Divide among 4 serving plates and enjoy.

MAKE IT A CARB-UP: *Replace half of the olive oil with water. Serve alongside the carb of your choice (find ideas on page 117, or visit healthfulpursuit.com/carbup to download the complimentary PDF "Carb-Up Recipes"). It's delicious with precooked and cooled white rice stirred into the salad in Step 3.*

STORE IT: *Keep in an airtight container in the fridge for up to 3 days.*

SERVE IT WITH: *To make this a complete meal, serve it on a bed of mixed salad greens.*

MAKE IT LOW-FODMAP: *Omit the garlic. Replace 2 tablespoons of the olive oil with 2 tablespoons of Garlic-Infused Oil (page 230).*

MAKE IT NIGHTSHADE-FREE: *Replace the grape tomatoes with your favorite chopped vegetables. A mixture of steamed and cooled cauliflower and broccoli is nice in this salad!*

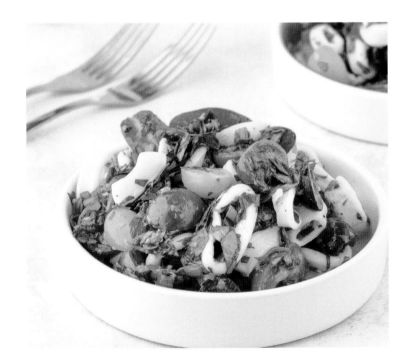

NUTRIENT INFORMATION (PER SERVING):

calories: 507 | calories from fat: 270 | total fat: 30g | saturated fat: 5.4g | cholesterol: 765mg

sodium: 1278mg | carbs: 4.3g | dietary fiber: 1.6g | net carbs: 2.7g | sugars: 1.8g | protein: 55g

RATIOS:

fat:	carbs:	protein:
54%	3%	43%

VERDE CAESAR SALAD WITH CRISPY CAPERS

PREP TIME: **10 minutes**   COOK TIME: **4 minutes**   SERVES: **4**

COCONUT-FREE • NUT-FREE   OPTIONS: EGG-FREE • LOW-FODMAP • VEGAN

Fat bombs come in all shapes and sizes, and this fat-filled salad is a perfect example. Coming from a diet culture that runs on dressing-less salads, or store-bought fat-free dressings, this fatty green salad will make you feel like a rebel with every bite. And I don't know about you, but when I was a kid, before I was told that dressing was "bad and fatty," the dressing was my favorite part of eating salad. So dig in to this green salad loaded with ketone-inducing MCT oil.

CRISPY CAPERS:

2 tablespoons refined avocado oil or refined olive oil

2 tablespoons capers, drained and patted dry

SALAD:

4 cups (140 g) arugula

¼ packed cup (20 g) fresh basil leaves, chopped

¼ packed cup (20 g) fresh cilantro leaves, chopped

¼ packed cup (10 g) fresh parsley leaves, chopped

¼ cup (37 g) hulled hemp seeds

½ cup (120 ml) Classic Caesar Dressing (page 224)

1. Place the avocado oil in a small frying pan over medium heat for 1 minute. Add the capers and fry until crispy, rotating every minute, about 4 minutes total. Transfer to a clean plate.

2. Place the arugula, herbs, and hemp seeds in a large bowl and toss to combine.

3. When ready to serve the salad, pour the Caesar dressing over the salad and toss to coat.

4. Divide the dressed salad among 4 salad bowls or plates and drop 2 teaspoons of crispy capers on top of each salad. Serve immediately.

MAKE IT LOW-FODMAP: *Follow the low-FODMAP instructions for the Classic Caesar Dressing.*

STORE IT: *Keep the components—crispy capers, salad, and dressing—in separate airtight containers in the fridge for up to 3 days. Follow Steps 3 and 4 to assemble the salad when ready to consume.*

PREP AHEAD: *Prepare the salad up to 2 days beforehand, keeping the components—crispy capers, salad, and dressing—separate. Follow Steps 3 and 4 to assemble the salad when ready to consume.*

SERVE IT WITH: *To make this a complete meal, top the salad with grilled and cooled chicken thighs or breasts. It tastes great with Rosemary Garlic Croutons (page 374).*

MAKE IT EGG-FREE/VEGAN: *Dress the salad with Vegan Caesar Dressing (page 224) instead of Classic Caesar Dressing.*

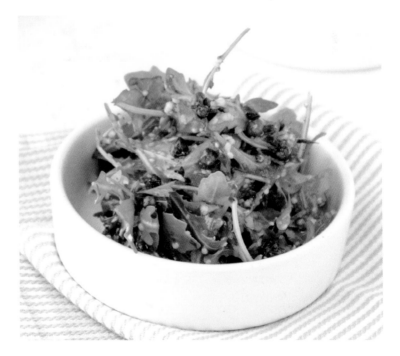

NUTRIENT INFORMATION (PER SERVING):

calories: 317 | calories from fat: 281 | total fat: 31.2g | saturated fat: 16.3g | cholesterol: 3mg

sodium: 263mg | carbs: 3.3g | dietary fiber: 1.9g | net carbs: 1.4g | sugars: 0.9g | protein: 5.8g

RATIOS:

fat:	carbs:	protein:
89%	4%	7%

GRILLED ROMAINE AND SCALLOP SALAD

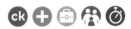

PREP TIME: **10 minutes**   COOK TIME: **5 minutes**   SERVES: **4**

COCONUT-FREE · EGG-FREE · LOW-FODMAP · NUT-FREE   OPTION: NIGHTSHADE-FREE

Kevin has always been really good at planning romantic nights out, accompanying me to beautiful restaurants where the food is good and the service is excellent. There's one restaurant in the city that we've been to a couple of times that makes a delicious grilled romaine and scallop salad. Topped with crushed bacon and a balsamic reduction, it's enough to make this low-carb girl weak in the knees! Because I love the challenge of recreating my favorite restaurant eats, this is my take on that delicious salad, made simpler because I like to spend as little time in the kitchen as possible.

Simplify this recipe even further by replacing the homemade seafood seasoning mixture with about 2¾ teaspoons of a store-bought variety.

SCALLOPS:

5 tablespoons refined avocado oil, divided

1 pound (455 g) wild bay scallops

1 teaspoon celery salt

½ teaspoon mustard powder

½ teaspoon red pepper flakes

¼ teaspoon ground black pepper

⅛ teaspoon ground allspice

⅛ teaspoon ground cloves

⅛ teaspoon ginger powder

⅛ teaspoon ground cardamom

⅛ teaspoon ground cinnamon

ROMAINE:

¼ cup (60 ml) refined avocado oil

2 tablespoons balsamic vinegar

1 tablespoon dried oregano leaves

½ teaspoon finely ground gray sea salt

½ teaspoon ground black pepper

2 heads romaine hearts (about 14 ounces/400 g), halved lengthwise

FOR SERVING:

¼ cup (20 g) finely chopped fresh cilantro

1. Preheat the grill to medium (350°F/177°C) or heat up a grill pan on the stovetop over medium heat. (Or you can broil the romaine rather than grill it, if you prefer.)

2. Prepare the scallops: Heat 3 tablespoons of the avocado oil in a large frying pan over medium heat. While the oil heats up, thoroughly dry the scallops, place them in a bowl, and drizzle with the remaining 2 tablespoons of avocado oil. In a small dish, combine the celery salt, mustard powder, red pepper flakes, black pepper, allspice, cloves, ginger powder, cardamom, and cinnamon. Sprinkle the spice mixture over the scallops and gently toss to coat.

3. Transfer the scallops to the hot frying pan and sear for 3 minutes, untouched, then turn them over and sear for another 2 minutes. Immediately remove the scallops from the pan and set at the back of the stove to keep warm.

4. Meanwhile, prepare the romaine: Combine the ¼ cup (60 ml) of avocado oil with the vinegar, oregano, salt, and pepper. Brush some of the dressing mixture onto the cut surface of the romaine heart halves. Place the romaine halves, cut side down, on the preheated grill or grill pan for 1 to 2 minutes, until grill marks appear. (If broiling the romaine, place an oven rack in the top position, turn the broiler to high, place the romaine halves cut side up on a rimmed baking sheet, then broil for 2 to 3 minutes, until the edges have turned golden.)

5. To serve, transfer the grilled romaine to a large serving plate. Top with the cooked scallops, then drizzle with the remaining dressing and sprinkle on the chopped cilantro.

STORE IT: *Keep in an airtight container in the fridge for up to 2 days.*

MAKE IT NIGHTSHADE-FREE: *Omit the red pepper flakes.*

MAKE IT A CARB-UP: *Reduce the amount of avocado oil to 2 tablespoons: 1 teaspoon for sautéing, 2 teaspoons for grilling, and 1 tablespoon for the dressing. Serve alongside the carb of your choice (find ideas on page 117, or visit healthfulpursuit.com/carbup to download the complimentary PDF "Carb-Up Recipes"). It's scrumptious with sautéed or roasted yams, kabocha squash, or grilled cassava.*

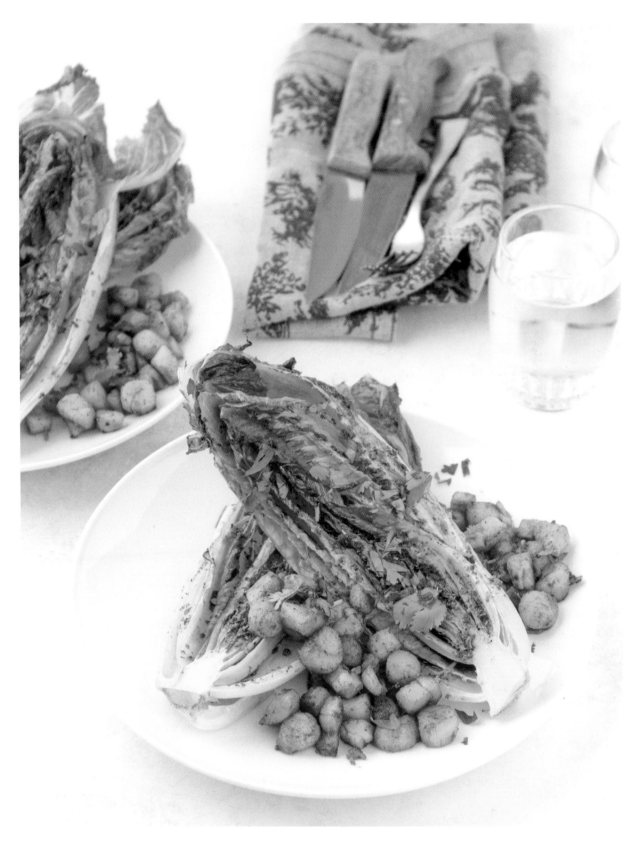

NUTRIENT INFORMATION (PER SERVING):

calories: 403 | calories from fat: 289 | total fat: 32.1g | saturated fat: 4.1g | cholesterol: 38mg

sodium: 430mg | carbs: 7.7g | dietary fiber: 1g | net carbs: 6.7g | sugars: 0g | protein: 20.7g

RATIOS:

fat: carbs: protein:

72% 8% 20%

SPINACH SALAD WITH FLANK STEAK

PREP TIME: **15 minutes, plus 24 hours to marinate steak**   COOK TIME: **12 minutes**   SERVES: **6**

COCONUT-FREE · EGG-FREE · NIGHTSHADE-FREE   OPTIONS: LOW-FODMAP · NUT-FREE

Flank steak is known as a particularly flavorful cut, but it's also known for its potentially chewy texture if not prepared properly. Sounds intimidating, right? Tackling flank steak always made me nervous, so I never, ever prepared it…until the day I made this recipe! And the cool part is, I only had to do it once to obtain perfection. Now, I'm not afraid of flank steak. In fact, it's part of our weekly rotation. It's that easy! The major requirement here is the marinating time. Don't shorten it; just don't.

Raw nuts are fine to use, but for health reasons, it's better to soak and roast them before using them in this recipe (see page 157).

STEAK:

3 tablespoons refined avocado oil

3 tablespoons fresh lemon juice

¼ teaspoon ground cloves

¼ teaspoon ground black pepper

1⅔ pounds (750 g) flank steak

SALAD:

8 cups (560 g) fresh spinach

2 cups (170 g) sliced red cabbage

1 cup (120 g) diced zucchini

½ cup (70 g) roughly chopped raw pecans

2 tablespoons capers

1 batch Red Wine Vinaigrette (page 227)

1. The day before you plan to enjoy this meal, marinate the steak: Place the avocado oil, lemon juice, ground cloves, and black pepper in a large casserole dish. Whisk to combine, then add the steak. Flip a couple of times to coat, then cover and place in the fridge for 24 hours.

2. When you're ready to prepare the recipe, place an oven rack in the top position. Set the broiler to high (if your oven broiler doesn't have a high setting, simply "broil" is fine). Place the marinated steak in a cast-iron pan or broiler pan lined with foil.

3. Broil the steak for 4 to 6 minutes per side, depending on the desired doneness. Eight minutes of total cooking time will yield medium-rare steak; 12 minutes, medium-done steak. Remove from the oven and let rest for 5 minutes.

4. Meanwhile, prepare the salad: Place all the ingredients, except the vinaigrette, in a large bowl. Pour the vinaigrette over the top and toss to combine. Divide the dressed salad equally among 6 plates.

5. Return to the steak: You will see pronounced muscle fibers running along the top of the steak. Set the steak on a cutting board with the muscle fibers running from left to right, and, using a sharp knife, cut the steak at a right angle to the grain, from the top down. Cutting in this manner makes the steak much more tender and enjoyable to eat.

6. Top the salads with the sliced steak and serve.

STORE IT: *Undressed salad and meat will keep in an airtight container for up to 3 days. Once dressed, the salad should be eaten right away, unless you're a lover of soupy salads.*

MAKE IT LOW-FODMAP: *Follow the low-FODMAP instructions for Red Wine Vinaigrette.*

MAKE IT NUT-FREE: *Replace the chopped pecans with the seed of your choice. Roasted pine nuts or hulled sunflower seeds would be nice in this recipe.*

NUTRIENT INFORMATION (PER SERVING):

calories: 568 | calories from fat: 388 | total fat: 43.1g | saturated fat: 8.7g | cholesterol: 69mg

sodium: 307mg | carbs: 6.5g | dietary fiber: 3.4g | net carbs: 3.1g | sugars: 2.1g | protein: 38.5g

RATIOS:

fat:	carbs:	protein:
68%	5%	27%

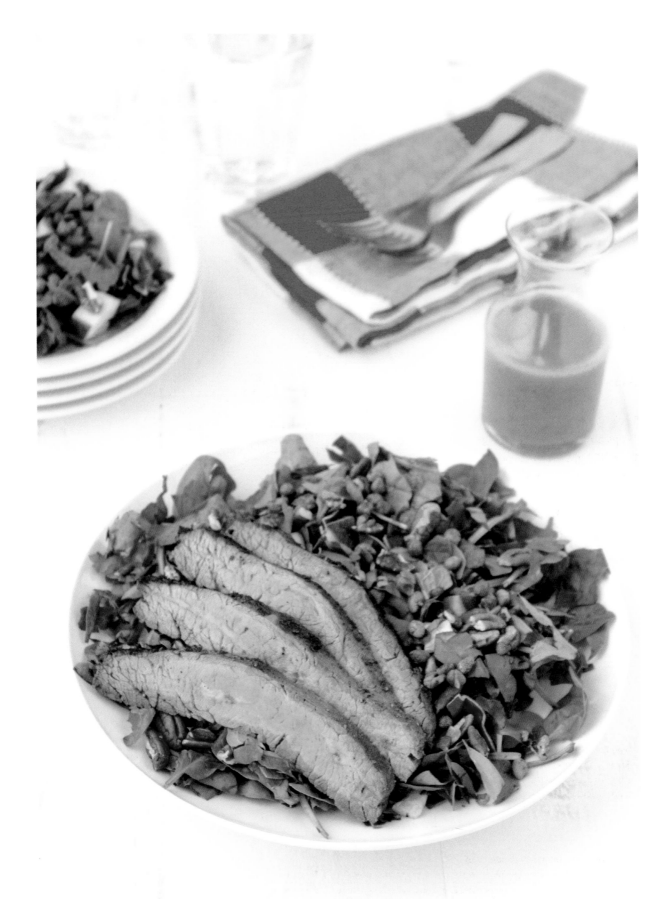

BERRY AVOCADO SALAD

PREP TIME: **10 minutes**   SERVES: **4**

COCONUT-FREE • EGG-FREE • NUT-FREE • VEGAN

This summery salad is perfect for your next barbecue, especially if you serve it as a side salad with a batch of Bendy Tortillas (page 370) filled with taco meat. If you're going to prepare this salad a couple of hours ahead of serving it, keep the avocado pits and place them in the salad—the pits will keep the cubed avocados from turning brown.

DRESSING:

2 tablespoons extra-virgin olive oil or refined avocado oil

1½ teaspoons fresh lime juice

1½ teaspoons chili powder

1 small clove garlic, minced

2 drops liquid stevia

Finely ground gray sea salt, to taste

SALAD:

2 large Hass avocados, skinned, pitted, and cubed (12 ounces/340 g flesh)

12 strawberries, cut into quarters or eighths (depending on size)

½ packed cup (30 g) fresh parsley, chopped

1 packed tablespoon fresh cilantro leaves, chopped

1 tablespoon finely diced white onion

STORE IT: *Best enjoyed immediately. However, you can store in airtight container in the fridge for up to 1 day if absolutely necessary.*

1. Place the ingredients for the dressing in a large bowl and whisk to combine. Add the salad ingredients and toss gently to coat.

2. Divide the salad among 4 bowls and serve immediately.

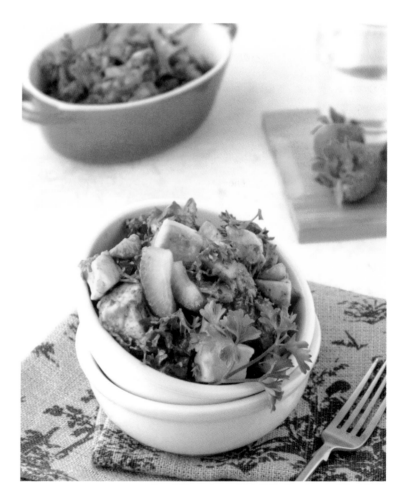

NUTRIENT INFORMATION (PER SERVING):

calories: 259 | calories from fat: 194 | total fat: 21.5g | saturated fat: 3.9g | cholesterol: 0mg

sodium: 73mg | carbs: 12.8g | dietary fiber: 9.9g | net carbs: 2.9g | sugars: 2g | protein: 3.5g

RATIOS:

fat:	carbs:	protein:
75%	20%	5%

MARINATED BOK CHOY SALAD

PREP TIME: **20 minutes + overnight**   SERVES: **6**

EGG-FREE · NIGHTSHADE-FREE · VEGAN   OPTIONS: COCONUT-FREE · NUT-FREE

I first made this salad back in 2007 and have been making it every week since. No joke. It's one of my favorite fridge-friendly recipes that packs well for lunches, road trips, or family barbecues.

After the bok choy has marinated overnight, this salad has a bit of liquid at the bottom. And the liquid is delicious! I love serving this salad alongside plain cauliflower rice (page 364), Creamy Mashed Turnips (page 382), or Roasted Brussels Sprouts with Walnut "Cheese" (page 388) so that the other vegetables soak up the liquidy goodness.

Raw nuts are fine to use, but for health reasons, it's better to soak and roast them before using them in this recipe (see page 157).

DRESSING:

⅓ cup (80 ml) extra-virgin olive oil or refined avocado oil

3 tablespoons MCT oil

3 tablespoons apple cider vinegar

2 tablespoons coconut aminos

4 small cloves garlic, minced

1 (2-inch/5-cm) piece fresh ginger root, minced

2 teaspoons prepared yellow mustard

¼ teaspoon finely ground gray sea salt

¼ teaspoon ground black pepper

2 drops liquid stevia

SALAD:

8 cups (900 g) chopped bok choy (about 1 large head)

⅓ cup (40 g) sliced raw almonds, divided

> STORE IT: *Keep in an airtight container in the fridge for up to 3 days.*
>
> PREP AHEAD: *Prepare the dressing up to 1 day before making the salad.*

1. Combine the ingredients for the dressing in a large bowl.

2. Add the bok choy and ¼ cup (30 g) of the sliced almonds. Toss to coat. Cover the bowl and place in the fridge for at least 12 hours, but not longer than 3 days.

3. When ready to serve, divide the salad among 6 bowls and sprinkle each salad with the remaining sliced almonds.

> SERVE IT WITH: *To make this a complete meal, top it with cooked ground pork. This salad tastes great paired with plain or Greek Cauliflower Rice (page 364).*
>
> MAKE IT COCONUT-FREE: *Replace the MCT oil with olive oil, unrefined canola oil, or refined avocado oil. Replace the coconut aminos with a wheat-free soy sauce, if you tolerate soy.*
>
> MAKE IT NUT-FREE: *Replace the sliced almonds with sunflower seeds or hulled hemp seeds.*

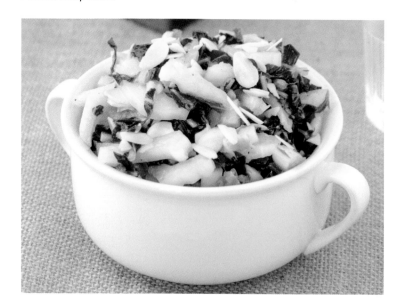

NUTRIENT INFORMATION (PER SERVING):

calories: 234 | calories from fat: 191 | total fat: 21.3g | saturated fat: 8.9g | cholesterol: 0mg

sodium: 201mg | carbs: 6.9g | dietary fiber: 2.4g | net carbs: 4.5g | sugars: 2.1g | protein: 3.7g

RATIOS:

fat: carbs: protein:

82%   12%   6%

CURRIED OKRA SALAD

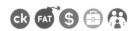

PREP TIME: **15 minutes** | COOK TIME: **15 minutes** | SERVES: **4**

EGG-FREE • NUT-FREE • VEGAN   OPTIONS: COCONUT-FREE • NIGHTSHADE-FREE

If you haven't had okra before, this salad is an awesome introduction. You can find okra in the produce section of many grocery stores, generally where the eggplants and lemongrass are kept. When cut, you may notice that they're a bit slimy. Don't let the sliminess deter you, it's normal!

If you don't have curry powder, or don't want to make your own, Garam Masala is also delicious in this salad.

FRIED OKRA:

¼ cup (55 g) plus 2 tablespoons coconut oil, divided

15 ounces (420 g) okra, trimmed and quartered lengthwise

SALAD:

¾ packed cup (60 g) fresh cilantro leaves, chopped

1 large tomato (about 2½ ounces/70 g), diced

½ small red onion, sliced (optional)

DRESSING:

⅓ cup (80 ml) extra-virgin olive oil, unrefined canola oil, or refined avocado oil

2 tablespoons fresh lemon juice

2 teaspoons Curry Powder (page 235)

¼ teaspoon finely ground gray sea salt

2 drops liquid stevia

---

1. Melt ¼ cup (55 g) of the coconut oil in a large frying pan over medium-high heat. Place half of the okra in the pan and fry for 6 to 8 minutes, until the pieces are browned. Transfer the browned okra pieces to a clean plate, add the remaining 2 tablespoons of oil to the pan, and repeat with the remaining okra.

2. Meanwhile, place the ingredients for the salad in a large bowl. After all the okra is browned, transfer it to the bowl with the salad.

3. In a separate small bowl, whisk together the ingredients for the dressing, then drizzle the dressing over the salad and toss to coat. Divide among 4 salad bowls and serve.

STORE IT: *Keep in an airtight container in the fridge for up to 3 days.*

PREP AHEAD: *Brown the okra and store it in an airtight container in the fridge for up to 1 day before preparing the salad. The dressing can be made up to 2 days ahead and stored in an airtight container in the fridge until ready to use.*

MAKE IT COCONUT-FREE: *Use lard in place of the coconut oil.*

MAKE IT NIGHTSHADE-FREE: *Replace the tomato with 1 medium zucchini, diced. Omit the dried chili peppers from the curry powder in the dressing.*

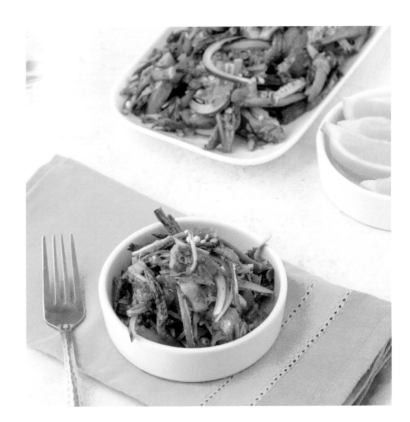

NUTRIENT INFORMATION (PER SERVING):

calories: 390 | calories from fat: 341 | total fat: 37.9g | saturated fat: 20.2g | cholesterol: 0mg

sodium: 152mg | carbs: 9.2g | dietary fiber: 4.6g | net carbs: 4.6g | sugars: 2.3g | protein: 3g

RATIOS:

fat:	carbs:	protein:
88%	9%	3%

SHAVED CUCUMBER AND SMOKED SALMON SALAD

PREP TIME: **10 minutes**   SERVES: **4**

EGG-FREE • NIGHTSHADE-FREE • NUT-FREE   OPTIONS: COCONUT-FREE • LOW-FODMAP • VEGAN

I enjoy salads that can be made into meals in less than ten minutes flat. This salad is one of the recipes that I go to time and time again. Once you've tried it, and fallen in love, make it with a batch of Zoodles (page 376) in place of the cucumber ribbons for a fun adjustment.

You could add 2 tablespoons of diced red onion to this recipe, if you enjoy onions. We're a pretty low-onion household so I always forget to add them. But I know this recipe would fabulous with them, or the same amount of sliced chives or green onions.

DRESSING:

⅓ cup (80 ml) full-fat coconut milk

Grated zest of ½ lemon

Juice of ½ lemon

¼ teaspoon finely ground gray sea salt

¼ teaspoon ground black pepper, plus more for garnish

SALAD:

2 English cucumbers, cut in half crosswise

8 ounces (225 g) smoked salmon, crumbled

2 packed tablespoons fresh dill, chopped, plus more for garnish

STORE IT: *Keep in an airtight container in the fridge for up to 1 day, straining the liquid from the cucumbers that have settled at the bottom of the container, before serving.*

PREP AHEAD: *Prepare the dressing up to 2 days before assembling the salad.*

SERVE WITH: *To make this a complete meal, double the smoked salmon and serve drizzled with 2 tablespoons of MCT oil per serving.*

MAKE IT COCONUT-FREE: *Replace the coconut milk with mayonnaise.*

MAKE IT LOW-FODMAP: *If you are super sensitive to coconut milk, replace the coconut milk with mayonnaise.*

MAKE IT VEGAN: *Replace the salmon with ½ cup hulled hemp seeds.*

1. Place the dressing ingredients in a large bowl and whisk to combine.

2. Take a cucumber and place it in your non-dominant hand. Hold it over the bowl with the dressing and, with the opposite hand, begin peeling the cucumber with a vegetable peeler.

3. Repeat the action until most of the cucumber has been peeled, and only a small, long core remains in your hand.

4. Repeat with the remaining cucumber halves.

5. Add the remaining salad ingredients and toss gently to coat.

6. Divide among 4 salad bowls and garnish with additional fresh dill and black pepper.

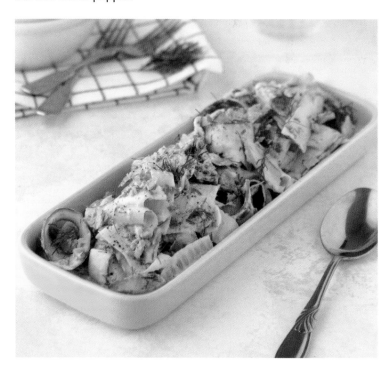

NUTRIENT INFORMATION (PER SERVING):
calories: 138 | calories from fat: 59 | total fat: 6.5g | saturated fat: 4.2g | cholesterol: 13mg
sodium: 1229mg | carbs: 6.7g | dietary fiber: 2.6g | net carbs: 4.1g | sugars: 2.7g | protein: 13.1g

RATIOS:

fat:	carbs:	protein:
43%	**19%**	**38%**

BACON-WRAPPED MINI MEATLOAVES

   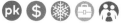

PREP TIME: **10 minutes**   COOK TIME: **about 30 minutes**   MAKES: **8 (8 servings)**

COCONUT-FREE • EGG-FREE • NUT-FREE   OPTION: LOW-FODMAP

You could make a classic meatloaf, or you could have fun with these small meatloaves, which require no cooling time after cooking before being sliced. Bake and enjoy quickly! Plus, they make really great leftovers, enjoyed hot or cold.

1 pound (455 g) ground beef (20% to 30% fat)

⅓ cup (22 g) nutritional yeast

¼ cup (60 ml) Kickin' Ketchup (page 223)

1 tablespoon prepared yellow mustard

¾ teaspoon finely ground gray sea salt

¼ teaspoon ground black pepper

8 strips bacon (about 8 ounces/240 g)

STORE IT: *Keep in an airtight container in the fridge for up to 4 days or in the freezer for up to 1 month.*

REHEAT IT: *Microwave until the desired temperature is reached. Or place in a covered casserole dish and reheat in a preheated 300°F (150°C) oven for 5 minutes, or until warmed through.*

THAW IT: *Allow to thaw completely in the fridge. Once defrosted, enjoy cold or use the reheating instructions above.*

SERVE IT WITH: *To make this a complete meal, serve alongside a green salad dressed with your favorite dressing or roasted vegetables drizzled with your favorite oil.*

This tastes great paired with Creamy Mashed Turnips (page 382) or served with dipping sauces, such as mayonnaise (page 220), Kickin' Ketchup (page 223), or mustard.

1. Preheat the oven to 350°F (177°C) and have on hand a large cast-iron frying pan.

2. Place the ground beef, nutritional yeast, ketchup, mustard, salt, and pepper in a medium-sized bowl. Using your hands, mix the ingredients together until well combined.

3. Divide the mixture into 8 equal portions. Take a portion and roll it between your hands to create a 3 by 1½-inch (7.5 by 4 cm) cylinder. Wrap one strip of bacon around the cylinder. Place the wrapped cylinder in the cast-iron pan with the loose bacon ends tucked underneath. Repeat with the remaining meat, spacing the wrapped cylinders at least ½ inch (1.25 cm) apart in the pan.

4. Once complete, transfer the mini meatloaves to the oven and bake for 30 minutes, or until the internal temperature reaches 165°F (74°C).

5. Set your oven broiler to high, keeping the oven rack in the middle of the oven. Broil the meatloaves for up to 2 minutes, just until the bacon has become crisp.

6. Remove the meatloaves from the oven and serve.

MAKE IT LOW-FODMAP: *Ensure that the mustard you are using is free of garlic and onions, or replace prepared mustard with 2 teaspoons of ground mustard mixed with 1 teaspoon of water. If you are very sensitive to FODMAP-rich foods, you may react to the sun-dried tomatoes in the Kickin' Ketchup if you enjoy more than one mini meatloaf.*

NUTRIENT INFORMATION (PER MINI MEATLOAF):

calories: 375 | calories from fat: 239 | total fat: 26.6g | saturated fat: 8.6g | cholesterol: 83mg
sodium: 986mg | carbs: 4.8g | dietary fiber: 2g | net carbs: 2.8g | sugars: 0.7g | protein: 29.2g

RATIOS:

fat:	carbs:	protein:
64%	**5%**	**31%**

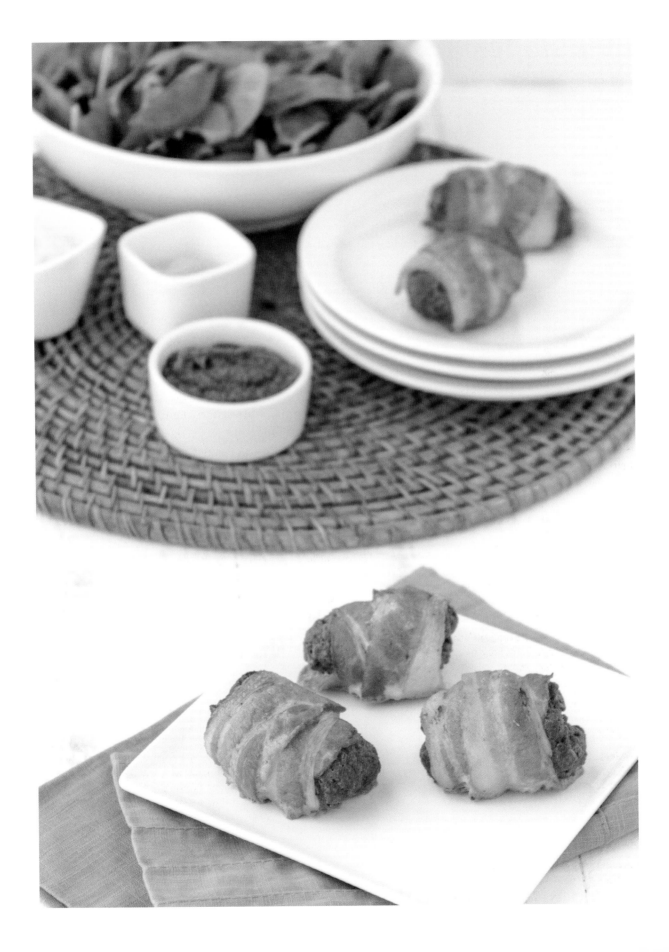

BEEF STROGANOFF

PREP TIME: **15 minutes**   COOK TIME: **1 hour**   SERVES: **8**

EGG-FREE · NIGHTSHADE-FREE · NUT-FREE   OPTIONS: COCONUT-FREE · LOW-FODMAP

I'm pleased, elated, and amazed that this beef stroganoff, without the use of starches, has one of the richest, most delicious gravies I've ever enjoyed. The key is in the gelatin!

I find the beef chuck roast easier to cut when it's still just slightly frozen.

⅔ cup (160 ml) beef bone broth (see page 152)

¼ cup (40 g) unflavored gelatin

2 pounds (910 g) beef chuck roast

1¼ teaspoons finely ground gray sea salt

½ teaspoon ground black pepper

½ cup (105 g) butter-infused coconut oil, melted

6 green onions, green parts only, finely chopped

2 teaspoons prepared yellow mustard

⅓ cup (80 ml) full-fat coconut milk

¼ cup (60 ml) white wine, such as Pinot Grigio, Sauvignon Blanc, or unoaked Chardonnay

8 white mushrooms (about 4 ounces/115 g), sliced

2 batches Zoodles (page 376), for serving

Sliced green onions, green part only, for garnish (optional)

1. Place the bone broth in a bowl. Sprinkle with the gelatin and set aside.

2. Melt the coconut oil in a large saucepan or deep-sided sauté pan over medium-high heat. Meanwhile, cut the chuck roast into ½ by 2-inch (1.25 by 5-cm) strips. Coat in the salt and pepper and transfer to the pan. Do not overcrowd the pan; cook in batches if needed.

3. Cook on medium-high heat for 3 minutes, flipping halfway through, until all pieces are browned.

4. Add the green onions and continue to cook for 3 minutes.

5. Whisk the broth mixture and, once smooth, add it to the pot along with the mustard. Cover and bring to a boil. Once boiling, reduce the heat to medium-low and simmer for 45 minutes, until the meat is tender. Then add the coconut milk, wine, and sliced mushrooms. Simmer, uncovered, for 15 minutes, or until the gravy has thickened.

6. Remove the pan from the heat and allow the stroganoff to sit, covered, for 15 minutes before serving. Divide the Zoodles among 8 bowls and ladle the stroganoff over the top. Garnish with sliced green onions, if desired.

STORE IT: *Keep in an airtight container in the fridge for up to 4 days or freeze the beef only for up to 1 month.*

REHEAT IT: *Microwave covered or place in a frying pan and fry on medium heat until the desired temperature is reached. If zoodles are stored with beef, this is okay.*

THAW IT: *Allow to thaw completely in the fridge. Once defrosted, use the reheating instructions above.*

PRESSURE-COOK IT: *In Step 2, transfer to a pressure cooker. In Step 3, set to the "sauté" setting and cook for 5 minutes, or until the meat is lightly browned. In Step 5, cover and set to high pressure for 20 minutes. Allow the pressure to release, then remove the lid. Add the coconut milk, wine, and sliced mushrooms, then set to "sauté" and cook for 10 to 15 minutes, until the gravy has thickened.*

MAKE IT COCONUT-FREE: *Replace the coconut oil with lard or ghee (if tolerated), and replace the coconut milk with your favorite nondairy milk.*

MAKE IT LOW-FODMAP: *Ensure you're using onion-free and garlic-free broth and mustard. If desired, replace the prepared mustard with 1 teaspoon of mustard powder mixed with 1 teaspoon of water. Omit the wine and mushrooms.*

NUTRIENT INFORMATION (PER SERVING):

calories: 598 | calories from fat: 427 | total fat: 47.5g | saturated fat: 26.2g | cholesterol: 117mg
sodium: 475mg | carbs: 5.7g | dietary fiber: 1.5g | net carbs: 4.2g | sugars: 2.3g | protein: 36.8g

RATIOS:

fat:	carbs:	protein:
72%	4%	24%

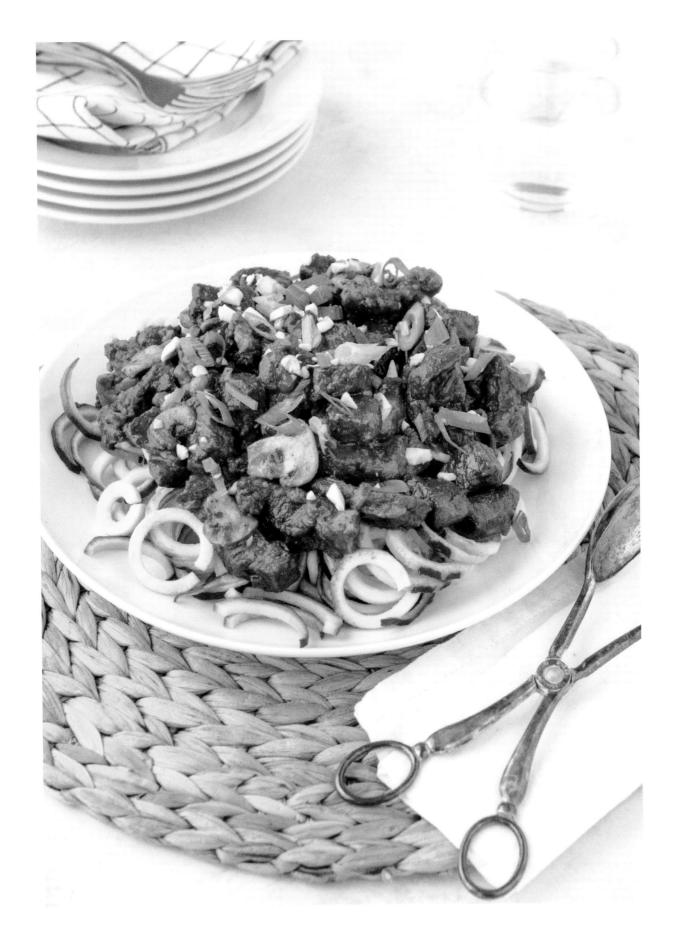

BOMBAY SLOPPY JOLENES

PREP TIME: **15 minutes**   COOK TIME: **40 minutes**   SERVES: **8**

EGG-FREE   OPTIONS: COCONUT-FREE • LOW-FODMAP • NUT-FREE

We all know and love sloppy joes. And while that recipe is a classic, sometimes classics need a little twist! If you enjoy ethnic-inspired dishes, look no further than these Sloppy Jolenes. Why Jolene? This recipe is prettier than your average Joe, so "Joe" just didn't fit here. The endive cups make enjoying this recipe a lot easier than soggy bread everywhere and meat sliding from your chin.

Raw nuts are fine to use, but for health reasons, it's better to soak and roast them before using them in this recipe (see page 157).

¼ cup (60 ml) plus 1½ teaspoons refined avocado oil or melted tallow

¼ cup (40 g) finely diced red onions

1 (2 by 1-in/5 by 2.5-cm) piece fresh ginger root, minced

2 small cloves garlic, minced

1 teaspoon cumin seeds

1 pound (455 g) ground beef (20% to 30% fat)

1⅔ cups (390 ml) sugar-free tomato sauce

¾ cup (180 ml) water

1 to 2 whole dried chilis, crushed

2 teaspoons Curry Powder (page 235)

1 teaspoon finely ground gray sea salt

½ teaspoon paprika

⅓ cup (57 g) raw macadamia nut halves

½ cup (120 ml) full-fat coconut milk

1 tablespoon apple cider vinegar

¼ cup (15 g) fresh cilantro leaves, chopped, plus more for garnish (optional)

4 endives, leaves separated, for serving

1. In a large saucepan on medium heat, place ¼ cup (60 ml) of the oil, onion, ginger, garlic, and cumin seeds. Cook for 2 to 3 minutes, until fragrant.

2. Add the ground beef and cook until no longer pink, about 8 minutes, stirring often to break the meat up into small clumps.

3. Add the tomatoes, water, crushed chilis, curry powder, salt, and paprika and stir. Cover partially, letting steam escape. Bring to a boil, reduce the heat to medium-low and simmer for 25 minutes.

4. Meanwhile, place the macadamia nuts and remaining 1½ teaspoons of oil in a frying pan. Roast on medium-low for 2 to 3 minutes, tossing frequently, until lightly golden.

5. Once the 25 minutes are up, add the coconut milk and vinegar to the meat mixture. Remove the lid and cook on medium-high heat for 5 minutes, until thickened.

6. Meanwhile, divide the endive leaves among 8 plates.

7. Transfer the roasted macadamia nuts and chopped cilantro into the meat mixture and stir to combine.

8. Using a spoon, transfer the Sloppy Jolene mixture to the endive leaves. Garnish with additional cilantro, if desired.

STORE IT: *Keep assembled Jolenes in an airtight container in the fridge for up to 4 days or freeze the meat only for up to 1 month.*

REHEAT IT: *Microwave the meat only until the desired temperature is reached. Or place in a covered casserole dish and reheat in a preheated 300°F (150°C) oven for 10 to 15 minutes, until warmed through. Or reheat in a saucepan, covered, on medium-low.*

THAW IT: *Allow to thaw completely in the fridge. Once defrosted, use the reheating instructions above, or enjoy cold in a salad.*

SERVE IT WITH: *To make this a complete meal, serve alongside sliced cucumber.*

MAKE IT COCONUT-FREE: *Replace the coconut milk with ⅓ cup (80 ml) of your favorite nondairy milk.*

MAKE IT LOW-FODMAP: *Replace the diced red onions with ½ cup (40 g) of chopped green onions, green parts only. Omit the garlic and replace 2 tablespoons of the avocado oil or tallow used in Step 1 with Garlic-Infused Oil (page 230), made with refined avocado oil.*

MAKE IT NUT-FREE: *Omit the macadamia nuts or replace with hulled sunflower seeds.*

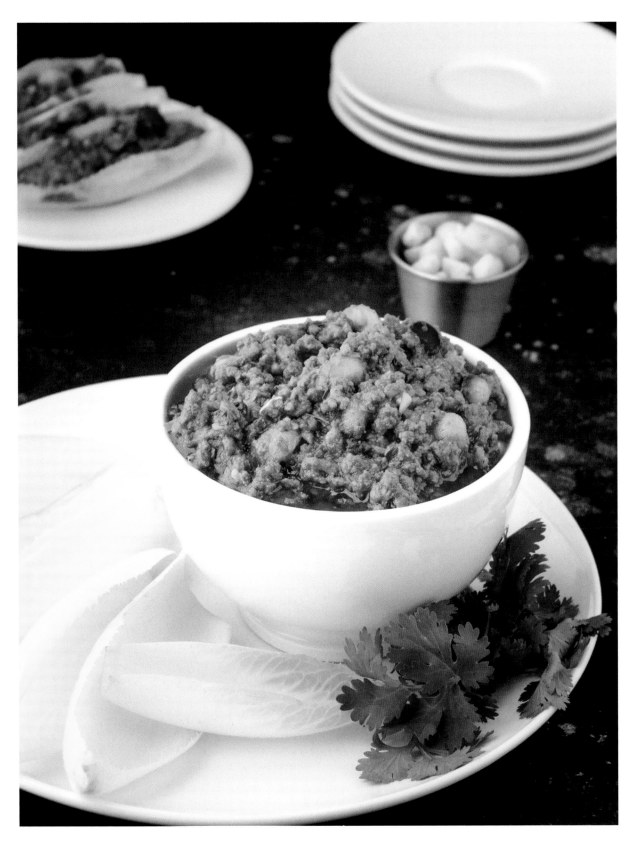

NUTRIENT INFORMATION (PER ⅓-CUP/180-G SERVING WITH ENDIVE LEAVES):

calories: 338 | calories from fat: 240 | total fat: 26.7g | saturated fat: 8.6g | cholesterol: 50mg

sodium: 693mg | carbs: 8.1g | dietary fiber: 2.8g | net carbs: 5.3g | sugars: 2.8g | protein: 16.4g

RATIOS:

fat:	carbs:	protein:
71%	10%	19%

CHILI-STUFFED AVOCADOS

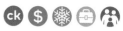

PREP TIME: **10 minutes**   COOK TIME: **30 minutes**   SERVES: **8**

COCONUT-FREE • EGG-FREE • NUT-FREE

When I make chili, I'm constantly cubing avocado and stirring it into the chili pot. One day, I thought how cool would it be if the chili was *in* the avocado. Well, this recipe is the result of that thought! And, it worked out fabulously.

My favorite way to enjoy these is with the chili spilling over the sides. While this makes the stuffed avocados way more fun to eat, it looks horribly messy and unappetizing, so the photo I took for this recipe has a little less chili stuffed into it than I personally like. If you're not serving fancy dinner guests, pack the avocados as much as you can! Messy is good!

2 tablespoons tallow or bacon grease

1 pound (455 g) ground beef (20% to 30% fat)

1 (14½-ounce/408-g/428-ml) can whole tomatoes with juices

1½ tablespoons chili powder

2 small cloves garlic, minced

2 teaspoons paprika

¾ teaspoon finely ground gray sea salt

¼ teaspoon ground cinnamon

2 tablespoons finely chopped fresh parsley

4 large Hass avocados, sliced in half, pits removed (leave skin on), for serving

1. Place the tallow into a large saucepan. Melt on medium heat before adding the ground beef. Cook until beef is no longer pink, 7 to 8 minutes, stirring often to break the meat up into small clumps.

2. Add the tomatoes, chili powder, garlic, paprika, salt, and cinnamon. Cover and bring to a boil on high heat. Once boiling, reduce the heat to medium-low and simmer for 20 to 25 minutes, with the cover slightly askew to let steam out.

3. Once thickened, remove from the heat and stir in the chopped parsley.

4. Place an avocado half on a small serving plate or on a platter if you plan to serve them family style. Scoop ⅓ scant cup (180 g) of chili into the hollow of the avocado, allowing the chili to spill over the sides, if need be. Repeat with remaining chili and avocados.

STORE IT: *Keep the meat only in an airtight container in the fridge for up to 4 days or in the freezer for up to 1 month. Use freshly sliced avocados for the leftover meat.*

REHEAT IT: *Microwave the meat only. Or place in a covered casserole dish and reheat in a preheated 300°F (150°C) oven for 10 to 15 minutes, until warmed through. Or reheat in a saucepan, covered, on medium-low.*

THAW IT: *Allow to thaw completely in the fridge. Once defrosted, enjoy cold or use the reheating instructions above.*

PRESSURE-COOK IT: *Place all the ingredients except the parsley and avocados in a pressure cooker. Seal and cook on high for 15 minutes. Allow the pressure to release, then remove the lid and proceed with Step 3.*

SERVE IT WITH: *Sliced cucumbers are a nice side with this dish.*

NUTRIENT INFORMATION (PER AVOCADO HALF WITH CHILI):

calories: 385 | calories from fat: 275 | total fat: 30.5g | saturated fat: 9.1g | cholesterol: 54mg

sodium: 251mg | carbs: 10.3g | dietary fiber: 7g | net carbs: 3.3g | sugars: 1.7g | protein: 17.2g

RATIOS:

fat: carbs: protein:

72%   10%   18%

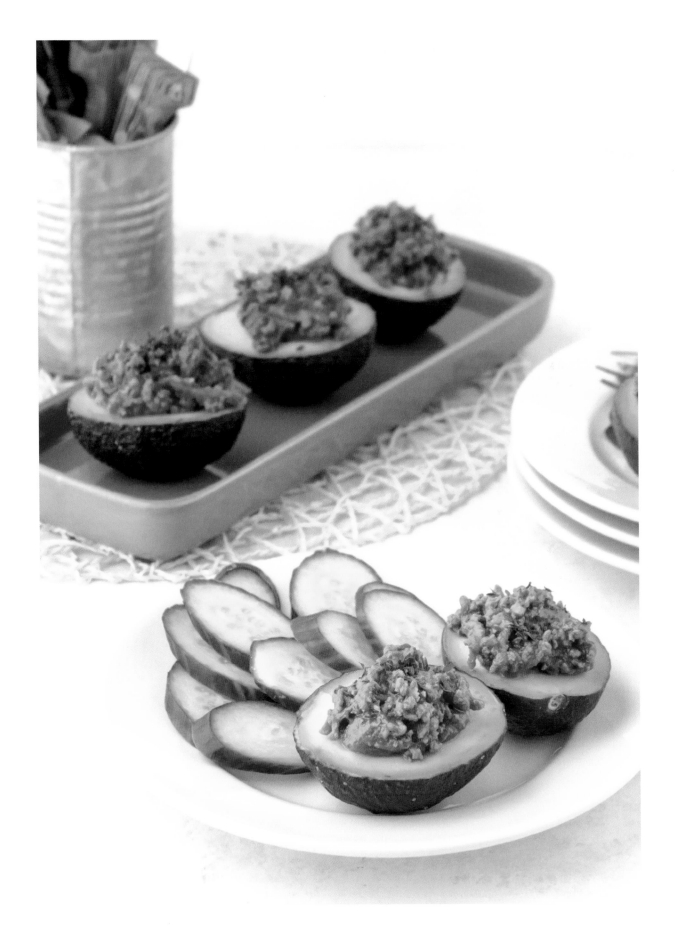

STEAK WITH TALLOW HERB BUTTER

PREP TIME: **10 minutes, plus 30 minutes to marinate steak**   COOK TIME: **4 to 8 minutes**   SERVES: **4**

COCONUT-FREE · EGG-FREE · NIGHTSHADE-FREE · NUT-FREE   OPTION: **LOW-FODMAP**

I'm an Albertan, so I grew up thinking that barbecuing in the dead of winter was totally commonplace. Turns out, normal people don't like trudging to their backyard when it's snowing to grill a steak. Weird. If you're one of these people, but also love enjoying a good steak when the weather isn't cooperating, this simple steak recipe is going to top your books. Everything is prepared and cooked in the kitchen, so you don't have to brave the cold for some good meat.

I chose to use beef strip loin for this recipe, but I've also used T-bone, porterhouse, and rib eye. Really, anything goes here.

You can prepare the tallow herb butter for any occasion. It's fabulous served with a batch of Crusty Sandwich Bread (page 366) or Classic Butter Biscuits (page 368), or dolloped on your favorite steamed vegetables.

13 ounces (370 g) boneless sirloin steak (aka strip steak or beef strip loin steak), about 1 inch (2.5 cm) thick

¾ teaspoon ground black pepper

¼ teaspoon garlic powder

¼ teaspoon finely ground gray sea salt

TALLOW HERB BUTTER:

¼ cup (52 g) tallow

1 sprig fresh thyme

1 sprig fresh rosemary

1 sprig fresh parsley

1 sprig fresh sage

STORE IT: *Keep in an airtight container in the fridge for up to 3 days or in the freezer for up to 1 month.*

REHEAT IT: *Place on a plate and microwave until the desired temperature is reached. Or place in a covered casserole dish and reheat in a preheated 300°F (150°C) oven for 10 minutes, or until warmed through.*

THAW IT: *Allow the steak to thaw completely in the fridge. Once defrosted, enjoy cold or use the reheating instructions above.*

PREP AHEAD: *Keep a batch of tallow herb butter in an airtight container in the fridge at all times. It will keep for several weeks in the fridge or several months in the freezer.*

SERVE IT WITH: *To make this a complete meal, serve alongside sautéed zucchini with fresh herbs. This tastes great paired with Potato Salad...That Isn't (page 386).*

1. Remove the steak from the fridge and place on a clean plate. Sprinkle the pepper, garlic powder, and salt over both sides of the steak. Wet your hands and rub the spices into the steak, on both sides, until a paste forms. If you require a bit more water, wet your hands again. Allow the coated steak to sit for 30 minutes.

2. Meanwhile, make the tallow herb butter: Melt the tallow in a small saucepan on medium heat. Add the remaining ingredients, cover, and reduce the heat to low. Simmer for 10 minutes. Once complete, strain the herbs and transfer the tallow herb butter back to the saucepan. Place the saucepan at the back of the stovetop, just to keep warm.

3. Ten minutes before the steak is ready, place an oven rack in the top position, place a large cast-iron frying pan on the rack, and turn the broiler on to high. (If your oven doesn't have a high/low setting for broil, simply set it to broil.)

4. Allow the cast-iron pan to heat up in the oven for 10 minutes. Wearing an oven mitt, remove the pan from the oven, leaving the broiler on. Place the pan on the stovetop and set the element to high.

5. Place the steak in the pan and sear for 30 seconds without moving it, then flip the steak over and sear the other side for 30 seconds. (Remember to use an oven mitt when touching the pan handle.)

6. Once seared, transfer the pan with the steak to the oven. Broil for 2 to 4 minutes, take the pan out of the oven and flip it, then return it to the oven to broil for another 2 to 4 minutes, depending on your desired doneness. (For medium-rare, cook for a total of 4 minutes; for medium, 5 minutes; for medium-well, 6 minutes; and for well-done, 8 minutes.)

MAKE IT LOW-FODMAP: *Omit the garlic powder.*

MAKE IT A CARB-UP: *Omit the herb butter and serve alongside the carb of your choice (find ideas on page 117, or visit healthfulpursuit.com/carbup to download the complimentary PDF "Carb-Up Recipes"). It's scrumptious with boiled potatoes, roasted cassava, or grilled delicata squash.*

7. Remove the pan from the oven and allow the steak to cool for 5 minutes.

8. Transfer to a cutting board to slice, divide among 4 plates, and drizzle with the tallow herb butter.

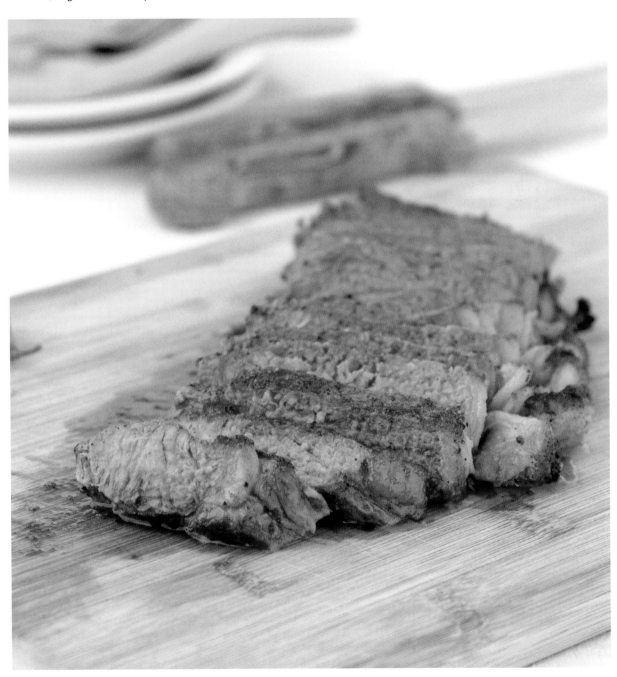

NUTRIENT INFORMATION (PER SERVING):

calories: 304 | calories from fat: 219 | total fat: 24.4g | saturated fat: 11g | cholesterol: 75mg

sodium: 163mg | carbs: 0.5g | dietary fiber: 0g | net carbs: 0.5g | sugars: 0g | protein: 20.5g

RATIOS:

fat:	carbs:	protein:
72%	1%	27%

MIND-BLOWING BURGERS

COCONUT-FREE • NUT-FREE   OPTIONS: EGG-FREE • LOW-FODMAP • NIGHTSHADE-FREE

The concept of mixing horseradish into your next batch of burger patties may sound a little weird, but it's anything but, I assure you. Whether you use this burger patty recipe or have one of your own, you must add horseradish to your next batch! The horseradish provides a slight kick without the need to rely on garlic or onions, and it keeps the patties moist, even if you accidentally overcook them a bit.

When purchasing horseradish, make sure to choose one that doesn't have loads of sugar! My favorite is Bubbies. If you want to get really crazy, use a horseradish that's made with beet powder. It'll make your burgers shine!

If you love barbecuing like I do, grill the patties to your liking. If barbecuing doesn't do it for you, I've included oven instructions as well.

BURGER PATTIES:

1 pound (455 g) ground beef (20% to 30% fat)

1 heaping tablespoon prepared horseradish

1½ teaspoons ground mustard

¼ teaspoon finely ground gray sea salt

¼ teaspoon ground black pepper

"BUNS":

1 medium eggplant, sliced into 3/8-inch (1-cm) thick rounds (about 10½ ounces/300 g edible portion)

3 tablespoons refined avocado oil or melted tallow

FIXINGS:

1 large Hass avocado, peeled, pitted, and mashed (about 6 ounces/170 g flesh)

6 tablespoons (90 ml) mayonnaise, homemade (page 220) or store-bought, or Kickin' Ketchup (page 223)

6 small lettuce leaves

> STORE IT: *Keep the assembled burgers in an airtight container in the fridge for up to 3 days. The patties only, cooked or raw, can be frozen for up to 1 month.*
>
> PREP AHEAD: *If you decide to prepare the patties ahead of time and store them in the freezer until use (this is great for camping), you can freeze them precooked, or freeze raw patties, placing a small square of parchment paper between each patty. My favorite way to store them this way is in coffee tins.*

1. Make the burgers: Preheat the oven to 375°F (190°C) and line a rimmed baking sheet with parchment paper or a silicone baking mat.

2. Place the burger patty ingredients in a medium-sized bowl. Mix with your hands until fully combined.

3. Divide the meat mixture into 6 equal portions, then shape into ½-inch (1.25-cm) thick patties.

4. Arrange the patties on the prepared baking sheet, leaving at least 1 inch (2.5 cm) of space between patties. Transfer to the oven and cook for 10 to 15 minutes, until the desired doneness is achieved. For medium-rare, cook for 10 minutes; for medium, 12 minutes; for medium-well, 14 minutes; and for well-done, 15 minutes.

5. Meanwhile, make the "buns": Place a large frying pan over medium-high heat. While the pan is heating up, place the eggplant slices in a bowl and drizzle them with avocado oil, turning them to ensure that the slices are evenly coated.

6. Transfer the coated eggplant slices to the frying pan. Sear for up to 1 minute per side, only until lightly golden. Repeat with the remaining slices, moving them to a cooling rack when done.

7. Assemble the burgers: Place an eggplant slice on a serving plate, top with a 1-ounce (28-g) scoop of mashed avocado, then place a patty on top, followed by a tablespoon of mayonnaise, a tablespoon of ketchup, a leaf of romaine, and a second eggplant slice. Repeat with the remaining fixings.

> VARIATION: GRILLED BURGERS. *Preheat a grill to medium-high, or 375°F (190°C). Complete Steps 2 and 3, then place the burgers on the hot grill. Cover the grill and cook for 3 minutes, then flip the burgers and cook for another 3 to 5 minutes. (For medium doneness, cook for a total of 6 minutes; for medium-well, 7 minutes; and for well-done, 8 minutes.) Continue with Steps 5 through 7.*

REHEAT IT: *To reheat the patties, microwave, covered, until the desired temperature is reached. Or place in a frying pan, cover, and fry on medium heat until the desired temperature is reached. Then assemble the burgers as described in Step 7.*

THAW IT: *If you froze the patties raw, allow them to thaw completely in the fridge. If you froze the patties after cooking, allow them to thaw completely in the fridge or reheat from frozen. Use the cooking or reheating instructions above.*

SERVE IT WITH: *This tastes great paired with Berry Avocado Salad (page 294), Zesty Nacho Cabbage Chips (page 252), or Avocado Fries with Dipping Sauce (page 378).*

MAKE IT EGG-FREE: *Use the egg-free variation of mayonnaise.*

MAKE IT LOW-FODMAP: *Follow the low-FODMAP instructions in the Kickin' Ketchup, and either limit the mashed avocado to ⅛ portion per serving (about 21 g), or omit completely and garnish with your favorite garlic-free sliced pickles.*

MAKE IT NIGHTSHADE-FREE: *Use butter lettuce or romaine lettuce cups in place of the eggplant buns. Alternatively, burgers are great served in NUCO Coconut Wraps. Top the burgers with mayonnaise instead of ketchup.*

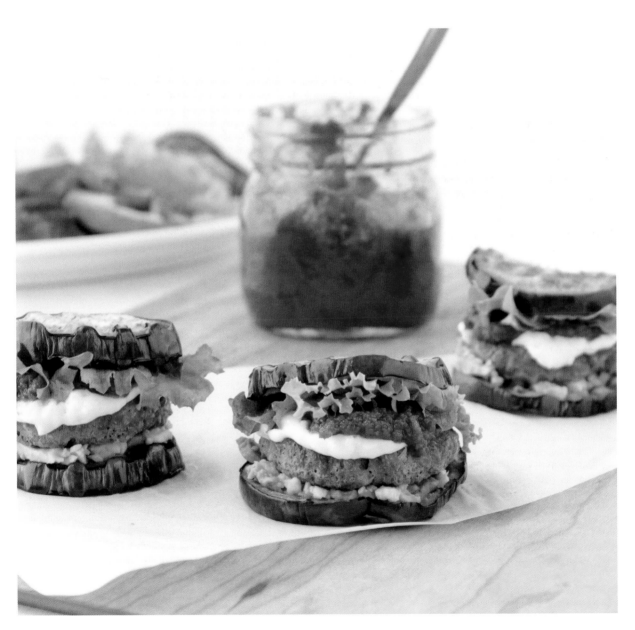

NUTRIENT INFORMATION (PER SERVING):

calories: 493 | calories from fat: 373 | total fat: 41.4g | saturated fat: 9.7g | cholesterol: 72mg

sodium: 341mg | carbs: 8.3g | dietary fiber: 4.4g | net carbs: 3.9g | sugars: 3.3g | protein: 21.7g

RATIOS:

fat:	carbs:	protein:
76%	7%	17%

ONE-POT HAMBURGER DINNER

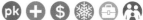

PREP TIME: **15 minutes** COOK TIME: **15 minutes** SERVES: **4**

COCONUT-FREE • EGG-FREE • NIGHTSHADE-FREE • NUT-FREE

When I have minimal time for dinner prep (which is most days), this is my go-to recipe. The husband loves it, I love it, the leftovers are freezable and microwavable, and it feels good on a cold night. To save even more time, I always keep a big container of riced cauliflower in the fridge.

- 1 pound (455 g) ground beef (20% to 30% fat)
- 4 cups (500 g) riced cauliflower florets (see page 163)
- ½ cup (120 ml) beef bone broth (see page 152)
- 1 tablespoon plus 1 teaspoon Italian Seasoning (page 234)
- 1½ teaspoons finely ground gray sea salt
- ¼ cup (17 g) nutritional yeast
- 1 tablespoon finely chopped fresh parsley
- 1 lemon, cut into wedges, for serving (optional)

1. Place the ground beef in a large frying pan over medium heat and cook until only slightly pink, stirring often to break it up into small clumps, 5 to 6 minutes.

2. Add the riced cauliflower, bone broth, Italian seasoning, and salt. Stir to combine, cover, and cook for 8 to 10 minutes, until the liquid has evaporated and the cauliflower rice is fork-tender.

3. Stir in the nutritional yeast and parsley. Divide among 4 plates and enjoy.

STORE IT: *Keep in an airtight container in the fridge for up to 3 days or in the freezer for up to 1 month.*

REHEAT IT: *Microwave until the desired temperature is reached. Or place in a covered casserole dish and reheat in a preheated 300°F (150°C) oven for 10 to 15 minutes, until warmed through. Or reheat in a frying pan, covered, on medium-low.*

THAW IT: *Allow to thaw completely in the fridge. Once defrosted, use the reheating instructions above, or enjoy cold in a salad.*

SERVE IT WITH: *To make this a complete meal, serve it on a bed of baby spinach.*

MAKE IT A CARB-UP: *Replace the riced cauliflower with 2 cups (300 g) of cooked white rice and strain some of the fat from the pan after completing Step 1.*

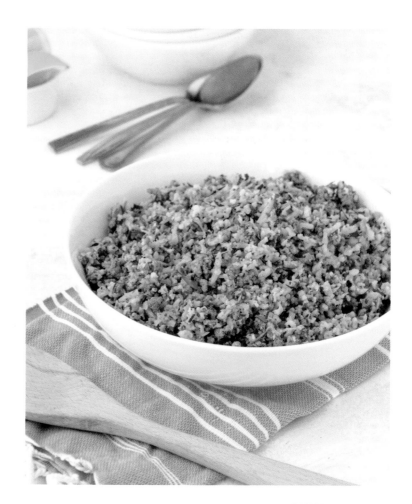

NUTRIENT INFORMATION (PER SERVING):

calories: 363 | calories from fat: 189 | total fat: 21.1g | saturated fat: 8g | cholesterol: 101mg

sodium: 897mg | carbs: 8.6g | dietary fiber: 4.2g | net carbs: 4.4g | sugars: 3g | protein: 34.6g

RATIOS:

fat:	carbs:	protein:
52%	**10%**	**38%**

ZUCCHINI ROLLS

PREP TIME: **10 minutes**　SERVES: **2**

COCONUT-FREE · EGG-FREE · NUT-FREE　OPTIONS: LOW-FODMAP · NIGHTSHADE-FREE

Leftover steak is the best for this recipe, but anything will do—your favorite sliced cooked beef, chicken, salmon, you name it. For the hot sauce, I used Yai's Thai chili garlic hot sauce. It's spicy, and it doesn't contain sugar or preservatives!

ROLLS:

1 medium zucchini (about 7 ounces/200 g)

1 cup (120 g) cooked beef strips

5 medium radishes, sliced thin

DIPPING SAUCE:

¼ cup (60 ml) extra-virgin olive oil or refined avocado oil

2 tablespoons hot sauce

2 teaspoons fresh lime juice

> STORE IT: *Keep in an airtight container in the fridge for up to 4 days.*
>
> SERVE IT WITH: *To make this a complete meal, serve the rolls with avocado slices drizzled with oil.*
>
> MAKE LOW-FODMAP/NIGHTSHADE-FREE: *Replace the dipping sauce with ⅓ cup (70 g) of Horseradish Sauce (page 262).*
>
> MAKE IT A CARB-UP: *Reduce the amount of sauce by half. In Step 2, add an additional filling of boiled and mashed sweet potatoes or yams.*

1. Place the zucchini on a cutting board and, using a vegetable peeler, peel long strips from the zucchini until it is next to impossible to create a full, long strip.

2. Place a zucchini strip on a cutting board, with a short end facing you. Place a couple of pieces of beef and 3 or 4 radish slices at the short end closest to you. Roll it up, then stab with a toothpick to secure. Repeat with the remaining zucchini strips, placing the completed rolls on a serving plate.

3. In a small serving dish, whisk together the dipping sauce ingredients. Serve the dipping sauce alongside the rolls.

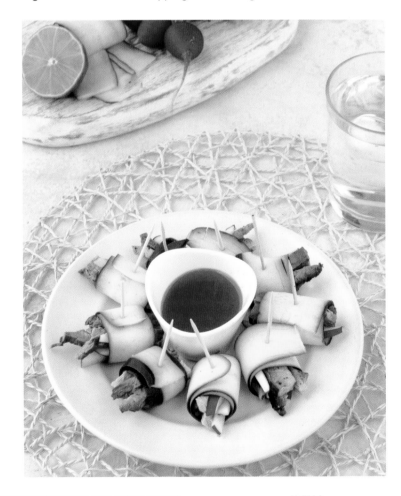

NUTRIENT INFORMATION (PER SERVING WITH 3 TABLESPOONS PLUS 1 TEASPOON SAUCE):
calories: 370 | calories from fat: 296 | total fat: 32.9g | saturated fat: 6.6g | cholesterol: 40mg
sodium: 422mg | carbs: 4g | dietary fiber: 1.1g | net carbs: 2.9g | sugars: 1.9g | protein: 14.4g

RATIOS:
fat: carbs: protein:
80% **4%** **16%**

MICHAEL'S PEPPERONI MEATZZA

PREP TIME: **20 minutes**   COOK TIME: **30 minutes**   SERVES: **6**

COCONUT-FREE   OPTIONS: LOW-FODMAP • NUT-FREE

After my solo trip to India, during which I lived in an ashram, jumped from waterfalls, and ate far too many carbs, I returned home, quit my job, and moved across the country to Montreal with my husband. The move to Montreal rekindled friendships and support systems that I never realized I had. Among them was a fabulous relationship I developed with my mom's cousin, Michael. Michael loves to cook, but gluten-free and dairy-free aren't in his vocabulary, and forget about Paleo or keto.

One Sunday, Michael and his wife had us over for a lunch of this delicious pepperoni "meatzza," completely free of all the things my body hates. I gobbled up a quarter of the meatzza during lunch, and they packaged up the rest for Kevin and me to share...but there was no sharing, let's be real. Here is the recipe Uncle Michael used, with a couple of twists because I couldn't resist.

My favorite pepperoni for this meatzza is fermented beef sticks from Paleovalley.

Refined avocado oil, for the pan

"CRUST":

1 pound (455 g) ground beef (20% to 30% fat)

⅓ cup (36 g) blanched almond flour

2 large eggs

1 tablespoon Italian Seasoning (page 234)

1 teaspoon finely ground gray sea salt

¼ teaspoon ground black pepper

"SAUCE":

½ cup (130 g) Kale Pâté (page 259)

1 tablespoon apple cider vinegar

TOPPING:

¾ cup (105 g) sliced pepperoni

STORE IT: *Keep in an airtight container in the fridge for up to 3 days or in the freezer for up to 1 month.*

REHEAT IT: *Microwave until the desired temperature is reached. Or place on a rimmed baking sheet and reheat in a preheated 300°F (150°C) oven for 10 minutes, or until warmed through.*

THAW IT: *Allow to thaw completely in the fridge. Once defrosted, use the reheating instructions above, or enjoy cold.*

PREP AHEAD: *Prepare the Kale Pâté up to 3 days before using it in this recipe.*

1. Preheat the oven to 425°F (220°C) and lightly grease a 9-inch (23-cm) pie pan with avocado oil.

2. Make the "crust": In a large bowl, combine the ground beef, almond flour, eggs, Italian seasoning, salt, and pepper with your hands until fully incorporated.

3. Transfer the meat mixture to the prepared pie pan. Use your hands to smooth it out in the bottom of the pan.

4. In a small bowl, combine the Kale Pâté with the vinegar. When fully mixed, spoon it onto the meat "crust" and spread it smooth with the back of the spoon, leaving a ½-inch (1.25-cm) border around the edge.

5. Lay the pepperoni slices on top of the pâté in a pretty pattern, or just toss them on.

6. Bake for 25 to 30 minutes, until the pepperoni has browned, the crust is pulling away from the edge of the pan, and the internal temperature of the crust reaches 165°F (74°C).

7. Allow the meatzza to rest in the pan for 10 minutes, then cut into 6 slices and serve.

SERVE IT WITH: *This meatzza tastes great paired with Verde Caesar Salad with Crispy Capers (page 289) or Porky Cabbage (page 385).*

MAKE IT LOW-FODMAP: *Ensure that the pepperoni you're using doesn't contain garlic or onions. Or you could use your favorite cold-cut meat or leftover pork or chicken slices in place of the pepperoni.*

MAKE IT NUT-FREE: *Use ground hulled sunflower seeds in place of the almond flour.*

NUTRIENT INFORMATION (PER SERVING):

calories: 446 | calories from fat: 315 | total fat: 35g | saturated fat: 9.9g | cholesterol: 148mg

sodium: 782mg | carbs: 4.1g | dietary fiber: 1.4g | net carbs: 2.7g | sugars: 0g | protein: 28.6g

RATIOS:

fat:	carbs:	protein:
71%	4%	25%

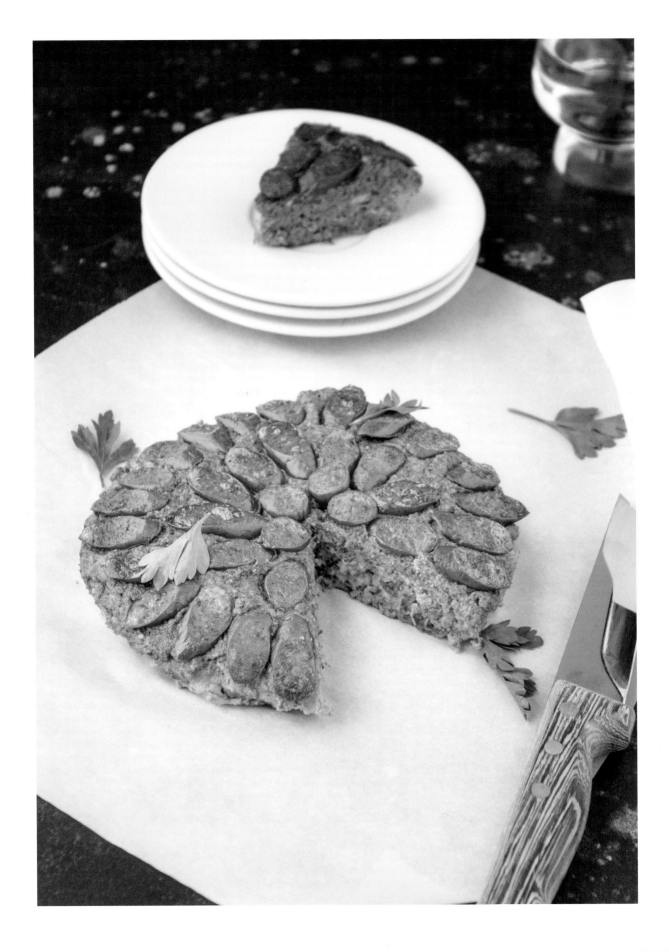

SHREDDED BEEF TACOS

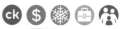

PREP TIME: **15 minutes**   COOK TIME: **4 to 8 hours**   SERVES: **8**

COCONUT-FREE · EGG-FREE · LOW-FODMAP · NIGHTSHADE-FREE · NUT-FREE

For years, I battled with intense acne. It wasn't until recently that I discovered nightshades were, in large part, contributing to my annoying acne. Once I removed nightshades from my diet, my skin became a lot clearer. But I enjoy the ease of shredded meat recipes since the meat can be repurposed for just about any dish. The problem is that there weren't many shredded beef, pork, or chicken recipes that don't contain nightshades...until now!

This recipe makes a lot of meat. And I don't blame you if you don't feel like having tacos every night for the next week. You can repurpose the shredded beef by adding the leftovers to a pan with your favorite veggies and fats, use it as the protein in a salad, or mix it with mayo and serve as a sandwich filling. The possibilities are endless!

Don't feel like spices? Don't add them! Sometimes my favorite way to prepare shredded beef is to simply cook it in beef bone broth. I call it "simple shredded beef." The same can be done with a whole chicken or pork shoulder in chicken bone broth. Same instructions, same tasty results. With the whole chicken, you have to pick through and find the bones, but it's fun...and delicious!

I've included both a set-it-and-forget-it slow cooker method and a hurry-up-and-get-it-done pressure cooker method for preparing this dish.

1 lime

1⅔ cups (390 ml) beef bone broth (see page 152)

2 tablespoons Garlic-Infused Oil (made with refined avocado oil) (page 230)

1 tablespoon ground cumin

1 tablespoon dried oregano leaves

1 teaspoon finely ground gray sea salt

½ teaspoon ground black pepper

¼ teaspoon ground cloves

3 pounds (1.4 kg) beef brisket or chuck roast

2 tablespoons granulated xylitol (optional)

SAUCE:

½ cup (105 g) mayonnaise, homemade (page 220) or store-bought

3 tablespoons Garlic-Infused Oil (made with refined avocado oil) (page 230)

FOR SERVING:

1 head butter lettuce, leaves separated, cleaned, and patted dry

8 radishes, finely diced

2 green onions, green parts only, thinly sliced

1. Juice the lime and save the juiced halves. Place the lime juice, bone broth, infused oil, cumin, oregano, salt, pepper, and cloves in a pressure cooker or slow cooker and whisk to combine. Add the reserved lime halves and beef brisket. Flip the brisket in the mixture to coat both sides.

2. If using a pressure cooker, seal the lid and cook on high for 4 hours. If using a slow cooker, cover and cook on high for 6 hours or low for 8 hours.

3. Strain the liquid from the meat, reserving the liquid. Transfer ⅔ cup (160 ml) of the reserved liquid back to the pressure cooker or slow cooker. Add the xylitol, if using. If using a pressure cooker, set it to "sauté." If using a slow cooker, set it to high. Cook, uncovered, for 5 minutes.

4. Meanwhile, make the sauce: In a small bowl, whisk together the mayonnaise and infused oil. For a pretty presentation, transfer the sauce to a piping bag or plastic baggie with a corner cut off.

5. After the brisket cooking liquid has reduced for 5 minutes, return the meat to the cooker and shred with 2 forks, mixing the shredded meat into the sauce.

6. To serve, divide the butter lettuce cups among 8 plates, then divide the shredded beef among the lettuce cups. Top with the radishes and green onions. Pipe the sauce on top or simply add a dollop to each taco with a small spoon. Enjoy!

VARIATION: KICKIN' SHREDDED BEEF TACOS.
If nightshades and FODMAP foods are not a concern for you, stir in ¾ cup (180 ml) of Kickin' Ketchup (page 223) when adding the xylitol.

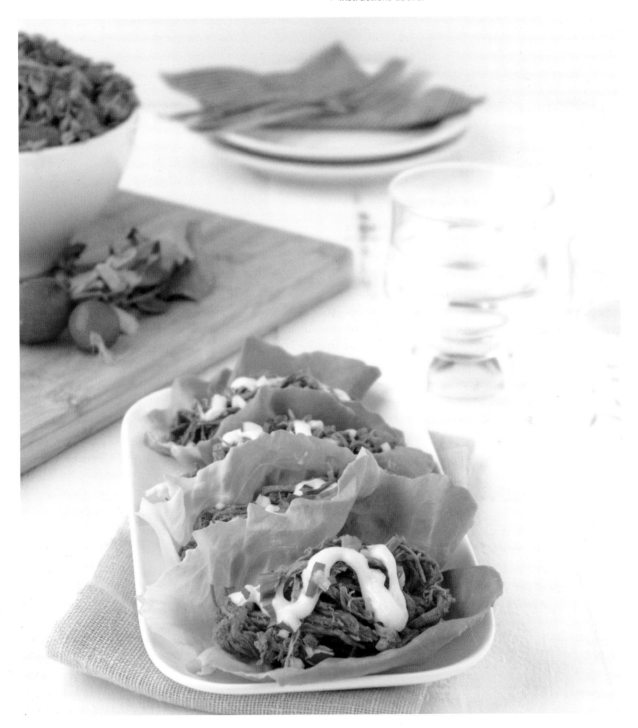

NUTRIENT INFORMATION (PER SERVING):

calories: 454 | calories from fat: 310 | total fat: 34.4g | saturated fat: 7.4g | cholesterol: 160mg

sodium: 541mg | carbs: 3.7g | dietary fiber: 0.8g | net carbs: 2.9g | sugars: 0.7g | protein: 32.5g

RATIOS:

fat:	carbs:	protein:
68%	**3%**	**29%**

COCONUT LAMB CURRY

PREP TIME: **25 minutes**   COOK TIME: **85 minutes**   SERVES: **8**

EGG-FREE • NUT-FREE   OPTION: NIGHTSHADE-FREE

There are days, albeit not too often, when I don't want anything to do with poultry, beef, pork, or seafood, but the sound of lamb gets me all sorts of hungry. This is the recipe I make on said occasions. Always prepared in my pressure cooker, it comes together lickety-split.

If the instructions for breaking open a coconut totally throw you off, it's a lot easier than it seems. And once you know how to open a fresh coconut, especially as a keto-er, you'll have the fresh stuff in your fridge all the time—it's that good. But if that doesn't sell you on the idea, you can replace the fresh coconut flesh in this recipe with ½ cup (50 g) of unsweetened shredded coconut.

1 small fresh coconut (about 1⅓ pounds/ 600 g)

1 cup (208 g) coconut oil

1 pound (455 g) boneless lamb cutlets, cut into 1-inch (2.5-cm) cubes

1 (13½-ounce/400-ml) can full-fat coconut milk

8 green onions, green parts only, sliced

2 tablespoons Curry Powder (page 235)

1 tablespoon apple cider vinegar

2 teaspoons yellow mustard seeds

1 teaspoon finely ground gray sea salt

¼ cup (20 g) finely chopped fresh cilantro

4 cups (500 g) riced cauliflower florets (see page 163), steamed, for serving

1. Preheat the oven to 375°F (190°C).

2. There are 3 holes at the top of a fresh coconut. Using a sharp knife, press into each of the holes until you find the weakest one. Your knife should go right through. Make a good-sized hole, set the coconut upside down on a glass, and allow the water to drain. Reserve the coconut water for smoothies (page 424).

3. Place the drained coconut on an unlined rimmed baking sheet, then bake for up to 10 minutes, until a crack forms on the outside.

4. Remove the coconut from the oven and wrap in a clean kitchen towel. Place the wrapped coconut in a garbage bag and find a hard surface to hit the coconut with. I use the concrete stairs outside my home.

5. Remove the coconut from the bag and peel the flesh away from the shell. Using a vegetable peeler, remove the brown skin from the white. Slice the white flesh into thin strips. The total yield from the coconut should be 2 cups (160 g) of strips.

6. Place the coconut strips, coconut oil, lamb pieces, coconut milk, green onions, curry powder, vinegar, mustard seeds, and salt in a large saucepan. Bring to a boil over medium-high heat. Reduce the heat to medium-low and simmer for 75 minutes, or until the coconut has softened and the lamb is tender.

7. Stir in the cilantro and serve over steamed riced cauliflower.

STORE IT: *Keep in an airtight container in the fridge for up to 4 days or in the freezer for up to 1 month. It is okay to store the rice with the lamb.*

REHEAT IT: *Microwave, covered, until the desired temperature is reached, or place in a saucepan and reheat on medium.*

THAW IT: *Allow to thaw completely in the fridge. Once defrosted, use the reheating instructions above.*

MAKE IT NIGHTSHADE-FREE: *Omit the dried chili peppers from the curry powder.*

PRESSURE-COOK IT: *Complete Steps 1 through 5, then place the coconut strips and the rest of the ingredients, except for the cilantro and riced cauliflower, in a pressure cooker. Seal the lid and set to high pressure for 30 minutes. Allow the pressure to release, then remove the lid and continue with Step 7.*

NUTRIENT INFORMATION (PER SERVING):

calories: 556 | calories from fat: 439 | total fat: 48.8g | saturated fat: 40.3g | cholesterol: 51mg

sodium: 315mg | carbs: 10g | dietary fiber: 4.3g | net carbs: 5.7g | sugars: 3.9g | protein: 19.3g

RATIOS:

fat:	carbs:	protein:
79%	7%	14%

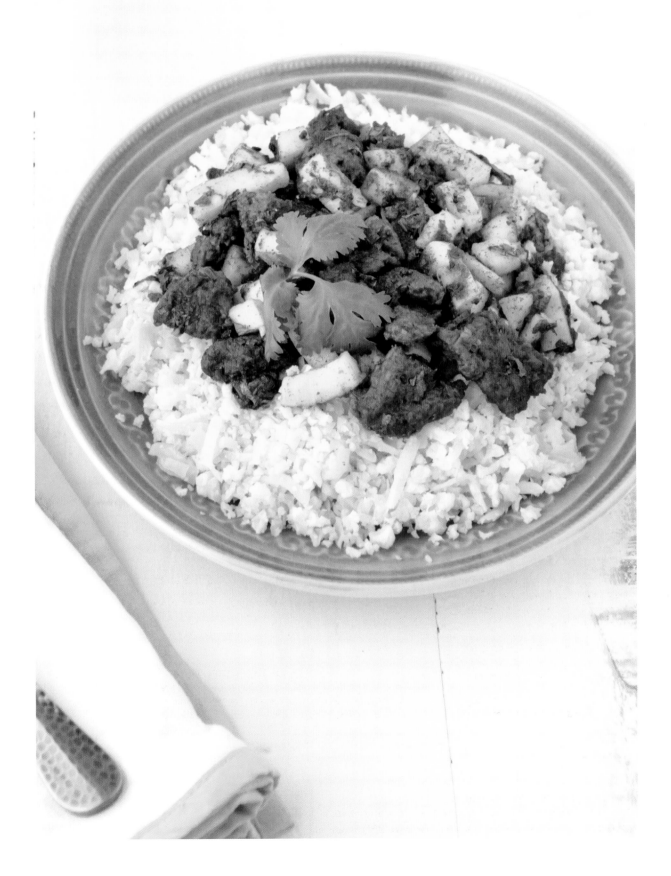

LAMB KEBABS

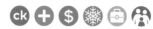

PREP TIME: **15 minutes**   COOK TIME: **15 minutes**   SERVES: **6**

EGG-FREE • NUT-FREE   OPTIONS: COCONUT-FREE • NIGHTSHADE-FREE

If you have extra time before enjoying this recipe, the tzatziki is best the day after it's made, after all the flavors have had a chance to meld overnight. But if you're like me and waiting for dinner is out of the question, the tzatziki is fine when freshly made. And you'll have day-old tzatziki for your leftovers. Win!

TZATZIKI:

1 cup (240 ml) coconut cream

1 (4-in/10-cm) piece English cucumber, grated

2 tablespoons extra-virgin olive oil

1 tablespoon apple cider vinegar

1 tablespoon finely chopped fresh dill

Grated zest of ½ lemon

Juice of ½ lemon

1 small clove garlic, minced

½ teaspoon finely ground gray sea salt

¼ teaspoon ground black pepper

KEBABS:

1 pound (455 g) ground lamb

¼ cup water

3 teaspoons Bahārāt Seasoning (page 233), divided

1 teaspoon finely ground gray sea salt

SPECIAL EQUIPMENT:

6 bamboo skewers, about 10 inches (25 cm) long

1. Preheat the oven to 375°F (190°C) and line a rimmed baking sheet with parchment paper or a silicone baking mat.

2. Place the skewers in a tall glass of water to soak for at least 30 minutes while you prepare the rest of the recipe.

3. Make the tzatziki: Place all the ingredients in a small bowl and stir to combine. Cover and place in the refrigerator.

4. Prepare the kebab meat: Place the lamb, water, 2 teaspoons of the Bahārāt seasoning, and salt in a medium-sized bowl. Combine with your hands until fully incorporated.

5. Divide the meat mixture into 6 portions and shape each portion into a cylinder about 6 inches (15 cm) long. Insert the skewers and reshape as necessary.

6. Sprinkle the skewers with the remaining 1 teaspoon of Bahārāt seasoning. Place on the baking sheet and bake until lightly golden, 10 minutes for medium-done kebabs or 15 minutes for well-done kebabs.

7. Divide the skewers and tzatziki among 6 plates and serve, using ¼ cup (60 ml) tzatziki per plate.

STORE IT: *Keep the kebabs in an airtight container in the fridge for up to 4 days or in the freezer for up to 1 month. Store the tzatziki in a separate airtight container in the fridge for up to 3 days.*

REHEAT IT: *Microwave the kebabs, covered, or reheat in a frying pan, covered, on medium heat until the desired temperature is reached.*

THAW IT: *Either allow the kebabs to thaw completely in the fridge or reheat directly from the freezer, using the reheating instructions above.*

SERVE IT WITH: *To make this a complete meal, serve the kebabs on a bed of greens. They also taste great paired with Marinated Bok Choy Salad (page 295).*

MAKE IT COCONUT-FREE: *Replace the coconut cream with the unsweetened dairy-free yogurt of your choice.*

MAKE IT NIGHTSHADE-FREE: *Replace the Bahārāt seasoning with one of the nightshade-free spice mixtures on pages 232 to 235.*

MAKE IT A CARB-UP: *Omit the tzatziki. Serve the kebabs alongside the carb of your choice (find ideas on page 117, or visit healthfulpursuit.com/carbup to download the complimentary PDF "Carb-Up Recipes"). They are fabulous with white rice.*

NUTRIENT INFORMATION (PER 1 SKEWER AND ¼ CUP/60 ML TZATZIKI):

calories: 274 | calories from fat: 206 | total fat: 22.9g | saturated fat: 14.1g | cholesterol: 54mg

sodium: 528mg | carbs: 3.1g | dietary fiber: 0.5g | net carbs: 2.6g | sugars: 0g | protein: 13.8g

RATIOS:

fat:	carbs:	protein:
75%	5%	20%

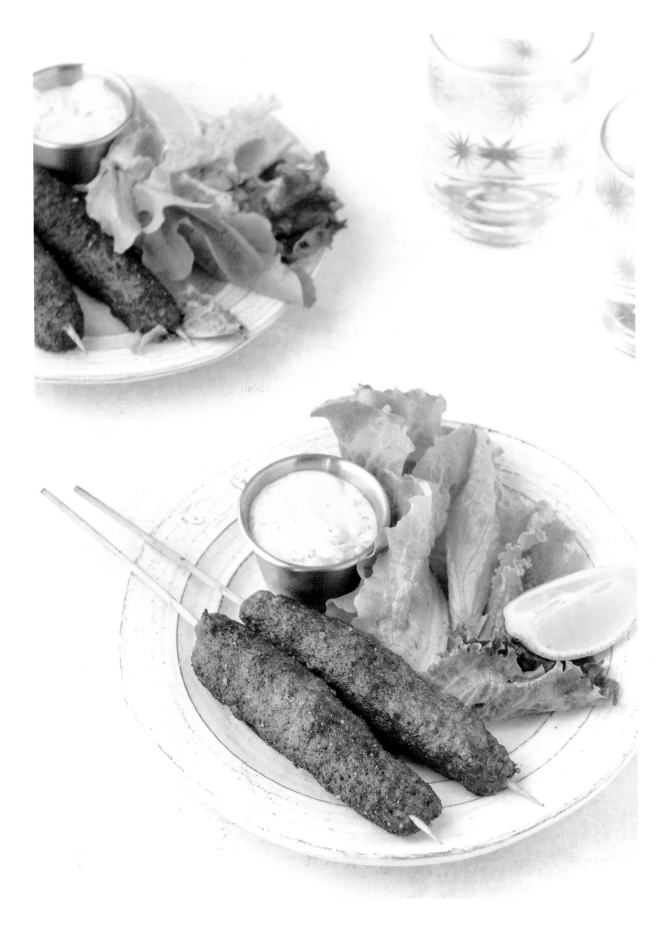

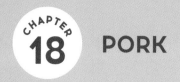
BACON MAC 'N' CHEESE

PREP TIME: **25 minutes**   COOK TIME: **50 minutes**   SERVES: **4**

COCONUT-FREE • NIGHTSHADE-FREE • NUT-FREE

This dish! While you may not think that a pasta-free, cheese-free mac 'n' cheese would be any good, I'd like for you to make this and have me prove you wrong. When I make this recipe again, I'm going to prepare it in single-serving ramekins so that each person gets their own and can't steal my portion! Yes, I'm speaking to you, dear husband....

Because this dish contains gelatin, it will congeal when chilled. Simply use the reheating instructions below to return it to cheesy goodness. It's pretty good at room temperature, though!

Coconut oil, for the dish

1 large head cauliflower (about 1⅔ pounds/750 g), cored and broken into ½-inch (1.25-cm) pieces

⅓ cup (22 g) finely chopped fresh parsley

6 strips bacon (about 6 ounces/170 g), cooked until crisp, then crumbled (reserve the grease)

2 cups (475 ml) unsweetened nondairy milk

2 tablespoons unflavored gelatin

1 tablespoon fresh lemon juice

1 teaspoon onion powder

1 teaspoon finely ground gray sea salt

¼ teaspoon garlic powder

⅓ cup (22 g) nutritional yeast

2 large eggs, beaten

2 teaspoons prepared yellow mustard

2 ounces (60 g) pork dust or ground pork rinds

STORE IT: *Keep in an airtight container in the fridge for up to 3 days.*

REHEAT IT: *Microwave until the desired temperature is reached. Or place in a covered casserole dish and reheat in a preheated 300°F (150°C) oven for 10 to 15 minutes, until warmed through. Or reheat in a frying pan, covered, on medium-low.*

1. Preheat the oven to 350°F (177°C) and grease a shallow 1½-quart (1.4-L) casserole dish with coconut oil. Set aside.

2. Place the cauliflower, parsley, and bacon in a large bowl and toss to combine.

3. Place the reserved bacon grease, milk, gelatin, lemon juice, onion powder, salt, and garlic powder in a medium-sized saucepan. Bring to a boil over medium heat, whisking occasionally. Once boiling, continue to boil for 5 minutes.

4. Whisk in the nutritional yeast, eggs, and mustard and gently cook for 3 minutes, whisking constantly.

5. Remove the saucepan from the heat and pour the "cheese" sauce over the cauliflower mixture. (If you've overcooked the sauce or didn't whisk it well enough, you may end up with small pieces of cooked egg; for an ultra-smooth sauce, pour the sauce through a fine-mesh strainer.) Toss with a spatula until all the cauliflower pieces are coated in the cheese sauce.

6. Transfer the coated cauliflower to the prepared casserole dish and smooth it out with the back of a spatula. Sprinkle the pork dust evenly over the top. Bake for 40 to 45 minutes, until the cauliflower is fork-tender, checking with a sharp knife on the edge of the casserole.

7. Allow to sit for 15 minutes before serving.

PREP AHEAD: *Prepare the cheese sauce up to 2 days in advance. Bring it to a light simmer before continuing with Step 5.*

SERVE IT WITH: *Add a dollop or two of mayonnaise.*

NUTRIENT INFORMATION (PER SERVING):

calories: 440 | calories from fat: 244 | total fat: 27g | saturated fat: 8.8g | cholesterol: 128mg

sodium: 973mg | carbs: 14.6g | dietary fiber: 6.6g | net carbs: 8g | sugars: 4.8g | protein: 34.6g

RATIOS:		
fat:	carbs:	protein:
55%	13%	32%

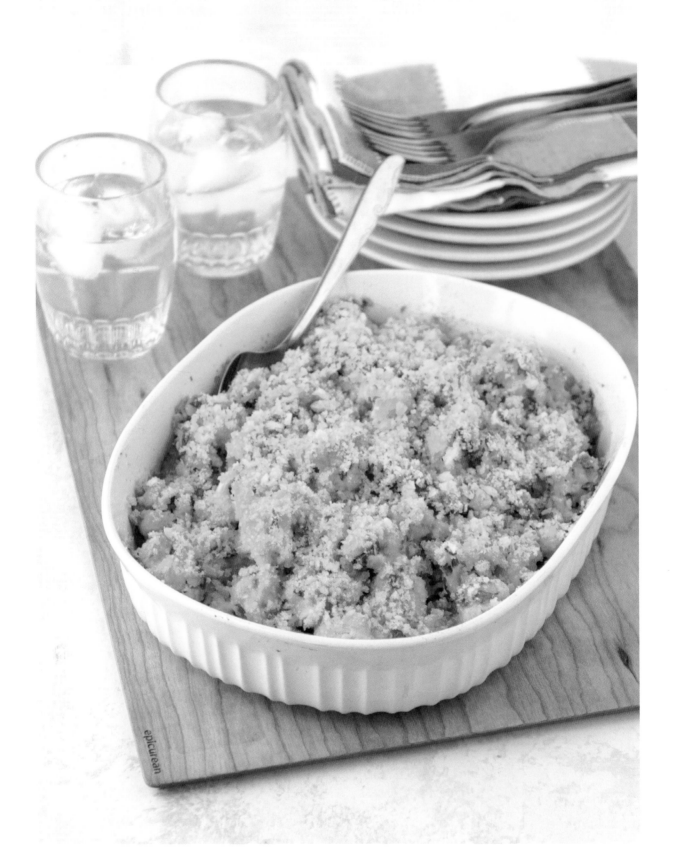

CHIPOTLE-SPICED MEATBALL SUBS

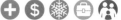

PREP TIME: **15 minutes**   COOK TIME: **35 minutes**   MAKES: **15 subs (15 servings)**

COCONUT-FREE • EGG-FREE • NUT-FREE

Who doesn't like meatballs? My favorite thing about meatballs is their versatility. You could use cabbage "buns," as I've outlined in this recipe. You could eat them on top of a slice of Crusty Sandwich Bread (page 366). You could let them cool slightly and serve them in romaine lettuce hearts. Or you could pile them on a bowl of mixed greens for an epic keto salad or use the leftovers in tomorrow's egg scramble!

I find it easiest to purchase a large head of cabbage and peel away the leaves in a non-uniform fashion. You're aiming for pieces about the size of your palm. Tear them away, then use the leftover cabbage for another recipe, such as Porky Cabbage (page 385).

MEATBALLS:

1⅔ pounds (750 g) ground pork

1 pound (455 g) ground chicken

½ cup (160 g) grated white onions

1½ teaspoons dried oregano leaves

1¼ teaspoons ground cumin

1 teaspoon finely ground gray sea salt

SAUCE:

2½ cups (600 ml) crushed tomatoes

½ cup (120 ml) refined avocado oil or melted chicken fat

⅔ cup (80 ml) chicken bone broth (see page 152)

1 tablespoon dried oregano leaves

1¼ teaspoons chipotle powder

1 teaspoon garlic powder

½ teaspoon onion powder

½ teaspoon smoked paprika

½ teaspoon finely ground gray sea salt

¼ teaspoon ground black pepper

FOR SERVING:

1 large head green cabbage

Finely chopped fresh cilantro (optional)

1. Preheat the oven to 350°F (177°C) and line a rimmed baking sheet with parchment paper or a silicone baking mat.

2. Place the ingredients for the meatballs in a large bowl. Mix with your hands until combined.

3. Wet your hands and pinch a 1½-tablespoon piece from the bowl, then roll it between your palms to form a ball. Place on the prepared baking sheet and repeat with the remaining meat mixture, making a total of 30 meatballs. Keeping your palms wet will help you shape the meatballs quicker.

4. Bake the meatballs for 25 to 30 minutes, until the internal temperature reaches 165°F (74°C).

5. Meanwhile, place the ingredients for the sauce in a large saucepan. Stir to combine, then cover, placing the lid slightly askew to allow steam to escape. Bring to a boil over medium-high heat, then reduce the heat to low and simmer for 20 minutes.

6. While the meatballs and sauce are cooking, remove 30 medium-sized leaves from the head of cabbage and lightly steam for 1 to 2 minutes.

7. Remove the meatballs from the oven and transfer to the saucepan with the sauce. Turn them to coat, cover, and cook on low for 5 minutes.

8. To serve, stack 2 cabbage leaves on top of one another, top with 2 meatballs, a dollop of extra sauce, and a sprinkle of cilantro, if using.

REHEAT IT: *Microwave the meatballs until the desired temperature is reached. Or place in a covered casserole dish and reheat in a preheated 300°F (150°C) oven for 10 to 15 minutes, until warmed through. Or reheat in a frying pan, covered, on medium-low.*

THAW IT: *Allow to thaw completely in the fridge. Once defrosted, enjoy cold in a salad or use the reheating instructions above.*

STORE IT: *Keep the subs (it's fine if they're already assembled) in an airtight container in the fridge for up to 3 days; the meatballs and/or sauce can be frozen for up to 1 month.*

SERVE IT WITH: *These meatballs are great with Bendy Tortillas (page 370).*

MAKE IT A CARB-UP: *Reduce the amount of avocado oil to ¼ cup (60 ml), omit the cabbage leaves, and replace with the carb of your choice (find ideas on page 117, or visit healthfulpursuit.com/carbup to download the complimentary PDF "Carb-Up Recipes"). It's fabulous with mashed sweet potatoes, yams, or potatoes.*

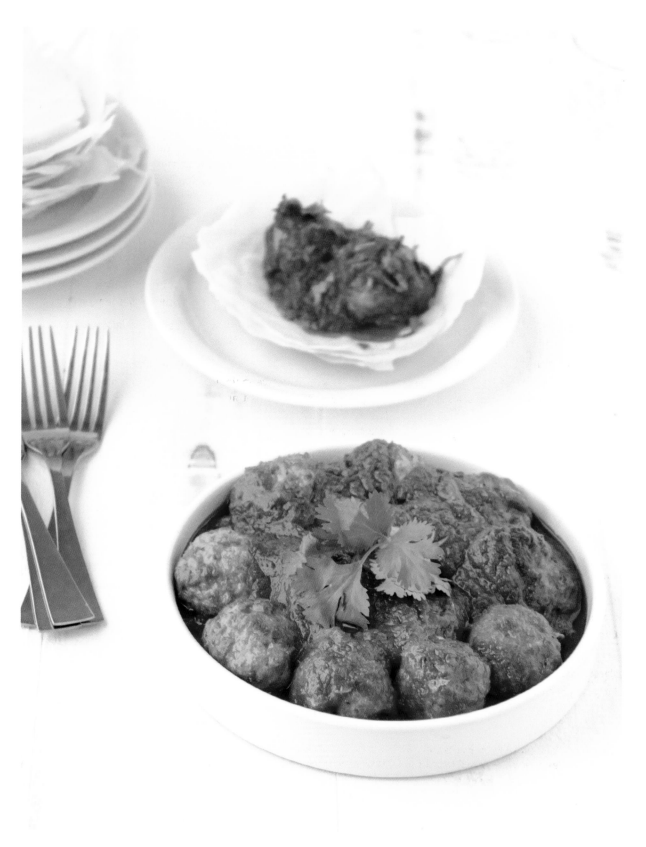

NUTRIENT INFORMATION (PER SUB):

calories: 253 | calories from fat: 151 | total fat: 16.8g | saturated fat: 4.3g | cholesterol: 52mg

sodium: 271mg | carbs: 7.9g | dietary fiber: 2.6g | net carbs: 5.3g | sugars: 4g | protein: 17.5g

RATIOS:

fat:	carbs:	protein:
60%	**12%**	**28%**

CRACKED-UP HAM SALAD SANDWICHES

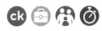

PREP TIME: **10 minutes**   MAKES: **8 sandwiches (serves 8)**

COCONUT-FREE · NIGHTSHADE-FREE   OPTIONS: EGG-FREE · NUT-FREE

There's nothing funny about a ham salad sandwich…unless it's got eggs, and then it's cracked up! Get it? But really, this combo of egg salad and ham salad is where it's at. Don't want to make a loaf of bread just to enjoy this recipe? I don't blame you. Roll the ham salad in collard leaves instead—it's unreal.

1¾ pounds (800 g) smoked ham, fully cooked

½ cup (105 g) mayonnaise, homemade (page 220) or store-bought

3 tablespoons prepared horseradish

2 tablespoons Dijon mustard

2 hard-boiled eggs, chopped

6 green onions, green parts only, sliced

3 radishes (about 3 ounces/85 g), finely diced

2 baby dill pickles, finely diced

1 celery stick, finely diced

FOR SERVING:

1 loaf Crusty Sandwich Bread (page 366), cut into 16 slices

Fresh parsley leaves or lettuce, torn (optional)

Pickles of choice

1. Cut the ham into large, rough chunks and place in a food processor or high-powered blender. Pulse for 20 to 30 seconds, until the desired consistency is reached.

2. Transfer the ham pieces to a large bowl. Add the mayonnaise, horseradish, mustard, hard-boiled eggs, green onions, radishes, pickles, and celery. Combine with a spatula until all the ham pieces are coated.

3. To serve, lay out a slice of bread on a cutting board, top it with pieces of parsley or lettuce, if using, and place ⅔ cup (175 g) of the ham salad on top. Top with a second slice of bread. Repeat with the remaining bread and meat to make a total of 8 sandwiches. Serve with pickles.

STORE IT: *Keep the sandwich components in separate airtight containers in the fridge for up to 4 days. Assembled sandwiches will keep for 2 days.*

PREP AHEAD: *Hard-boil the eggs up to 3 days before preparing this recipe and keep them in the fridge, unpeeled. The bread can be made up to 3 days in advance, or you can bake it a month ahead and freeze it. The mayo can be made up to 5 days ahead.*

MAKE IT EGG-FREE: *Use egg-free mayonnaise variation, omit the hard-boiled eggs, and serve the salad on romaine lettuce leaves.*

MAKE IT NUT-FREE: *Omit the bread and serve the ham salad on romaine lettuce leaves.*

NUTRIENT INFORMATION (PER SANDWICH):
calories: 509 | calories from fat: 333 | total fat: 37g | saturated fat: 6.1g | cholesterol: 207mg
sodium: 1404mg | carbs: 11.9g | dietary fiber: 7.9g | net carbs: 4g | sugars: 2.2g | protein: 32g

RATIOS:
fat:	carbs:	protein:
66%	9%	25%

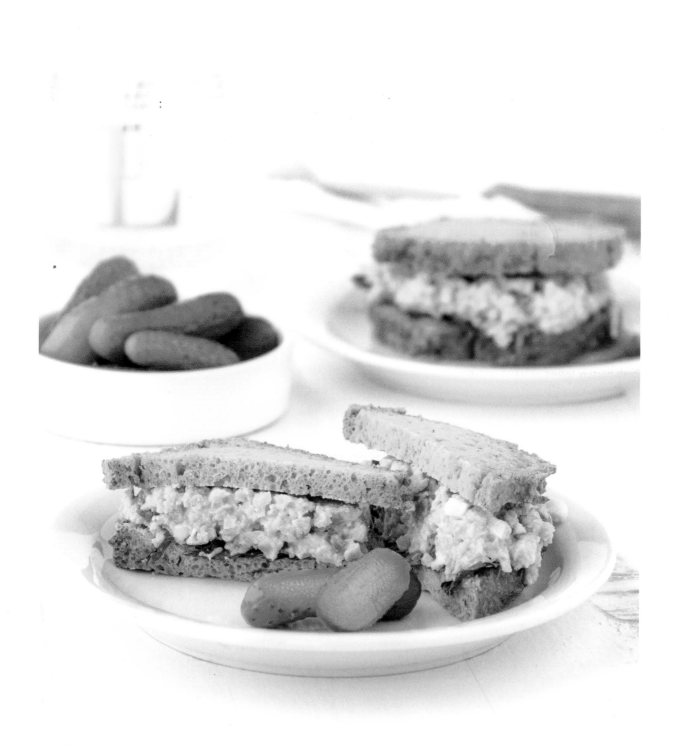

HERB-CRUSTED PORK CHOPS

PREP TIME: **15 minutes**   COOK TIME: **24 minutes**   SERVES: **6**

LOW-FODMAP • NIGHTSHADE-FREE • NUT-FREE   OPTION: COCONUT-FREE

You could cook a boring old pork chop and slather it with mayonnaise, or you could make this recipe and feel fancy as you cut into your crusted chop. (I still highly recommend that you slather it with mayonnaise.) If you have an extra-large frying pan that can accommodate all six chops at once without crowding, feel free to fry the chops in one batch, using the full ½ cup of oil; otherwise, you will need to fry them in two batches, as described below.

6 boneless center-cut pork chops (5½ ounces/155 g each)

2 teaspoons finely ground gray sea salt

½ teaspoon ground black pepper

½ cup (120 ml) refined avocado oil or melted coconut oil, divided, for the pan

DRY HERB COATING:

3 ounces (85 g) pork dust or ground pork rinds

1 teaspoon dried parsley

1 teaspoon dried ground sage

½ teaspoon dried marjoram or oregano leaves

½ teaspoon dried rosemary leaves

½ teaspoon dried thyme leaves

WET COATING:

2 large eggs

Finely chopped fresh parsley, for garnish (optional)

1. Season the chops on both sides with the salt and pepper and set aside.

2. Pour ¼ cup of the oil into a large frying pan and set over medium heat. While the oil is heating, prepare the coatings.

3. Combine the ingredients for the dry herb coating in a pie dish. Crack the eggs into a medium-sized bowl and whisk them.

4. Dip a chop into the whisked eggs, allowing the excess to drip off. Then place the wet chop in the dry herb coating and turn it to coat, shaking off the excess. Transfer the coated chop to the preheated pan and repeat with 2 more chops. Cook the chops for 5 to 6 minutes per side, until the internal temperature reaches 165°F (74°C). Transfer the cooked chops to a clean plate.

5. Discard the used oil and wipe the pork rind pieces from the pan. Pour the remaining ¼ cup of oil into the pan. Coat and cook the remaining 3 chops by following Step 4.

6. Sprinkle the fried chops with chopped parsley, if desired, and serve.

STORE IT: *Keep in an airtight container in the fridge for up to 4 days or in the freezer for up to 1 month.*

REHEAT IT: *Microwave until the desired temperature is reached. Or place in a covered casserole dish and reheat in a preheated 300°F (150°C) oven for 5 to 10 minutes, until warmed through. Or reheat in a frying pan, covered, on medium-low.*

THAW IT: *Allow to thaw completely in the fridge. Once defrosted, enjoy cold in a salad or use the reheating instructions above.*

SERVE IT WITH: *Make it a complete meal by adding a slather of mayonnaise. These chops taste great paired with Greek Cauliflower Rice (page 364), Herbed Radishes (page 384), or Creamy Mashed Turnips (page 382).*

MAKE IT COCONUT-FREE: *Use avocado oil.*

MAKE IT A CARB-UP: *Reduce the amount of avocado oil to ¼ cup (60 ml). Serve alongside the carb of your choice (find ideas on page 117, or visit healthfulpursuit.com/carbup to download the complimentary PDF "Carb-Up Recipes"). It's delicious with mashed potatoes and gravy made with tapioca starch.*

NUTRIENT INFORMATION (PER SERVING):
calories: 471 | calories from fat: 272 | total fat: 30.2g | saturated fat: 6.9g | cholesterol: 163mg
sodium: 731mg | carbs: 0.4g | dietary fiber: 0g | net carbs: 0.4g | sugars: 0g | protein: 49.4g

RATIOS:
fat: | carbs: | protein:
58% | **1%** | **41%**

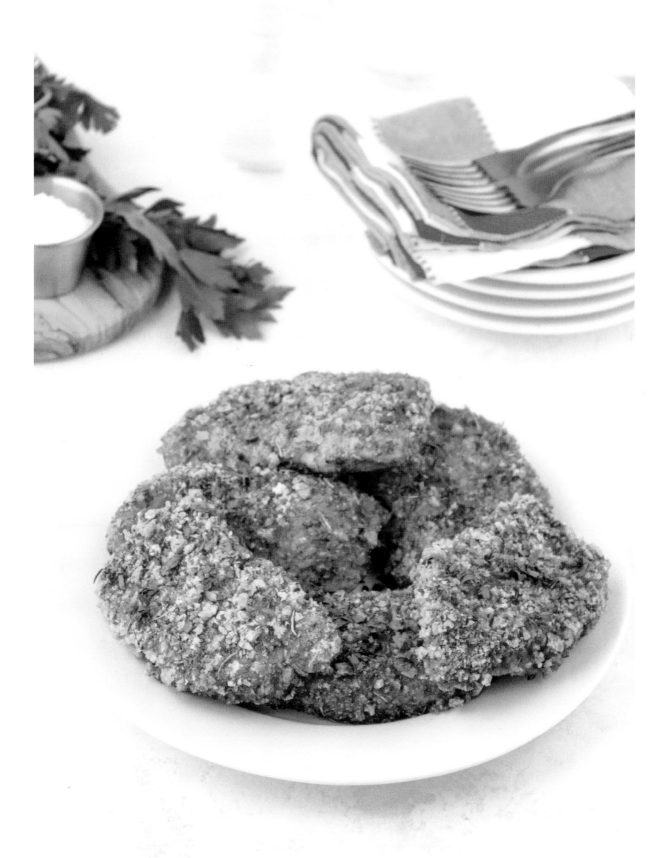

KUNG PAO PORK

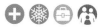

PREP TIME: **15 minutes**   COOK TIME: **10 minutes**   SERVES: **4**

EGG-FREE   OPTIONS: COCONUT-FREE · LOW-FODMAP · NIGHTSHADE-FREE · NUT-FREE

There's nothing quite like stir-fry on a busy weeknight, and if you haven't paired stir-fry with a chilled salad, now's the time! If cold foods aren't in line with the current season, cauliflower rice (page 364) is really good with this dish.

STIR-FRIED PORK:

2 tablespoons refined avocado oil or hazelnut oil

1 pound (455 g) pork stir-fry pieces

4 small cloves garlic, minced

1 (1-inch/2.5-cm) piece fresh ginger root

2 to 4 dried chilis

2 tablespoons coconut aminos

2 teaspoons apple cider vinegar

2 drops liquid stevia

¼ cup (40 g) roasted cashews, roughly chopped

SALAD DRESSING:

2 tablespoons unsweetened smooth almond butter

2 tablespoons refined avocado oil or hazelnut oil

1 tablespoon plus 1 teaspoon apple cider vinegar

1 tablespoon toasted sesame oil

1 tablespoon coconut aminos

FOR SERVING:

1 cucumber, spiral sliced (see page 154)

½ bunch fresh cilantro (about 1 ounce/ 28 g), chopped

1. If you want to marinate the pork before cooking, place all the ingredients for the stir-fry, except the cashews, in a large casserole dish. Toss to coat, then refrigerate for at least 1 hour and up to 12 hours.

2. To prepare the stir-fry: Place a medium-sized frying pan over medium heat. If you didn't marinate the pork, pour the oil into the hot pan and wait until the oil is hot, about 1 minute, then add the remaining stir-fry ingredients. If you did marinate the pork, add the marinated stir-fry ingredients, including the marinating juices, to the hot pan. Cook for 10 minutes, stirring frequently, or until the pork is cooked through. Remove from the heat and stir in the chopped cashews.

3. Meanwhile, make the salad dressing: Place the ingredients for the dressing in a small bowl and whisk to combine.

4. Place the spiral-sliced cucumber and cilantro on a serving platter and toss quickly. Place the stir-fried pork on the platter, next to the salad, and drizzle the salad and pork with the dressing.

STORE IT: *Keep in an airtight container in the fridge for up to 3 days or freeze the meat only for up to 1 month.*

REHEAT IT: *Microwave the meat until the desired temperature is reached. Or place in a covered casserole dish and reheat in a preheated 300°F (150°C) oven for 10 to 15 minutes, until warmed through. Or reheat in a frying pan, covered, on medium-low.*

THAW IT: *Allow to thaw completely in the fridge. Once defrosted, enjoy cold with the salad and dressing or use the reheating instructions above.*

MAKE IT COCONUT-FREE: *Replace the coconut aminos with a wheat-free soy sauce, if you tolerate soy.*

MAKE IT LOW-FODMAP: *Omit the garlic and replace the avocado oil in the stir-fry with Garlic-Infused Oil (page 230) made with refined avocado oil. Replace the cashews with roasted hulled sunflower seeds. If you are very, very sensitive to the FODMAPs in almonds, you could replace the almond butter with unsweetened sunflower seed butter.*

MAKE IT NIGHTSHADE-FREE: *Omit the dried chilis.*

MAKE IT NUT-FREE: *Replace the cashews with roasted hulled sunflower seeds and the almond butter with unsweetened sunflower seed butter. Use avocado oil rather than hazelnut oil.*

MAKE IT A CARB-UP: *Reduce the amount of pork to ½ pound (225 g). Omit the oil in the stir-fried pork and immediately place the marinade in the hot pan. Omit the cashews. Omit the avocado or hazelnut oil from the dressing, using only the 1 tablespoon of toasted sesame oil in the dressing. Serve alongside the carb of your choice (find ideas on page 117, or visit healthfulpursuit.com/carbup to download the complimentary PDF "Carb-Up Recipes"). It's scrumptious with spiral-sliced and roasted sweet potatoes, roasted cassava, or delicata squash.*

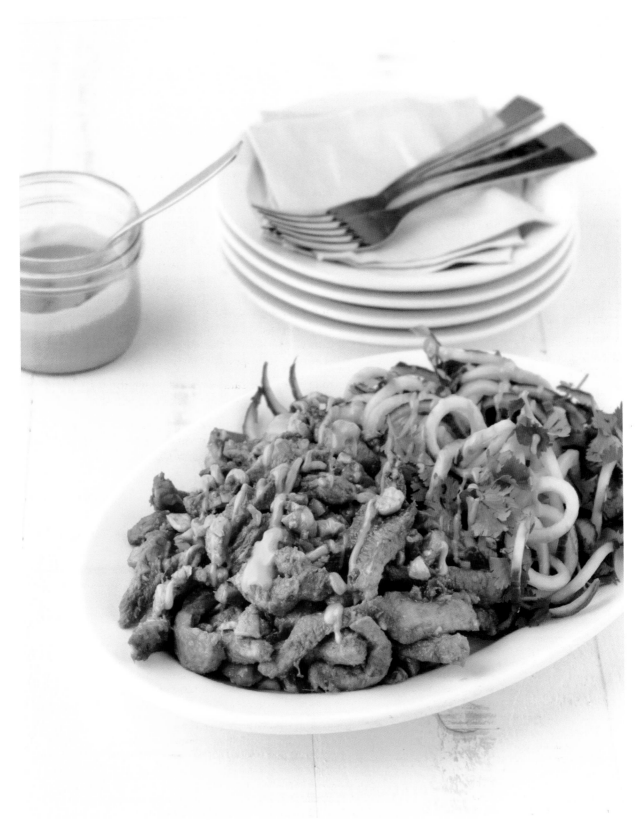

NUTRIENT INFORMATION (PER SERVING):

calories: 453 | calories from fat: 292 | total fat: 32.4g | saturated fat: 5.7g | cholesterol: 65mg

sodium: 81mg | carbs: 12g | dietary fiber: 2.1g | net carbs: 9.9g | sugars: 2.2g | protein: 28.4g

RATIOS:

fat:	carbs:	protein:
64%	11%	25%

PART 4: RECIPES   329

SALT AND PEPPER RIBS

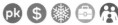

PREP TIME: **10 minutes, plus time to rest overnight** COOK TIME: **35 minutes to 4 hours 15 minutes** SERVES: **8**

COCONUT-FREE • EGG-FREE • NUT-FREE OPTIONS: LOW-FODMAP • NIGHTSHADE-FREE

This is my favorite way to enjoy ribs of any kind. I'm sure you could speed up the process, but I wouldn't recommend it. This recipe involves three steps: first you cook the ribs in a pressure cooker or slow cooker, then you let them rest overnight in the fridge, and finally you give them a nice charred exterior under the broiler or on the grill. If you're up for it, let the ribs kiss the flames! I do about 2 to 4 minutes per side, just to heat them up and develop the flavor. Depending on what part of the world you live in, the type of pork ribs used in this recipe may be called "pork side ribs" or "riblets."

3⅓ pounds (1.5 kg) country-style pork ribs

2 cups (475 ml) chicken bone broth (see page 152), or more as needed

1 tablespoon finely ground gray sea salt

2 teaspoons ground black pepper

1 batch Kickin' Ketchup (page 223), for serving (optional)

STORE IT: *Keep in an airtight container in the fridge for up to 4 days or in the freezer for up to 1 month.*

REHEAT IT: *Microwave until the desired temperature is reached. Or place in a covered casserole dish and reheat in a preheated 300°F (150°C) oven for 10 to 15 minutes, until warmed through. Or cut into individual rib pieces and reheat in a frying pan, covered, on medium-low.*

THAW IT: *Allow to thaw completely in the fridge. Once defrosted, use the reheating instructions above.*

PREP AHEAD: *The cooked ribs will keep in their cooking liquid in the fridge for up to 48 hours before being finished in the oven or on the grill.*

SERVE IT WITH: *To make this a complete meal, serve the ribs with a green salad, drizzled with your favorite dressing. These taste great paired with Potato Salad…That Isn't (page 386), Porky Cabbage (page 385), or Pesto Zoodles (page 381).*

1. Stand the ribs up around the inside wall of a pressure cooker or slow cooker, keeping the same side of the ribs facing outward. Add enough broth to come halfway up the sides of the ribs.

2. If using a pressure cooker, seal the lid and cook on high pressure for 15 minutes (for riblets) or 25 minutes (for full side ribs). If using a slow cooker, cook on low for 4 hours or on high for 2 hours. The ribs are perfectly cooked when the meat is tender but is still firmly attached to the bone; make sure to remove the ribs before the meat falls off the bones.

3. Transfer the cooked ribs and cooking liquid to a shallow baking dish. Once cool, cover and refrigerate overnight.

4. When ready to cook the ribs, preheat a grill to medium heat (350°F/177°C) or, if using the oven, place an oven rack in the top position and preheat the oven to 400°F (205°C).

5. Remove the ribs from the fridge. There will be hardened fats all around them. Slather the fats on the meaty top of each rib. Coat the ribs all over in the salt and pepper.

6. If finishing the ribs in the oven, place them on an unlined rimmed baking sheet and cook for 10 minutes, just until heated through. Then turn the broiler to low if that is an option; otherwise, simply "broil" is fine. Broil for 5 to 7 minutes, just until crisp.
If finishing the ribs on the grill, place the ribs in the preheated grill and cook for 1 to 2 minutes per side to heat them up and give them a crispy exterior.

7. Transfer to a serving plate and dig in!

MAKE IT LOW-FODMAP: *Use the low-FODMAP variation of the Kickin' Ketchup, or simply omit the ketchup.*

MAKE IT NIGHTSHADE-FREE: *Omit the ketchup.*

NUTRIENT INFORMATION (PER SERVING):

calories: 374 | calories from fat: 238 | total fat: 26.5g | saturated fat: 0g | cholesterol: 0mg

sodium: 752mg | carbs: 0.5g | dietary fiber: 0g | net carbs: 0.5g | sugars: 0g | protein: 33.3g

RATIOS:

fat:	carbs:	protein:
64%	**1%**	**35%**

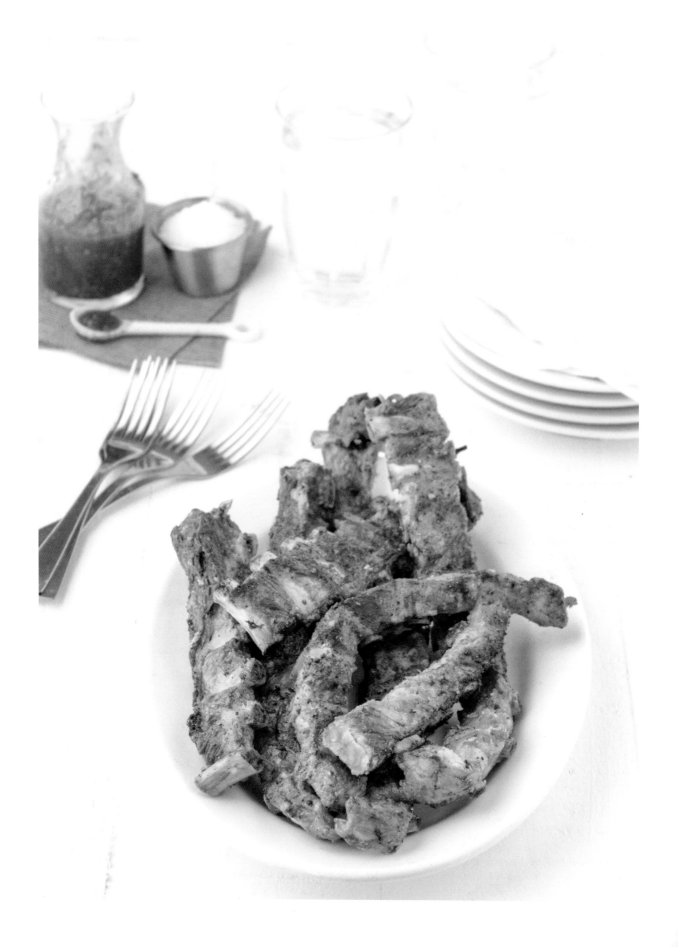

SHOULDER CHOPS WITH LEMON-THYME GRAVY

PREP TIME: **30 minutes**   COOK TIME: **40 minutes**   SERVES: **6**

EGG-FREE • LOW-FODMAP • NIGHTSHADE-FREE • NUT-FREE

Have you ever had a pork steak? Well, it's not called a "steak," exactly, but it may as well be. It's a steak! And it's great. I make pork steaks all the time, and I always use this recipe. Having grown up on pork chops and thinking that the chop was the only part of a pig you could eat, making pork steaks somehow feels…exclusive—rebellious even!

¼ cup (60 ml) refined avocado oil or melted coconut oil, for frying

2½ pounds (1.2 kg) bone-in pork shoulder blade chops (aka shoulder chops, blade steaks, or pork shoulder steaks), about ½ inch (1.25 cm) thick

1½ teaspoons finely ground gray sea salt, divided

1 teaspoon ground black pepper

⅓ cup (80 ml) white wine, such as Pinot Grigio, Sauvignon Blanc, or unoaked Chardonnay

2 tablespoons unflavored gelatin

Grated zest of 1 lemon

Juice of 1 lemon

1 teaspoon dried thyme leaves

⅔ cup (160 ml) full-fat coconut milk

1. Place the oil in a large frying pan over high heat. While the oil is heating, sprinkle 1 teaspoon of the salt and the pepper on both sides of the chops. Place the chops in the hot oil and sear for 4 minutes per side. Transfer the seared chops to a clean plate.

2. Remove the pan from the heat. Leaving the fat in the pan, add the wine, gelatin, lemon zest, lemon juice, thyme, and remaining ½ teaspoon of salt. Whisk to combine.

3. Return the chops to the frying pan. Cover and cook over medium-low heat for 30 minutes, flipping them halfway through cooking.

4. Place an oven rack in the top position and turn on the broiler to low, if that is an option (if not, simply "broil" is fine). Place the chops in an oven-safe pan (I like to use cast iron) and set the pan on the top rack of the oven. Broil the chops for 3 minutes per side, or until just browned. Allow to rest for 5 minutes.

5. Meanwhile, add the coconut milk to the liquid in the frying pan. Cook over medium heat for 15 minutes, whisking occasionally, until slightly thickened.

6. If serving individually instead of family style, remove the bones from each chop and divide the steaks into 6 servings. Serve the chops drizzled with the gravy.

STORE IT: *Keep in an airtight container in the fridge for up to 4 days or in the freezer for up to 1 month.*

REHEAT IT: *Microwave until the desired temperature is reached. Or place in a covered casserole dish and reheat in a preheated 300°F (150°C) oven for 5 to 10 minutes, until warmed through. Or reheat in a frying pan, covered, on medium-low.*

SERVE IT WITH: *To make this a complete meal, serve it alongside your favorite steamed vegetables. I used broccoli for this shot, but steamed cabbage or sautéed chard would be great, too!*

NUTRIENT INFORMATION (PER SERVING WITH 2½ TABLESPOONS GRAVY):
calories: 511 | calories from fat: 369 | total fat: 40.9g | saturated fat: 14.9g | cholesterol: 118mg
sodium: 658mg | carbs: 2.5g | dietary fiber: 0g | net carbs: 2.5g | sugars: 0g | protein: 33.3g

RATIOS:
fat: carbs: protein:
72%   2%   26%

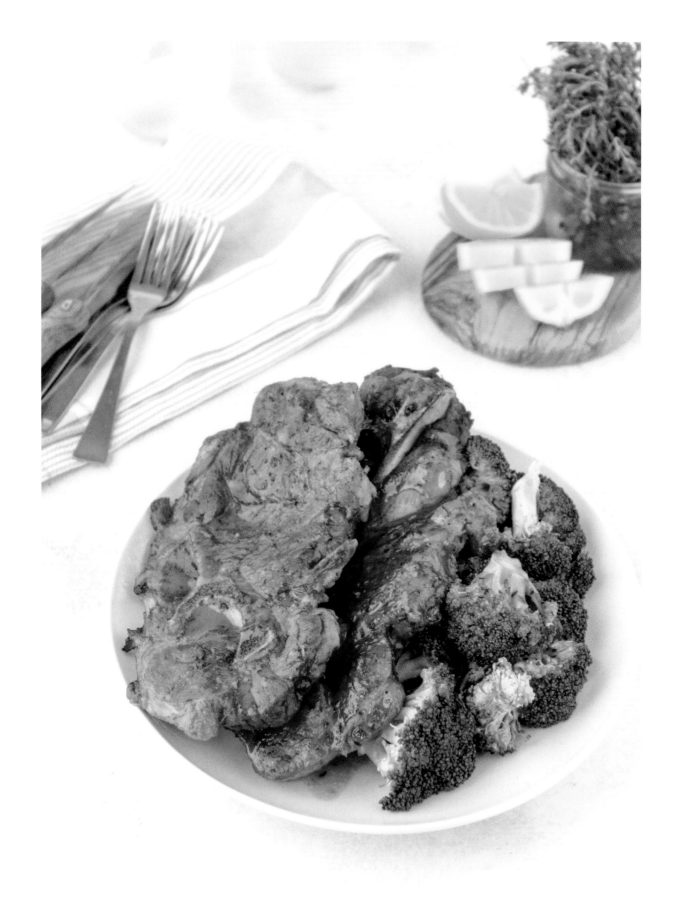

STUFFED PORK ROAST WITH HERB GRAVY

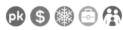

PREP TIME: **15 minutes**   COOK TIME: **1 hour 40 minutes**   SERVES: **8**

COCONUT-FREE · EGG-FREE · LOW-FODMAP · NIGHTSHADE-FREE · NUT-FREE

You can use any high-fat cut of boneless meat you'd like for this recipe. A butterflied beef tenderloin, pork shoulder roast, or pork loin would also work. I like using boneless pork rib roast as I find it doesn't need to be marinated, making this recipe really quick to prep. While "rib roast" suggests that there are ribs in the cut, you can get rib roasts from your local grocer or butcher without the bone.

For this recipe, the roast needs to be butterflied, or cut open like a book. Unless you have a really good knife and confidence in cutting a slab of meat perfectly, I suggest that you ask your butcher to butterfly the roast for you. Because I'm a klutz in the kitchen, I ask my butcher to cut the roast so that it opens "like a book" so that I can stuff and roll it; they do a perfect job, and I get to keep all my fingers!

For the pork rinds, I crush a 2-ounce (56-g) bag of Bacon's Heir Rosemary and Sea Salt Pork Clouds. The rosemary flavor takes the stuffing to a whole new level.

2 pounds (910 g) boneless pork rib roast, butterflied

1 tablespoon refined avocado oil, for the pan

2 cups (475 ml) chicken bone broth (see page 152)

1 teaspoon tapioca starch, for the gravy

STUFFING:

1 bunch fresh parsley (about 2 ounces/ 55 g), chopped

3 tablespoons refined avocado oil or refined olive oil

2 ounces (57 g) pork dust or ground pork rinds (see note, above)

1 tablespoon Italian Seasoning (page 234)

1 teaspoon finely ground gray sea salt

1 teaspoon ground black pepper

HERB COATING:

3 tablespoons refined avocado oil or refined olive oil

2 teaspoons Italian Seasoning (page 234)

1 teaspoon finely ground gray sea salt

½ teaspoon ground black pepper

SPECIAL EQUIPMENT:

3 pieces cotton twine, 16 inches (40.5 cm) each

STORE IT: *Keep in an airtight container in the fridge for up to 4 days or in the freezer for up to 1 month.*

1. Preheat the oven to 325°F (163°C).

2. Place the roast on a cutting board and lay it flat, with a short end facing you. Combine the ingredients for the stuffing in a medium-sized bowl. Spread the stuffing over the surface of the roast, pushing it all the way to the two long edges and the short end nearest to you, leaving about one-quarter on the farthest, short end free from stuffing. Roll it up like a sushi roll and tie together with twine.

3. Heat 1 tablespoon of avocado oil in a large cast-iron frying pan or other oven-safe pan over medium-high heat. Meanwhile, combine the ingredients for the herb coating and coat the roast on all sides.

4. Transfer the coated roast to the hot pan and sear on all sides, 2 minutes per section. Once seared, pour the chicken broth into the pan around the roast. Transfer the pork to the oven and roast for 1½ hours, or until the internal temperature reaches 165°F (74°C) and the top has browned really nicely.

5. Transfer the roast to a cutting board to rest while you make the gravy. Set the pan over medium-high heat. Sprinkle in the tapioca starch and simmer, whisking constantly, until thickened, about 2 minutes.

6. Slice the roast into 8 pieces, transfer to a serving plate, and drizzle with the gravy, or serve the gravy on the side.

REHEAT IT: *Microwave until the desired temperature is reached. Or place in a covered casserole dish and reheat in a preheated 300°F (150°C) oven for 10 to 15 minutes, until warmed through. Or reheat in a frying pan, covered, on medium-low.*

THAW IT: *Allow to thaw completely in the fridge. Once defrosted, enjoy cold in a salad or use the reheating instructions above.*

SERVE IT WITH: *To make this a complete meal, serve alongside your favorite roasted vegetables.*

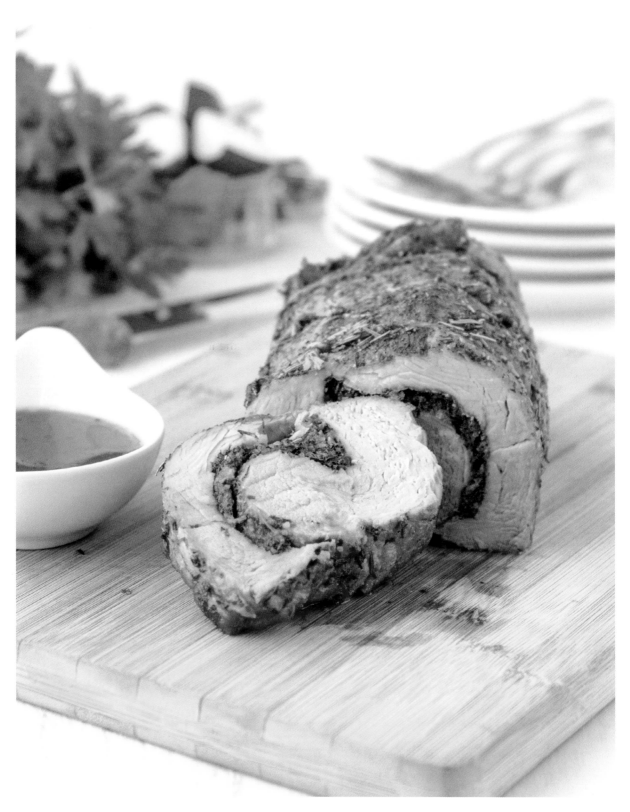

NUTRIENT INFORMATION (PER SERVING WITH 1½ TABLESPOONS GRAVY):

calories: 434 | calories from fat: 270 | total fat: 30.1g | saturated fat: 8.4g | cholesterol: 95mg

sodium: 794mg | carbs: 1.1g | dietary fiber: 0g | net carbs: 1.1g | sugars: 0g | protein: 39.7g

RATIOS:

fat:	carbs:	protein:
62%	**1%**	**37%**

BAKED OLIVE CHICKEN

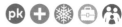

PREP TIME: **20 minutes**   COOK TIME: **about 50 minutes**   SERVES: **8**

COCONUT-FREE • EGG-FREE • NIGHTSHADE-FREE • NUT-FREE   OPTION: **LOW-FODMAP**

This meal strategy is often the one I turn to when I'm in a rush to prepare dinner but still want something warm and homemade. While I've chosen to prepare this dish with a Mediterranean flair, you can place just about anything in the pan before adding the chicken. And it doesn't even have to be chicken! I've made this meal with turkey thighs, salmon, steak, and pork chops wrapped in bacon. Instead of fennel and onions, try chopped cabbage for the base. It's a fabulous alternative, as is zucchini, celery, squash, or braising greens.

BASE:

1 lemon

½ cup (120 ml) refined avocado oil or melted chicken fat

1 large fennel bulb (about 10½ ounces/ 300 g), sliced thinly

2 small white onions, sliced

2 (13½-ounce/400-ml) cans pitted kalamata olives

⅔ cup (40 g) fresh parsley, roughly chopped

8 small cloves garlic or 4 large cloves garlic, minced

Leaves from 2 sprigs fresh rosemary

1 teaspoon finely ground gray sea salt

½ teaspoon ground black pepper

4 bone-in, skin-on chicken breasts (about 2 pounds/910 g)

1 tablespoon Greek Seasoning (page 232) or Italian Seasoning (page 234)

½ teaspoon finely ground gray sea salt

½ teaspoon ground black pepper

1. Preheat the oven to 375°F (190°C).

2. Make the base: Juice the lemon and cut the juiced halves into thirds. Place the lemon juice, lemon wedges, and the rest of the ingredients for the base in a large bowl. Toss to combine, then transfer to a large roasting pan or cast-iron pan.

3. Place the chicken breasts on top and sprinkle with the Greek or Italian seasoning and ½ teaspoon each of salt and pepper.

4. Bake for 45 to 55 minutes, until the internal temperature of the chicken reaches 165°F (74°C) and the juices run clear.

5. Remove the pan from the oven, transfer the chicken to a cutting board, and cut each breast in half. Remove the lemon pieces from the olive mixture, then divide the mixture, including the juices, among 8 large, shallow soup bowls. Top with a halved chicken breast and dig in.

STORE IT: *Keep in an airtight container in the fridge for up to 4 days or in the freezer for up to 1 month.*

REHEAT IT: *Microwave, covered, until the desired temperature is reached or reheat in a frying pan, covered, on medium.*

THAW IT: *Allow to thaw completely in the fridge. Once defrosted, use the reheating instructions above.*

MAKE IT LOW-FODMAP: *Use Italian seasoning. Replace the fennel bulb, onions, and olives with 2 large zucchinis and 1 medium eggplant, cut into rounds. Replace 2 tablespoons of the avocado oil with Garlic-Infused Oil (page 230) made with refined avocado oil.*

MAKE IT A CARB-UP: *Omit the avocado oil and use boneless, skinless chicken breasts. Serve alongside the carb of your choice (find ideas on page 117, or visit healthfulpursuit.com/carbup to download the complimentary PDF "Carb-Up Recipes"). It's amazing with a bowl of fresh fruit as a simple dessert.*

NUTRIENT INFORMATION (PER SERVING):

calories: 463 | calories from fat: 234 | total fat: 26g | saturated fat: 4.5g | cholesterol: 130mg

sodium: 952mg | carbs: 13.3g | dietary fiber: 4.3g | net carbs: 9g | sugars: 1.7g | protein: 43.9g

RATIOS:

fat: 51%   carbs: 11%   protein: 38%

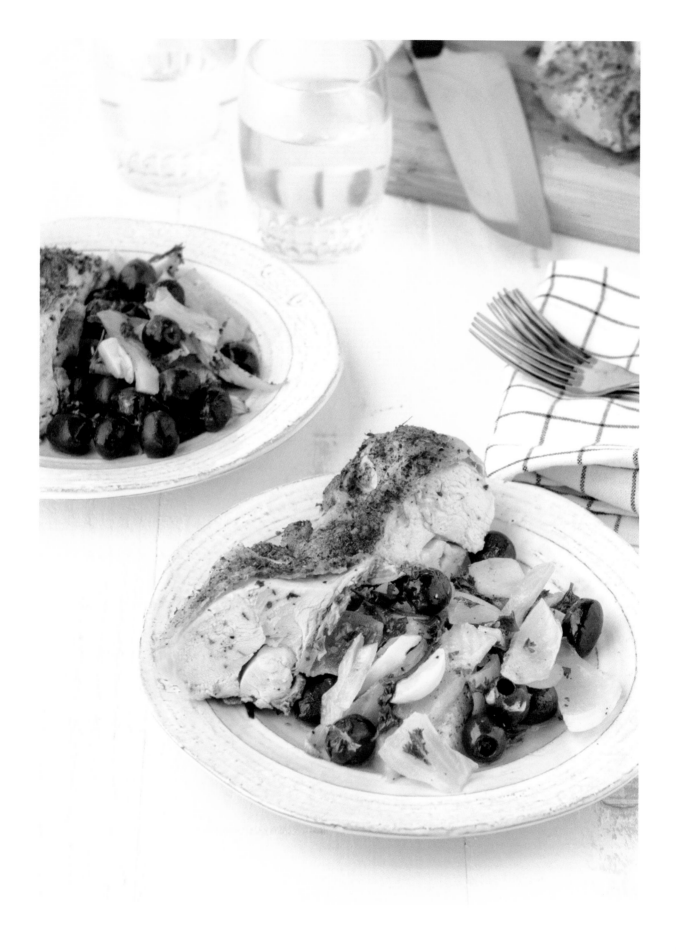

BALSAMIC TURKEY THIGHS

    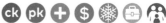

PREP TIME: 5 minutes, plus at least 1 hour to marinate   COOK TIME: 1 hour   SERVES: 8

COCONUT-FREE · EGG-FREE · LOW-FODMAP · NIGHTSHADE-FREE · NUT-FREE

The real goodness (and crispy skin!) happens when I use NUCO's balsamic-style coconut vinegar for this marinade. The vinegar is fermented coconut syrup, so it has natural sugars that lightly crystallize and crisp the thickest of skin, making it a fabulous addition to your next marinade!

¼ cup (60 ml) balsamic vinegar (see above)

¼ cup (60 ml) refined avocado oil or refined olive oil

1 tablespoon Dijon mustard

2 teaspoons finely ground gray sea salt

1 teaspoon Italian Seasoning (page 234)

2½ pounds (1.2 kg) bone-in, skin-on turkey thighs

1. Place the vinegar, oil, mustard, salt, and seasoning in a large casserole dish or resealable plastic bag. Mix thoroughly. Add the turkey thighs and cover. Marinate in the refrigerator for 1 hour or up to 24 hours.

2. When ready to cook, preheat the oven to 350°F (177°C). Lay the turkey thighs on an unlined rimmed baking sheet or cast-iron pan. Bake for 55 to 60 minutes, until the internal temperature reaches 165°F (74°C) and the juices run clear.

3. Turn the oven broiler to high. (If your oven does not offer that option, simply "broil" is fine.) Broil for 3 to 5 minutes, until browned. Allow to rest for 5 minutes before slicing and serving.

STORE IT: *Keep in an airtight container in the fridge for up to 4 days or in the freezer for up to 1 month.*

REHEAT IT: *Microwave, covered, until the desired temperature is reached. Or place in a covered casserole dish and reheat in a preheated 300°F (150°C) oven for 10 to 15 minutes, until warmed through. Or reheat in a frying pan, covered, on medium.*

THAW IT: *Allow to thaw completely in the fridge. Once defrosted, use the reheating instructions above, or enjoy cold on a salad.*

PREP AHEAD: *Begin marinating the turkey thighs up to 24 hours before cooking.*

SERVE IT WITH: *To make this a complete meal, serve it with an arugula salad with crushed roasted hazelnuts, balsamic vinegar, and olive oil. It also tastes great paired with Pesto Zoodles (page 381).*

MAKE IT A CARB-UP: *Serve alongside the carb of your choice (find ideas on page 117, or visit healthfulpursuit.com/carbup to download the complimentary PDF "Carb-Up Recipes"). It's scrumptious with a green salad tossed with sliced grapes and apples.*

NUTRIENT INFORMATION (PER SERVING):
calories: 333 | calories from fat: 224 | total fat: 24.9g | saturated fat: 0.9g | cholesterol: 0mg
sodium: 491mg | carbs: 0.2g | dietary fiber: 0g | net carbs: 0.2g | sugars: 0g | protein: 27.1g

RATIOS:
fat:	carbs:	protein:
67%	0%	33%

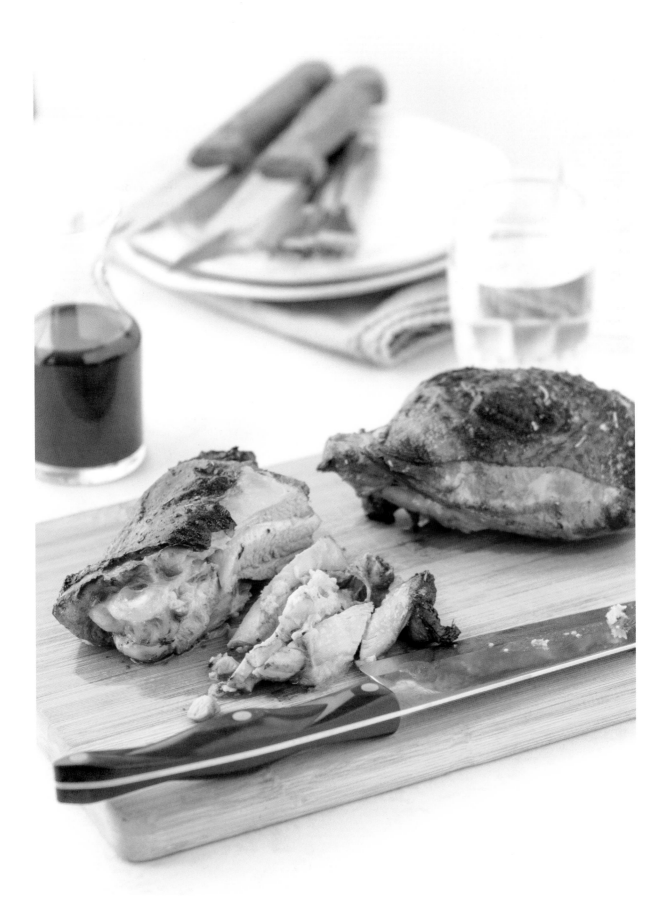

BUTTER CHICKEN

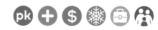

PREP TIME: **10 minutes**   COOK TIME: **45 minutes**   SERVES: **4**

EGG-FREE   OPTIONS: LOW-FODMAP • NUT-FREE

One of the many highlights of my trip to India was taking an all-day cooking class in south India with a couple of travel pals. We learned how to make some of our newfound favorite southern Indian dishes, including aloo palak, dhal aloo kofta, baingan bharta, and pineapple payasam. While butter chicken is less Indian than it is North American, I've taken what I learned in the class and translated it into this dish. If you want to go all out, you can make your own garam masala by toasting whole spices and grinding them to a powder (look for recipes online), or you can skip all that and go for the quickest route (which is what I do), which is to use a premade garam masala blend.

⅓ cup (70 g) coconut oil

1⅓ pounds (600 g) boneless, skinless chicken thighs, cubed

½ cup (70 g) sliced yellow onions

2 small cloves garlic, minced

1 (1-in/2.5-cm) piece fresh ginger root, grated

1 (14½-ounce/400-g/428-ml) can diced tomatoes

1 cup (240 ml) chicken bone broth (see page 152)

1 bay leaf

1 tablespoon garam masala or Curry Powder (page 235)

1 teaspoon ground cumin

1 teaspoon finely ground gray sea salt

½ teaspoon ground coriander

¼ teaspoon ground cloves

⅛ teaspoon ground black pepper

⅛ teaspoon ground cardamom

⅓ cup (80 ml) full-fat coconut milk

3 tablespoons blanched almond flour

1 tablespoon fresh lemon juice

Handful of fresh cilantro, roughly chopped, for garnish

Sliced green onions, for garnish

> STORE IT: *Keep in an airtight container in the fridge for up to 4 days or in the freezer for up to 1 month.*

1. Melt the coconut oil in a large saucepan or deep sauté pan over medium-high heat. Add the cubed chicken to the pan and cook for 10 minutes, or until the chicken is no longer pink.

2. Add the onions, garlic, and ginger and continue to cook for 5 minutes, until fragrant.

3. Add the tomatoes, bone broth, bay leaf, garam masala, cumin, salt, coriander, cloves, pepper, and cardamom and give everything a stir. Cover and bring to a boil, then reduce the heat to low and lightly simmer for 20 minutes.

4. Stir in the coconut milk, almond flour, and lemon juice. Increase the heat to medium-high and cook for 5 minutes, until slightly thickened.

5. Remove the bay leaf. Divide the chicken and sauce among 4 serving bowls. Top with cilantro and green onions and enjoy.

REHEAT IT: *Microwave, covered, until the desired temperature is reached; place in a covered casserole dish and reheat in a preheated 300°F (150°C) oven for 10 to 15 minutes, until warmed through; or reheat in a frying pan, covered, on medium.*

THAW IT: *Allow to thaw completely in the fridge. Once defrosted, use the reheating instructions above.*

PRESSURE-COOK IT: *Complete Steps 1 and 2 in a pressure cooker, using the sauté function. Add the ingredients listed in Step 3, then seal the lid and set to high pressure for 10 minutes. Allow the pressure to release, then remove the lid. Continue with the recipe, using the sauté function to complete Step 4.*

SERVE IT WITH: *This dish tastes great paired with Coconut Cauliflower Rice or plain cauliflower rice (both on page 364).*

MAKE IT LOW-FODMAP: *Replace the sliced yellow onions with sliced green onions, green parts only. Replace the garlic and 2 tablespoons of the coconut oil with 2 tablespoons of Garlic-Infused Oil (page 230) made with refined avocado oil. Use only the green part of the onion for garnish.*

MAKE IT NUT-FREE: *Omit the almond flour.*

MAKE IT A CARB-UP: *Reduce the amount of coconut oil to 1 tablespoon. Serve alongside the carb of your choice (find ideas on page 117, or visit healthfulpursuit.com/carbup to download the complimentary PDF "Carb-Up Recipes"). It's amazing with spiral-sliced parsnips (see page 154), grilled pineapple, or microwaved acorn squash.*

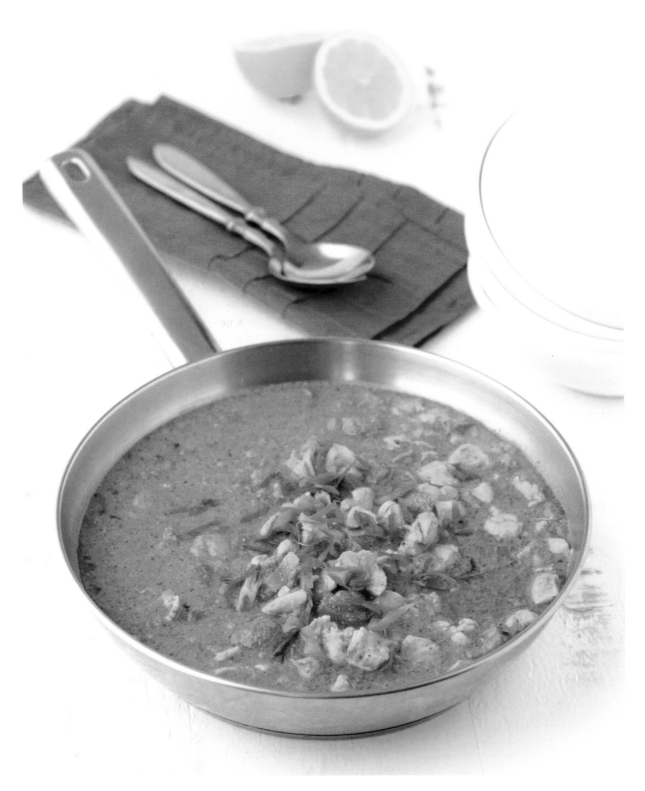

NUTRIENT INFORMATION (PER SERVING):

calories: 450 | calories from fat: 281 | total fat: 31.3g | saturated fat: 20.5g | cholesterol: 126mg

sodium: 716mg | carbs: 7.6g | dietary fiber: 2.2g | net carbs: 5.4g | sugars: 3.5g | protein: 34.4g

RATIOS:

fat: carbs: protein:

63% **7%** **30%**

CHICKEN ALFREDO

PREP TIME: **15 minutes**   COOK TIME: **35 minutes**   SERVES: **4**

NIGHTSHADE-FREE • NUT-FREE   OPTIONS: COCONUT-FREE • LOW-FODMAP

If you accidentally include some egg whites in the egg yolk mixture, or slightly overcook the egg yolks, and the alfredo sauce starts to get all chunky on you, you can strain it through a fine-mesh strainer.

4 bone-in, skin-on chicken thighs (about 1⅓ pounds/600 g)

2 teaspoons finely ground gray sea salt

2 teaspoons ground black pepper

ALFREDO SAUCE:

1 cup (240 ml) nondairy milk

¼ cup (52 g) coconut oil

2 teaspoons apple cider vinegar

2 tablespoons Garlic-Infused Oil (page 230), made with refined avocado oil

¼ teaspoon finely ground gray sea salt

½ teaspoon ground black pepper

6 large egg yolks

1 batch Zoodles or Doodles (page 376), for serving

Chopped fresh parsley, for garnish (optional)

1. Preheat the oven to 400°F (205°C). Place the chicken thighs in a cast-iron frying pan or on an unlined rimmed baking sheet. Season the chicken with 2 teaspoons of salt and 2 teaspoons of pepper. Roast for 30 minutes, or until the internal temperature reaches 165°F (74°C) and the juices run clear. Remove from the oven and allow to sit for 5 minutes.

2. Meanwhile, make the sauce: Place the milk, coconut oil, vinegar, infused oil, ¼ teaspoon salt, and ½ teaspoon pepper in a small saucepan over medium heat. Bring to a boil, then reduce the heat to low.

3. In a medium-sized heatproof bowl, lightly whisk the egg yolks. Slowly add the hot milk mixture to the yolks, whisking continuously. Once a third of the milk mixture is in the egg bowl, transfer the egg mixture to the saucepan, whisking nonstop. Continue to cook over low heat, stirring constantly, for 1 minute.

4. Divide the noodles among 4 dinner plates. Place a chicken thigh on each plate and drizzle the sauce over the top. Garnish with parsley, if desired, and serve.

STORE IT: *Keep the sauce and the noodles in separate airtight containers in the fridge for up to 4 days.*

REHEAT IT: *Microwave, covered, until the desired temperature is reached. Or place in a covered casserole dish and reheat in a preheated 300°F (150°C) oven for 10 to 15 minutes, until warmed through. Or reheat in a frying pan, covered, on medium.*

PREP AHEAD: *Use 15½ ounces (445 g) of cooked chicken.*

MAKE IT COCONUT-FREE: *Replace the coconut oil with refined avocado oil, melted lard, or ghee (if tolerated).*

MAKE IT LOW-FODMAP: *Avoid using cashew or pistachio milk.*

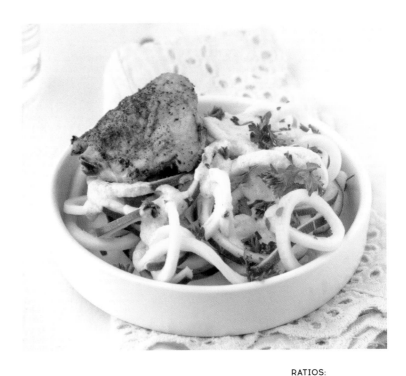

NUTRIENT INFORMATION (PER SERVING):

calories: 651 | calories from fat: 506 | total fat: 56.2g | saturated fat: 25.4g | cholesterol: 462mg

sodium: 1226mg | carbs: 5.6g | dietary fiber: 1.7g | net carbs: 3.9g | sugars: 1.9g | protein: 30.8g

RATIOS:

fat:	carbs:	protein:
78%	3%	19%

ONE-POT CHICKEN DINNER

PREP TIME: **10 minutes**   COOK TIME: **about 20 minutes**   SERVES: **4**

COCONUT-FREE • EGG-FREE • LOW-FODMAP • NIGHTSHADE-FREE   OPTION: **NUT-FREE**

You don't have to toast the walnuts, but they sure taste delicious when you do! Raw walnuts are fine to use, but for health reasons it's better to soak and roast them before using them in this recipe (see page 157).

¼ cup (52 g) lard

10½ ounces (300 g) boneless, skinless chicken thighs, thinly sliced

8 strips bacon (about 8 ounces/225 g), chopped

4 cups (470 g) sliced green or red cabbage

1 tablespoon dried oregano leaves

1 teaspoon finely ground gray sea salt

½ teaspoon ground black pepper

½ cup (56 g) raw walnut pieces, roasted

1 tablespoon apple cider vinegar

1. Melt the lard in a large saucepan or frying pan over medium-high heat. Once melted, add the sliced chicken and chopped bacon. Cook until the chicken is no longer pink, about 10 minutes.

2. Add the sliced cabbage, oregano, salt, and pepper. Cover, reduce the heat to medium-low, and cook until the cabbage is fork-tender, about 6 minutes.

3. Add the walnuts and vinegar. Cover and cook for another 5 minutes.

4. Divide the mixture among 4 serving bowls and enjoy!

STORE IT: *Keep in an airtight container in the fridge for up to 3 days.*

REHEAT IT: *Microwave, covered, until the desired temperature is reached. Or place in a covered casserole dish and reheat in a preheated 300°F (150°C) oven for 10 to 15 minutes, until warmed through; or reheat in a frying pan, covered, on medium.*

PRESSURE-COOK IT: *Complete Step 1 in a pressure cooker using the sauté function. Add the rest of the ingredients plus ¼ cup (60 ml) of chicken bone broth (see page 152). Seal the lid and cook on high pressure for 2 minutes. Allow the pressure to release, then remove the lid and serve.*

SERVE IT WITH: *To make this a complete meal, top it with sliced avocado.*

MAKE IT NUT-FREE: *Replace the walnuts with hulled hemp seeds.*

MAKE IT A CARB-UP: *Omit the lard. Cook the bacon in the saucepan until the fat has rendered, about 5 minutes. Add the chicken and cook until no longer pink, about 10 minutes. Pick up with Step 2 above. Serve alongside the carb of your choice (find ideas on page 117, or visit healthfulpursuit.com/carbup to download the complimentary PDF "Carb-Up Recipes"). It's delicious with fried spiral-sliced potatoes.*

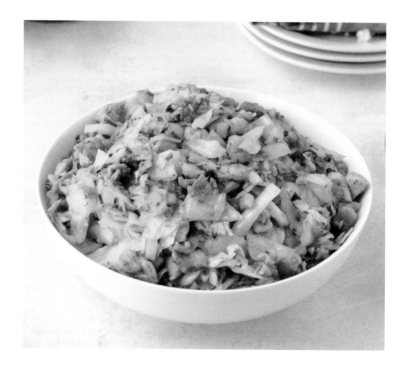

NUTRIENT INFORMATION (PER SERVING):

calories: 592 | calories from fat: 446 | total fat: 49.6g | saturated fat: 14.8g | cholesterol: 116mg

sodium: 952mg | carbs: 10.5g | dietary fiber: 4.3g | net carbs: 6.2g | sugars: 4.7g | protein: 25.9g

RATIOS:

fat:	carbs:	protein:
75%	7%	18%

CHICKEN POT PIE CRUMBLE

PREP TIME: **25 minutes**   COOK TIME: **45 minutes**   SERVES: **4**

NIGHTSHADE-FREE • NUT-FREE

You could make a chicken pot pie topped with a smooth crust. You'd spend a lot of time making the dough, kneading it, rolling it, and getting frustrated when it inevitably tears. Or you could make a crumble and shave 30 minutes off the total preparation time. I vote the latter…and I'm sure you do, too.

Coconut oil, for the dish

FILLING:

¼ cup (55 g) coconut oil or duck fat

1 pound (455 g) boneless, skinless chicken thighs, cubed

⅓ cup (55 g) diced celery

¼ cup (45 g) diced white onions

¼ cup (40 g) diced carrots

2 small cloves garlic, minced

1 small head cauliflower

2 cups (475 ml) chicken bone broth (see page 152)

¾ teaspoon finely ground gray sea salt

½ teaspoon onion powder

CRUMBLE:

1 tablespoon hot cauliflower cooking liquid (from above)

¼ cup plus 2 tablespoons (40 g) coconut flour

¼ cup (55 g) coconut oil

1 large egg

½ teaspoon garlic powder

½ teaspoon onion powder

1. Preheat the oven to 350°F (177°C) and grease a shallow 1½-quart (1.4-L) casserole dish with coconut oil.

2. Make the filling: Melt the coconut oil in a frying pan over medium heat. Add the chicken and sauté for 10 minutes, or until cooked through. Add the celery, onions, carrots, and garlic and continue to cook for 5 minutes. Remove from the heat.

3. Meanwhile, break up the cauliflower into large florets (you should have about 14 ounces/400 g of florets) and place them in a saucepan with the broth. Cover and bring to a boil over high heat. Reduce the heat to medium-low and simmer for 15 minutes, until the cauliflower is fork-tender. Transfer the cauliflower and ½ cup (120 ml) of the cooking liquid (reserve the rest for later) to a blender. Add the salt and onion powder and blend on high until smooth, about 1 minute.

4. Pour the cauliflower cream into the frying pan with the chicken pieces. Stir to combine, then transfer to the prepared casserole dish.

5. Make the crumble: Place 1 tablespoon of the hot cauliflower cooking liquid, the coconut flour, coconut oil, egg, garlic powder, and onion powder in a medium-sized bowl. Combine with your hands until the mixture forms a ball.

6. Crumble the dough over the top of the filling, distributing it evenly. Bake for 25 to 30 minutes, until the top is golden. Serve immediately.

STORE IT: *Keep in an airtight container in the fridge for up to 3 days.*

REHEAT IT: *Microwave until the desired temperature is reached, or place in a covered casserole dish and reheat in a preheated 300°F (150°C) oven for 10 to 15 minutes, until warmed through. (Note: To prevent breakage, never place a chilled glass or ceramic dish directly from the fridge into a hot oven.)*

PREP AHEAD: *Following Step 3, prepare the cauliflower cream up to 2 days before making the rest of the recipe. Remember to reserve 1 tablespoon of the cooking liquid for the crumble and heat it up before using it in Step 5. If you forget to reserve the cooking liquid, use 1 tablespoon of hot chicken bone broth or hot water.*

NUTRIENT INFORMATION (PER SERVING):

calories: 474 | calories from fat: 312 | total fat: 34.7g | saturated fat: 26.6g | cholesterol: 137mg

sodium: 359mg | carbs: 10.3g | dietary fiber: 4.8g | net carbs: 5.5g | sugars: 2.5g | protein: 30g

RATIOS:

fat:	carbs:	protein:
66%	**9%**	**25%**

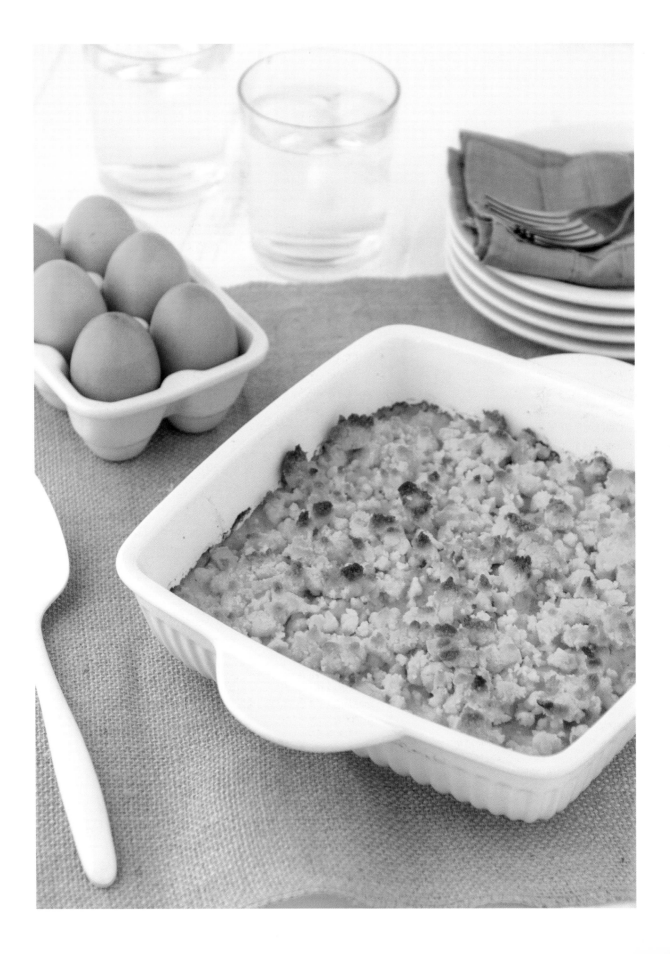

GREEK CHICKEN WITH GRAVY AND ASPARAGUS

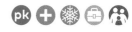

PREP TIME: **15 minutes**   COOK TIME: **1½ hours**   SERVES: **6**

EGG-FREE • NIGHTSHADE-FREE • NUT-FREE   OPTION: COCONUT-FREE

When I'm pressed for time but craving a hearty meal that helps me wind down after a stressful week, this roast chicken does the trick every time. Depending on what you have on hand or how much effort you want to put into it, you can change the ingredients used to stuff the chicken, as well as the herbs used to season the chicken. My other go-to combination (and an even simpler one) is salt and pepper sprinkled over the top and pieces of green apple and fresh parsley stuffed inside. A bit of juice from the apples is added to the drippings as the chicken cooks, and the apples keep the meat really moist. A win every time!

My family has always prepared giblet gravy. When I make this kind of gravy for guests, they think it's the oddest thing. But using the giblets makes the gravy taste so, so good, not to mention boosting the nutrients, that I wouldn't dream of doing it another way! You could, however, replace the giblet cooking liquids with an equal amount of chicken bone broth to save time, or if your chicken didn't come with the giblets!

1 (3½-pound/1.6-kg) whole chicken, giblets removed and reserved

3 tablespoons refined avocado oil or melted coconut oil

1½ tablespoons Greek Seasoning (page 232)

1 apple, roughly chopped

Handful of fresh parsley

6 sprigs fresh oregano

6 sprigs fresh thyme

4 small cloves garlic

GRAVY:

Giblets (from above)

3 tablespoons melted duck fat

1 teaspoon tapioca starch

1 pound (455 g) asparagus, tough ends removed, for serving

1. Preheat the oven to 350°F (177°C). Set the chicken in a roasting pan or large cast-iron frying pan. Coat all sides of the bird with the oil, then top with the Greek seasoning. Stuff the bird with the apple, parsley, oregano, thyme, and garlic. Roast for 1 hour 15 minutes, or until the internal temperature in the thigh reaches 165°F (74°C) and the juices run clear.

2. While the bird is cooking, cook the giblets: Place the giblets in a small saucepan and cover with about 1½ cups (350 ml) of water, then cover the pan with a lid and bring to a boil. Reduce the heat to low and simmer for 30 minutes. Strain the giblet pieces, reserving the flavorful cooking liquid. Discard the giblets.

3. About 10 minutes before the bird is done, steam the asparagus.

4. When the chicken is done, remove it from the oven and transfer the bird to a serving platter. Remove the stuffing and surround the chicken with the steamed asparagus.

5. Place the roasting pan on the stovetop over medium heat. Add ½ cup (120 ml) of the giblet cooking liquid and the melted duck fat to the pan and whisk to combine. Add the tapioca starch and continue to whisk until the gravy has thickened.

6. Drizzle the gravy over the bird or serve on the side.

STORE IT: *Keep in an airtight container in the fridge for up to 4 days or in the freezer for up to 1 month.*

REHEAT IT: *Microwave, covered, or place in a frying pan, cover, and warm over medium heat until the desired temperature is reached.*

THAW IT: *Allow to thaw completely in the fridge. Once defrosted, use the reheating instructions above.*

MAKE IT COCONUT-FREE: *Use avocado oil.*

MAKE IT A CARB-UP: *Omit the gravy or save it for another meal. Do not coat the bird with oil. Serve the chicken alongside the carb of your choice (find ideas on page 117, or visit healthfulpursuit.com/carbup to download the complimentary PDF "Carb-Up Recipes"). It's fabulous with grilled cassava, boiled green plantains, or roasted jicama.*

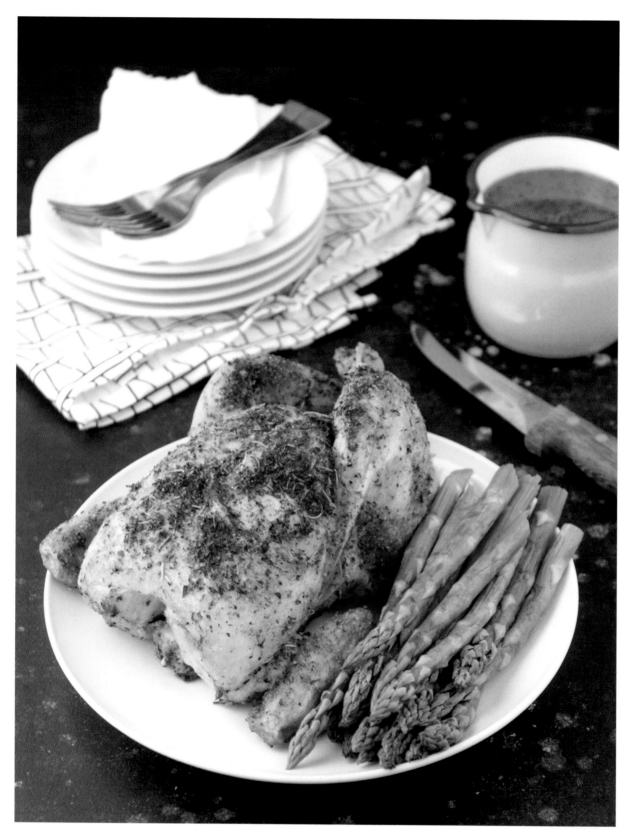

NUTRIENT INFORMATION (PER SERVING WITH 2 TABLESPOONS GRAVY):

calories: 580 | calories from fat: 366 | total fat: 40.7g | saturated fat: 11.9g | cholesterol: 231mg

sodium: 248mg | carbs: 3.8g | dietary fiber: 1.9g | net carbs: 1.9g | sugars: 1.5g | protein: 49.7g

RATIOS:

fat: carbs: protein:

63%   **3%**   **34%**

ORANGE-GLAZED ROASTED DUCK

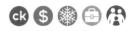

PREP TIME: **15 minutes**   COOK TIME: **1½ hours**   SERVES: **6**

COCONUT-FREE • EGG-FREE • NIGHTSHADE-FREE • NUT-FREE   OPTION: LOW-FODMAP

My mom is obsessed with duck. During a visit last summer, she taught me to how roast a duck perfectly, thanks to a gorgeous recipe from one of her favorite chefs that she'd adapted to cut the prep time in half. While Mom loves to cook, she doesn't enjoy spending countless hours in the kitchen. When I started planning the poultry chapter for this book, it was a no-brainer to include this recipe!

1 (5-pound/2.3-kg) whole duck, giblets removed

1 orange

4 fresh thyme sprigs

Handful of fresh parsley

2¼ teaspoons finely ground gray sea salt, divided

1 teaspoon ground coriander

¾ teaspoon ground black pepper

½ teaspoon ground cumin

¾ cup (180 ml) chicken bone broth (see page 152), divided

¼ cup white wine, such as Pinot Grigio, Sauvignon Blanc, or unoaked Chardonnay

⅓ cup (53 g) confectioners'-style erythritol

2 tablespoons apple cider vinegar

SPECIAL EQUIPMENT:

Cotton twine

STORE IT: *Keep in an airtight container in the fridge for up to 4 days or in the freezer for up to 1 month.*

REHEAT IT: *Microwave, covered, until the desired temperature is reached. Or place in a covered casserole dish and reheat in a preheated 300°F (150°C) oven for 10 to 15 minutes, until warmed through; or reheat in a frying pan, covered, on medium.*

THAW IT: *Allow to thaw completely in the fridge. Once defrosted, enjoy cold on a salad or use the reheating instructions above.*

---

1. Preheat the oven to 475°F (245°C).

2. Using a microplane or fine grater, zest the orange, then cut the orange in half. Juice one half and cut the other half into wedges. Set the zest and juice aside. Stuff the orange wedges and thyme and parsley sprigs into the duck cavity. Tie the legs together with cotton twine and set the duck in a cast-iron pan or small roasting pan.

3. Sprinkle 2 teaspoons of the salt, the coriander, pepper, and cumin all over the outside of the duck. Roast for 30 minutes.

4. Put the reserved orange juice in a bowl along with ½ cup (120 ml) of the bone broth and the wine. After the duck has roasted for 30 minutes, lower the heat to 350°F (177°C) and pour the broth mixture into the pan. Bake for an additional 50 to 60 minutes, until the internal temperature reaches 165°F (74°C). If you want crispy skin, set the broiler to high, move the rack to the top position, and broil for 5 minutes, or until the skin has crisped up. Remove from the oven and transfer the roasted duck to a cutting board.

5. Make the glaze: Place the remaining ¼ cup (60 ml) of bone broth, erythritol, vinegar, and remaining ¼ teaspoon salt in the pan with the drippings. Set over medium-low heat and whisk continuously until the erythritol has dissolved. Add the reserved orange zest. Whisk continuously for 5 minutes, until the glaze has thickened.

6. Slice the duck and place on a serving plate. Drizzle with the orange glaze, or serve the glaze on the side in a gravy boat.

SERVE IT WITH: *To make this a complete meal, serve it on a large bed of spinach, drizzling the glaze over the greens as well.*

MAKE IT LOW-FODMAP: *Replace the erythritol with 5 drops of liquid stevia.*

NUTRIENT INFORMATION (PER SERVING WITH 2 TABLESPOONS GLAZE):

calories: 458 | calories from fat: 337 | total fat: 37.4g | saturated fat: 12.4g | cholesterol: 116mg

sodium: 776mg | carbs: 3.9g | dietary fiber: 0.8g | net carbs: 3.1g | sugars: 2.9g | protein: 26.4g

RATIOS:

fat:	carbs:	protein:
74%	3%	23%

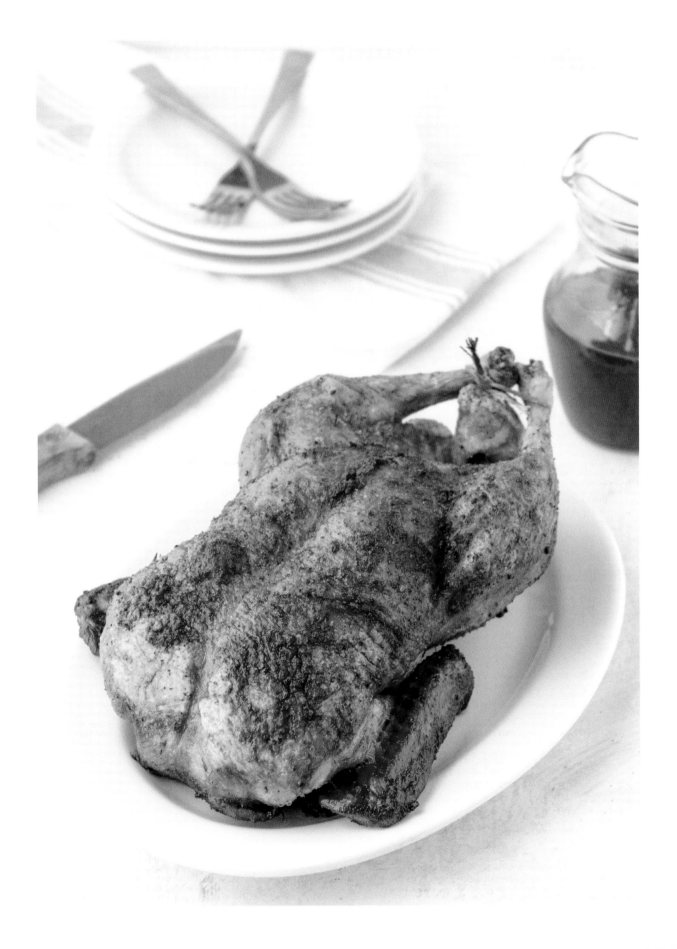

SUNFLOWER CHICKEN WINGS WITH BOK CHOY

PREP TIME: **10 minutes**   COOK TIME: **40 minutes**   SERVES: **6**

EGG-FREE • NUT-FREE   OPTIONS: COCONUT-FREE • LOW-FODMAP • NIGHTSHADE-FREE

Just about any type of chicken works for this recipe! I like wings because they take time to eat, and they're fun. But bone-in chicken thighs or breasts are fabulous, too!

SAUCE:

½ cup (40 g) sliced green onions, green parts only

⅓ cup (80 ml) refined avocado oil or refined olive oil

⅓ cup (80 ml) chicken bone broth (see page 152)

¼ cup (70 g) unsweetened sunflower seed butter

1½ tablespoons coconut aminos

1 tablespoon apple cider vinegar

1 tablespoon fresh lime juice

1 teaspoon fish sauce

¼ teaspoon red pepper flakes

2 pounds (900 g) chicken drumettes and/or wings

BOK CHOY:

3 tablespoons refined avocado oil or refined olive oil

1 large bok choy (about 18 ounces/ 525 g), sliced

2 teaspoons Shichimi Seasoning (page 234)

STORE IT: *Keep in an airtight container in the fridge for up to 3 days.*

REHEAT IT: *Microwave, covered, until the desired temperature is reached. Or place in a covered casserole dish and reheat in a preheated 300°F (150°C) oven for 10 to 15 minutes, until warmed through. Or reheat in a frying pan on medium.*

MAKE IT COCONUT-FREE: *Replace the coconut aminos with a wheat-free soy sauce, if you tolerate soy.*

1. Preheat the oven to 375°F (190°C).

2. Place the ingredients for the sauce in a large bowl. Whisk to combine. Add the chicken and toss to coat.

3. Transfer the coated chicken to a large casserole dish or cast-iron pan. Bake for 30 minutes, then raise the oven temperature to 425°F (220°C) and bake for another 10 minutes.

4. Meanwhile, make the bok choy: Heat the 3 tablespoons of oil in a frying pan over medium-high heat for 1 minute. Add the sliced bok choy and Shichimi seasoning to the hot oil and sauté for 5 minutes, until fork-tender.

5. Divide the bok choy among 6 dinner plates and top with the chicken wings.

MAKE IT LOW-FODMAP: *Replace the Shichimi seasoning with one of the low-FODMAP spice mixtures on pages 232 to 235.*

MAKE IT NIGHTSHADE-FREE: *Omit the red pepper flakes. Replace the Shichimi seasoning with one of the nightshade-free spice mixtures on pages 232 to 235.*

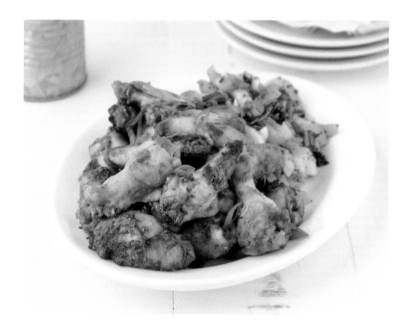

NUTRIENT INFORMATION (PER SERVING):

calories: 584 | calories from fat: 433 | total fat: 48.2g | saturated fat: 9.7g | cholesterol: 116mg

sodium: 653mg | carbs: 6.2g | dietary fiber: 1.1g | net carbs: 5.1g | sugars: 1.2g | protein: 31.4g

RATIOS:

fat:	carbs:	protein:
74%	4%	22%

WALDORF-STUFFED TOMATOES

  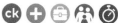

PREP TIME: **10 minutes**   SERVES: **4**

COCONUT-FREE   OPTIONS: EGG-FREE • LOW-FODMAP • NIGHTSHADE-FREE • NUT-FREE

Everything about this recipe makes me happy. It's creamy, it's quick, and it's ready to rock your lunch kit any day of the work week. Feel free to swap out the cooked chicken with just about anything—steak, pork chops, turkey, you name it!

Raw walnuts are fine to use, but for health reasons it's better to soak and roast them before using them in this recipe (see page 157).

SALAD:

2⅓ cups (300 g) diced cooked skin-on chicken thighs

1 cup (170 g) diced celery

½ cup (105 g) mayonnaise, homemade (page 220) or store-bought

½ cup (75 g) diced red apples

½ cup (60 g) raw walnut pieces, roasted

1 tablespoon plus 1 teaspoon fresh lemon juice

¼ teaspoon finely ground gray sea salt

1 drop liquid stevia

4 hothouse tomatoes (about 1 pound/ 455 g), for serving

¼ cup (17 g) chopped fresh parsley, for garnish

1. Place the ingredients for the salad in a large bowl. Toss to coat and set aside.

2. Place the tomatoes on a cutting board. Cut a circle around the top of each tomato as you would with a pumpkin. Remove the tops and, using a small spoon, spoon out and discard the guts.

3. Fill the hollowed-out tomatoes with the Waldorf salad and garnish with parsley.

MAKE IT NIGHTSHADE-FREE: *Use romaine lettuce leaves instead of tomatoes.*

MAKE IT NUT-FREE: *Replace the walnuts with roasted hulled sunflower seeds.*

MAKE IT A CARB-UP: *Replace the chicken thighs with skinless chicken breasts, reduce the amount of mayonnaise to ¼ cup (52 g), and omit the walnuts. Add ½ cup (115 g) of raisins in Step 1.*

STORE IT: *Keep in an airtight container in the fridge for up to 3 days.*

MAKE IT EGG-FREE: *Use egg-free mayonnaise.*

MAKE IT LOW-FODMAP: *Reduce the amount of celery to ¼ cup (42 g) and replace the apples with 2 tablespoons of unsweetened dried cranberries, chopped.*

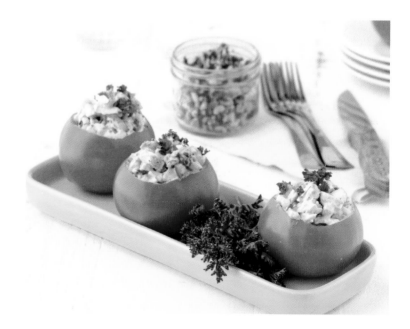

NUTRIENT INFORMATION (PER STUFFED TOMATO):

calories: 507 | calories from fat: 374 | total fat: 41.6g | saturated fat: 7.3g | cholesterol: 80mg

sodium: 364mg | carbs: 10.5g | dietary fiber: 3.6g | net carbs: 6.9g | sugars: 6.1g | protein: 22.6g

RATIOS:

fat:	carbs:	protein:
74%	8%	18%

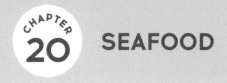
LOBSTER PIE

PREP TIME: **15 minutes**   COOK TIME: **35 minutes**   SERVES: **6**

LOW-FODMAP • NIGHTSHADE-FREE • NUT-FREE   OPTION: COCONUT-FREE

This comforting meal is an adaptation of the beloved shepherd's pie. Swap the meat for lobster, the gravy for cream sauce, and the seasonal veggies for a bunch of green onions, and you're all set! You could also use leeks in place of the green onions. That was my original plan for this dish, but every grocery store in my little town was sold out of leeks, so green onions it was!

FILLING:

¼ cup (52 g) coconut oil

2 cups (160 g) chopped green onions, green parts only

2½ cups (450 g) chopped cooked lobster meat

¼ cup (60 ml) full-fat coconut milk

¼ cup (18 g) chopped fresh dill

½ teaspoon finely ground gray sea salt

TOPPING:

3 cups (475 g) roughly chopped turnips, steamed

¼ cup (60 ml) full-fat coconut milk

2 tablespoons coconut oil

½ teaspoon finely ground gray sea salt

¼ teaspoon ground black pepper

3 large egg yolks

1. Preheat the oven to 400°F (205°C).

2. Make the filling: Place ¼ cup (52 g) of coconut oil and the green onions in a large frying pan over medium heat. Sauté the onions in the oil for 5 minutes. Add the lobster meat, ¼ cup coconut milk, dill, and ½ teaspoon salt and sauté for another 2 minutes. Transfer the mixture to a shallow 1½-quart (1.4-L) casserole dish.

3. Make the topping: Place the steamed turnips, ¼ cup (60 ml) coconut milk, 2 tablespoons coconut oil, ¼ teaspoon salt, and the pepper in a blender or food processor or the bowl of a stand mixer. Pulse or whip until mashed but with a bit of chunkiness remaining. Add the egg yolks and mix until just combined.

4. Spread the mashed turnips evenly over the lobster mixture in the casserole dish. Using a fork, fluff the turnip topping until little peaks form.

5. Bake for 25 minutes, or until the top turns light golden. Remove from the oven and serve!

STORE IT: *Keep in an airtight container in the fridge for up to 3 days.*

REHEAT IT: *Microwave, covered, until the desired temperature is reached. Or place in a covered casserole dish and reheat in a preheated 300°F (150°C) oven for 10 to 15 minutes, until warmed through. Or reheat in a frying pan on medium.*

SERVE IT WITH: *This dish tastes great paired with Classic Butter Biscuits (page 368).*

MAKE IT COCONUT-FREE: *Replace the coconut oil with ghee, if tolerated, or refined avocado oil. Replace the coconut milk with ⅓ cup (80 ml) of your favorite nondairy milk, divided in use equally between Steps 2 and 3.*

NUTRIENT INFORMATION (PER SERVING):

calories: 301 | calories from fat: 185 | total fat: 20.6g | saturated fat: 16.3g | cholesterol: 158mg

sodium: 737mg | carbs: 10.4g | dietary fiber: 2.5g | net carbs: 7.9g | sugars: 4g | protein: 18.4g

RATIOS:

fat:	carbs:	protein:
62%	14%	24%

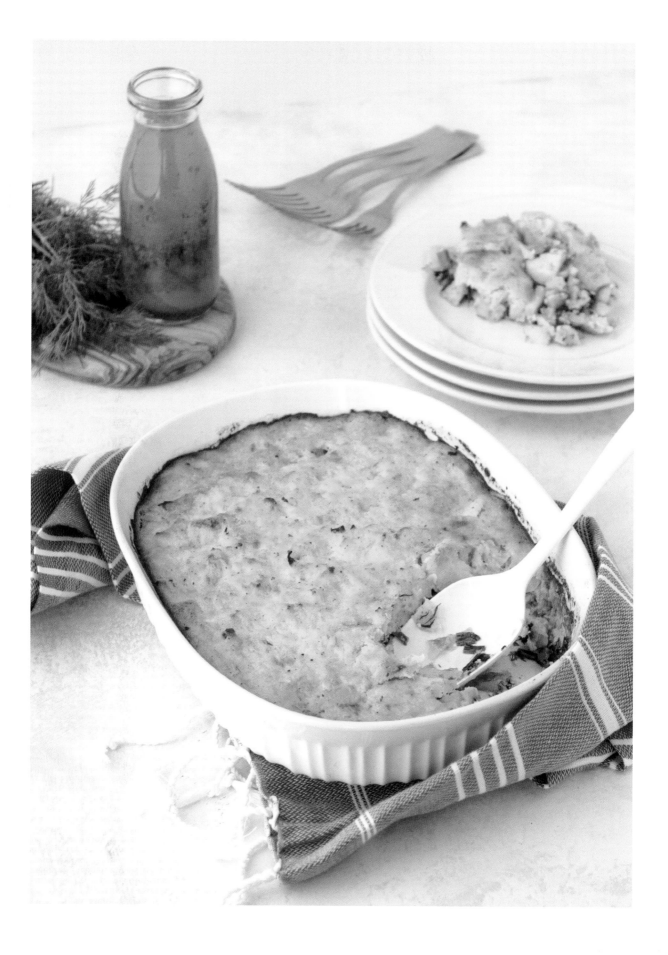

CRAB TACOS

PREP TIME: **5 minutes**   MAKES: **8 tacos (4 servings)**

COCONUT-FREE • NUT-FREE   OPTION: LOW-FODMAP

If you think I prepped and steamed a bunch of crabs, cracked them open, pulled out the meat, and then made this recipe, you've got me all wrong, my friend. First, I would never spend that long on a recipe unless it was a cake—then I'd spend three hours if that meant I'd get to eat it. Second, handling a bunch of crustaceans couldn't be further from what I ever, ever want to do with my time.

Luckily, we live in a modern era where you can buy precooked crab leg meat at the grocery store, ready to be devoured sans steaming, cracking, or pulling. Win! I found cooked crab leg meat in the fresh seafood section of my local grocer.

1 cup (230 g) cooked crab leg meat

2 small tomatoes, diced

⅓ cup (55 g) diced radishes

Juice of 1 lime

3 tablespoons extra-virgin olive oil

3 tablespoons finely chopped green bell pepper

2 tablespoons finely chopped yellow bell pepper

2 tablespoons finely chopped fresh cilantro, plus more for garnish

2 tablespoons Sriracha sauce

1 tablespoon finely chopped fresh mint

¼ teaspoon finely ground gray sea salt

8 Bendy Tortillas (page 370), for serving

1. Place all the ingredients except the tortillas in a large bowl. Toss to combine.

2. Divide the crab mixture evenly among the 8 tortillas. Garnish with additional cilantro, if using, and serve.

STORE IT: *Keep the tortillas separate from the filling. Store in the fridge for up to 3 days.*

PREP AHEAD: *Prepare the tortillas beforehand, storing according to the instructions on page 370.*

SERVE IT WITH: *To make this a complete meal, top the tacos with sliced avocado. They taste great paired with Berry Avocado Salad (page 294) or Avocado Fries with Dipping Sauce (page 378).*

MAKE IT LOW-FODMAP: *Be sure to check for garlic and onions in the Sriracha sauce. Alternatively, you can use chili sauce.*

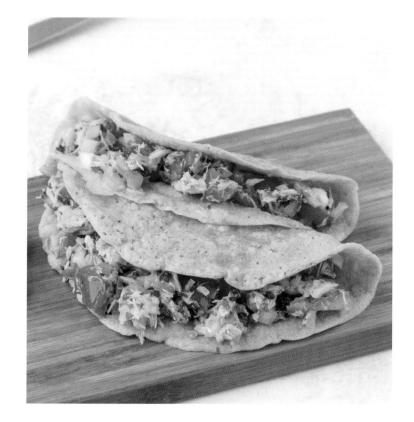

NUTRIENT INFORMATION (PER 2 TACOS):

calories: 297 | calories from fat: 176 | total fat: 19.5g | saturated fat: 4.4g | cholesterol: 129mg

sodium: 747mg | carbs: 5.5g | dietary fiber: 1.1g | net carbs: 4.4g | sugars: 3.4g | protein: 24.9g

RATIOS:

fat:	carbs:	protein:
60%	**7%**	**33%**

STUFFED TROUT

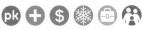

PREP TIME: **5 minutes** · COOK TIME: **20 minutes** · SERVES: **4**

COCONUT-FREE · EGG-FREE · LOW-FODMAP · NIGHTSHADE-FREE · NUT-FREE

My mom deserves all the credit for this recipe. Truth be told, seafood isn't my forte. I enjoy eating it from time to time, but my mom is the seafood aficionado of the family. In fact, she knows how to cook a lot of less-common proteins, like duck and lamb. I'm a ranch-loving, small-town-dwelling girl who eats beef. Chicken is my "seafood." So when Mom and I were discussing the seafood chapter, she recommended that I stuff trout with, well, everything that's in this recipe. Really, this is my mom's recipe that she was gracious enough to share with me so that I could share it with you. And hey, it's pretty good!

2 (7-ounce/200-g) head-off, gutted trout

2 tablespoons refined avocado oil or melted coconut oil

2 teaspoons dried dill weed

1 teaspoon dried thyme leaves

½ teaspoon ground black pepper

¼ teaspoon finely ground gray sea salt

½ lemon, sliced

1 green onion, green part only, sliced in half lengthwise

1. Preheat the oven to 400°F (205°C).

2. Place the fish in a large cast-iron frying pan or on an unlined rimmed baking sheet and coat with the oil. In a small bowl, mix together the dried herbs, pepper, and salt. Sprinkle the fish—top, bottom, and inside—with the herb mixture.

3. Open up the fish and place the lemon and green onion slices inside. Lay it flat on the pan or baking sheet and transfer to the oven. Bake for up to 20 minutes, until the desired doneness is reached.

4. Cut the fish in half before transferring to a serving platter.

STORE IT: *Keep in an airtight container in the fridge for up to 4 days or in the freezer for up to 1 month.*

REHEAT IT: *Microwave, covered, until the desired temperature is reached; place in a covered casserole dish and reheat in a preheated 300°F (150°C) oven for 5 to 10 minutes, until warmed through; or place in a frying pan with oil and reheat on medium.*

THAW IT: *Allow to thaw completely in the fridge. Once defrosted, use the reheating instructions above.*

SERVE IT WITH: *This fish tastes great paired with Berry Avocado Salad (page 294) or Kale Pâté (page 259).*

MAKE IT A CARB-UP: *Reduce the amount of oil to 1 tablespoon. Serve alongside the carb of your choice (find ideas on page 117, or visit healthfulpursuit.com/carbup to download the complimentary PDF "Carb-Up Recipes"). It's scrumptious with grilled apricots or pears.*

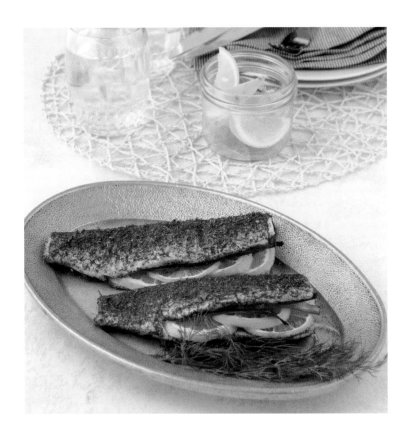

NUTRIENT INFORMATION (PER SERVING):

calories: 219 | calories from fat: 108 | total fat: 12g | saturated fat: 2g | cholesterol: 74mg

sodium: 186mg | carbs: 0.9g | dietary fiber: 0g | net carbs: 0.9g | sugars: 0g | protein: 26.9g

RATIOS:		
fat:	carbs:	protein:
49%	2%	49%

CRISPY SALMON STEAKS WITH SWEET CABBAGE

PREP TIME: **10 minutes**   COOK TIME: **40 minutes**   SERVES: **4**

COCONUT-FREE • EGG-FREE • NIGHTSHADE-FREE   OPTIONS: **LOW-FODMAP • NUT-FREE**

I was destined to be keto. From the time I could make my own food choices, I lived for sauerkraut, cabbage, and high-fat fish—all keto-friendly delicacies. This simple entrée, perfect for a weeknight meal, is a breeze to put together. And if you feel like steak or chicken instead of fish, no problem! The sweet cabbage also goes great with Balsamic Turkey Thighs (page 338) or the flank steak from the recipe on page 292.

SWEET CABBAGE:

¼ cup (60 ml) refined avocado oil or macadamia nut oil

⅓ cup (55 g) sliced red onions

4 cups (470 g) sliced red cabbage

⅓ cup (80 ml) red wine, such as Pinot Noir, Merlot, or Cabernet Sauvignon

¼ cup (60 ml) chicken bone broth (see page 152)

1 tablespoon balsamic vinegar

½ teaspoon finely ground gray sea salt

¼ teaspoon ground black pepper

SALMON:

4 salmon steaks (6 ounces/170 g each)

3 tablespoons refined avocado oil or macadamia nut oil

Finely ground gray sea salt and ground black pepper

2 tablespoons chopped fresh parsley, for garnish

1. Prepare the cabbage: Place ¼ cup (60 ml) of avocado oil and the red onions in a large frying pan over medium heat. Sauté the onions for 5 minutes. Add the sliced cabbage and continue to cook for 5 minutes, or until lightly wilted. Add the wine, bone broth, vinegar, salt, and pepper. Cover, reduce the heat to medium-low, and cook for 25 minutes. During the last 5 minutes of cooking, remove the lid and continue to cook, uncovered, to allow some of the juices to evaporate.

2. Meanwhile, place an oven rack in the top position and set the broiler to low. (If your oven doesn't have a low broil setting, just "broil" is fine.)

3. Place the salmon steaks on an unlined rimmed baking sheet or in a large cast-iron frying pan. Drizzle with 3 tablespoons of avocado oil and sprinkle with salt and pepper. For medium-done steaks, still slightly translucent in the center, broil for 9 minutes; for fully cooked steaks, opaque throughout, broil for 12 minutes.

4. Divide the cabbage among 4 plates, top each plate with a salmon steak, and serve garnished with parsley.

STORE IT: *Keep in an airtight container in the fridge for up to 3 days or in the freezer for up to 1 month.*

REHEAT IT: *Microwave, covered, until the desired temperature is reached; place in a covered casserole dish and reheat in a preheated 300°F (150°C) oven for 10 to 15 minutes, until warmed through; or reheat in a frying pan on medium.*

THAW IT: *Allow to thaw completely in the fridge. Once defrosted, use the reheating instructions above.*

SERVE IT WITH: *This dish tastes great paired with Kale Pâté (page 259).*

MAKE IT LOW-FODMAP: *Omit the onions and replace 2 tablespoons of the avocado oil used in Step 1 with Garlic-Infused Oil (page 230) made with avocado oil.*

MAKE IT NUT-FREE: *Use avocado oil.*

MAKE IT A CARB-UP: *Reduce the amount of oil to 1½ teaspoons in Step 1 and 1½ teaspoons in Step 3. Serve sprinkled with 2 cups (435 g) of fresh blackberries.*

NUTRIENT INFORMATION (PER SERVING):

calories: 485 | calories from fat: 310 | total fat: 34.5g | saturated fat: 4.6g | cholesterol: 75mg

sodium: 499mg | carbs: 8.3g | dietary fiber: 3.3g | net carbs: 5g | sugars: 4.4g | protein: 35.2g

RATIOS:

fat:	carbs:	protein:
64%	**7%**	**29%**

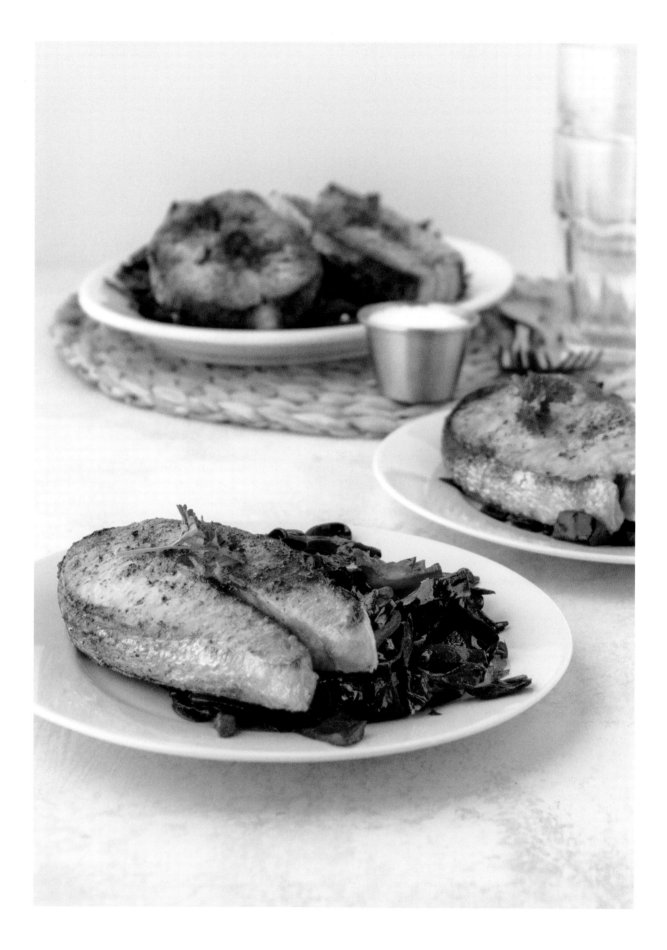

PROSCIUTTO-WRAPPED FISH FILLETS WITH MEDITERRANEAN VEGETABLES

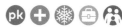

PREP TIME: **15 minutes**   COOK TIME: **30 minutes**   SERVES: **6**

COCONUT-FREE • EGG-FREE • NIGHTSHADE-FREE   OPTIONS: LOW-FODMAP • NUT-FREE

The prosciutto will tear as you wrap the fish, but don't worry, the casserole will still turn out lovely! Raw nuts are fine to use, but for health reasons, it's better to soak the pecans before using them in this recipe (see page 157).

VEGETABLES:

10½ ounces (300 g) endive or radicchio, roughly chopped

6 canned artichoke hearts

½ cup (70 g) raw pecan halves

⅓ cup (80 ml) refined avocado oil or melted lard

4 green onions, green parts only, chopped

Juice of 1 lime

1 (1-in/2.5-cm) piece fresh ginger root, grated

Leaves from 1 sprig fresh tarragon

½ teaspoon finely ground gray sea salt

¼ teaspoon ground black pepper

FISH:

1 pound (455 g) trout, tilapia, or catfish fillets

Finely ground gray sea salt and ground black pepper

9 ounces (255 g) thinly sliced prosciutto

FOR GARNISH (OPTIONAL):

Fresh parsley leaves

Lime wedges

1. Preheat the oven to 350°F (177°C).

2. In a large bowl, place the ingredients for the vegetables. Toss to coat before transferring to a shallow 1½-quart (1.4-L) casserole dish.

3. Place the fish fillets on a clean surface. Sprinkle with salt and pepper. One at a time, wrap each fillet with 2 or 3 pieces of prosciutto. Once wrapped, place on top of the endive mixture.

4. Bake for 30 minutes, or until the sides of the casserole start to brown and the fish flakes with a fork.

5. Divide the fish and vegetables among 6 plates and garnish with fresh parsley and lime wedges, if desired. Serve!

STORE IT: *Keep in an airtight container in the fridge for up to 3 days. Wrapped fish only can be frozen for up to 1 month.*

REHEAT IT: *Microwave, covered, until the desired temperature is reached; place in a covered casserole dish and reheat in a preheated 300°F (150°C) oven for 10 to 15 minutes, until warmed through; or reheat in a frying pan, covered, on medium.*

THAW IT: *Allow the wrapped fish to thaw completely in the fridge. Once defrosted, use the reheating instructions above.*

VARIATION: PROSCIUTTO-WRAPPED SHRIMP WITH MEDITERRANEAN VEGETABLES. *Follow the recipe as written, but replace the fish fillets with 1 pound of jumbo shrimp, peeled and deveined, and tear each piece of prosciutto into a couple of pieces before wrapping the shrimp. Cook for 20 minutes, or until the casserole starts to brown around the edges.*

MAKE IT LOW-FODMAP: *Replace the artichoke hearts with 1 celeriac, chopped, or a couple of handfuls of chopped kale or chopped radishes.*

MAKE IT NUT-FREE: *Omit the pecans.*

MAKE IT A CARB-UP: *Reduce the amount of oil to 3 tablespoons. Serve alongside the carb of your choice (find ideas on page 117, or visit healthfulpursuit.com/carbup to download the complimentary PDF "Carb-Up Recipes"). It's delicious with white rice, roasted parsnips, or steamed yams.*

NUTRIENT INFORMATION (PER SERVING):

calories: 436 | calories from fat: 265 | total fat: 29.5g | saturated fat: 4.4g | cholesterol: 78mg

sodium: 772mg | carbs: 10g | dietary fiber: 5.5g | net carbs: 4.5g | sugars: 1.3g | protein: 32.6g

RATIOS:		
fat:	carbs:	protein:
61%	**9%**	**30%**

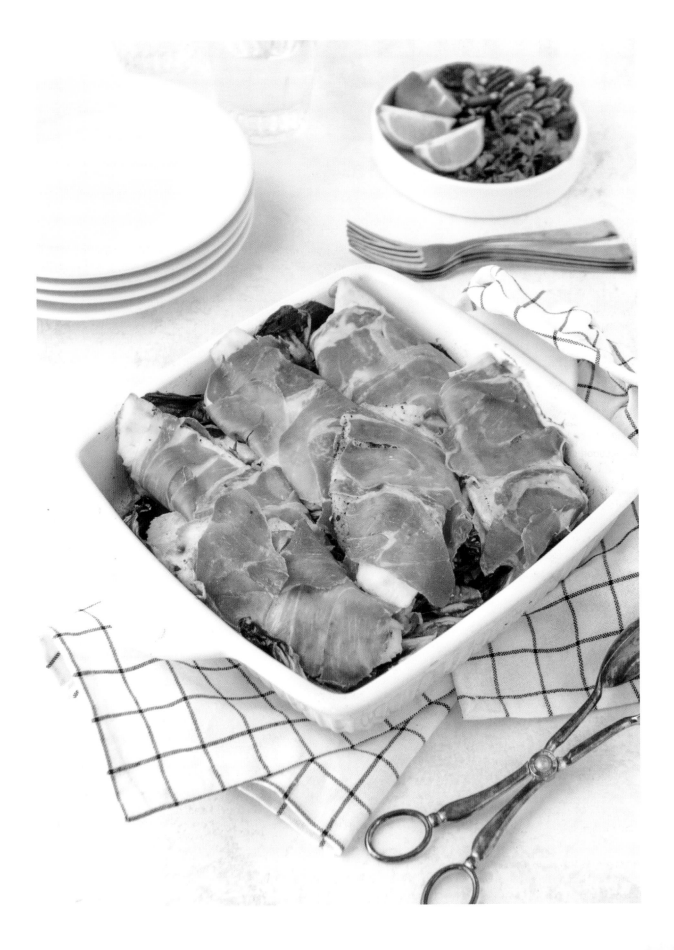

SALMON CAKES WITH DILL CREAM SAUCE

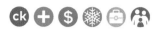

PREP TIME: **5 minutes**   COOK TIME: **about 15 minutes (based on cooking in 2 batches)**   SERVES: **4**

LOW-FODMAP • NIGHTSHADE-FREE   OPTIONS: COCONUT-FREE • NUT-FREE

I've been making this recipe for a very long time. It's changed over the years, getting simpler and simpler to the point where it became blended salmon with egg, fried in oil. Nothing fancy, but so good and fatty! You can dress up these cakes any way you like—add more fresh herbs like parsley or chopped vegetables such as celery, or spice it up with a seasoning mixture (see pages 232 to 235).

Don't worry about bones in the canned salmon. In fact, if you can find canned salmon with bones, it's even better—keeping the bones in there pumps up the nutrient profile of this recipe! They'll be pulverized when making the batter, so you don't have to worry about choking. If the canned salmon you're using has a lot of salt in it, omit the salt called for in this recipe.

¼ cup (60 ml) refined avocado oil or macadamia nut oil, for the pan

SALMON CAKES:

2 (7½-ounce/213-g) cans salmon, drained

2 large eggs

2 tablespoons roughly chopped fresh dill

Juice of ½ lemon

½ teaspoon finely ground gray sea salt

DILL CREAM SAUCE:

1 cup (240 ml) coconut cream

Juice of ½ lemon

2 teaspoons finely chopped fresh dill

½ teaspoon ground black pepper

1. Warm the oil in a large frying pan over medium heat for 2 minutes.

2. Meanwhile, make the salmon cakes: Place the salmon, eggs, dill, lemon juice, and salt in a high-powered blender or food processor and blend until smooth. Spoon about 3 tablespoons of the mixture into your palm, roll it into a ball, and flatten it like a burger patty. Repeat with the remaining salmon mixture, making a total of 8 patties.

3. Pan-fry the cakes in the hot oil for 3 to 5 minutes on the first side, then turn them over and fry for 3 minutes on the second side, just until lightly golden. Transfer to a cooling rack. You may have to fry the cakes in batches if your pan isn't large enough to fit them without overcrowding.

4. Meanwhile, prepare the dill cream sauce: Place all the sauce ingredients in a medium-sized bowl and stir to combine.

5. Divide the fried cakes among 4 plates, drizzle with the cream sauce, and dig in!

STORE IT: *Keep the cakes and sauce in separate airtight containers in the fridge for up to 4 days or freeze the cakes only for up to 1 month.*

REHEAT IT: *Microwave, covered, until the desired temperature is reached; place in a covered casserole dish and reheat in a preheated 300°F (150°C) oven for 10 to 15 minutes, until warmed through; or place in a frying pan with oil and reheat on medium.*

THAW IT: *Allow to thaw completely in the fridge. Once defrosted, use the reheating instructions above.*

SERVE IT WITH: *This tastes great paired with Potato Salad…That Isn't (page 386) or Pesto Zoodles (page 381).*

MAKE IT COCONUT-FREE: *Replace the coconut cream with mayonnaise.*

MAKE IT NUT-FREE: *Use avocado oil or coconut oil.*

MAKE IT A CARB-UP: *Reduce the amount of dill cream sauce by half. Serve alongside the carb of your choice (find ideas on page 117, or visit healthfulpursuit.com/carbup to download the complimentary PDF "Carb-Up Recipes"). It's fabulous with sautéed jicama.*

NUTRIENT INFORMATION (PER 2 CAKES AND ¼ CUP/60 ML SAUCE):

calories: 459 | calories from fat: 337 | total fat: 37.4g | saturated fat: 16.4g | cholesterol: 140mg

sodium: 331mg | carbs: 4.7g | dietary fiber: 1.6g | net carbs: 3.1g | sugars: 2.5g | protein: 25.8g

RATIOS:

fat:	carbs:	protein:
73%	4%	23%

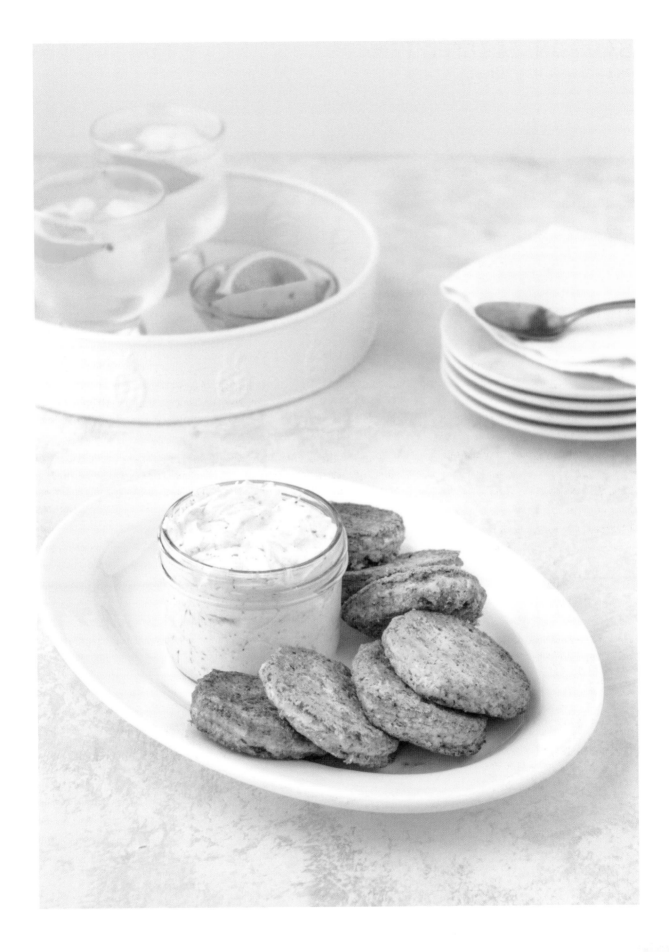

SARDINE FRITTER WRAPS

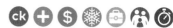

PREP TIME: **5 minutes**   COOK TIME: **8 minutes (based on cooking in 2 batches)**   MAKES: **8 wraps (4 servings)**

COCONUT-FREE   OPTIONS: LOW-FODMAP • NIGHTSHADE-FREE • NUT-FREE

I know, I say that sardines are among the healthiest fish…but I can't bring myself to enjoy them unless they're made into fritters. I don't know what it is about these fish, but I can't eat them like others do, mashed up with mayonnaise. No way! If you're like me and can't enjoy sardines straight from the can, you need to prepare these fritters. Of course, you'll put mayo on them when they're done…duh!

If you use sardines that are packed with lots of salt, omit the salt in this recipe.

⅓ cup (80 ml) refined avocado oil, for frying

FRITTERS:

2 (4.375-ounce/125-g) cans sardines, drained

½ cup (55 g) blanched almond flour

2 large eggs

2 tablespoons finely chopped fresh parsley

2 tablespoons finely diced red bell pepper

2 cloves garlic, minced

½ teaspoon finely ground gray sea salt

¼ teaspoon ground black pepper

FOR SERVING:

8 romaine lettuce leaves

1 small English cucumber, sliced thin

8 tablespoons (105 g) mayonnaise, homemade (page 220) or store-bought

Thinly sliced green onions

1. Pour the avocado oil into a large frying pan. Heat on medium for a couple of minutes.

2. Meanwhile, prepare the fritters: Place the fritter ingredients in a medium-sized bowl and stir to combine, being careful not to mash the heck out of the sardines. Spoon about 1 tablespoon of the mixture into the palm of your hand and roll it into a ball, then flatten it like a burger patty. Repeat with the remaining fritter mixture, making a total of 16 small patties.

3. Fry the fritters in the hot oil for 2 minutes per side, then transfer to a cooling rack. You may have to fry the fritters in batches if your pan isn't large enough to fit them all without overcrowding.

4. Meanwhile, divide the lettuce leaves among 4 dinner plates. Top with the sliced cucumber. When the fritters are done, place 2 fritters on each leaf. Top with a dollop of mayonnaise, sprinkle with sliced green onions, and serve!

STORE IT: *Keep in an airtight container in the fridge for up to 3 days or freeze the fritters only for up to 1 month.*

REHEAT IT (FRITTERS ONLY): *Microwave, covered, until the desired temperature is reached; place in a covered casserole dish and reheat in a preheated 300°F (150°C) oven for 10 to 15 minutes, until warmed through; or reheat in a frying pan, covered, on medium.*

THAW IT: *Allow to thaw completely in the fridge. Once defrosted, use the reheating instructions above.*

MAKE IT LOW-FODMAP: *Replace the minced garlic with ¼ cup (20 g) of finely chopped green onions, green parts only. Use only the green part of the onion for garnish.*

MAKE IT NIGHTSHADE-FREE: *Replace the bell pepper with finely diced radish.*

MAKE IT NUT-FREE: *Use hulled hemp seeds in place of the almond flour.*

MAKE IT A CARB-UP: *Reduce the amount of mayonnaise to ¼ cup (52 g). Instead of frying the fritters, bake them on a parchment-lined rimmed baking sheet for 15 minutes at 350°F (177°C), or until lightly golden. Serve alongside the carb of your choice (find ideas on page 117, or visit healthfulpursuit.com/carbup to download the complimentary PDF "Carb-Up Recipes"). These wraps are delicious with grilled kabocha squash or roasted yams.*

NUTRIENT INFORMATION (PER 2 WRAPS):
calories: 612 | calories from fat: 499 | total fat: 55.5g | saturated fat: 7.6g | cholesterol: 192mg

sodium: 731mg | carbs: 5.5g | dietary fiber: 1.9g | net carbs: 3.6g | sugars: 1.8g | protein: 22.5g

RATIOS:

fat:	carbs:	protein:
81%	**4%**	**15%**

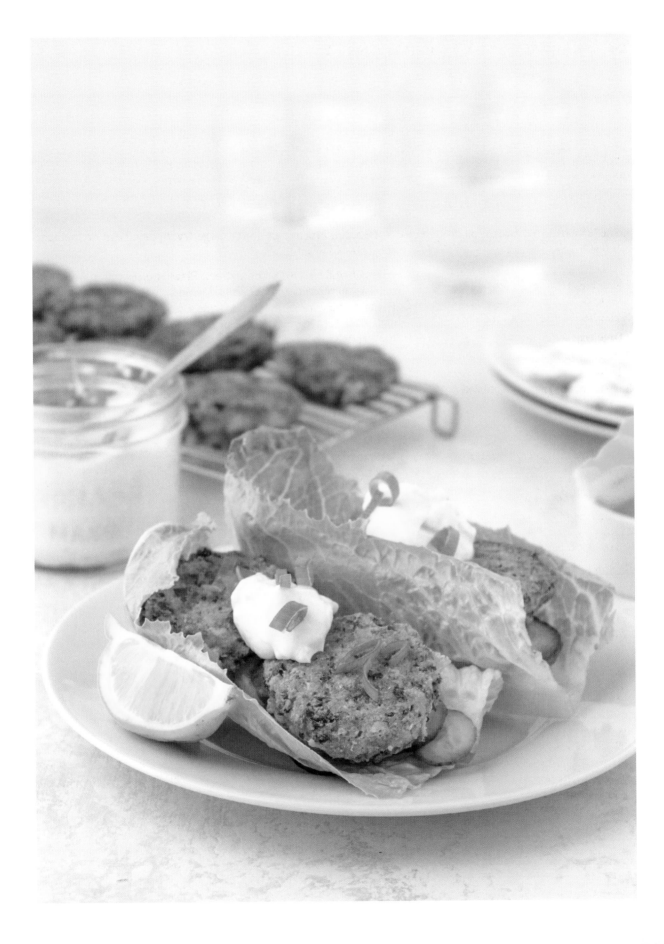

SIDES & ACCOMPANIMENTS

CAULIFLOWER RICE

PREP TIME: **15 minutes**   COOK TIME: **15 minutes**   SERVES: **4**

EGG-FREE • NIGHTSHADE-FREE • NUT-FREE   OPTIONS: COCONUT-FREE • VEGAN

If you haven't made cauliflower rice before, you're missing out. This is a super-simple side dish that everyone in the family will love. Nowadays, you can go to your local grocery store and find riced cauliflower in the frozen foods section, but if you want to save a couple of bucks, making it on your own is super-easy and a pretty good workout. Once you've separated the florets from the stem, begin grating them on the large holes of a box grater, or use the grater attachment for your food processor (the medium size, if you have a choice). Just avoid creating super-small shreds, as the size can impact the finished dish.

With any cauliflower rice recipe, make sure that you don't cook it too long, which leads to mushiness. As soon as the cauliflower is fork-tender, it is ready to go!

⅓ cup (69 g) lard

4 cups (500 g) riced cauliflower florets

1 cup (240 ml) chicken bone broth (see page 152)

½ teaspoon finely ground gray sea salt

1. Place the lard in a large frying pan over medium heat. When melted, add the remaining ingredients. Cover and cook for 8 to 10 minutes, until the rice has softened.

2. Remove the lid and cook for another 5 minutes, or until the liquid has evaporated.

3. Divide the rice among 4 small bowls and serve.

STORE IT: *Keep in an airtight container in the fridge for up to 3 days.*

REHEAT IT: *Microwave, covered, or place in a frying pan and fry over medium heat until the desired temperature is reached.*

PREP AHEAD: *Rice the cauliflower up to 3 days in advance and store in the fridge.*

VARIATION: GREEK CAULIFLOWER RICE. *Simply replace the salt with 2 tablespoons of Greek seasoning (page 232).*

VARIATION: COCONUT CAULIFLOWER RICE. *Melt ¼ cup (55 g) of coconut oil in a large frying pan over medium heat. Add 2 cloves of garlic, minced, ½ small red onion, minced, and 1 teaspoon of minced fresh ginger and cook for 1 minute. Add 4 cups (500 g) of riced cauliflower, 1 cup (240 ml) of full-fat coconut milk, ½ teaspoon of finely ground gray sea salt, and ½ teaspoon of ground cardamom. Cover and cook for 8 to 10 minutes, until the rice has softened. Remove the lid and cook for another 5 minutes, or until the liquid has evaporated. Divide the rice among 4 small bowls and serve sprinkled with a pinch of ground black pepper.*

SERVE IT WITH: *To make this a complete meal, top it with grilled chicken. It also tastes great paired with Lamb Kebabs (page 318), Kung Pao Pork (page 328), and Baked Olive Chicken (page 336).*

MAKE IT COCONUT-FREE: *Make the plain or Greek version.*

MAKE IT VEGAN: *Replace the lard with avocado oil and the chicken bone broth with vegetable stock.*

MAKE IT A CARB-UP: *Reduce the amount of lard to 2 tablespoons and replace the riced cauliflower with 2 cups (300 g) of cooked white rice.*

NUTRIENT INFORMATION (PER SERVING OF PLAIN CAULIFLOWER RICE):

calories: 200 | calories from fat: 155 | total fat: 17.2g | saturated fat: 6.7g | cholesterol: 16mg

sodium: 137mg | carbs: 6.6g | dietary fiber: 3.1g | net carbs: 3.5g | sugars: 3g | protein: 4.6g

RATIOS:

fat: carbs: protein:

78%   **13%**   **9%**

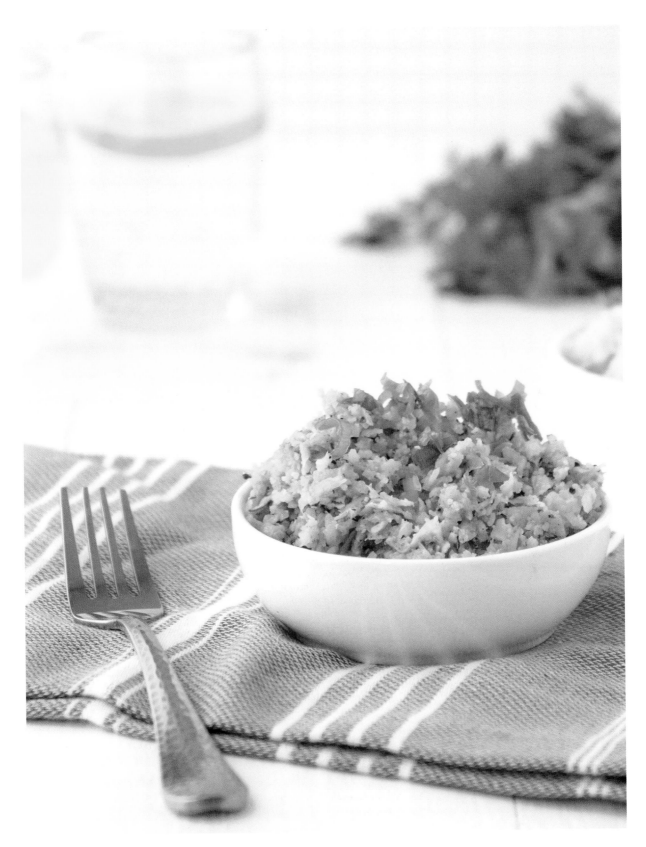

NUTRIENT INFORMATION (PER SERVING OF COCONUT CAULIFLOWER RICE):

calories: 281 | calories from fat: 233 | total fat: 25.8g | saturated fat: 22.8g | cholesterol: 0mg

sodium: 344mg | carbs: 11.5g | dietary fiber: 3.7g | net carbs: 7.8g | sugars: 4.9g | protein: 3.9g

RATIOS:

fat:	carbs:	protein:
79%	16%	5%

CRUSTY SANDWICH BREAD

PREP TIME: 20 minutes, plus 1 hour to cool   COOK TIME: 1 hour   MAKES: one 8½ by 4½-inch/21 by 11-cm loaf (16 slices)

COCONUT-FREE • NIGHTSHADE-FREE

There are a lot of bread recipes in this book. Not because I eat a lot of bread—in fact, before nailing this recipe, I hadn't had bread in over a year—but because I figured that if you're new to eating keto or you want your whole family on board, you'll appreciate having a bunch of bread recipes to choose from. I remember how much I yearned for all things bread when I first started keto—so I get it!

All Germans I know, including my husband, are quite picky about their bread, and they all love this crusty loaf. That's how I know it's good. This fluffy bread makes the perfect sandwich and holds together fabulously well for Sunday brunch French toast. (If you're planning to use this bread for French toast, use a butter-infused refined olive oil instead of one infused with savory ingredients, such as herbs or garlic.)

The type of almond butter you use in this recipe has a huge impact on the result. Use only unsweetened smooth almond butter made from blanched almonds. My favorite brand for this recipe is Barney Butter. For the infused olive oil, I used a Tuscan herb–infused refined olive oil. (Being refined, it can withstand higher heat; read more about this on page 137.) You can use any infused flavor, from garlic to rosemary or harissa. Psyllium husks can be found in the bulk bin section at many health food stores. Psyllium is sold as husks or powdered. This recipe uses husks to create a beautiful rise in the bread.

½ cup (42 g) psyllium husks

1 teaspoon baking powder

½ teaspoon finely ground gray sea salt

¾ cup (210 g) unsweetened smooth almond butter (made with blanched almonds)

5 large eggs

¼ cup (60 ml) infused refined olive oil (see note above)

⅓ cup (80 ml) water

¼ cup (40 g) unflavored gelatin

STORE IT: *The bread is best stored as a loaf, unsliced, on the counter in a sealed plastic bag for up to 3 days. Store slices in an airtight container in the freezer for up to 1 month.*

REHEAT IT: *Toast it!*

THAW IT: *Place the slices on a cooling rack and allow to defrost completely before using, or toast them from frozen.*

SERVE IT WITH: *To make this a complete meal, sandwich mayonnaise, cooked bacon, avocado, arugula, and a slice of tomato between two slices.*

MAKE IT A CARB-UP: *Find carb ideas on page 117, or visit healthfulpursuit.com/ carbup to download the PDF "Carb-Up Recipes." Try it toasted and slathered with boiled berries or topped with sliced bananas or grilled peaches.*

1. Preheat the oven to 350°F (177°C) and line an 8½ by 4½-inch (21 by 11-cm) loaf pan with parchment paper, leaving the ends draped over the sides for easy lifting.

2. In a small bowl, stir together the psyllium husks, baking powder, and salt until incorporated.

3. Place the almond butter, eggs, and oil in the bowl of a stand mixer fitted with the flat beater attachment (or in a mixing bowl if using a hand mixer) and mix until combined. Remove the bowl from the stand and set aside.

4. Place the water in a small saucepan and sprinkle the gelatin on top. Do not stir. After 5 minutes, turn the burner on to medium and whisk until the gelatin has dissolved and the mixture resembles goo. Continue to whisk until the mixture is smooth, then add it to the almond butter mixture and mix by hand with a spatula until smooth.

5. Transfer the dry ingredients to the wet and mix with the spatula until incorporated. The dough will be very sticky.

6. Using a rubber spatula, scrape the dough into the prepared loaf pan and smooth out the top as best you can. (Don't stress about it too much; this bread rises so well that clumps here and there won't affect the end result.) Bake for 1 hour, or until the top begins to brown and a toothpick inserted in the middle comes out clean.

7. Using the overhanging parchment paper, immediately remove the loaf from the pan and place it on a cooling rack. Remove the parchment paper.

8. Allow the loaf to sit for at least 1 hour before slicing. Using a serrated knife, cut evenly into 16 slices.

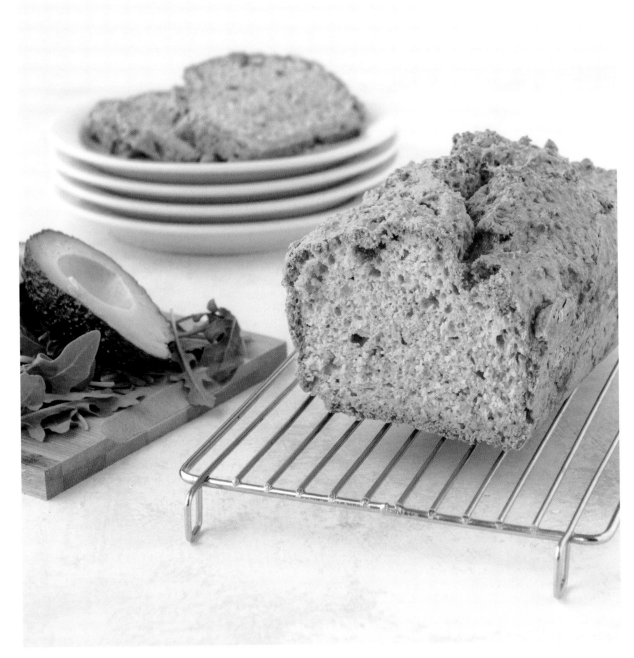

NUTRIENT INFORMATION (PER SLICE):

calories: 151 | calories from fat: 103 | total fat: 11.5g | saturated fat: 1.7g | cholesterol: 58mg

sodium: 83mg | carbs: 4.7g | dietary fiber: 3.5g | net carbs: 1.2g | sugars: 0g | protein: 7.1g

RATIOS:

fat: carbs: protein:

69% **12%** **19%**

CLASSIC BUTTER BISCUITS

PREP TIME: **15 minutes, plus 1 hour to cool**   COOK TIME: **25 minutes**   MAKES: **12 biscuits (12 servings)**

EGG-FREE • LOW-FODMAP • NIGHTSHADE-FREE • NUT-FREE

Once this dough is ready to be shaped into biscuits, it will not want to stick together, because the gelatin is setting as you work. I like to separate the dough into balls, press the balls of dough on the counter between my palms, and roll them out with the support of the counter.

These biscuits are fabulous with gravy or almond butter. The leftovers are delicious cut in half crosswise and toasted, then slathered with coconut oil.

¾ cup (180 ml) water

3 tablespoons unflavored gelatin

1½ cups (150 g) coconut flour

¾ teaspoon baking powder

¾ teaspoon finely ground gray sea salt

½ cup (120 ml) full-fat coconut milk

6 tablespoons (80 g) coconut oil

1 tablespoon apple cider vinegar

¾ cup (160 g) coconut oil, for serving

1. Preheat the oven to 375°F (190°C) and line a baking sheet with parchment paper or a silicone baking mat.

2. Place the water in a small saucepan and sprinkle the gelatin on top. Do not stir. After 5 minutes, turn on the burner to medium and bring the mixture to a light boil, stirring occasionally. Once the mixture is smooth, set aside. If it begins to cool, it will begin to solidify. If that happens, simply reheat to break it down again to liquid form.

3. Meanwhile, place the coconut flour, baking powder, and salt in the bowl of a stand mixer fitted with the flat beater attachment or in a mixing bowl (if using a hand mixer). Mix until combined.

4. Add the coconut milk, coconut oil, vinegar, and gelatin mixture and mix until the batter is combined and sticky. (You want it sticky; if you mix too long, it will no longer be sticky.)

5. Working quickly, divide the batter into 12 balls, about ¼ cup in size, and place them on a clean counter. Pressing with the palm of your hand, flatten and shape the balls into biscuits, about 1½ inches (4 cm) thick, rotating with your palm until the biscuits are the desired shape.

6. Place the biscuits on the prepared baking sheet, leaving ½ inch (1.25 cm) of space between them.

7. Bake the biscuits for 20 to 25 minutes, until the tops crack and begin to turn golden.

8. Allow the biscuits to cool on the baking sheet for 1 hour. Enjoy each biscuit with 1 tablespoon of coconut oil.

STORE IT: *Keep in an airtight container on the counter for up to 3 days or freeze for up to 1 month.*

REHEAT IT: *Cut a room-temperature biscuit in half crosswise and plop it into the toaster, or add to a pan with coconut oil and fry on medium-low heat until golden on both sides.*

THAW IT: *Set on the counter until thawed, about 30 minutes.*

SERVE IT WITH: *To make this a complete meal, slice a biscuit in half and top each half with a sunny-side-up egg. Cover in cheese sauce (page 218) or leftover Lemon-Thyme Gravy (page 332). These biscuits also taste great with Early-Day Jambalaya (page 242).*

MAKE IT A CARB-UP: *Instead of coconut oil, serve with the carb of your choice (find ideas on page 117, or visit healthfulpursuit.com/carbup to download the complimentary PDF "Carb-Up Recipes"). These biscuits are amazing smeared with boiled pears, roasted apples, or raw berries.*

NUTRIENT INFORMATION (PER BISCUIT):

calories: 266 | calories from fat: 218 | total fat: 24.2g | saturated fat: 21.3g | cholesterol: 0mg

sodium: 147mg | carbs: 7.6g | dietary fiber: 4.5g | net carbs: 3.1g | sugars: 1.1g | protein: 4.4g

RATIOS:

fat:	carbs:	protein:
82%	11%	7%

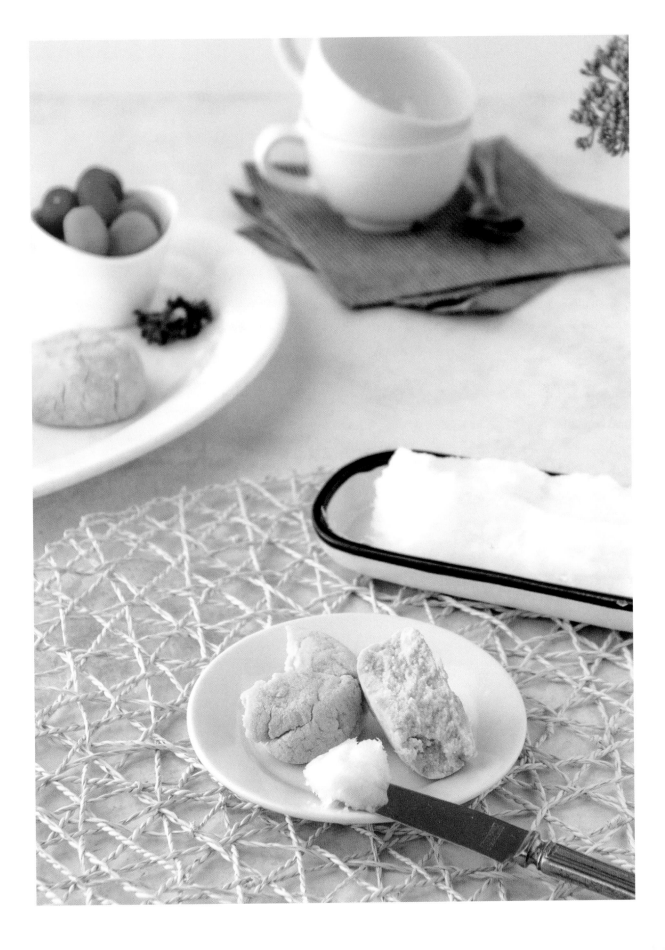

BENDY TORTILLAS

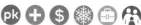

PREP TIME: **5 minutes**   COOK TIME: **3 hours (using one pan), plus time to cool pan between batches**   MAKES: **12 tortillas (12 servings)**

COCONUT-FREE • LOW-FODMAP • NUT-FREE   OPTION: NIGHTSHADE-FREE

It's a fluke that this recipe even exists. I'd been in the kitchen for days, attempting to create a simple tortilla recipe, when a bag of pork rinds fell into the sink. As they got wet, they became gummy and stuck to the bottom of the sink. Then it dawned on me that the wet pork rinds were doing exactly what I wanted the tortilla batter to do: get sticky without the use of starch. And boom! A company named Bacon's Heir makes pork dust, a flour-like product that you can find online. Alternatively, you can make your own pork dust by roughly grinding pork rinds in a blender until they are the size and texture of breadcrumbs. If the pork rinds you're using contain salt, herbs, or spices, omit the Seasoning Salt or sea salt from this recipe.

To make a successful batch of Bendy Tortillas, follow the key steps outlined below. Like, for real; you have to follow these steps or you'll end up with crispy, burnt tortillas that don't bend, and you'll be frustrated.

· You'll need an 8-inch (20 cm) nonstick frying pan (I use a ceramic-coated pan). If you want to save loads of time, have more than one nonstick frying pan on hand so that you can cook multiple tortillas at once. I have three pans, so a batch of tortillas takes me under an hour to prepare.

· If you notice that the edges of your tortillas are crisping or browning, the heat is too high. The key to all this is patience. Low heat and a longer cooking time create the best tortilla. This allows the ingredients to "gum" together, resulting in the perfect bendy tortilla.

· It's imperative that you spread the batter thinly in the bottom of the pan. This helps the tortillas cook evenly and ensures that you don't end up with tortillas that have an omelet-like texture. Spreading the batter thin is easy to do when you add it to a cool pan; however, if you add the batter to a hot pan, it will instantly begin cooking, making it difficult to maneuver and form a perfect circle. This is why the pan must be cooled between batches (and why having more than pan comes in handy).

1⅓ cups (85 g) pork dust or roughly ground pork rinds

1¼ cups (300 ml) water

3 large eggs

1 tablespoon Seasoning Salt (page 235) or ½ teaspoon finely ground gray sea salt (optional)

STORE IT: *Keep in an airtight container in the fridge for up to 3 days or store in an airtight container in the freezer, separated by sheets of parchment paper, for up to 1 month.*

REHEAT IT: *Place in a frying pan and heat on medium for 30 seconds per side.*

THAW IT: *Allow to thaw in the container, uncovered, for 1 hour. Once thawed, remove the parchment paper and they are ready to use.*

1. Place all the ingredients in a blender and blend until smooth. Transfer to a medium-sized bowl and set beside the stove.

2. Scoop 3 tablespoons of the batter into an 8-inch (20-cm) nonstick frying pan. Spread the batter evenly with the back of a spoon or by rotating the pan until the batter reaches the edges. Don't allow the batter to go too far up the sides of the pan or it will burn. Once the batter is spread evenly, cover the pan and set over medium-low to low heat, closer to low.

3. Cook until the tortilla is easy to flip and lightly browned on the underside, 7 to 10 minutes. Flip the tortilla and cook, covered, for an additional 6 to 8 minutes, until lightly browned.

4. Transfer the tortilla to a cooling rack. Remove the pan from the heat and allow it to cool for a couple of minutes before repeating with the remaining batter. As the batter sits between batches, it will thicken slightly; that's okay. If the batter gets too thick to spread easily, add a couple of drops of water until it reaches a similar consistency to when you initially prepared it.

SERVE IT WITH: *To make this a complete meal, fill a tortilla with your favorite protein and drizzle it with mayonnaise. These tortillas are great for Crab Tacos (page 354) or Shredded Beef Tacos (page 314).*

MAKE IT NIGHTSHADE-FREE: *Use finely ground gray sea salt instead of Seasoning Salt.*

MAKE IT A CARB-UP: *Serve alongside the carb of your choice (find ideas on page 117, or visit healthfulpursuit. com/carbup to download the complimentary PDF "Carb-Up Recipes"). These tortillas are delicious filled with roasted sweet potatoes or sautéed delicata squash.*

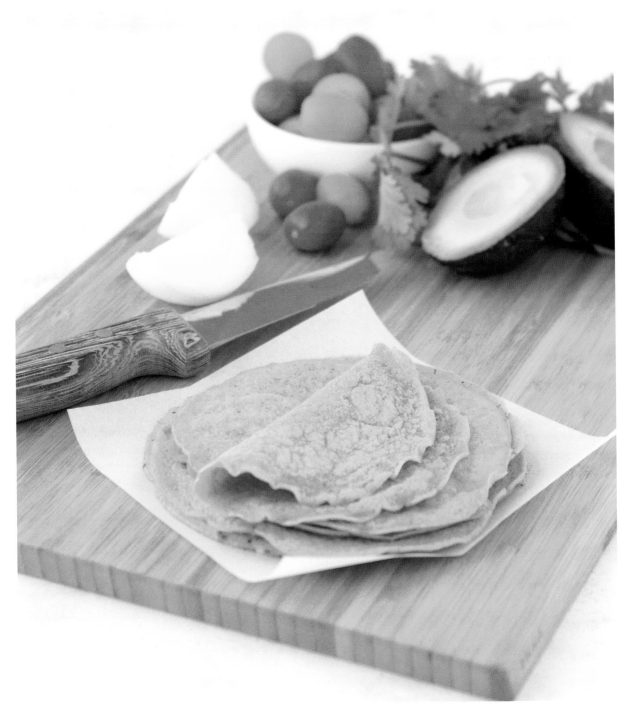

NUTRIENT INFORMATION (PER TORTILLA):

calories: 67 | calories from fat: 34 | total fat: 3.8g | saturated fat: 1.4g | cholesterol: 49mg

sodium: 263mg | carbs: 0.1g | dietary fiber: 0g | net carbs: 0.1g | sugars: 0g | protein: 8.2g

RATIOS:

fat:	carbs:	protein:
51%	1%	48%

OLIVE & TOMATO
FLAXSEED FOCACCIA

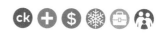

PREP TIME: 15 minutes, plus 1 hour to cool   COOK TIME: 25 minutes   MAKES: one 13 by 9-inch (33 by 23-cm) focaccia (18 servings)

NUT-FREE • VEGETARIAN   OPTIONS: COCONUT-FREE • EGG-FREE • NIGHTSHADE-FREE • VEGAN

I use this recipe as a delivery system for additional fat. Slathered with mayonnaise, coconut oil, ghee, or grass-fed butter (if you can tolerate the latter two), it's a fabulous way to boost the fat in your day.

If you'd like an extra-thick focaccia bread that's about 1½ inches (4 cm) thick, prepare the recipe without the olives and tomatoes in an 8-inch (20-cm) square baking pan and bake for an additional 2 to 5 minutes. Once cool, cut into 12 squares. The Classic and the Olive & Tomato versions can also be cut in half crosswise and used as the base for sandwiches!

The egg-free version should be made in the larger baking pan, and it's best without the olive and tomato topping. The bread doesn't rise as well without eggs; it's a thinner, denser bread that's perfect for sandwiches. Cut it into squares and use them as "bread slices" for your next keto sandwich creation.

DRY INGREDIENTS:

2 cups (260 g) roughly ground flax seeds

1 tablespoon baking powder

1 tablespoon Italian Seasoning (page 234)

1 teaspoon finely ground gray sea salt

WET INGREDIENTS:

5 large eggs

½ cup (120 ml) water

⅓ cup (80 ml) refined avocado oil

TOPPINGS:

12 grape tomatoes, halved lengthwise

10 pitted olives, halved lengthwise

FOR SERVING:

18 tablespoons (234 g) mayonnaise, homemade (page 220) or store-bought, or coconut oil

STORE IT: *Keep in an airtight container in the fridge for up to 3 days. To freeze it, transfer the squares to an airtight container and freeze for up to 1 month.*

REHEAT IT: *Place in a frying pan and add your favorite heat-friendly oil. Cover and cook on medium heat for 1 to 2 minutes, until toasted.*

THAW IT: *Unwrap and place on the counter to thaw for 1 hour.*

1. Place an oven rack in the center of the oven. Preheat the oven to 350°F (177°C) and line a 13 by 9-inch (33 by 23-cm) baking pan with parchment paper, leaving some paper hanging over the sides for easy lifting.

2. Place the ground flax seeds, baking powder, Italian seasoning, and salt in a large bowl. Stir to combine.

3. Place the eggs, water, and avocado oil in a blender. Blend until frothy, about 30 seconds.

4. Pour the egg mixture into the bowl with the dry ingredients and mix with a spatula until incorporated. Allow the batter to sit for 3 minutes.

5. Transfer the batter to the prepared pan and smooth out the top with the back of the spatula.

6. Scatter the tomato and olive halves over the top of the focaccia, pressing each in lightly so the tops are nearly flush with the batter.

7. Bake for 23 to 25 minutes, until the top begins to turn golden and a toothpick inserted in the middle comes out clean.

8. Immediately transfer the focaccia to a cooling rack, using the parchment paper flaps to lift it from the pan. Carefully peel the parchment from the bottom.

9. Let the focaccia cool for 1 hour. Cut into 18 squares and serve each piece with 1 tablespoon of mayonnaise or coconut oil.

NUTRIENT INFORMATION (PER SQUARE OF CLASSIC FOCACCIA WITH 1 TABLESPOON MAYO):

calories: 225 | calories from fat: 182 | total fat: 20.2g | saturated fat: 3.1g | cholesterol: 57mg

sodium: 200mg | carbs: 4.7g | dietary fiber: 3.9g | net carbs: 0.8g | sugars: 0g | protein: 4.4g

RATIOS:

fat:	carbs:	protein:
83%	9%	8%

SERVE IT WITH: *The egg-free version is a fabulous accompaniment to Vegan Cream of Broccoli Soup (page 282).*

MAKE IT COCONUT-FREE: *Serve with mayo, not coconut oil.*

MAKE IT EGG-FREE/VEGAN: *Make the Egg-Free Flaxseed Focaccia.*

MAKE IT NIGHTSHADE-FREE: *Make the Classic Flaxseed Focaccia.*

MAKE IT A CARB-UP: *Make the Classic Flaxseed Focaccia and omit the mayo for serving. Instead, serve it with the carb of your choice (find ideas on page 117, or visit healthfulpursuit.com/carbup to download the PDF "Carb-Up Recipes"). It's amazing with boiled cherries or berries or sautéed bananas.*

VARIATION: CLASSIC FLAXSEED FOCACCIA. *Omit the tomatoes and olives and skip Step 6.*

VARIATION: EGG-FREE FLAXSEED FOCACCIA. *Place 1¼ cups (300 ml) of water in a small saucepan and sprinkle 5 tablespoons (50 g) of unflavored gelatin on top. Do not stir. Allow to sit for 5 minutes. Meanwhile, complete Steps 1 and 2 of the main recipe. After 5 minutes, turn on the burner to medium, bring the gelatin to a light simmer, and continue to heat just until the gelatin dissolves, stirring occasionally. Add the avocado oil, stir, then pour the mixture into the bowl with the dry ingredients. (The eggs are omitted from the wet ingredients.) Using a spatula, mix the dry and wet ingredients together until the batter is smooth. Immediately transfer the batter to the lined baking pan, omitting the tomato and olive toppings, and bake for 30 minutes, or until the sides begin to crisp and the top is golden and firm to the touch. (Do not allow the batter to sit as outlined in Step 4 of the main recipe.) Remove the bread from the pan, keeping it attached to the parchment. Place on a cooling rack to cool in the parchment for 2 hours before cutting into squares. Serve with coconut oil or egg-free mayonnaise.*

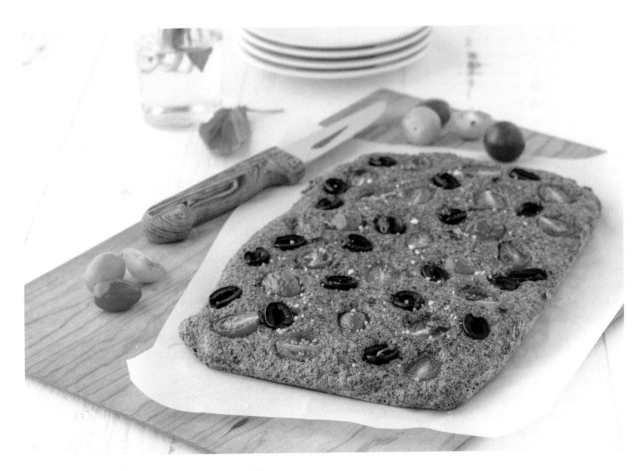

NUTRIENT INFORMATION
(PER SQUARE OF OLIVE & TOMATO FOCACCIA WITH 1 TABLESPOON MAYO):

calories: 222 | calories from fat: 184 | total fat: 20.4g | saturated fat: 3.1g | cholesterol: 57mg

sodium: 220mg | carbs: 5.1g | dietary fiber: 4.1g | net carbs: 1g | sugars: 0g | protein: 4.5g

RATIOS:
fat: carbs: protein:
83% 9% 8%

NUTRIENT INFORMATION
(PER SQUARE OF EGG-FREE FOCACCIA WITH 1 TABLESPOON COCONUT OIL):

calories: 242 | calories from fat: 202 | total fat: 22.4g | saturated fat: 12.9g | cholesterol: 1mg

sodium: 116mg | carbs: 4.6g | dietary fiber: 3.9g | net carbs: 0.7g | sugars: 0g | protein: 5.1g

RATIOS:
fat: carbs: protein:
84% 8% 8%

ROSEMARY GARLIC CROUTONS

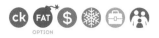

PREP TIME: **65 minutes**   COOK TIME: **50 minutes**   MAKES: **64 croutons (8 servings)**

COCONUT-FREE • NIGHTSHADE-FREE • VEGETARIAN   OPTIONS: EGG-FREE • LOW-FODMAP • VEGAN

This is my go-to recipe for croutons. It requires two steps: first you make the bread, and then you cut the bread into croutons and rebake them. But it's worth the work! I like to keep these croutons in the freezer for quick access when a salad needs a little pick-me-up.

These croutons are chia seed–based, so this recipe is a good option if you're craving something bread-like but you don't tolerate flax seeds (which form the base of my focaccia recipe on page 372). If you can't handle flax, you can even skip the step of making the croutons and use the bread to make sandwiches, sliced horizontally. For the best bread-like texture, however, I suggest that you stick to the flax seed–based focaccia recipe when you're craving focaccia and use this recipe when you're craving croutons. You'll have the best of both worlds!

DRY INGREDIENTS:

½ cup (55 g) ground chia seeds

⅓ cup (40 g) blanched almond flour

2 teaspoons dried rosemary leaves

1½ teaspoons garlic powder

1 teaspoon baking powder

½ teaspoon finely ground gray sea salt

¼ teaspoon ground black pepper

WET INGREDIENTS:

½ cup (120 ml) refined avocado oil

4 large eggs

TOPPINGS:

2 tablespoons refined avocado oil

Finely ground gray sea salt

STORE IT: *Keep croutons or bread in an airtight container on the counter for up to 1 week, or freeze for up to 1 month.*

THAW IT: *Use the croutons straight from the freezer. For bread, set it on the counter to thaw for 1 hour.*

SERVE IT WITH: *These croutons taste great on Shaved Cucumber and Smoked Salmon Salad (page 297).*

MAKE IT A FAT BOMB/GREAT FOR ADAPTING: *Make the bread variation and eat it topped with coconut oil or ghee.*

MAKE IT LOW-FODMAP: *Replace the garlic powder with 2 teaspoons of Italian seasoning (page 234).*

1. Preheat the oven to 350°F (177°C) and line a 13 by 9-inch (33 by 23-cm) baking pan with parchment paper, leaving enough paper hanging over the sides for easy lifting.

2. Place the dry ingredients in a large bowl. Stir to combine.

3. Add the wet ingredients and mix with a spatula until incorporated. The batter will be similar to muffin batter.

4. Pour the batter into the prepared pan and smooth out the top with the back of the spatula. Place on the middle rack of the oven and bake for 20 to 25 minutes, until the top begins to turn lightly golden and a toothpick inserted in the middle comes out clean.

5. Immediately remove the bread from the pan and place it on a cutting board. Reduce the oven temperature to 300°F (150°C).

6. Cut the bread into ½-inch (1.25-cm) cubes. Transfer the cubes to an unlined rimmed baking sheet, then drizzle with 2 tablespoons of avocado oil and sprinkle with additional salt. Turn the cubes with your fingers, being careful not to break them, to evenly coat them in the oil and salt.

7. Bake the croutons until crisp and browned, 30 to 40 minutes. Watch carefully, as they can burn quickly toward the end of the baking time.

8. Allow to cool completely before using or storing.

VARIATION: ROSEMARY GARLIC BREAD. *Complete Steps 1 through 4. Immediately remove the bread from the pan and place it on a cooling rack. Carefully peel the parchment from the bottom and allow the bread to cool for 1 hour. To serve, cut it into 18 slices and slather each piece with 1 tablespoon of melted coconut oil or ghee.*

NUTRIENT INFORMATION (PER SLICE OF BREAD WITH 1 TABLESPOON COCONUT OIL OR GHEE):

calories: 212 | calories from fat: 201 | total fat: 22.4g | saturated fat: 12.6g | cholesterol: 41mg

sodium: 83mg | carbs: 2.2g | dietary fiber: 1.5g | net carbs: 0.7g | sugars: 0g | protein: 2.5g

RATIOS:

fat:	carbs:	protein:
92%	**4%**	**4%**

MAKE IT EGG-FREE/VEGAN: *This adaptation works well for croutons, but it doesn't work for the Rosemary Garlic Chia Bread because the bread does not rise and tastes gummy. To make, replace the eggs with ¾ cup (180 ml) of warm water mixed with 2 tablespoons plus 2 teaspoons of ground chia seeds.*

Allow the mixture to sit for 5 minutes before using it in place of the eggs in Step 3. Follow the rest of the instructions as written, except in Step 4 increase the baking time to 30 minutes. When cutting the bread into croutons in Step 7, use a very sharp knife. The bread will be sticky, but just keep going!

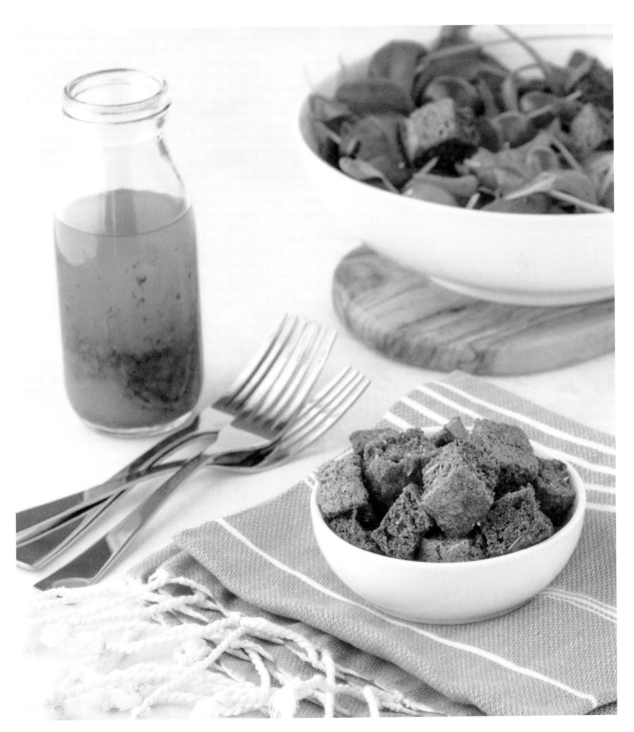

NUTRIENT INFORMATION (PER 8 CROUTONS):

calories: 263 | calories from fat: 220 | total fat: 24.5g | saturated fat: 3.4g | cholesterol: 93mg

sodium: 185mg | carbs: 5g | dietary fiber: 3.4g | net carbs: 1.6g | sugars: 0.5g | protein: 5.5g

RATIOS:

fat:	carbs:	protein:
84%	8%	8%

ZOODLES AND DOODLES

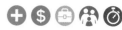

PREP TIME: **5 minutes** COOK TIME: – MAKES: **4 cups (4 servings)**

COCONUT-FREE • EGG-FREE • LOW-FODMAP • NIGHTSHADE-FREE • NUT-FREE • VEGAN

I usually eat Zoodles and Doodles raw or barely cooked. If you like your noodles warmed or you're interested in tender noodles for your dish, head on over to page 154, where I explain how to heat various spiral-sliced vegetables, including zucchini and daikon.

These low-carb noodles aren't just great for pasta-based dishes. Use them as the base for your next salad, chop and add them to soup right before serving, use them as a taco filling, or scatter them on the bottom of your plate before serving up your next meal. I always like to have a batch in the fridge for a quick vegetable infusion to just about any meal.

If you do not own a spiral slicer (known commonly as a spiralizer) and still want to make vegetable noodles, you can make noodle ribbons with a vegetable peeler. For more on making noodles out of your favorite vegetables and fruits, turn to page 154.

FOR ZOODLES:

2 medium zucchinis (about 7 ounces/ 200 g each), green or yellow

FOR DOODLES:

1 medium daikon (about 14 ounces/ 400 g)

1. If you have a spiral slicer, slice a zucchini or daikon into noodles, following the manufacturer's instructions.

To make noodles using a vegetable peeler, take a zucchini or daikon in your non-dominant hand. Hold it over a bowl and, with the opposite hand, begin peeling the zucchini or daikon. How far you go down the zucchini/daikon will determine the length of the ribbons. If you want shorter ribbons, simply drag the vegetable peeler across a shorter section of the zucchini/daikon. Repeat until most of the zucchini/daikon has been peeled and only a small, long core remains in your hand.

2. If making Zoodles, repeat with the second zucchini.

3. Use immediately or store as directed at left.

STORE IT: *Keep in the refrigerator in a plastic bag with the air squeezed out or in another airtight container for up to 3 days.*

SERVE IT WITH: *To make this a complete meal, slather the noodles with meat sauce.*

MAKE IT A CARB-UP: *Follow the instructions for preparing spiral-sliced fruits, sweet potatoes, potatoes, and/or other starchy roots on page 154.*

NUTRIENT INFORMATION (PER SERVING OF ZOODLES):

calories: 16 | calories from fat: 2 | total fat: 0.2g | saturated fat: 0g | cholesterol: 0mg
sodium: 0mg | carbs: 3.3g | dietary fiber: 1.1g | net carbs: 2.2g | sugars: 1.7g | protein: 1.2g

RATIOS:

fat:	carbs:	protein:
9%	67%	24%

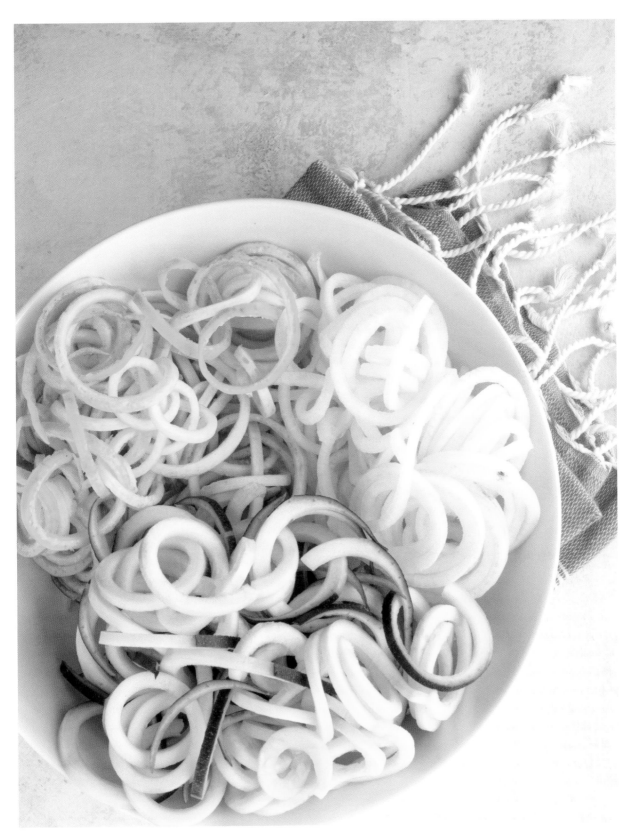

NUTRIENT INFORMATION (PER SERVING OF DOODLES):

calories: 20 | calories from fat: 0 | total fat: 0g | saturated fat: 0g | cholesterol: 0mg

sodium: 20mg | carbs: 4g | dietary fiber: 2g | net carbs: 2g | sugars: 2g | protein: 2g

RATIOS:

fat:	carbs:	protein:
0%	67%	33%

AVOCADO FRIES
WITH DIPPING SAUCE

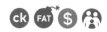

PREP TIME: **10 minutes**   COOK TIME: **16 minutes (if cooked in two batches)**   SERVES: **4**

COCONUT-FREE • NUT-FREE • VEGETARIAN   OPTIONS: EGG-FREE • NIGHTSHADE-FREE • VEGAN

A couple of weeks after embarking on my keto journey all those years ago, I discovered the goodness of keto fries. I was camping, and all I had on hand was avocados, oil, mayonnaise, and salt. From these four ingredients, I came up with something absolutely delightful. While I love them when they're made over an open flame, these keto-friendly fries are pretty tasty when made in a frying pan at home, too. Be sure to use an avocado oil that's labeled as safe for high-heat cooking. If you're in need of more guidance on cooking oils, turn to page 135.

FRIES:

2 large Hass avocados, peeled and pitted (6 ounces/170 g flesh)

½ teaspoon Seasoning Salt (page 235)

3 tablespoons refined avocado oil

DIPPING SAUCE:

¼ cup (52 g) mayonnaise, homemade (page 220) or store-bought

¾ teaspoon Seasoning Salt (page 235)

¼ teaspoon apple cider vinegar

FOR GARNISH:

⅛ teaspoon dried parsley

⅛ teaspoon ground black pepper

> **MAKE IT EGG-FREE/VEGAN:** *Use egg-free mayonnaise.*
>
> **MAKE IT NIGHTSHADE-FREE:** *Replace the Seasoning Salt with Italian seasoning (page 234) and use ¼ teaspoon of finely ground gray sea salt in Step 1.*

1. Make the fries: Cut the avocados lengthwise into frylike strips (4 or 5 strips or "fries" per avocado half). Lay the strips on a clean surface and dust with ½ teaspoon Seasoning Salt, covering all surfaces.

2. Place the avocado oil in a large frying pan and turn the heat to medium. Heat for 1 minute.

3. Add the avocado strips to the hot oil and fry until golden on one side, about 4 minutes. (Fry them in two batches if needed to avoid overcrowding the pan.) Carefully flip each strip over and repeat until all the strips are golden on all sides. Transfer the completed fries to a clean plate and repeat with any remaining uncooked fries.

4. Meanwhile, prepare the dipping sauce: In a small bowl, combine the mayonnaise with the ¾ teaspoon Seasoning Salt and the vinegar.

5. Once all the fries are done, sprinkle with the parsley and pepper. Serve with the dipping sauce and enjoy immediately.

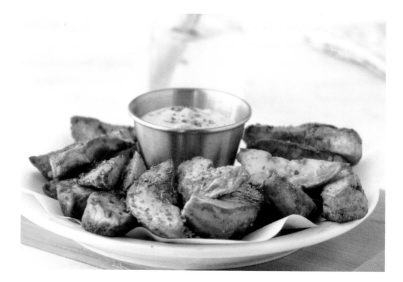

NUTRIENT INFORMATION (PER 5 FRIES WITH 1 TABLESPOON OF SAUCE):
calories: 355 | calories from fat: 309 | total fat: 34.4g | saturated fat: 5.7g | cholesterol: 5mg
sodium: 304mg | carbs: 8.6g | dietary fiber: 8.5g | net carbs: 0.1g | sugars: 0g | protein: 2.8g

RATIOS:
fat:	carbs:	protein:
87%	**10%**	**3%**

SHICHIMI COLLARDS

PREP TIME: **15 minutes**   COOK TIME: **15 minutes**   SERVES: **4**

EGG-FREE • VEGAN   OPTIONS: COCONUT-FREE • NUT-FREE

This dish works fabulously with an equal amount of Swiss chard as well. Making the switch would make each serving lower in overall carbohydrates, but would also decrease the fiber.

Raw sesame seeds are fine to use, but for health reasons, it's better to soak and roast them before using them in this recipe (see page 157).

¼ cup (60 ml) refined avocado oil or hazelnut oil

½ red onion, sliced thin

2 bunches collards (about 18 ounces/ 510 g), stems removed, roughly chopped

1 tablespoon Shichimi Seasoning (page 234)

2 tablespoons coconut aminos

1 teaspoon apple cider vinegar

¼ green bell pepper, sliced thin

Finely ground gray sea salt

Sesame seeds, for garnish (optional)

1. Place the avocado oil and sliced red onion in a frying pan. Cook on medium-low heat for 10 minutes, until lightly browned.

2. Add the collards, Shichimi seasoning, coconut aminos, and vinegar. Cover and cook on medium-low for 5 minutes, or until the greens are bright and lightly wilted.

3. Add the bell pepper and salt to taste.

4. Divide among 4 small serving bowls and sprinkle with sesame seeds, if desired.

MAKE IT COCONUT-FREE: *Replace the coconut aminos with a wheat-free soy sauce, if you tolerate soy.*

MAKE IT NUT-FREE: *Use avocado oil.*

MAKE IT A CARB-UP: *Reduce the amount of avocado oil to 2 tablespoons and serve alongside the carb of your choice (find ideas on page 117, or visit healthfulpursuit.com/carbup to download the complimentary PDF "Carb-Up Recipes").*

STORE IT: *Keep in an airtight container in the fridge for up to 3 days.*

REHEAT IT: *Microwave, covered, or place in a frying pan, uncovered, over medium heat until the desired temperature is reached.*

SERVE IT WITH: *To make this a complete meal, top it with sliced hard-boiled eggs. This dish also tastes great paired with Salt and Pepper Ribs (page 330).*

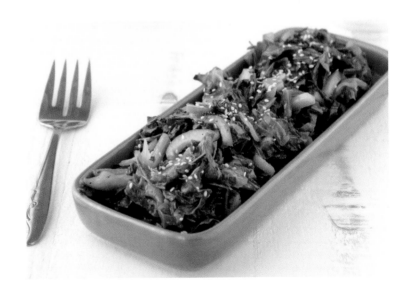

NUTRIENT INFORMATION (PER SERVING):

calories: 184 | calories from fat: 132 | total fat: 14.6g | saturated fat: 2.1g | cholesterol: 0mg

sodium: 674mg | carbs: 9.9g | dietary fiber: 4.9g | net carbs: 5g | sugars: 1.2g | protein: 3.3g

RATIOS:

fat:	carbs:	protein:
71%	21%	8%

CREAMY BAKED ASPARAGUS

PREP TIME: **5 minutes**   COOK TIME: **20 minutes**   SERVES: **4**

COCONUT-FREE • NIGHTSHADE-FREE • NUT-FREE   OPTIONS: EGG-FREE • VEGAN • VEGETARIAN

This dish is fabulous for a family get-together, especially if members of said family don't believe that keto foods can possibly taste good. The recipe combines a couple of simple ingredients for big-time flavor, and the dairy-free ranch dressing brings about longtime digestive happiness.

A company called Bacon's Heir makes pork dust, a breadcrumb-like product that you can find online. Alternatively, you can make your own pork dust by roughly grinding pork rinds in a blender until they have the texture of coarse breadcrumbs. If the pork rinds you're using contain salt, herbs, or spices, omit the salt that's sprinkled on the dish before baking.

1 pound (455 g) asparagus, tough ends removed

1 cup (240 ml) Ranch Dressing (page 226)

½ cup (32 g) pork dust or roughly ground pork rinds

Pinch of finely ground gray sea salt

Chopped fresh parsley, for garnish (optional)

1. Preheat the oven to 375°F (190°C). Place the asparagus spears in a medium-sized casserole dish.

2. Evenly distribute the ranch dressing over the top of the asparagus, then coat them with the pork dust. Sprinkle with the salt.

3. Bake for 18 to 20 minutes, until the top is lightly golden.

4. Serve immediately, garnished with fresh parsley, if desired.

STORE IT: *Keep in an airtight container in the fridge for up to 3 days.*

REHEAT IT: *Microwave, covered, or place in a frying pan and reheat, covered, over medium heat until the desired temperature is reached.*

PREP AHEAD: *Prepare the ranch dressing up to 2 days in advance.*

SERVE IT WITH: *To make this a complete meal, serve it alongside your favorite cut of beef. This dish tastes great paired with Steak with Tallow Herb Butter (page 306).*

MAKE IT EGG-FREE: *Prepare the egg-free variation of the ranch dressing.*

MAKE IT VEGETARIAN: *Replace the pork dust with coarsely ground almond flour.*

MAKE IT VEGAN: *Prepare the egg-free variation of the ranch dressing. Replace the pork dust with coarsely ground almond flour.*

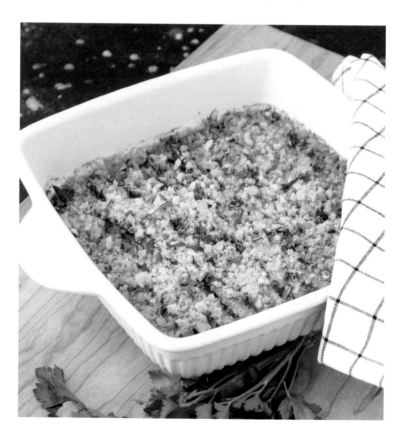

NUTRIENT INFORMATION (PER SERVING):

calories: 292 | calories from fat: 228 | total fat: 25.3g | saturated fat: 6.8g | cholesterol: 12mg

sodium: 429mg | carbs: 5.7g | dietary fiber: 2.6g | net carbs: 3.1g | sugars: 2.5g | protein: 10.4g

RATIOS:

fat:	carbs:	protein:
78%	**8%**	**14%**

PESTO ZOODLES

PREP TIME: **15 minutes, plus at least 8 hours to soak almonds**   SERVES: **6**

COCONUT-FREE • EGG-FREE • NIGHTSHADE-FREE • VEGAN   OPTION: NUT-FREE

I'm known as the pâté girl, and whether you call 'em pâtés or pestos or dips or spreads, I make and enjoy them all. All my friends know that I love turning nuts, seeds, and fresh herbs—and sometimes even fresh leafy vegetables like spinach, kale, and cabbage—into pestos like this one. You can enjoy this pesto on just about anything! In the summer, my favorite way to eat it is tossed with Zoodles or Doodles (page 376), and in the winter, I slather it on roasted meats and vegetables.

HERB PESTO:

4 ounces (115 g) fresh basil (about 2 cups leaves and stems)

¾ cup (120 g) raw almonds, soaked overnight, then drained and rinsed

¾ cup (45 g) fresh parsley leaves

1 small clove garlic, minced if not using a high-powered blender

3 tablespoons extra-virgin olive oil or refined avocado oil

2 tablespoons apple cider vinegar

1 tablespoon fresh lemon juice

1 or 2 drops liquid stevia (optional)

¼ teaspoon finely ground gray sea salt

FOR SERVING:

1 batch Zoodles or Doodles (page 376)

Freshly ground black pepper

> STORE IT: *If possible, store the pesto separate from the noodles in airtight containers in the fridge for up to 5 days. When ready to serve, coat the noodles. Coated noodles can be stored in an airtight container in the fridge for up to 3 days.*
>
> PREP AHEAD: *Prepare the pesto up to 2 days before serving.*
>
> SERVE IT WITH: *To make this a complete meal, top the Pesto Zoodles with grilled salmon. These noodles also taste great paired with Stuffed Pork Roast with Herb Gravy (page 334).*
>
> MAKE IT NUT-FREE: *Replace the almonds with ½ cup (75 g) of hulled hemp seeds.*
>
> MAKE IT A CARB-UP: *Follow the carb-up instructions in the Zoodles and Doodles recipe.*

1. Make the pesto: Remove the leaves from the basil. Place the leaves along with the rest of the ingredients for the pesto in a high-powered blender or food processor fitted with the "S" blade and pulse just until chunky. You can either continue processing for a smooth pesto or stop while there are still chunks of almonds.

2. Place the Zoodles in a mixing bowl. Transfer the pesto to the bowl with the noodles and toss with your fingers to coat.

3. Divide the coated noodles among 6 small serving bowls and sprinkle with ground black pepper before serving.

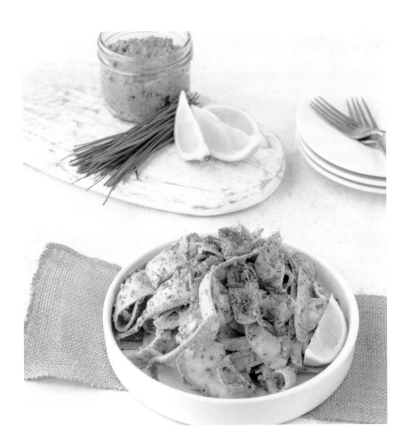

NUTRIENT INFORMATION (PER SERVING):

calories: 161 | calories from fat: 119 | total fat: 13.3g | saturated fat: 1.5g | cholesterol: 0mg

sodium: 109mg | carbs: 6g | dietary fiber: 2.8g | net carbs: 3.2g | sugars: 1.8g | protein: 4.2g

RATIOS:

fat:	carbs:	protein:
75%	15%	10%

CREAMY MASHED TURNIPS

EGG-FREE • NIGHTSHADE-FREE • NUT-FREE   OPTIONS: COCONUT-FREE • LOW-FODMAP • VEGAN

These mashed turnips have 63 percent less carbohydrates than an equal portion of classic mashed potatoes. They're delicious with gravy and all the classic fixings but won't give you the carb hangover, blood sugar spikes, or cravings that mashed potatoes do. While it's a festive dish, it is simple enough for everyday meals, and the leftovers will fare well in your lunch the next day.

4 large turnips (about 2¼ pounds/1 kg), cubed

2 tablespoons refined avocado oil, melted tallow, or ghee (if tolerated)

6 small cloves garlic, peeled

2 teaspoons dried thyme leaves

1 teaspoon finely ground gray sea salt

⅔ cup (160 ml) heated full-fat coconut milk

FOR GARNISH (OPTIONAL):

Freshly ground black pepper

Chopped fresh parsley

1. Preheat the oven to 375°F (190°C).

2. Place the cubed turnips, avocado oil, garlic cloves, thyme, and salt on an unlined rimmed baking sheet. Toss with your hands to coat the turnips.

3. Roast the turnips for 25 to 30 minutes, flipping them every 10 minutes, until they are soft and browned.

4. Transfer the roasted turnips to a blender or food processor. Add the hot coconut milk and pulse 5 to 10 times, until the desired consistency is reached.

5. Transfer to a 1-quart (950-ml) serving dish and serve sprinkled with freshly ground pepper and chopped parsley. If not serving immediately, cover to keep warm.

STORE IT: *Keep in an airtight container in the fridge for up to 3 days.*

REHEAT IT: *Microwave, covered, or place in a frying pan, add a dollop of lard or a drizzle of avocado oil, and fry on medium heat until the desired temperature is reached.*

PREP AHEAD: *Roast the turnips up to 2 days ahead. When ready to prepare the recipe, heat the turnips using the reheating instructions above and pick up at Step 4.*

SERVE IT WITH: *To make this a complete meal, serve it alongside roasted chicken. This dish also tastes great paired with Balsamic Turkey Thighs (page 338).*

MAKE IT COCONUT-FREE: *Replace the coconut milk with the nondairy milk of your choice. I like unsweetened almond milk.*

MAKE IT LOW-FODMAP: *Omit the garlic and reduce the amount of avocado oil to 1 tablespoon. After placing the roasted turnips in the blender in Step 4, add 3 tablespoons of Garlic-Infused Oil (page 230) made with olive oil. If you are super-sensitive to coconut milk, use another nondairy milk instead.*

MAKE IT VEGAN: *Use avocado oil.*

MAKE IT A CARB-UP: *Replace the turnips with your favorite type of potato. Reduce the amount of avocado oil to 1 tablespoon and the coconut milk to ¼ cup (60 ml).*

NUTRIENT INFORMATION (PER SERVING):

calories: 93 | calories from fat: 55 | total fat: 6.1g | saturated fat: 3.4g | cholesterol: 0mg
sodium: 261mg | carbs: 8.2g | dietary fiber: 1.9g | net carbs: 6.3g | sugars: 4.6g | protein: 1.3g

RATIOS:

fat:	carbs:	protein:
60%	**35%**	**5%**

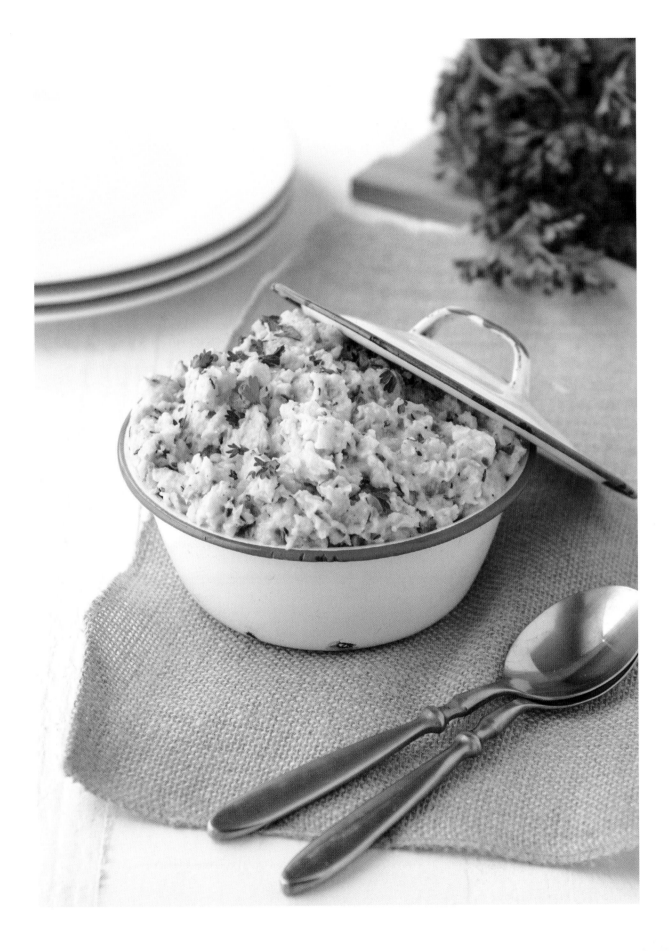

HERBED RADISHES

PREP TIME: **10 minutes**   COOK TIME: **15 minutes**   SERVES: **2**

COCONUT-FREE • EGG-FREE • LOW-FODMAP • NIGHTSHADE-FREE • NUT-FREE   OPTION: **VEGAN**

I love having a batch of these radishes in the fridge for quick lunch assembly. They're great tossed into a salad or served alongside your favorite meat dish. My favorite recipe to pair with these tasty radishes is Bacon-Wrapped Mini Meatloaves (page 298).

3 tablespoons lard

14 ounces (400 g) radishes (about 2 bunches), quartered

⅛ teaspoon finely ground gray sea salt

⅛ teaspoon ground black pepper

2 tablespoons sliced fresh chives

1 tablespoon chopped fresh herbs, such as thyme and/or rosemary

1. Heat the lard in a large frying pan over medium heat until melted. Add the quartered radishes, salt, and pepper. Cover and cook for 5 minutes, or until softened.

2. Remove the lid and cook for another 7 minutes, stirring frequently, or until the pieces begin to brown.

3. Add the chives and fresh herbs and toss to combine. Reduce the heat to medium-low and continue to cook for 2 minutes.

4. Remove from the heat, divide among 4 small bowls, and serve.

STORE IT: *Keep in an airtight container in the fridge for up to 3 days.*

REHEAT IT: *Microwave, covered, or place in a frying pan and heat, covered, on medium until the desired temperature is reached.*

SERVE IT WITH: *To make this a complete meal, serve it alongside browned ground beef seasoned with your favorite spice mixture (pages 232 to 235). This dish also tastes great paired with Balsamic Turkey Thighs (page 338).*

MAKE IT VEGAN: *Replace the lard with coconut oil.*

MAKE IT A CARB-UP: *Reduce the lard to 1 tablespoon and replace the radishes with beets.*

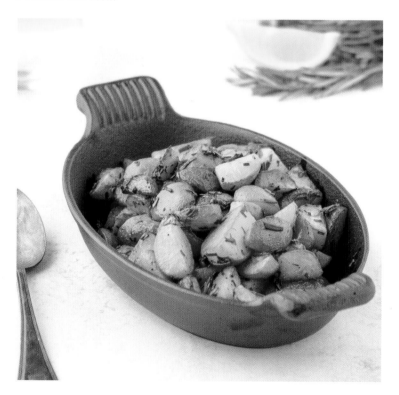

NUTRIENT INFORMATION (PER SERVING):

calories: 223 | calories from fat: 174 | total fat: 19.3g | saturated fat: 7.6g | cholesterol: 18mg

sodium: 173mg | carbs: 6.6g | dietary fiber: 0.6g | net carbs: 6g | sugars: 5.6g | protein: 5.8g

RATIOS:

fat:	carbs:	protein:
78%	12%	10%

PORKY CABBAGE

PREP TIME: **10 minutes**   COOK TIME: **25 minutes**   SERVES: **4**

COCONUT-FREE · EGG-FREE · LOW-FODMAP · NIGHTSHADE-FREE · NUT-FREE

Cabbage and bacon were meant to be together forever. The bacon-and-avocado combination wins every time in my book, but cabbage plus bacon is the next best thing. And hey, if you wanted to get crazy, you could add sliced avocado to this dish and enjoy the best of both worlds.

I like using green cabbage in this recipe so that you can see the bacon, but purple cabbage tastes just as wonderful. If you cut the cabbage thin enough, this recipe doubles as an awesome sandwich filling.

6 strips bacon (about 6 ounces/170 g)

4 cups (470 g) sliced green cabbage

½ teaspoon finely ground gray sea salt

⅛ teaspoon ground black pepper

> STORE IT: *Keep in an airtight container in the fridge for up to 3 days.*
>
> REHEAT IT: *Microwave, covered, or place in a frying pan and heat, covered, over medium heat until the desired temperature is reached.*
>
> PREP AHEAD: *Prepare the bacon bits up to a month ahead and store in an airtight container in the freezer. When ready to use, simply add to the recipe in Step 5. In Step 2, melt 3 tablespoons plus 1 teaspoon of bacon grease in the frying pan before adding the cabbage, salt, and pepper.*

1. Place the bacon in a large frying pan over medium heat and cook until crisp, flipping it over halfway through. When crisp, remove the bacon from the pan and place on a plate to cool.

2. Keep the bacon grease in the pan and add the sliced cabbage, salt, and pepper. Cover and cook, stirring frequently, for 10 minutes, or until softened and lightly translucent.

3. Remove the lid and cook for another 5 minutes, stirring frequently, until the liquid evaporates and the cabbage begins to brown lightly.

4. Meanwhile, break up the cooled bacon into bits.

5. Add the bacon bits to the pan with the cabbage. Remove from the heat and toss to combine. Divide among 4 small bowls and serve.

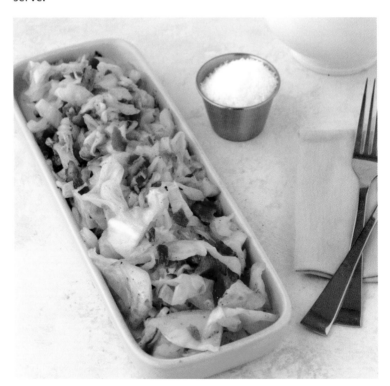

NUTRIENT INFORMATION (PER SERVING):

calories: 215 | calories from fat: 156 | total fat: 17.4g | saturated fat: 5.8g | cholesterol: 30mg

sodium: 552mg | carbs: 7.6g | dietary fiber: 2.8g | net carbs: 4.8g | sugars: 4.2g | protein: 6.9g

RATIOS:

fat:	carbs:	protein:
73%	14%	13%

POTATO SALAD…THAT ISN'T

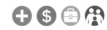

PREP TIME: **25 minutes**   COOK TIME: **10 minutes**   SERVES: **6**

COCONUT-FREE • NIGHTSHADE-FREE • NUT-FREE • VEGETARIAN   OPTIONS: EGG-FREE • VEGAN

A Paleo and keto "potato" salad…with no potatoes at all! It's made with clean low-carb, keto ingredients and can be made vegan, too.

Pickle juice is the pickling liquid that comes in the bottle of your favorite brand of pickles. This is the secret ingredient that's made my dad's potato salad famous among our family and friends for decades. The key to a good "potato" salad, like this one, is pickle juice. Trust me.

When I'm making this recipe and I don't have time to let the cauliflower bits cool on the counter or chill in the fridge, I transfer the steamed cauliflower to a baking sheet and place it in the freezer to cool. By the time I've prepped the rest of the salad, the cauliflower is at the perfect temperature!

1 large head cauliflower (about 1¾ pounds/800 g), stem removed

6 large eggs, hard-boiled

⅓ cup (13 g) fresh parsley leaves, chopped

6 baby dill pickles, diced

6 green onions, green parts only, sliced

DRESSING:

Cooked egg yolks (from hard-boiled eggs, above)

½ cup (105 g) mayonnaise, homemade (page 220) or store-bought

3 tablespoons pickle juice

2 tablespoons Dijon mustard

¼ teaspoon finely ground gray sea salt

⅛ teaspoon ground black pepper

1. Chop the cauliflower into bite-sized pieces. Steam the cauliflower pieces until softened but not mushy. Set aside to cool to room temperature.

2. Meanwhile, separate the yolks and whites from the hard-boiled eggs. Chop the whites and transfer to a large bowl. Place the yolks in a blender or food processor.

3. To make the dressing: To the blender or food processor with the egg yolks, add the mayonnaise, pickle juice, mustard, salt, and pepper. Blend on medium speed until smooth.

4. Transfer the dressing to the bowl with the chopped egg whites, then add the cooled cauliflower pieces, parsley leaves, pickles, and green onions. Toss to coat.

5. Serve right away or cover and transfer to the fridge to cool completely, about 4 hours, before serving. To serve, divide the salad among 6 bowls.

STORE IT: *Keep in an airtight container in the fridge for up to 3 days.*

PREP AHEAD: *The dressing and salad can be made up to 2 days ahead, stored separately, and tossed just before serving.*

SERVE IT WITH: *To make this a complete meal, serve it alongside roasted chicken thighs. This salad also tastes great paired with Mind-Blowing Burgers (page 308).*

MAKE IT EGG-FREE/VEGAN: *Omit the hard-boiled eggs and use egg-free mayonnaise.*

MAKE IT A CARB-UP: *Replace the cauliflower with raw boiling potatoes. Cube the potatoes and place them in a large pot. Cover with water and bring to a boil; continue to boil until fork-tender, about 15 minutes. Drain and set aside to cool to room temperature. Prepare the rest of the salad as instructed, beginning with Step 2.*

NUTRIENT INFORMATION (PER SERVING):
calories: 189 | calories from fat: 128 | total fat: 14.2g | saturated fat: 2.7g | cholesterol: 145mg
sodium: 401mg | carbs: 8g | dietary fiber: 3.6g | net carbs: 4.4g | sugars: 3.5g | protein: 7.3g

RATIOS:
fat: carbs: protein:
68%   **17%**   **15%**

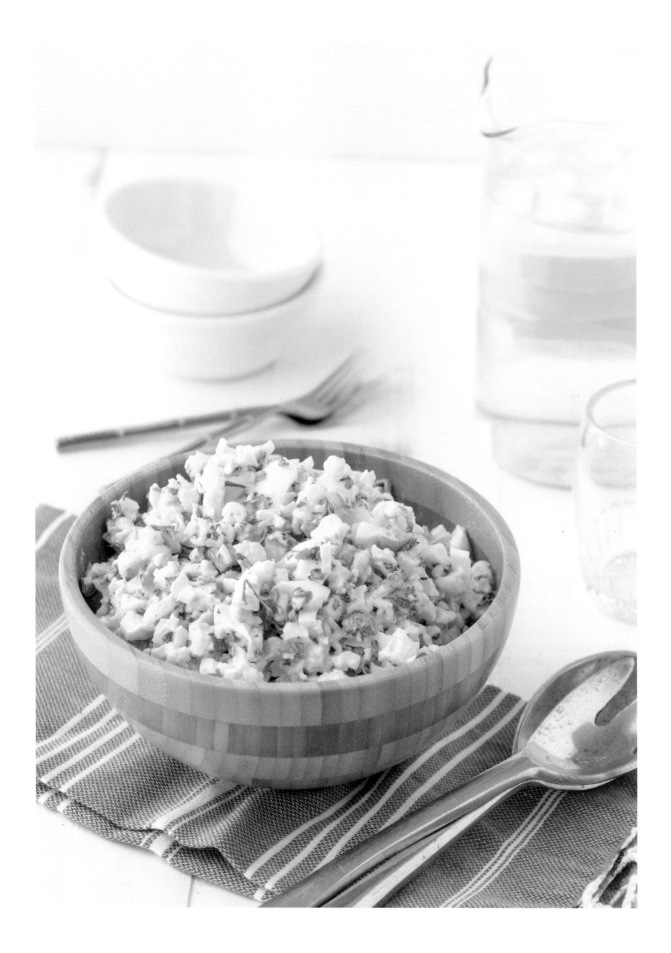

ROASTED BRUSSELS SPROUTS WITH WALNUT "CHEESE"

PREP TIME: **20 minutes**   COOK TIME: **25 minutes**   SERVES: **8**

EGG-FREE · NIGHTSHADE-FREE   OPTIONS: COCONUT-FREE · VEGAN

This is my favorite recipe in this entire book. I just can't stop making it, eating it, and making more of it. If you try only one recipe from *The Keto Diet*, please let it be this one—especially if you're a lover of nutritional yeast, as I am. Nutritional yeast is a deactivated yeast product that tastes similar to cheese but is 100 percent dairy-free. Paired with the ingredients in this recipe, you cannot go wrong.

When roasting the Brussels sprouts, rogue leaves will burn; just pick them out when you transfer the Brussels sprouts to the "cheese" bowl. And don't think you need to reheat this dish when using it as leftovers. I love these roasted Brussels sprouts with walnut cheese even more when they're cold.

ROASTED BRUSSELS SPROUTS:

5 cups (600 g) trimmed and halved Brussels sprouts

¼ cup (60 ml) melted lard, tallow, or coconut oil

½ teaspoon finely ground gray sea salt

¼ teaspoon ground black pepper

Leaves from 3 sprigs fresh thyme, or ¼ teaspoon dried thyme leaves

WALNUT "CHEESE":

¾ cup (85 g) raw walnut pieces, soaked for 24 hours, then drained, rinsed, and finely chopped

3 tablespoons extra-virgin olive oil or refined avocado oil

⅓ cup (22 g) nutritional yeast

2 teaspoons fresh lemon juice

½ teaspoon Dijon mustard

¼ teaspoon onion powder

¼ teaspoon garlic powder

Pinch of finely ground gray sea salt

Pinch of ground black pepper

EXTRAS:

½ packed cup (32 g) fresh parsley leaves, finely chopped

2 tablespoons extra-virgin olive oil or refined avocado oil

1 tablespoon fresh lemon juice

Finely ground gray sea salt

1. To roast the Brussels sprouts: Preheat the oven to 375°F (190°C). Place the Brussels sprouts, melted fat, salt, pepper, and thyme leaves on an unlined rimmed baking sheet and toss to coat with your hands. Roast for 20 to 25 minutes, flipping the sprouts every 10 minutes, until they are golden.

2. Meanwhile, make walnut "cheese": Place all the ingredients for the cheese in a large bowl and stir to combine.

3. Once the Brussels sprouts are done, transfer them to the bowl with the walnut cheese. Add the chopped parsley, olive oil, lemon juice, and salt to taste.

4. Divide among 8 small bowls and serve.

STORE IT: *Keep in an airtight container in the fridge for up to 3 days.*

REHEAT IT: *Microwave, covered, or place in a frying pan, add a dollop of lard or a drizzle of avocado oil, cover, and fry over medium heat until the desired temperature is reached.*

PREP AHEAD: *Prepare the "cheese" up to 1 day before using in the recipe.*

SERVE IT WITH: *To make this a complete meal, add it to your favorite salad. This dish tastes great paired with Michael's Pepperoni Meatzza (page 312).*

MAKE IT COCONUT-FREE: *Use lard or tallow.*

MAKE IT VEGAN: *Use coconut oil.*

NUTRIENT INFORMATION (PER SERVING):

calories: 263 | calories from fat: 200 | total fat: 22.2g | saturated fat: 4.5g | cholesterol: 6mg

sodium: 204mg | carbs: 9.9g | dietary fiber: 4.3g | net carbs: 5.6g | sugars: 2.1g | protein: 5.8g

RATIOS:

fat:	carbs:	protein:
76%	15%	9%

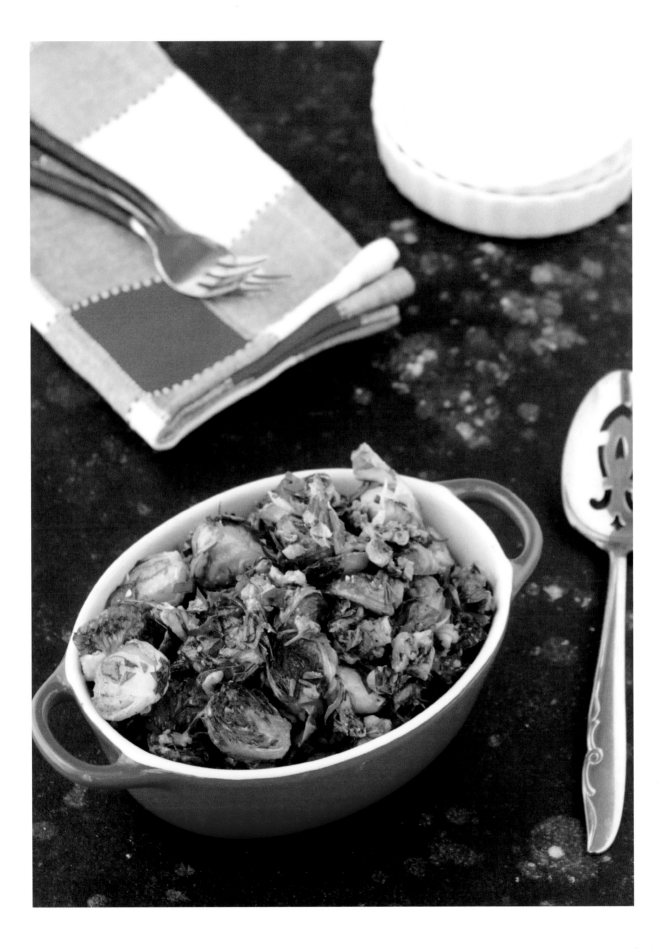

CHAPTER 22

SWEET TOOTH SNACKS & DESSERTS

COCONUT MOUNDS

PREP TIME: 20 minutes, plus at least 45 minutes to chill   MAKES: 18 bars (18 servings)

EGG-FREE • NIGHTSHADE-FREE • VEGAN   OPTION: NUT-FREE

As I was taking the photographs, I kept saying to myself how in love with this recipe I was. Of all the recipes in this book, this one's my favorite! If you love those classic store-bought treats—you know the ones I'm referring to—then you're going to love these! And they are high in fat to boot, which means that eating these will help you get into ketosis. Oh, the world we live in. Enjoy!

2⅔ cups (240 g) unsweetened shredded coconut

1 batch Sweetened Condensed Coconut Milk (page 415), heated just until lukewarm

¼ cup (60 ml) melted coconut oil or ghee (if tolerated)

1 tablespoon plus 1 teaspoon confectioners'-style erythritol

1 teaspoon vanilla extract or powder

¼ teaspoon finely ground gray sea salt

36 almonds, roasted

½ cup (112 g) stevia-sweetened chocolate chips, melted

SPECIAL EQUIPMENT:

Silicone mold(s) with 18 (1-ounce/30-ml) rectangular cavities (optional)

STORE IT: *Keep in an airtight container in the fridge for up to 3 days or in the freezer for up to 1 month.*

THAW IT: *Set on the counter until thawed, about 15 minutes.*

PREP AHEAD: *Prepare the condensed milk up to 3 days before making the mounds and warm it before use in Step 2. Roast almonds in bulk and keep in the freezer for up to 3 months for quicker meal prep.*

MAKE IT NUT-FREE: *Omit the roasted almonds.*

1. Line a rimmed baking sheet with parchment paper or a silicone baking mat. Or have on hand a silicone mold with 18 (1-ounce/30-ml) rectangular cavities.

2. Place the shredded coconut, condensed milk, coconut oil, erythritol, vanilla, and salt in a large bowl. Toss to ensure that each piece of coconut is coated.

3. If using a baking sheet, scoop up 2 tablespoons of the mixture and use your hands to press it into a barlike shape, then place it on the lined baking sheet. Repeat with the rest of the dough. If using a silicone mold, press 2 tablespoons of the mixture into each cavity. Regardless of method, be sure to press down on the mixture to compact it.

4. Place the baking sheet or mold in the fridge to set for at least 30 minutes.

5. Remove from the fridge. If using a silicone mold, gently remove the bars from the mold and place on a sheet of parchment paper or a silicone baking mat.

6. Place 2 almonds atop each bar, then drizzle the melted chocolate over the top.

7. Return to the fridge to set for 15 minutes. Enjoy!

NUTRIENT INFORMATION (PER BAR):
calories: 204 | calories from fat: 168 | total fat: 18.7g | saturated fat: 15.1g | cholesterol: 0mg
sodium: 41mg | carbs: 6.6g | dietary fiber: 3.3g | net carbs: 3.3g | sugars: 1.4g | protein: 2.2g

RATIOS:
fat: carbs: protein:
83%   13%   4%

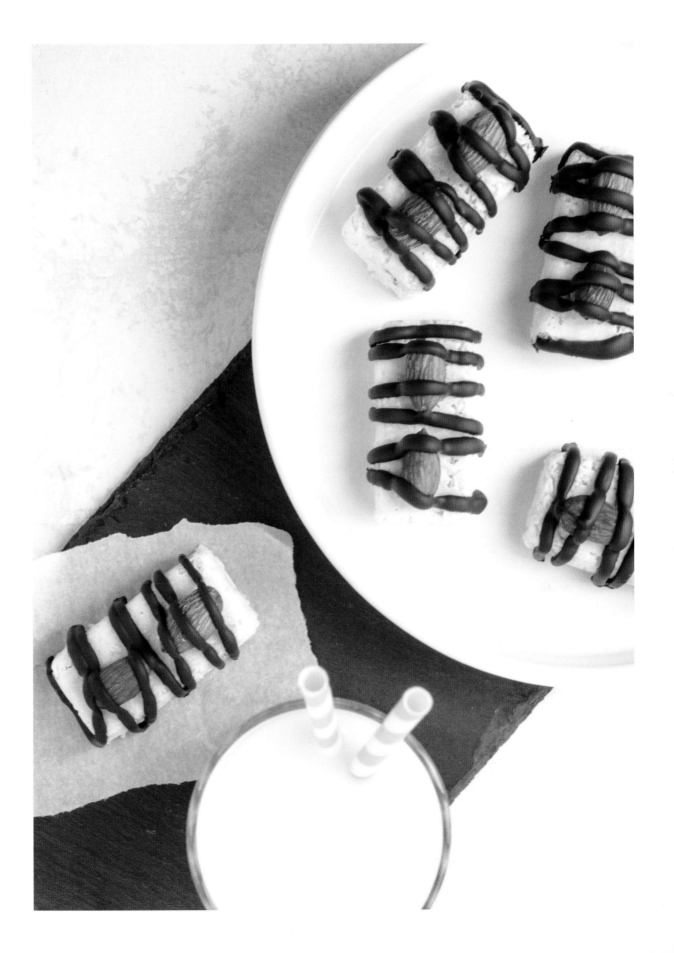

ALMOND CHAI TRUFFLES

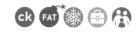

PREP TIME: **20 minutes, plus at least 30 minutes to chill**   MAKES: **10 truffles (10 servings)**

COCONUT-FREE • EGG-FREE • LOW-FODMAP • NIGHTSHADE-FREE • VEGAN   OPTION: NUT-FREE

Unlike other fat bombs, these guys travel well without melting at room temperature, making them great for lunches. I've given you two flavor options; which you choose depends on your preference or food allergies. If you leave the truffle mixture in the fridge too long and it gets too firm, don't worry; simply set it on the counter and wait until it is easy to mold into balls. The key is to mash up the truffle mixture with a fork before you start rolling it into balls, which will remove any large chunks that would make it difficult to roll. When you start rolling the mixture between your palms, don't worry too much about making the truffles perfectly circular, because the topping will cover most imperfections. But remember to clean your hands after preparing each ball or you'll have a sticky mess in your topping bowl!

½ cup (140 g) unsweetened smooth almond butter

¼ cup plus 2 tablespoons (90 g) cacao butter, melted

1 tablespoon plus 1 teaspoon chai spice (recipe below)

1 tablespoon confectioners'-style erythritol or 2 to 4 drops liquid stevia

½ teaspoon vanilla extract or powder

Pinch of finely ground gray sea salt

3 tablespoons almonds, roasted

SPECIAL EQUIPMENT:

10 mini paper liners (optional)

1. Combine the almond butter, cacao butter, chai spice, erythritol, vanilla, and salt in a medium-sized bowl and stir to combine. Place in the fridge to set for 30 to 45 minutes, until firm yet still pliable.

2. Meanwhile, put the roasted almonds in a small baggie, seal, and cover with a kitchen towel. Bash with a mallet or the bottom of a mug until the pieces are no larger than ⅛ inch (3 mm). Pour the pieces into a small bowl.

3. Line a rimmed baking sheet with parchment paper or a silicone baking mat.

4. Remove the truffle mixture from the fridge and break it up with a fork until no clumps larger than a pencil eraser remain. Scoop up a tablespoon of the mixture and roll it quickly between your palms, then place it in the bowl with the roasted almond pieces and toss to coat. Once coated, transfer to the prepared baking sheet. Clean your hands so as not to transfer the almond pieces to the truffle mixture. Repeat with the remaining dough, making 10 truffles total.

5. Serve the truffles in mini paper liners, if desired. They are best when consumed at room temperature.

STORE IT: *Keep in an airtight container in the fridge for up to 2 weeks or in the freezer for up to 1 month.*

THAW IT: *Set on the counter until thawed, about 15 minutes.*

MAKE IT NUT-FREE: *Prepare the Coconut Chai Truffles variation.*

VARIATION: COCONUT CHAI TRUFFLES. *Use ½ cup (130 g) of coconut butter in place of the almond butter, use ¼ cup plus 2 tablespoons (90 ml) of melted coconut oil in place of the cacao butter, and use ⅓ cup (33 g) of roasted unsweetened shredded coconut in place of the almonds.*

VARIATION: MAKE-YOUR-OWN CHAI SPICE. *For variety, use this homemade chai spice as a replacement for cinnamon in your favorite cinnamon-flavored recipes. Combine the following ingredients in a small jar and shake: 2 teaspoons of ground cinnamon, 2 teaspoons of ground cloves, 2 teaspoons of ground cardamom, 1 teaspoon of ground coriander, 1 teaspoon of ginger powder, ½ teaspoon of ground white pepper, and a pinch of finely ground gray sea salt. Makes 3 tablespoons.*

NUTRIENT INFORMATION (PER ALMOND CHAI TRUFFLE):

calories: 196 | calories from fat: 165 | total fat: 18.4g | saturated fat: 7.2g | cholesterol: 0mg

sodium: 16mg | carbs: 3.9g | dietary fiber: 2.4g | net carbs: 1.5g | sugars: 0.6g | protein: 3.7g

RATIOS:

fat:	carbs:	protein:
85%	8%	7%

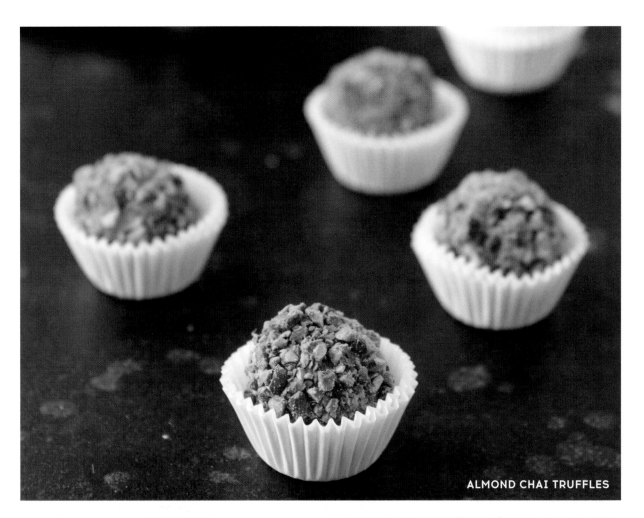

ALMOND CHAI TRUFFLES

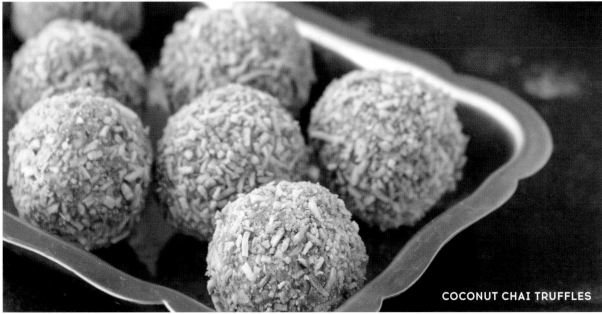

COCONUT CHAI TRUFFLES

NUTRIENT INFORMATION (PER COCONUT CHAI TRUFFLE):

calories: 147 | calories from fat: 137 | total fat: 15.2g | saturated fat: 13.5g | cholesterol: 0mg

sodium: 16mg | carbs: 3.2g | dietary fiber: 2.3g | net carbs: 0.9g | sugars: 0.7g | protein: 0.7g

RATIOS:

fat:	carbs:	protein:
90%	8%	2%

BACON FUDGE

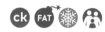

PREP TIME: **10 minutes, plus 1 hour to chill**   COOK TIME: **5 minutes**   SERVES: **4**

COCONUT-FREE • EGG-FREE • NIGHTSHADE-FREE • NUT-FREE   OPTION: **LOW-FODMAP**

Bacon and chocolate is a winning combination. Don't believe me? Check the Internet. It's everywhere! But not like this. If you've been busy cooking lots of bacon (and something tells me you have) and you're not sure what to do with all the leftover bacon grease, this recipe will be your saving grace. In fact, my guess is that you'll love it so much, you'll cook bacon just to have grease to make this fudge! The consistency of this fudge is bang on. And it makes the fattiest of fat bombs in all the land. To make this recipe, you will need a mold with a total volume capacity of 12 ounces (350 ml). You can make the fudge pieces in any size or shape you like. To make four large pieces of fudge, as shown, you will need a mold with four 3-ounce (90-ml) cavities. I used a large silicone ice cube tray (called "icebergs") to create four large pieces.

½ cup (70 g) bacon grease, melted

¼ cup (60 g) cacao butter

¼ cup (20 g) cacao powder

3 tablespoons confectioners'-style erythritol

1 teaspoon vanilla extract or powder

⅛ teaspoon finely ground gray sea salt

SPECIAL EQUIPMENT:

Silicone mold with four 3-ounce (90-ml) cavities or a total volume capacity of 12 ounces (350 ml)

1. Place all the ingredients in a small bowl and whisk continuously until the erythritol has dissolved, about 5 minutes.

2. Pour the mixture into a silicone mold. Set the mold in the fridge to firm up for 1 hour. The fudge is best enjoyed after softening on the counter for about 30 minutes.

MAKE LOW-FODMAP: *Use 2 to 4 drops of liquid stevia instead of erythritol. Start with 2 drops and adjust to taste as you're making the recipe.*

VARIATION: PEPPERMINT BACON FUDGE. *Decrease the amount of vanilla extract or powder to ½ teaspoon and add ½ teaspoon of peppermint extract.*

STORE IT: *Keep in an airtight container in the fridge for up to 1 week or in the freezer for up to 1 month.*

THAW IT: *Set on the counter until thawed, about 45 minutes.*

PREP AHEAD: *Render fat from bacon ahead of time. You'll need 13 ounces (370 g) of bacon to yield the ½ cup (70 g) of grease needed for this recipe. Keep the bacon grease in an airtight container in the fridge for up to 1 week or in the freezer for up to 1 month. If you're looking for a recipe that uses lots of bacon and will leave you with lots of grease, try Bacon Crackers (page 254).*

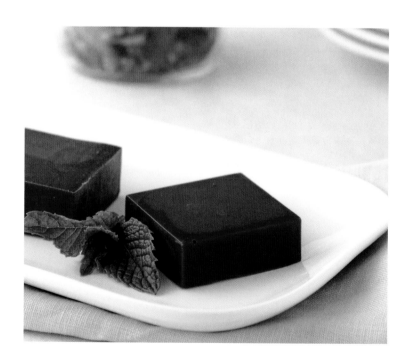

NUTRIENT INFORMATION (PER SERVING):

calories: 412 | calories from fat: 396 | total fat: 44g | saturated fat: 21.9g | cholesterol: 27mg
sodium: 117mg | carbs: 2.5g | dietary fiber: 1.5g | net carbs: 1g | sugars: 0g | protein: 1.5g

RATIOS:

fat:	carbs:	protein:
97%	1%	2%

CARDAMOM ORANGE BARK

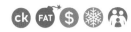

PREP TIME: **15 minutes, plus at least 1 hour to chill**   SERVES: **6**

EGG-FREE · NIGHTSHADE-FREE · VEGAN   OPTIONS: COCONUT-FREE · LOW-FODMAP · NUT-FREE

Bark is one of my favorite late-night keto snacks because it's quick to whip together, making high-fat snacking a breeze. Immediately after dinner, I'll combine the ingredients for this recipe and pop the bark in the freezer while we tidy up. By the time everything's been put away and we're ready for the following day, the bark is ready to chow down on! If you want to get crazy, sprinkle a handful of stevia-sweetened chocolate chips over the top of the bark before popping it in the fridge or freezer to set—because a little chocolate is never a bad thing.

Raw walnuts are fine, but for health reasons it's better to soak and roast them before using them in this recipe (see page 157).

¾ cup (180 ml) melted coconut oil

2 tablespoons confectioners'-style erythritol

2 teaspoons ginger powder

1¾ teaspoons ground cardamom

½ teaspoon vanilla extract or powder

½ teaspoon orange extract

⅛ teaspoon finely ground gray sea salt

⅔ cup (75 g) raw walnut pieces, roasted

1. Place all the ingredients except the walnuts in a blender. Blend on high for 20 seconds, until everything is incorporated and the erythritol has dissolved.

2. Add the roasted walnuts and pulse briefly, until they're broken into small chunks about ¼ inch (6 mm) in size.

3. Transfer the mixture to an 8-inch (20-cm) square pan lined with parchment paper or a silicone baking mat and chill in the fridge for 2 hours or in the freezer for 1 hour.

4. Remove the sheet of bark from the pan and transfer to a clean surface. Using the tip of a butter knife, break the bark into rough pieces, starting in the middle and working your way out. Try to break the bark into 6 large pieces (for easy portioning) or several smaller pieces. Enjoy!

STORE IT: *Keep in an airtight container in the fridge for up to 2 weeks or in the freezer for up to 2 months.*

THAW IT: *Enjoy straight from the freezer or allow to thaw for 1 to 2 minutes before consuming.*

MAKE IT COCONUT-FREE: *Replace the coconut oil with cacao butter or ghee, if tolerated.*

MAKE IT LOW-FODMAP: *Use 2 to 4 drops of liquid stevia instead of erythritol.*

MAKE IT NUT-FREE: *Replace the walnuts with roasted hulled sunflower seeds.*

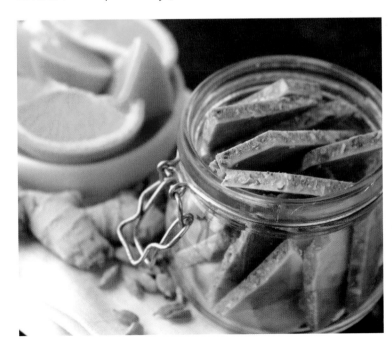

NUTRIENT INFORMATION (PER SERVING):

calories: 334 | calories from fat: 316 | total fat: 35.1g | saturated fat: 24.4g | cholesterol: 0mg

sodium: 51mg | carbs: 2.4g | dietary fiber: 1g | net carbs: 1.4g | sugars: 0g | protein: 2.1g

RATIOS:

fat:	carbs:	protein:
95%	3%	2%

CARROT CAKE

PREP TIME: **45 minutes, plus 8 hours to chill**   COOK TIME: **35 minutes**   MAKES: one two-layer 9-inch (23-cm) round cake (16 servings)

EGG-FREE · NIGHTSHADE-FREE · NUT-FREE

Last year, we hosted a surprise party for my mom's sixtieth birthday. Combined, our family is allergic to nuts, seeds, eggs, dairy, grains, gluten, and sugar, and I was tasked with making a cake that everyone could enjoy. Enter the allergen-free carrot cake! The key to this recipe is resting the cake layers overnight. I think it has everything to do with allowing the gelatin to set. The dairy-free cream cheese frosting also benefits from sitting in the fridge overnight. The advantage to this approach is that on the day of serving, the cake comes together in a snap. The end result is a moist, dense cake filled with classic carrot cake flavors.

CAKE:

1 cup (240 ml) water

¼ cup (40 g) unflavored gelatin

1 cup (100 g) coconut flour

½ cup (65 g) arrowroot starch

1½ teaspoons ground cinnamon

1½ teaspoons baking soda

½ teaspoon finely ground gray sea salt

1 cup (240 ml) melted coconut oil

⅔ cup (155 g) granulated xylitol

¾ teaspoon vanilla extract

⅔ cup (120 g) shredded carrots, lightly packed

FROSTING:

1 (13½-ounce/400-ml) can coconut cream, chilled for at least 12 hours, or cream from 2 (13½-ounce/400-ml) cans full-fat coconut milk, chilled for at least 12 hours (see tip, page 414)

3 tablespoons confectioners'-style erythritol

2½ teaspoons apple cider vinegar

2 teaspoons fresh lemon juice

¼ teaspoon vanilla extract

STORE IT: *Wrap the frosted cake in plastic wrap and keep in the fridge for up to 3 days. Freeze unfrosted cake layers for up to 2 weeks.*

THAW IT: *Set the cake layers on the counter until thawed, about 30 minutes. Frost the cake after thawing.*

1. Preheat the oven to 325°F (163°C). Grease two 9-inch (23-cm) round cake pans with coconut oil, then line the bottoms with parchment paper.

2. Place the water in a small saucepan. Sprinkle the gelatin on top. Do not stir. After 5 minutes, turn the heat to medium and bring the mixture to a light boil, stirring occasionally. Once the mixture is smooth, set aside. If it begins to cool, it will start to solidify. Simply heat to liquefy again before using in Step 5.

3. Place the coconut flour, arrowroot starch, cinnamon, baking soda, and salt in the bowl of a stand mixer fitted with the flat beater attachment or in a mixing bowl (if using a hand mixer). Mix until combined.

4. In a separate bowl, whisk together the hot gelatin, melted coconut oil, xylitol, and vanilla until smooth.

5. Turn on the mixer to medium-low speed and transfer the wet mixture to the dry. Once combined, squeeze the juices from the shredded carrots by placing them in a clean kitchen cloth and wringing out over the sink. Add to the bowl and mix to combine.

6. Divide the batter between the prepared pans, smoothing out the tops with oiled or damp hands. Bake for 33 to 35 minutes, until a toothpick inserted in the middle comes out clean.

7. Allow the cakes to cool in the pans for 30 minutes, then transfer to cooling racks to cool completely. Wrap in plastic wrap and transfer to the fridge overnight.

8. To prepare the frosting, place the coconut cream in a high-powered blender or in the bowl of a stand mixer fitted with the whisk attachment. If using a blender, cover, turn it to low, and slowly increase the speed until you reach medium. Stay at medium speed until the coconut milk has thickened to the consistency of whipped cream, about 30 seconds. If using a stand mixer, whisk for 30 seconds, or until fluffy.

9. Add the remaining frosting ingredients, blending or whisking until combined. Transfer to an airtight container and allow to firm up in the fridge overnight.

NUTRIENT INFORMATION (PER SERVING):

calories: 239 | calories from fat: 180 | total fat: 20g | saturated fat: 17.8g | cholesterol: 0mg

sodium: 224mg | carbs: 11.2g | dietary fiber: 2.7g | net carbs: 8.5g | sugars: 0.9g | protein: 3.5g

RATIOS:

fat:	carbs:	protein:
75%	19%	6%

PREP AHEAD: *Prepare the cake layers and freeze for up to 2 weeks before thawing and frosting.*

SERVE IT WITH: *This cake tastes great with Vanilla Ice Cream (page 410).*

10. To assemble, remove the cake from the fridge 30 minutes before you plan to frost and serve it. Place the first cake layer on a large plate and cover the top with frosting. Place the second cake layer on top and frost the sides and top of the cake. Transfer to the freezer for 10 minutes if the frosting gets too soupy. You can keep the cake in the freezer for up to 20 minutes before serving.

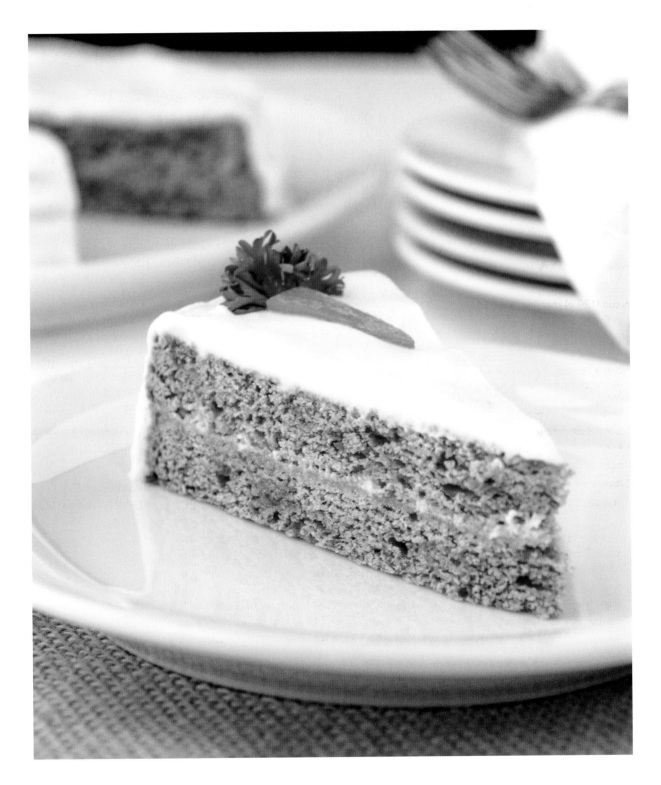

ST. LOUIS GOOEY "BUTTER" CAKE

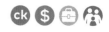

PREP TIME: **55 minutes**   COOK TIME: **22 minutes**   MAKES: **one 13 by 9-inch (33 by 23-cm) sheet cake (18 servings)**

NIGHTSHADE-FREE • VEGETARIAN

This is the cake for your next barbecue, family get-together, or tea date with the girls. No one will believe that it's low-carb, at only 1.8 grams per slice. And that's a good-sized slice, too. After you've prepared the batter, you'll probably think that it's not enough. Don't be be worried that you did something wrong; the cake will rise slightly while it bakes, but it isn't a particularly tall cake. And no worries about not serving the cake right away. It gets even gooier when it sits overnight—and more delicious, if you ask me.

- ¾ cup (85 g) blanched almond flour, plus more for the pan
- 1 teaspoon baking powder
- ½ teaspoon finely ground gray sea salt
- ¼ cup (52 g) coconut oil, plus more for the pan
- ¾ cup (120 g) confectioners'-style erythritol, plus more for dusting
- 5 large eggs, at room temperature
- 1½ teaspoons vanilla extract
- 1 batch Sweetened Condensed Coconut Milk, heated until lukewarm (page 415)

STORE IT: *Cover in plastic wrap and refrigerate for up to 3 days.*

PREP AHEAD: *Prepare the condensed milk up to 3 days before baking the cake. Warm it before use in Step 7.*

1. Preheat the oven to 350°F (177°C). Lightly grease a 13 by 9-inch (33 by 23-cm) glass or metal baking pan with a dab of coconut oil, then dust with a handful of almond flour. Set aside.

2. In a small bowl, whisk together the almond flour, baking powder, and salt.

3. In the bowl of a stand mixer fitted with the flat beater attachment or in a mixing bowl (if using a hand mixer), whip the coconut oil on medium speed until fluffy, about 1 minute.

4. Decrease the speed to low and slowly add the erythritol over 1 minute. Then add the eggs one at a time and mix thoroughly until combined.

5. Add the vanilla and mix to combine. Then, with the mixer running on low speed, slowly add the flour mixture in 3 batches. When just combined, turn off the mixer.

6. Pour the batter into the prepared pan and bake for 20 to 22 minutes, until the cake is light golden and a toothpick inserted in the middle comes out clean. Allow to cool in the pan for 30 minutes.

7. When the cake is cool, poke the top all over with a fork or skewer. Pour the warmed condensed milk over the top.

8. The cake can be served immediately but is best when allowed to sit in the fridge for a day, covered in plastic wrap. For the best consistency, remove the chilled cake from the fridge 30 minutes before you plan to serve it. Slice into eighteen 1¾ by 3-inch (4.5 by 7.6-cm) pieces and dust with confectioners'-style erythritol.

SERVE IT WITH: *This cake tastes great paired with Fatty Green Tea (page 419), Iced Omega Tea (page 420), or Rocket Fuel Latte (page 428).*

NUTRIENT INFORMATION (PER SERVING):

calories: 119 | calories from fat: 98 | total fat: 10.9g | saturated fat: 6.8g | cholesterol: 52mg
sodium: 91mg | carbs: 1.8g | dietary fiber: 0.5g | net carbs: 1.3g | sugars: 0.7g | protein: 3.3g

RATIOS:

fat:	carbs:	protein:
83%	**6%**	**11%**

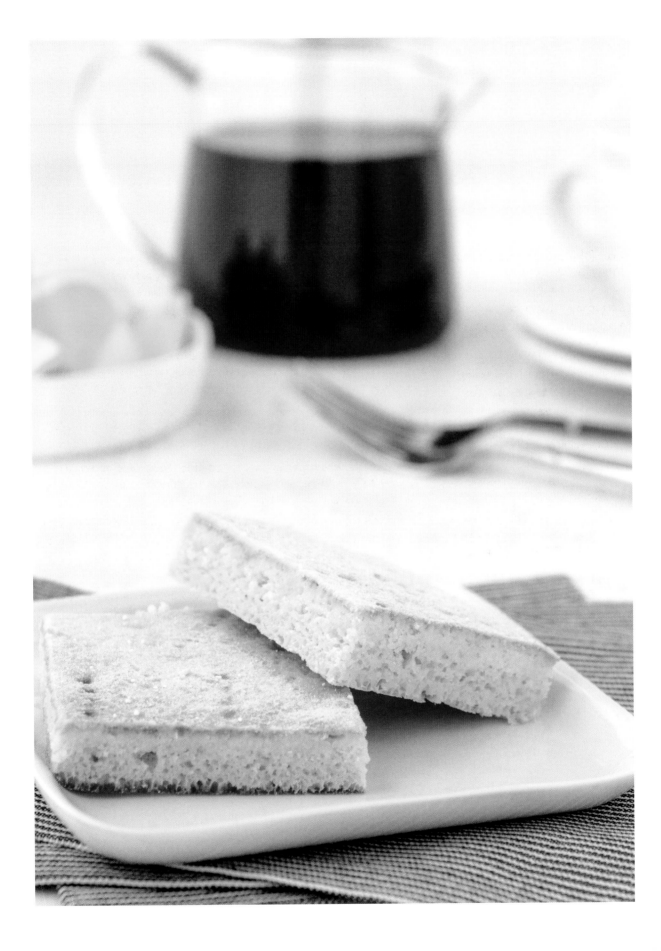

RHUBARB MICROWAVE CAKES

PREP TIME: **5 minutes**   COOK TIME: **about 2 minutes**   MAKES: **2 small cakes (2 servings)**

COCONUT-FREE · NIGHTSHADE-FREE · VEGETARIAN   OPTION: NUT-FREE

If you smother these cakes with nut or seed butter or top them with Vanilla Ice Cream (page 410) or Coconut Whipped Cream (page 414), you will change the ratios of the dish and make it an awesome Classic Keto treat! If you can't find or don't like rhubarb, you can replace it with ¼ cup (45 g) of blueberries or ¼ cup (50 g) of diced strawberries. In either case, the cook time will need to be increased to 3 to 3½ minutes.

1 large egg

3 tablespoons refined avocado oil or macadamia nut oil

1 tablespoon plus 1 teaspoon confectioners'-style erythritol (see note below)

¼ teaspoon vanilla extract or powder

¼ cup (32 g) roughly ground flax seeds

1 teaspoon ground cinnamon

¼ teaspoon ground nutmeg

¼ teaspoon baking powder

1 (2½-in/6.5-cm) piece rhubarb, diced

1 to 2 fresh strawberries, hulled and sliced, for garnish (optional)

1. Place the egg, oil, erythritol, and vanilla in a small bowl. Whisk to combine.

2. In a separate small bowl, place the flax seeds, cinnamon, nutmeg, and baking powder. Stir to combine, then add to the bowl with the wet ingredients.

3. Add the diced rhubarb to the bowl and stir until coated.

4. Divide the mixture between two 8-ounce (240-ml) ramekins, coffee cups, or other small microwave-safe containers. Microwave for 2 to 2½ minutes, until a toothpick inserted in the middle comes out clean. Garnish with strawberry slices, if desired.

NOTE: *Erythritol is the preferred sweetener for this dessert; however, if you do not tolerate erythritol, feel free to substitute 6 drops of liquid stevia.*

STORE IT: *Cover with plastic wrap and keep in the fridge for 2 days.*

REHEAT IT: *Microwave for a couple of seconds until warmed, or enjoy cold.*

SERVE IT WITH: *These cakes taste great paired with Vanilla Ice Cream (page 410) or Coconut Whipped Cream (page 414).*

MAKE IT NUT-FREE: *Use avocado oil.*

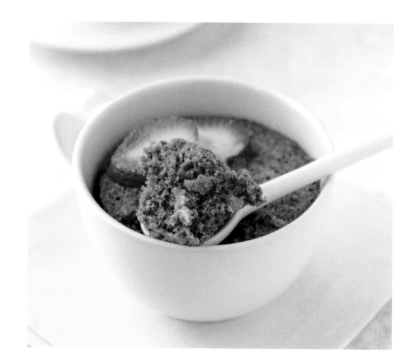

NUTRIENT INFORMATION (PER CAKE):

calories: 303 | calories from fat: 250 | total fat: 27.8g | saturated fat: 4.1g | cholesterol: 82mg

sodium: 37mg | carbs: 7.3g | dietary fiber: 5.5g | net carbs: 1.8g | sugars: 0.9g | protein: 6g

RATIOS:

fat:	carbs:	protein:
82%	10%	8%

NO-BAKE N'OATMEAL CHOCOLATE CHIP COOKIES

PREP TIME: **20 minutes, plus 30 minutes to chill**   MAKES: **14 cookies (14 servings)**

EGG-FREE • NIGHTSHADE-FREE • NUT-FREE • VEGAN   OPTION: COCONUT-FREE

Stevia-sweetened chocolate chips from Lily's brand are the answer to your low-carb baking prayers. My favorite way to use them is in these no-bake cookies or in a batch of Cardamom Orange Bark (page 395).

1¼ cups (185 g) hulled hemp seeds

¼ cup (60 ml) melted coconut oil or cacao butter

½ teaspoon vanilla extract or powder

½ teaspoon ground cinnamon

2 drops liquid stevia

¼ cup (56 g) stevia-sweetened chocolate chips

STORE IT: *Keep in an airtight container in the fridge for up to 1 week or in the freezer for up to 1 month.*

THAW IT: *Set on the counter until thawed, about 15 minutes.*

SERVE IT WITH: *These cookies taste great paired with a Fat-Burning Golden Milkshake (page 416) or Rocket Fuel Latte (page 428).*

MAKE IT COCONUT-FREE: *Use cacao butter or ghee, if tolerated, instead of coconut oil.*

1. Line a baking sheet with parchment paper or a silicone baking mat.

2. Put the hemp seeds, coconut oil, vanilla, cinnamon, and stevia in a medium-sized bowl. Stir to combine.

3. Transfer the mixture to a blender or food processor and pulse, just lightly, 1 second per pulse, three times. After the third pulse, pinch some dough with your fingers. If it holds together nicely, you're ready to move on. If not, pulse again until the dough holds together.

4. Fold the chocolate chips into the dough.

5. Using a round tablespoon (or a 1-tablespoon cookie scoop/melon baller), scoop up the dough, packing it firmly into the tablespoon. Transfer the scoop to the prepared baking sheet. Repeat with the remaining dough, making 14 cookies.

6. Chill for 30 minutes before consuming. These cookies are best served chilled, straight from the fridge.

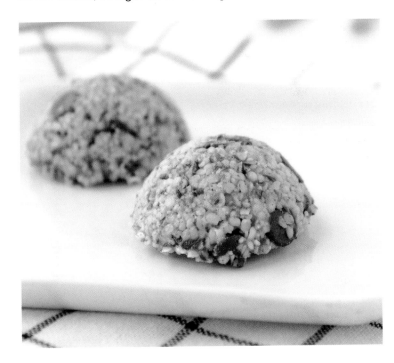

NUTRIENT INFORMATION (PER COOKIE):

calories: 126 | calories from fat: 97 | total fat: 10.8g | saturated fat: 4.7g | cholesterol: 0mg

sodium: 0mg | carbs: 2.6g | dietary fiber: 1.9g | net carbs: 0.7g | sugars: 0g | protein: 4.7g

RATIOS:

fat:	carbs:	protein:
77%	8%	15%

NO-NUTS BROWNIES

PREP TIME: 20 minutes, plus 30 minutes to cool   COOK TIME: 30 minutes   MAKES: 16 brownies (16 servings)

EGG-FREE · NIGHTSHADE-FREE · NUT-FREE   OPTION: COCONUT-FREE

There are three types of brownies: fudgy (fudge-like with a moist chocolate interior), chewy (not as fudgy but still rich, and a bit more crumbly), and fluffy (cake-like with a moist crumb). The fact that I've classified them should tell you just how serious I am about brownies. Freshly baked, these brownies are fudgy; after being stored in the fridge, they lean toward chewy. If you opt to serve them without the whipped cream topping, they are also coconut-free! If you want to go way, way overboard, you could top them with homemade marshmallows (page 412).

½ cup (120 ml) water

2 tablespoons unflavored gelatin

1 cup (260 g) tahini

¼ cup (60 ml) refined avocado oil or melted ghee (if tolerated)

¾ cup (120 g) confectioners'-style erythritol

⅔ cup (53 g) cacao powder

¼ teaspoon finely ground gray sea salt

¼ teaspoon baking powder

OPTIONAL TOPPINGS:

1 cup (240 ml) Coconut Whipped Cream, sweetened and chocolate-flavored (page 414)

Extra cacao powder, for dusting

STORE IT: *Keep in an airtight container in the fridge for up to 1 week or in the freezer for up to 1 month. For the best consistency, leave out on the counter for 30 minutes before enjoying.*

THAW IT: *Set on the counter until thawed, about 30 minutes.*

MAKE IT COCONUT-FREE: *Omit the Coconut Whipped Cream topping.*

1. Preheat the oven to 350°F (177°C) and line an 8-inch (20-cm) square baking pan with parchment paper, with the ends draped over the sides for easy lifting.

2. Place the water in a small saucepan. Sprinkle the gelatin on top. Do not stir. After 5 minutes, turn the heat to medium and bring the mixture to a light boil, stirring occasionally. Once the mixture is smooth, set aside. If the mixture begins to cool, it will begin to solidify. Simply reheat to liquefy before using in Step 4.

3. Put the tahini and avocado oil in the bowl of a stand mixer or a mixing bowl (if using a hand mixer). Mix with the flat beater (or hand mixer) until combined.

4. Add the hot gelatin liquid, erythritol, cacao powder, salt, and baking powder. Stir until just combined.

5. Transfer the brownie batter to the prepared pan and press down with your palms to even it out.

6. Bake for 25 to 30 minutes, until the corners are crisp and a toothpick inserted in the middle comes out clean.

7. Allow the brownies to cool in the pan for 30 minutes, then cut into 16 squares.

8. If desired, top each brownie with a tablespoon-sized dollop of whipped cream just before serving, then dust with cacao powder.

NUTRIENT INFORMATION (PER BROWNIE, WITHOUT TOPPINGS):

calories: 161 | calories from fat: 124 | total fat: 13.8g | saturated fat: 2.2g | cholesterol: 0mg

sodium: 45mg | carbs: 3.7g | dietary fiber: 3g | net carbs: 0.7g | sugars: 0g | protein: 5.6g

RATIOS:

fat:	carbs:	protein:
77%	9%	14%

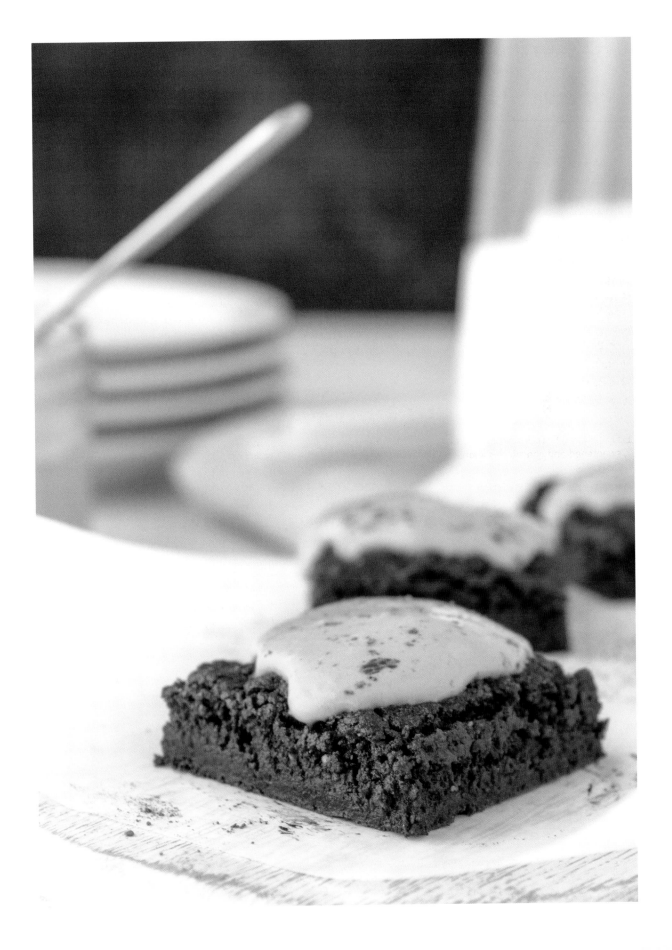

JELLY PIE JARS

PREP TIME: **20 minutes, plus 1 hour to rest**   COOK TIME: **about 15 minutes**   MAKES: **eight 4-ounce (120-ml) servings**

NIGHTSHADE-FREE   OPTIONS: COCONUT-FREE • LOW-FODMAP • VEGETARIAN

These jars bring pie to the table without the need to roll out dough or stress about filling overflow. It's a win-win! The keys to success in making the layers super-concise are to press the pie filling down before baking and to allow the jars and jam filling to cool before assembly. I know, it's tempting to get everything into the jar and chow down, but it's worth the wait!

Coconut oil, for the jars

PIE BASE:

1 cup (110 g) blanched almond flour

1 tablespoon plus 1½ teaspoons whisked egg (about ½ large egg)

1 tablespoon lard

2 drops liquid stevia

¼ teaspoon ground cinnamon

Pinch of finely ground gray sea salt

JAM FILLING:

1½ heaping cups (260 g) fresh blackberries

⅓ cup (80 ml) water

1½ teaspoons vanilla extract

3 drops liquid stevia

¼ cup (38 g) chia seeds

1½ teaspoons balsamic vinegar

ALMOND BUTTER TOPPING:

¾ cup (210 g) unsweetened smooth almond butter

¼ cup (60 ml) melted coconut oil or ghee (if tolerated)

1 teaspoon ground cinnamon

2 to 4 drops liquid stevia

FOR GARNISH (OPTIONAL):

16 to 24 fresh blackberries

1. Preheat the oven to 325°F (163°C). Grease eight 4-ounce (120-ml) mason jars with a dab of coconut oil and set on a rimmed baking sheet.

2. To prepare the base, place the ingredients for the base in a large bowl and mix with a fork until fully combined.

3. Divide the dough evenly among the jars, pressing it in firmly and evening it out with your fingers. Place the jars back on the baking sheet and bake for 15 to 17 minutes, until the tops are golden. Remove from the oven and allow to cool completely, at least 30 minutes. Meanwhile, make the filling.

4. To prepare the jam filling, place the blackberries, water, vanilla, and stevia in a medium-sized saucepan. Cook, covered, over medium heat for 5 minutes.

5. Reduce the heat to low and add the chia seeds and balsamic vinegar. Cook, uncovered, for another 3 to 4 minutes, stirring frequently, until the mixture has thickened. Transfer the mixture to a heat-safe bowl and set aside to cool to room temperature, at least 30 minutes.

6. To prepare the almond butter topping, place the topping ingredients in a small bowl and whisk to combine.

7. To assemble, divide the cooled jam filling among the jars, being sure to keep the layer as flat as possible. Then add the almond butter topping, pouring it in slowly to avoid spillover. Transfer the assembled jars to the fridge to cool for 30 minutes.

8. Before serving, top each jar with 2 or 3 blackberries, if desired. Enjoy!

STORE IT: *Seal the mason jars with their lids and place in the fridge for up to 3 days or freeze for up to 1 month. (If freezing, do not garnish the jars with the berries.)*

THAW IT: *Set on the counter until thawed, about 15 minutes.*

PREP AHEAD: *Prepare the pie base up to 3 days ahead by following Steps 1 through 3, then store in the fridge. Prepare the jam filling up to 1 day ahead by following Steps 4 and 5 and store in an airtight container.*

MAKE IT COCONUT-FREE: *Replace the coconut oil with ghee (if tolerated) or hazelnut oil.*

MAKE LOW-FODMAP: *Replace the almond butter with sunflower seed butter. The almond flour used in the pie base comes out to about 2 tablespoons per serving, so it should be okay depending on your tolerance.*

MAKE IT VEGETARIAN: *Replace the lard with coconut oil.*

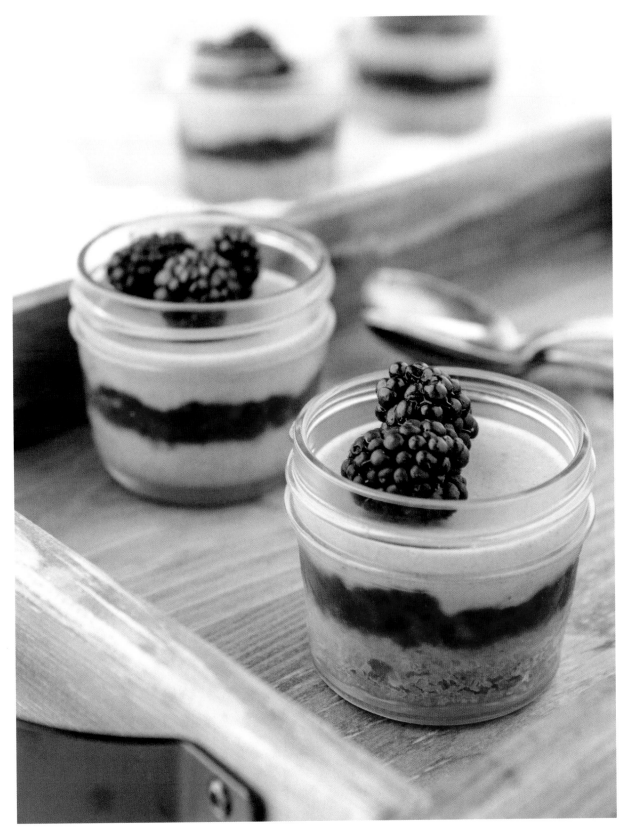

NUTRIENT INFORMATION (PER JAR):

calories: 388 | calories from fat: 290 | total fat: 32.2g | saturated fat: 8.9g | cholesterol: 13mg

sodium: 27mg | carbs: 13.1g | dietary fiber: 8.9g | net carbs: 4.2g | sugars: 3g | protein: 11.1g

RATIOS:

fat:	carbs:	protein:
75%	13%	12%

ICED TEA LEMONADE GUMMIES

PREP TIME: **10 minutes, plus 1 hour to chill**   COOK TIME: **5 minutes**   MAKES: **thirty-six 1-inch (2.5-cm) square gummies (4 servings)**

COCONUT-FREE • EGG-FREE • NIGHTSHADE-FREE • NUT-FREE   OPTION: **LOW-FODMAP**

Chowing down on gummies is my favorite thing to do when fat bombs just aren't hitting the spot. If you're a candy fanatic like I am, you may find solace in homemade gummies. Although I use a silicone mold to shape the gummies, it isn't necessary. You can also use a 13 by 9-inch (33 by 23-cm) pan and cut the gummies into 36 small squares once set. How many gummies this recipe makes depends entirely on the size of the mold you use. Not sure which tea to choose for this recipe? My favorite is Tulsi Sweet Rose Tea from Organic India.

¾ cup (180 ml) boiling water

3 tea bags

¼ cup (40 g) unflavored gelatin

¾ cup (180 ml) fresh lemon juice

2 tablespoons confectioners'-style erythritol or granulated xylitol

SPECIAL EQUIPMENT:

Silicone mold(s) with 36 (½-ounce/15-ml) cavities

STORE IT: *Keep in an airtight container in the fridge for up to 5 days.*

MAKE IT LOW-FODMAP: *Use 2 to 4 drops of liquid stevia instead of erythritol or xylitol.*

VARIATION: MATCHA LEMONADE GUMMIES. *Replace the tea bags with 1 tablespoon of matcha powder (pictured below).*

1. Set the silicone mold(s) on a rimmed baking sheet.

2. Place the boiling water in a heat-safe mug and steep the tea according to type, following the suggested steep time on the package. Once complete, remove the tea bags and wring out as much liquid from the bags as possible. Sprinkle the gelatin over the tea and set aside.

3. Pour the lemon juice into a small saucepan. Add the erythritol and bring to a light simmer over medium heat, about 5 minutes.

4. Once at a light simmer, remove the pan from the heat. Whisk the tea mixture until the gelatin dissolves, then pour it into the hot lemon juice mixture. Whisk to combine.

5. Pour the hot mixture into the mold(s) and transfer the baking sheet to the fridge to set for at least 1 hour. Once firm, remove the gummies from the mold(s) and enjoy!

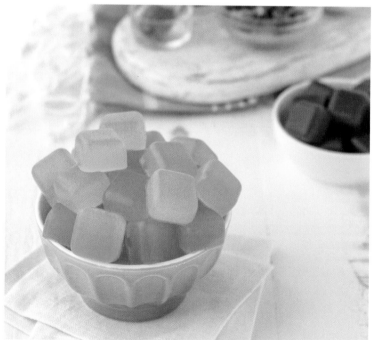

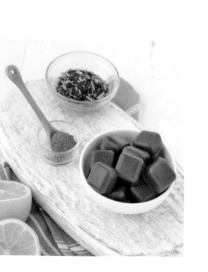

NUTRIENT INFORMATION (PER 9 GUMMIES, MADE WITH ERYTHRITOL):

calories: 48 | calories from fat: 3 | total fat: 0.4g | saturated fat: 0g | cholesterol: 0mg

sodium: 9mg | carbs: 1g | dietary fiber: 0g | net carbs: 1g | sugars: 1g | protein: 10.2g

RATIOS:

fat:	carbs:	protein:
8%	8%	84%

LEMON DROPS

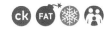

PREP TIME: **5 minutes, plus 1 hour to chill**   MAKES: **20 drops (4 servings)**

EGG-FREE • NIGHTSHADE-FREE • NUT-FREE • VEGAN   OPTIONS: COCONUT-FREE • LOW-FODMAP

If you love lemon, you're going to go crazy over these fat bombs! Whether you make them in a silicone mold or candy mold or opt to pour the mixture into an 8-inch (20-cm) square baking pan and then break it into 20 pieces once hardened, you won't be disappointed. I like to add magnesium powder for a nutrient boost. The magnesium powder I prefer is Natural Calm from Natural Vitality, available at major grocery and health food stores. It has a raspberry-lemon flavor that adds a sour kick, almost like a sour lollipop. But you can totally make this recipe without it. I just love the sourness!

¼ cup (60 ml) melted (but not hot) cacao butter

¼ cup (60 ml) melted (but not hot) coconut oil

1½ teaspoons confectioners'-style erythritol

2 teaspoons lemon-flavored magnesium powder (optional)

1 teaspoon lemon extract

SPECIAL EQUIPMENT:

Silicone mold(s) with 20 (½-ounce/15-ml) round cavities

1. Set the silicone mold(s) on a baking sheet.

2. Place the cacao butter, coconut oil, and erythritol in a small bowl. Whisk until the erythritol has dissolved.

3. If using magnesium powder, add it to the bowl along with the lemon extract. Whisk to combine.

4. Pour the mixture into the silicone mold(s), distributing the amount evenly between the 20 molds. Transfer the baking sheet to the fridge to harden for 1 hour.

5. Once hardened, remove the lemon drops from the molds and enjoy! Serve directly from the fridge.

STORE IT: *Keep in an airtight container in the fridge for up to 2 weeks or in the freezer for up to 2 months.*

THAW IT: *Enjoy straight from the freezer or allow to thaw for 1 to 2 minutes before consuming.*

MAKE IT COCONUT-FREE: *Replace the coconut oil with ghee, if tolerated.*

MAKE IT LOW-FODMAP: *Use 2 to 4 drops of liquid stevia instead of erythritol.*

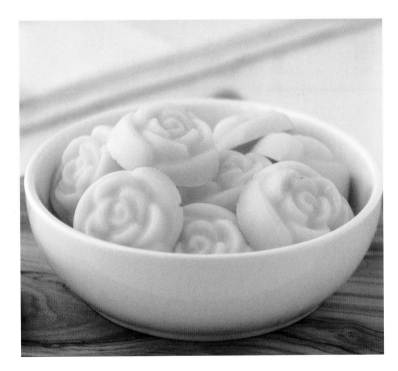

NUTRIENT INFORMATION (PER 5 DROPS):

calories: 258 | calories from fat: 258 | total fat: 28.6g | saturated fat: 22.2g | cholesterol: 0mg

sodium: 0mg | carbs: 0.2g | dietary fiber: 0g | net carbs: 0.2g | sugars: 0g | protein: 0g

RATIOS:

fat:	carbs:	protein:
100%	0%	0%

CHOCOLATE-COVERED COFFEE BITES

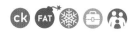

PREP TIME: **10 minutes, plus at least 1 hour to chill**   MAKES: **8 bites (8 servings)**

COCONUT-FREE • EGG-FREE • NIGHTSHADE-FREE

The instant coffee you use will have a large impact on this recipe, so choose wisely!

BITES:

¼ cup plus 2 tablespoons (90 g) cacao butter

½ cup (75 g) macadamia nuts, roasted

1 tablespoon confectioners'-style erythritol or 1 or 2 drops liquid stevia

½ teaspoon instant coffee (medium or light roast, regular or decaf)

2 tablespoons collagen peptides

CHOCOLATE TOPPING:

¼ cup (56 g) stevia-sweetened chocolate chips, melted

GARNISH:

About ¼ teaspoon large flake sea salt

SPECIAL EQUIPMENT:

Silicone mold with eight 1-ounce (30-ml) semispherical cavities

STORE IT: *Keep in an airtight container in the fridge for up to 2 weeks or in the freezer for up to 2 months.*

THAW IT: *Enjoy straight from the freezer, or allow the bites to thaw for 15 minutes before consuming.*

1. Place the cacao butter, macadamia nuts, erythritol, and instant coffee in a high-powered blender or food processor. Blend on high speed until the nuts have broken down quite a bit but are still chunky, about 20 seconds.

2. Add the collagen and pulse to combine.

3. Using a spoon, scoop and press the mixture into 8 cavities of a silicone mold. Place the mold in the fridge for 2 hours or in the freezer for 1 hour, until the bites are set.

4. Meanwhile, line a baking sheet with parchment paper or a silicone baking mat and set aside.

5. Remove the mold from the fridge or freezer and pop out the bites onto the prepared baking sheet. Drizzle the melted chocolate over the top, then sprinkle each bite with a pinch of salt. Return the bites to the fridge until the chocolate is set, about 10 minutes. Enjoy!

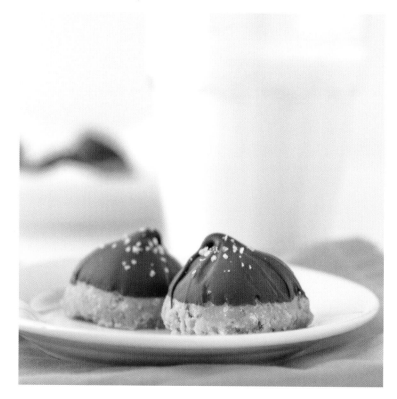

NUTRIENT INFORMATION (PER BITE):

calories: 213 | calories from fat: 183 | total fat: 20.4g | saturated fat: 10.2g | cholesterol: 0mg

sodium: 89mg | carbs: 3.8g | dietary fiber: 1.8g | net carbs: 2g | sugars: 0g | protein: 3.6g

RATIOS:

fat:	carbs:	protein:
86%	7%	7%

STRAWBERRY BUTTER BITES

PREP TIME: **10 minutes, plus 1 hour to chill**   MAKES: **12 bites (12 servings)**

EGG-FREE • NIGHTSHADE-FREE • NUT-FREE • VEGAN   OPTION: **LOW-FODMAP**

Since I went keto, my favorite snack has been nut or seed butter with berries. A couple of months ago, I realized that I could keep mounds of nut or seed butter and strawberries on hand for easy snacking without having to reach into the jar with a spoon and slather the butter all over the berries one by one. If you like this combination, too, you're going to love this easy recipe! Sometimes I don't even wait for the bites to chill.

½ cup (135 g) unsweetened sunflower seed butter

¼ cup (60 ml) melted coconut oil

2 teaspoons confectioners'-style erythritol

Pinch of finely ground gray sea salt (if the sunflower seed butter is unsalted)

8 fresh strawberries, hulled and diced

STORE IT: *Keep in an airtight container in the fridge for up to 3 days.*

MAKE IT LOW-FODMAP: *Use 2 to 4 drops of liquid stevia instead of erythritol.*

1. Line a baking sheet with parchment paper or a silicone baking mat.

2. Place the sunflower seed butter and melted coconut oil in the bowl of a stand mixer or a mixing bowl (if using a hand mixer). Mix with the flat beater (or hand mixer) on medium speed until well combined.

3. Add the erythritol and salt, if using, and mix until incorporated.

4. Add the diced strawberries and mix until combined.

5. One tablespoon at a time, drop the dough on the prepared baking sheet. Place in the fridge to chill for 1 hour. Enjoy!

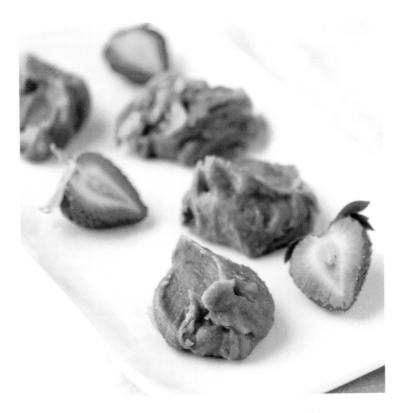

NUTRIENT INFORMATION (PER BITE):

calories: 111 | calories from fat: 89 | total fat: 9.9g | saturated fat: 4.6g | cholesterol: 0mg

sodium: 52mg | carbs: 3.1g | dietary fiber: 1.5g | net carbs: 1.6g | sugars: 1.5g | protein: 2.4g

RATIOS:

fat:	carbs:	protein:
80%	11%	9%

VANILLA ICE CREAM

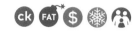

PREP TIME: **about 30 minutes, plus 3½ hours to chill and freeze**   MAKES: **3 cups (672 g) (6 servings)**

NIGHTSHADE-FREE · VEGETARIAN   OPTION: **NUT-FREE**

If you don't have an ice cream maker but you do have patience, any ice cream recipe can be made with a large bowl, a fork, and a blender or food processor. After preparing and chilling the ice cream mixture, pour it into a large bowl. Place in the freezer for 30 minutes, stir with the fork, and repeat until the mixture is hard yet still mixable. The length of time this will take will depend on the volume of the mixture—this recipe makes 3 cups, so it'll take about 3 hours to set and 6 stirs. If the mixture has hardened too much, you can transfer the chunks to a high-powered blender or food processor and pulse until smooth. Just don't let it turn into an ice cube or it will be very difficult to revert to ice cream.

1 (13½-ounce/400-ml) can full-fat coconut milk

6 large egg yolks

2 teaspoons vanilla extract or powder

½ cup (120 ml) melted (but not hot) coconut oil

2 tablespoons granulated xylitol

Pinch of finely ground gray sea salt

OPTIONAL TOPPING:

2 tablespoons sliced blanched almonds, roasted

SPECIAL EQUIPMENT:

Ice cream maker (optional; see above)

1. Place an airtight, lidded 32-ounce (950-ml) or larger freezer-safe glass container, loaf pan, or bowl in the freezer.

2. Place all the ingredients in a blender and blend on high speed until smooth.

3. Transfer the mixture to an airtight container such as a mason jar and place in the fridge to chill for 2 hours.

4. Once ready to churn, add the mixture to an ice cream maker and churn following the manufacturer's instructions.

5. Transfer the churned ice cream to the chilled container (if using a loaf pan, line it with parchment paper first). Cover with the lid and place back in the freezer for at least 1½ hours before serving.

6. When ready to serve, set the ice cream on the counter to soften for 5 to 10 minutes. Garnish each serving with a teaspoon of roasted almonds, if desired.

STORE IT: *Keep in the freezer for up to 2 weeks.*

PREP AHEAD: *Blend the ingredients and set in the fridge up to 2 days before churning.*

SERVE IT WITH: *This ice cream tastes great paired with No-Nuts Brownies (page 402).*

MAKE IT NUT-FREE: *Omit the roasted almond topping.*

NUTRIENT INFORMATION (PER ½-CUP/112-G SERVING, WITHOUT ALMOND TOPPING):
calories: 356 | calories from fat: 326 | total fat: 36.2g | saturated fat: 29.7g | cholesterol: 210mg
sodium: 52mg | carbs: 3.7g | dietary fiber: 0g | net carbs: 3.7g | sugars: 1.2g | protein: 3.8g

RATIOS:
fat: carbs: protein:
92% **4%** **4%**

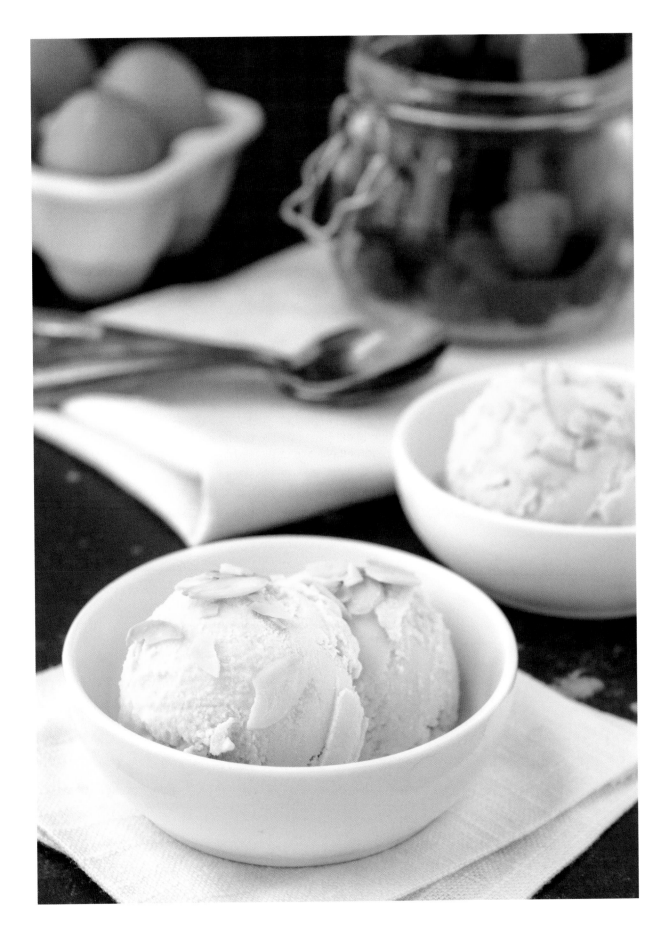

TOASTED COCONUT MARSHMALLOWS

PREP TIME: **15 minutes, plus 1 to 2 hours to set** COOK TIME: **15 minutes** MAKES: **64 marshmallows (16 servings)**

EGG-FREE • NIGHTSHADE-FREE • NUT-FREE OPTION: COCONUT-FREE

I'm just as amazed as you are that marshmallows can be part of a keto diet. While I wouldn't use marshmallows as your go-to snack (they're pretty devoid of nutrients aside from the gelatin), they just might do the trick if you're looking to satisfy a sweet tooth and a fat bomb isn't cutting it! Now, if you beat the mixture too long, the fluff will become stiff and difficult to spread, leading to odd-shaped marshmallows. And because they don't contain sugar, they can't be toasted like regular marshmallows.

½ cup (50 g) toasted unsweetened shredded coconut, divided

1 cup (240 ml) water, divided

3 tablespoons unflavored gelatin

1 cup (160 g) confectioners'-style erythritol

2 teaspoons vanilla extract

¼ teaspoon finely ground gray sea salt

STORE IT: *Keep in an airtight container in the pantry for 2 to 3 weeks or in the freezer for up to 1 month.*

THAW IT: *Set on the counter until thawed, about 30 minutes.*

SERVE IT WITH: *These marshmallows taste great in a Rocket Fuel Latte (page 428) or atop No-Nuts Brownies (page 402).*

VARIATION: PLAIN MARSHMALLOWS. *Omit the coconut.*

VARIATION: CACAO-DUSTED MARSHMALLOWS. *Omit the coconut. After cutting the marshmallows into squares, place 2 tablespoons of cacao powder in a bowl. Add the marshmallows and toss until coated.*

1. Line an 8-inch (20-cm) square pan with parchment paper, with the ends draped over the sides for easy lifting. Sprinkle ¼ cup (25 g) of the toasted coconut into the pan, spreading it evenly.

2. Affix the whisk attachment to a hand mixer or stand mixer.

3. Place ½ cup (120 ml) of the water in the bowl of your mixer and sprinkle the gelatin on top. Do not stir. Simply leave it to sit as you prepare everything else.

4. In a small saucepan, combine the remaining ½ cup (120 ml) of water, erythritol, vanilla, and salt. Turn the heat to medium and stir occasionally until the mixture begins to boil rapidly and almost spills over. Ensure that it doesn't spill over by removing it from the heat. Then reduce the heat to low and keep the mixture at a low boil for 5 minutes.

5. Transfer the hot liquid to the bowl with the gelatin. Turn the mixer to high speed and beat for 6 to 7 minutes, until the mixture thickens to a spreadable consistency, similar to that of marshmallow fluff. If you beat it too long, it will stiffen and will no longer be easily spreadable.

6. Once thickened, transfer the mixture to the prepared pan and sprinkle the remaining ¼ cup (25 g) of toasted coconut on top.

7. Smooth the marshmallow fluff with the back of a spatula. Alternatively, you can grease your palms with a dollop of coconut oil and spread the fluff with your hands.

8. Allow the marshmallows to sit at room temperature for 1 to 2 hours, until firm, then cut into 1-inch (2.5-cm) squares and enjoy.

NUTRIENT INFORMATION (PER 4 MARSHMALLOWS):

calories: 30 | calories from fat: 18 | total fat: 2g | saturated fat: 1.8g | cholesterol: 0mg

sodium: 36mg | carbs: 0.8g | dietary fiber: 0.5g | net carbs: 0.3g | sugars: 0g | protein: 2.1g

RATIOS:

fat:	carbs:	protein:
61%	11%	28%

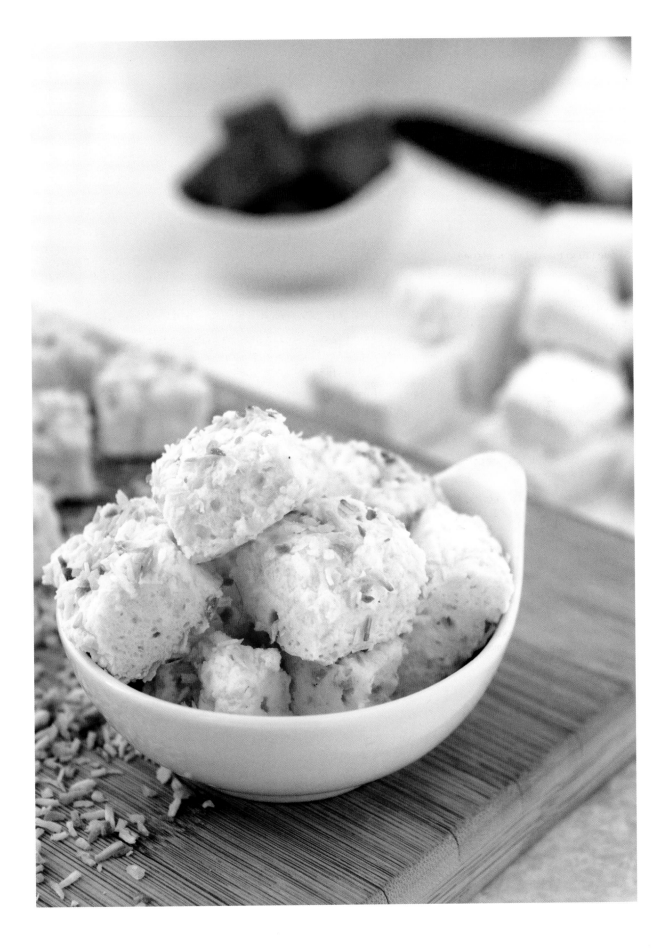

COCONUT WHIPPED CREAM

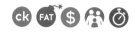

PREP TIME: **5 minutes**   MAKES: **1¾ cups (475 ml) (7 servings)**

EGG-FREE • NIGHTSHADE-FREE • NUT-FREE • VEGAN

The first time I prepared a batch of coconut whipped cream, I used it to top Paleo-friendly strawberry shortcakes. I was skeptical, but I had heard that coconut cream makes the best dairy-free whipped cream, so I gave it a whirl. Boy, was I impressed with how thick it was after a quick blend! You can get coconut cream from a can of high-quality full-fat coconut milk, or you can buy canned coconut cream. If using coconut milk, the higher the fat content, the more success you'll have. You will need to chill the cans of coconut milk for at least 12 hours before making whipped cream. As the milk chills, the cream separates from the coconut water and rises to the top of the can. Keep this whipped cream plain, or jazz it up with sweetener and flavorings. It's your choice!

1 (13½-ounce/400-ml) can coconut cream, chilled, or cream from 2 (13½-ounce/400-ml) cans full-fat coconut milk, chilled for at least 12 hours (see Tip below)

OPTIONAL ADDITIONS:

1 tablespoon confectioners'-style erythritol

1 teaspoon vanilla extract

2 tablespoons cacao powder

1. Place the coconut cream in a blender or the bowl of a stand mixer fitted with the whisk attachment. If using a blender, cover, turn the speed to low, and slowly increase the speed until you reach medium. Stay at medium speed until the coconut milk has thickened to the consistency of whipped cream, about 30 seconds if using a high-powered blender. If using a stand mixer, whisk for 30 seconds, or until fluffy. Stop here if you want your whipped cream plain and unsweetened. Continue to Step 2 for a sweetened and flavored option.

2. To make sweetened, vanilla-flavored whipped cream, add the erythritol and vanilla. To make sweetened, chocolate-flavored whipped cream, add the erythritol, vanilla, and cacao powder. Cover and blend for another 10 seconds, until the ingredients are thoroughly combined.

TIP: HOW TO EXTRACT THE CREAM FROM A CAN OF COCONUT MILK. *Take a can of full-fat coconut milk that's been chilled for at least 12 hours and gently flip it over. Open the bottom of the can (now on top) with a can opener and drain the watery liquid, leaving the cream. Scrape the cream out of the can and use as directed.*

STORE IT: *Keep in an airtight container in the fridge for up to 3 days.*

SERVE IT WITH: *Use the whipped cream as the base for a keto parfait. Simply top, or layer, with a handful of berries, nuts, seeds, or citrus zest, or all four, and serve in pretty glasses to impress guests.*

This whipped cream tastes great paired with No-Nuts Granola with Clusters (page 246) or Rocket Fuel Frappé Coffee (page 430).

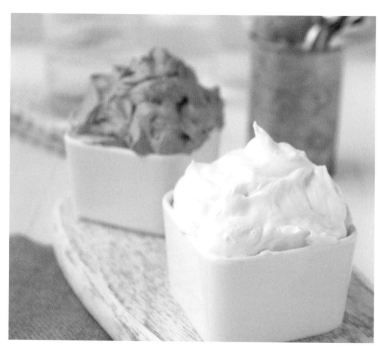

NUTRIENT INFORMATION (PER ¼-CUP/60-ML SERVING OF THE SWEETENED VANILLA-FLAVORED VERSION):

calories: 116 | calories from fat: 104 | total fat: 11.6g | saturated fat: 10.6g | cholesterol: 0mg

sodium: 14mg | carbs: 1.9g | dietary fiber: 0g | net carbs: 1.9g | sugars: 1g | protein: 1g

RATIOS:

fat:	carbs:	protein:
90%	**7%**	**3%**

SWEETENED CONDENSED COCONUT MILK

PREP TIME: **less than 5 minutes**   COOK TIME: **35 minutes**   MAKES: **¾ cup (180 ml) (12 servings)**

EGG-FREE • NIGHTSHADE-FREE • NUT-FREE • VEGAN

In addition to being the star of the show in St. Louis Gooey "Butter" Cake (page 398) and Coconut Mounds (page 390), this condensed milk is great in just about any keto-friendly dessert or fat bomb, upping the richness without adding carbs. Use this milk in your next batch of fat fudge and in ice creams, puddings, and pies. I bet it would taste pretty fantastic drizzled on brownies, too!

1 (13½-ounce/400-ml) can full-fat coconut milk

2 tablespoons confectioners'-style erythritol

Place all the ingredients in a small saucepan and bring to a rapid boil over medium-high heat. Reduce the heat and simmer lightly for 32 to 35 minutes, until the milk has thickened and reduced by about half. Use immediately in a recipe that calls for it, or let it cool and store in the fridge for later use.

STORE IT: *Keep in an airtight container in the fridge for up to 3 days.*

REHEAT IT: *Heat in a saucepan or in the microwave just until warm to the touch, or enjoy cold.*

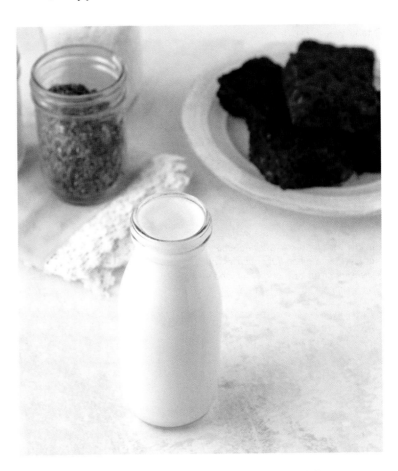

NUTRIENT INFORMATION (PER 2-TABLESPOON SERVING):

calories: 68 | calories from fat: 61 | total fat: 6.8g | saturated fat: 6.2g | cholesterol: 0mg

sodium: 8mg | carbs: 1.1g | dietary fiber: 0g | net carbs: 1.1g | sugars: 0.6g | protein: 0.6g

RATIOS:

fat:	carbs:	protein:
75%	13%	12%

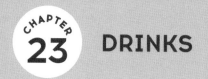

DRINKS

FAT-BURNING GOLDEN MILKSHAKE

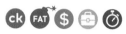

PREP TIME: **5 minutes**   MAKES: **one 13-ounce (385-ml) serving**

EGG-FREE • NIGHTSHADE-FREE • NUT-FREE • VEGAN   OPTION: **LOW-FODMAP**

This recipe is known as the "Fat Burning Shake" on my blog, HealthfulPursuit.com. In the online version, I add 1 teaspoon of my favorite magnesium powder (Natural Calm) to the cold or hot version and promote it as a fabulous bedtime snack. If you decide to add magnesium, do so after blending and heating (if desired); otherwise, the magnesium will fizz and you'll have staining turmeric all over everything. Add it to the blended drink, give it a little shake, and you're good to go. I highly recommend using fresh turmeric and ginger root in this recipe; they add a great depth of flavor and pack more of a nutritional punch.

1½ cups (350 ml) nondairy milk

2 tablespoons MCT oil or melted coconut oil

1 (3-in/7.5-cm) piece fresh turmeric root, peeled, or ¾ teaspoon turmeric powder

1 (½-in/1.25-cm) piece fresh ginger root, peeled, or ½ teaspoon ginger powder

¼ teaspoon ground cinnamon, plus more for sprinkling

¼ teaspoon vanilla extract or powder

2 to 4 drops liquid stevia

Pinch of finely ground Himalayan rock salt

2 ice cubes

1. Place all the ingredients in a high-powered blender. (*Note:* If your blender is not a high-powered one, grate or mince the turmeric and ginger roots before adding them to the blender, or use powdered turmeric and ginger.) Blend on high speed for 10 to 30 seconds. The longer the mixture is blended, the stronger the turmeric and ginger flavor will be, especially if using fresh roots.

2. Pour the milkshake into a glass, sprinkle with cinnamon, and enjoy.

STORE IT: *Keep in an airtight container in the fridge for up to 3 days. If consuming it cold, give it a little shake before serving.*

SERVE IT WITH: *To make this milkshake a complete meal, add ¼ cup (40 g) of collagen peptides or protein powder. For the hot milk version, add 2 tablespoons of unflavored gelatin or protein powder.*

MAKE IT LOW-FODMAP: *Avoid using cashew or pistachio milk.*

VARIATION: FAT-BURNING GOLDEN HOT MILK. *Use coconut oil rather than MCT oil and omit the ice cubes. Complete Step 1, then transfer the blended mixture to a small saucepan and bring to a light simmer over medium heat, stirring occasionally, about 8 minutes. Pour into a mug, sprinkle with cinnamon, and enjoy.*

NUTRIENT INFORMATION (MADE WITH FRESH ROOTS):
calories: 351 | calories from fat: 316 | total fat: 35.2g | saturated fat: 35g | cholesterol: 0mg
sodium: 177mg | carbs: 6.9g | dietary fiber: 1.4g | net carbs: 5.5g | sugars: 0g | protein: 1.6g

RATIOS:
fat: carbs: protein:
92%   6%   2%

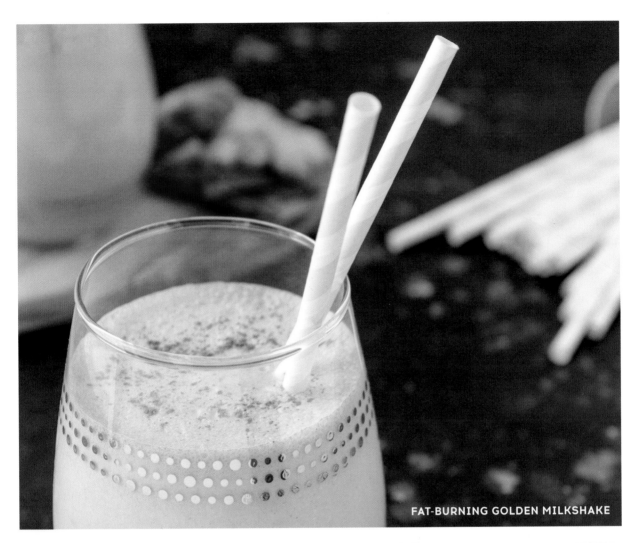

FAT-BURNING GOLDEN MILKSHAKE

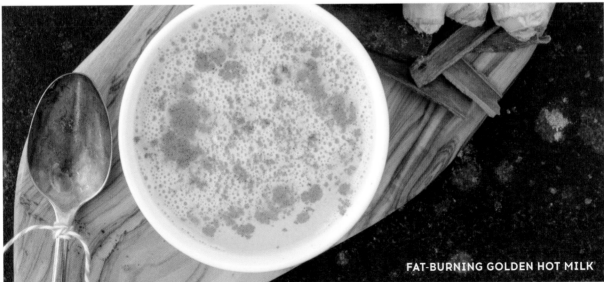

FAT-BURNING GOLDEN HOT MILK

NUTRIENT INFORMATION (MADE WITH POWDERED TURMERIC AND GINGER):

calories: 356 | calories from fat: 316 | total fat: 35.2g | saturated fat: 35g | cholesterol: 0mg

sodium: 177mg | carbs: 5.3g | dietary fiber: 0.8g | net carbs: 4.5g | sugars: 0g | protein: 1.7g

RATIOS:

fat:	carbs:	protein:
92%	6%	2%

ACV ICED TEA

PREP TIME: **5 minutes** MAKES: **one 16-ounce (475-ml) serving**

COCONUT-FREE · EGG-FREE · LOW-FODMAP · NUT-FREE · VEGAN OPTION: **NIGHTSHADE-FREE**

Since I love everything vinegar, it's no surprise to find a vinegar-based drink in this book. Don't be scared—this tea tastes amazing, and the concept is as versatile as they come. Play around with using your favorite teas as the base for this recipe and be amazed at how good you feel after drinking it! ACV Iced Tea is fabulous for balancing blood sugar, clearing your skin, and boosting digestion. I like to sip on it between meals or in the morning after a carb-up.

2 cups (475 ml) chilled brewed tea (rooibos is my favorite for this recipe)

1 tablespoon apple cider vinegar

8 drops liquid stevia

2 to 4 ice cubes, for serving

1. Place all the ingredients except the ice in a 16-ounce (475-ml) or larger glass jar, such as a mason jar. Cover and give it a little shake.

2. When ready to consume, transfer to a large drinking glass and add the ice.

STORE IT: *Keep in an airtight container in the fridge for up to 3 days.*

PREP AHEAD: *Brew the tea, let it cool, and store it in the fridge for up to 3 days.*

MAKE IT NIGHTSHADE-FREE: *Replace the rooibos tea, which is a nightshade, with another type, such as green, black, white, or herbal.*

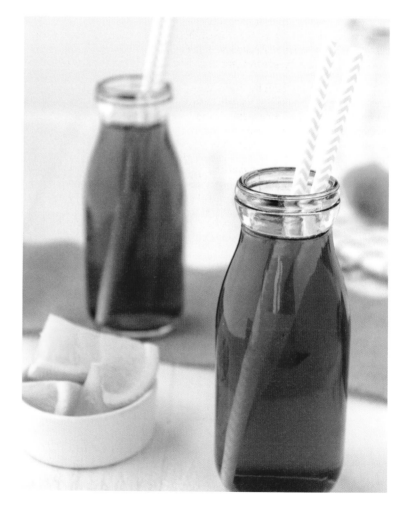

NUTRIENT INFORMATION:

calories: 3 | calories from fat: 0 | total fat: 0g | saturated fat: 0g | cholesterol: 0mg

sodium: 0mg | carbs: 0.8g | dietary fiber: 0g | net carbs: 0.8g | sugars: 0g | protein: 0g

RATIOS:

fat:	carbs:	protein:
0%	0%	0%

FATTY GREEN TEA

PREP TIME: **5 minutes**   MAKES: **two 17-ounce (500-ml) servings**

EGG-FREE • LOW-FODMAP • NIGHTSHADE-FREE • NUT-FREE

Made with decaf tea, this is my go-to drink when I'm still a bit hungry come bedtime but too tired to make a concerted effort in the kitchen. The longer the tea is blended, the stronger the ginger flavor will be. If you're serious about ginger, you could even leave the ginger pulp in the drink! I'm not that hardcore, but my husband loves Fatty Green Tea unstrained, with the pulp.

4 cups (950 ml) hot brewed green tea (decaf or regular)

2 tablespoons unflavored gelatin

2 tablespoons coconut oil or MCT oil

2 tablespoons peeled and chopped fresh ginger root

2 tablespoons fresh lemon juice

6 to 8 drops liquid stevia

1. Place all the ingredients in a blender and blend on high speed for 10 to 30 seconds. The longer the mixture is blended, the stronger the ginger flavor will be.

2. Place a fine-mesh strainer over a heat-safe pitcher, such as a teapot. Pour the blended tea mixture through the strainer, catching the ginger pulp.

3. Divide the tea between 2 mugs and enjoy.

STORE IT: *Keep in an airtight container in the fridge for up to 3 days. Fatty Green Tea becomes gummy when cold because of the gelatin, so it must be reheated (see below).*

REHEAT IT: *Scoop the Fatty Green Tea into a saucepan and bring to a light simmer over medium heat, stirring often. Or you can heat the tea in the microwave until the desired temperature is reached.*

PREP AHEAD: *Brew the tea and keep it in the fridge for up to 3 days. When ready to prepare the drink, reheat the tea on the stovetop or in the microwave, then add it to the blender with the other ingredients.*

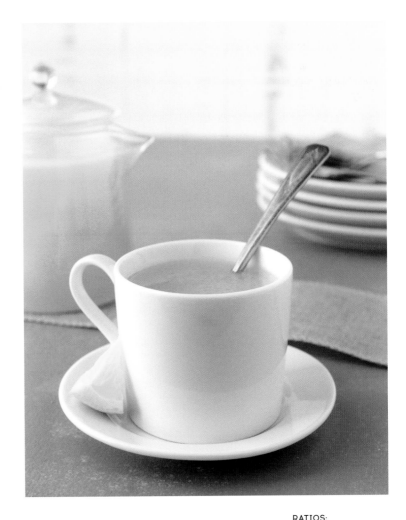

NUTRIENT INFORMATION (PER SERVING):

calories: 186 | calories from fat: 126 | total fat: 14g | saturated fat: 12g | cholesterol: 0mg

sodium: 5mg | carbs: 4.6g | dietary fiber: 0.7g | net carbs: 3.9g | sugars: 0.5g | protein: 10.5g

RATIOS:

fat:	carbs:	protein:
68%	**10%**	**22%**

ICED OMEGA TEA

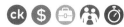

EGG-FREE • LOW-FODMAP • NIGHTSHADE-FREE • NUT-FREE   OPTION: **VEGAN**

When it comes to getting your daily dose of omegas, drinking this iced tea is a lot more fun than swallowing a handful of pills. There are a bunch of flavored omega oils on the market. My favorites are Barlean's Omega Swirl fish and flax oils. Choose your favorite flavor and run with it! If you're FODMAP sensitive, be sure to check the ingredients of the oil before using.

5 cups (1.2 L) chilled brewed green tea

¼ cup (60 ml) flavored flax oil or fish oil blend

¼ cup (40 g) collagen peptides or protein powder

¼ cup (60 ml) MCT oil

8 to 10 drops liquid stevia (optional)

8 ice cubes, for serving

2 fresh strawberries, sliced in half lengthwise, for garnish

STORE IT: *Keep in an airtight container in the fridge for up to 3 days.*

PREP AHEAD: *Brew the tea, let it cool, and store it in the fridge for up to 3 days.*

1. Place the green tea, fish oil, collagen, MCT oil, and stevia, if using, in a blender. Blend on high speed for 20 seconds, until combined.

2. Divide the tea among four 10-ounce (300-ml) or larger glasses, drop 2 ice cubes into each glass, and gently place a strawberry half on top.

| MAKE IT VEGAN: *Use flax oil and a plant-based protein powder.*

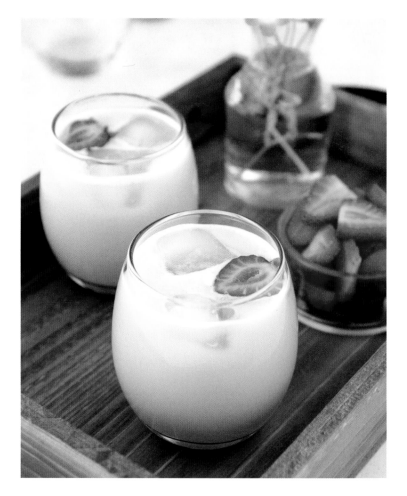

NUTRIENT INFORMATION (PER SERVING):

calories: 211 | calories from fat: 172 | total fat: 19.1g | saturated fat: 15.5g | cholesterol: 36mg

sodium: 29mg | carbs: 5.1g | dietary fiber: 0g | net carbs: 5.1g | sugars: 0g | protein: 4.7g

RATIOS:

fat:	carbs:	protein:
81%	**10%**	**9%**

KETO COLADA

PREP TIME: **5 minutes**   MAKES: **four 8-ounce (240-ml) servings**

EGG-FREE • NIGHTSHADE-FREE • NUT-FREE • VEGAN

I surveyed the Healthful Pursuit community, and 99 percent of respondents said that the only booze-based drink they needed in their keto lives was a piña colada. Honestly? I didn't think this drink was going to be as good as it ended up being. Don't sketch out on the apple cider vinegar; it brings an unexpected life to the flavors. Make it virgin for the kids or when you're first adapting to the keto lifestyle and don't want to have alcohol. (For more on alcohol on the keto diet, turn to page 119.)

I use Barlean's Omega Swirl flax oil in this recipe. It's an omega oil that's sweetened with xylitol, free of artificial flavors and colors, and non-GMO.

1⅓ cups (315 ml) full-fat coconut milk

2 ounces (60 ml) dark rum (optional)

2 tablespoons piña colada–flavored omega oil

2 tablespoons MCT oil

2 teaspoons apple cider vinegar

4 to 8 drops liquid stevia

4 cups (640 g) ice cubes

NOTE: *I use a high-powered blender to make this recipe. If you're using a regular blender, you will likely get a smoother result if you crush the ice before adding it to the blender. Do so by placing the ice cubes in a bag, wrapping the bag in a kitchen towel, and hitting it with a mallet.*

1. Place all the ingredients in a blender. Blend on high speed until the ice is crushed and the mixture is smooth. You may have to start and stop your blender, pushing the ingredients into the blades.

2. Divide the drink among four 8-ounce (240-ml) glasses and enjoy immediately.

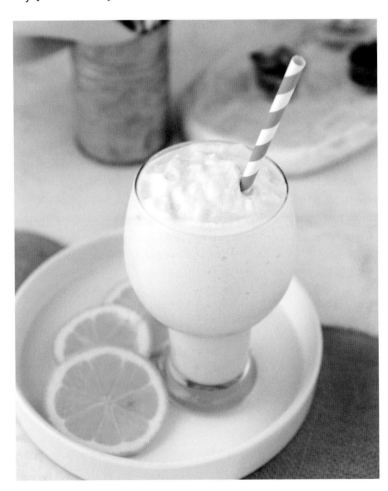

NUTRIENT INFORMATION (PER SERVING):

calories: 256 | calories from fat: 230 | total fat: 25.5g | saturated fat: 22.4g | cholesterol: 18mg

sodium: 20mg | carbs: 5.2g | dietary fiber: 0g | net carbs: 5.2g | sugars: 1.3g | protein: 1.3g

RATIOS:

fat:	carbs:	protein:
90%	8%	2%

KETO LEMONADE

PREP TIME: **3 minutes**   MAKES: **one 36-ounce (1.1-L) serving**

COCONUT-FREE • EGG-FREE • LOW-FODMAP • NIGHTSHADE-FREE • NUT-FREE • VEGAN

Meant to be sipped throughout the day, this lemonade is perfect for preventing the dreaded keto flu because of its epic amount of naturally occurring electrolytes. If you sip on this lemonade while you're adapting, you'll be set. If you're not familiar with aloe vera juice and want to give it a try, start with 1 tablespoon and work your way up. My gut feels fantastic when I add aloe vera juice to my Keto Lemonade, and yours may, too! You can find bottled aloe vera juice at most health food stores and drugstores. My favorite brand is Lily of the Desert. If you need protein, add a couple of scoops of collagen as well.

4 cups (950 ml) water

⅓ cup (80 ml) fresh lemon juice

1 to 4 tablespoons aloe vera juice, from the inner fillet (optional)

¼ teaspoon finely ground Himalayan rock salt

4 to 6 drops liquid stevia (optional)

1 cup (160 g) ice cubes, for serving

Fresh mint leaves, for garnish (optional)

1 lemon, sliced thin, for serving (optional)

> STORE IT: *Keep in an airtight container in the fridge for up to 3 days.*
>
> VARIATION: KETO LIMEADE. *Replace the lemon juice with lime juice.*

1. Place the water, lemon juice, aloe vera juice (if using), salt, and stevia (if using) in a liquid-safe container such as a mason jar. Cover and give it a little shake.

2. When ready to drink the lemonade, transfer to a drinking glass and add ice. If desired, top with a couple of mint leaves and serve with lemon slices.

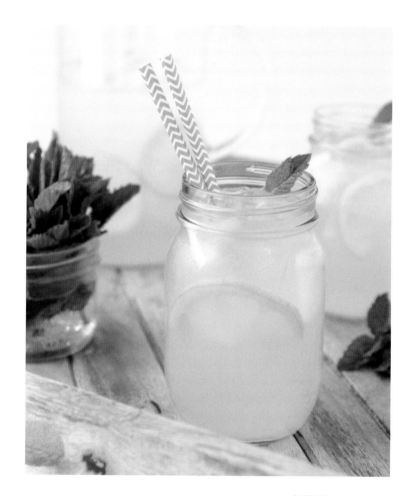

NUTRIENT INFORMATION:

calories: 20 | calories from fat: 6 | total fat: 0.7g | saturated fat: 0.7g | cholesterol: 0mg

sodium: 6mg | carbs: 2.7g | dietary fiber: 0g | net carbs: 2.7g | sugars: 1.7g | protein: 0.7g

RATIOS:

fat:	carbs:	protein:
32%	54%	14%

KETO MILKSHAKE

PREP TIME: **5 minutes**   MAKES: **one 20-ounce (600-ml) serving**

NIGHTSHADE-FREE • NUT-FREE   OPTION: EGG-FREE

I created this recipe while I was writing this very book! There were periods of such intensity that I literally didn't have time to eat. While my body didn't mind the full-day fasts, my brain started to. So I threw my favorite ingredients into the blender, and with a few adjustments over time, the Keto Milkshake was born. It is the most epic of meal replacements, fit for your keto lifestyle. Add a handful of spinach if you're game; it makes the color of the milkshake a little funky but doesn't affect the taste at all. *Note:* This recipe uses a raw egg yolk. If you not comfortable consuming raw eggs, follow the egg-free option below.

2 cups full-fat coconut milk

½ large Hass avocado, peeled and pitted (3 ounces/85 g flesh)

2 tablespoons cacao powder

2 tablespoons MCT oil

1 large egg yolk (optional)

2 ice cubes

6 to 8 drops liquid stevia or 2 teaspoons confectioners'-style erythritol

½ teaspoon vanilla extract or powder

Pinch of finely ground Himalayan rock salt

¼ cup (40 g) collagen peptides or protein powder

STORE IT: *Keep in an airtight container in the fridge for up to 1 day.*

MAKE IT EGG-FREE: *Replace the egg yolk with 1 tablespoon of the nut or seed butter of your choice.*

1. Place the coconut milk, avocado, cacao powder, MCT oil, egg yolk, ice cubes, sweetener, vanilla, and salt in a blender. Blend on low, slowing increasing the speed until you reach high. Stay at high speed for 30 seconds, until the ice is crushed and the mixture is smooth.

2. Add the collagen and blend for another 10 seconds.

3. Transfer to a glass and enjoy!

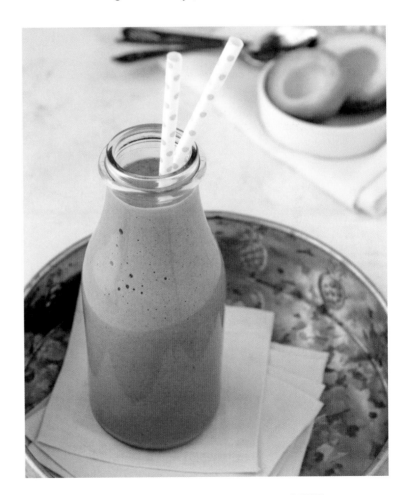

NUTRIENT INFORMATION:
calories: 889 | calories from fat: 757 | total fat: 84.3g | saturated fat: 62.9g | cholesterol: 210mg
sodium: 314mg | carbs: 7.8g | dietary fiber: 4g | net carbs: 3.8g | sugars: 0g | protein: 24.7g

RATIOS:
fat: carbs: protein:
85%   4%   11%

Five years ago, smoothies were everything to me—my friends still call me the Green Smoothie Queen. While you won't see me downing a blended concoction of my favorite ingredients these days, smoothies can have a place in your high-fat eating style. Follow these instructions for making high-fat, low-carb smoothies!

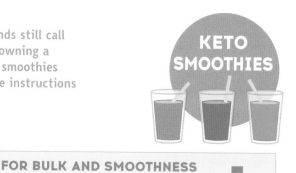

KETO SMOOTHIES

FOR SWEETNESS

Lemon
Lime
Alcohol-free stevia
Alcohol-free vanilla extract (¼ teaspoon)
Blackberries
Blueberries
Cranberries
Raspberries
Strawberries

FOR BULK AND SMOOTHNESS

Avocado
MCT oil
Liquid coconut oil
Macadamia nut oil
Hulled hemp seeds
Almond butter, unsweetened smooth
Cashews*
Macadamia nuts*
Chia seeds
Flax seeds
Sunflower seeds*
Tahini
Coconut meat
Cauliflower, steamed until fork-tender, drained, and cooled
Grass-fed collagen peptides

*Optional: follow the soaking instructions on page 157.

LIQUIDS

Iced coffee
Iced green or herbal tea
Full-fat coconut milk, unsweetened
Lite coconut milk
Water
Water with 1 to 2 tablespoons fresh lemon juice
Water with 1 to 2 tablespoons fresh lime juice
Water with 1 to 2 tablespoons apple cider vinegar
1¾ cups (175 ml) water with ¼ cup (60 g) almond yogurt, unsweetened
1¾ cups (175 ml) water with ¼ cup (60 g) coconut yogurt, unsweetened
Kombucha
Water kefir
Almond milk, unsweetened

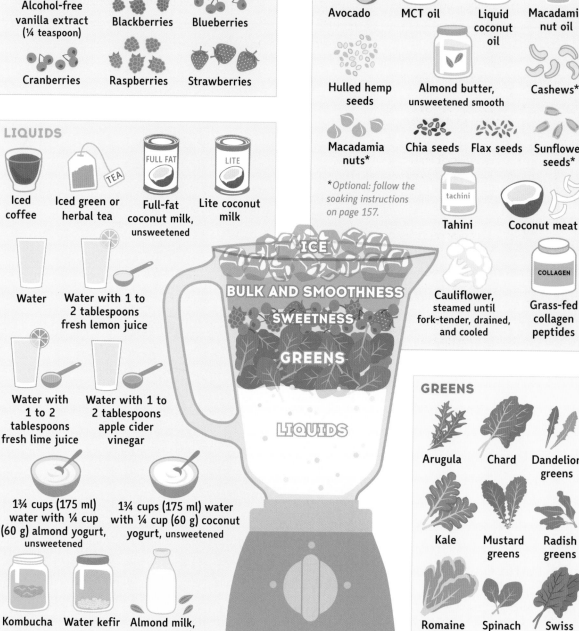

ICE

BULK AND SMOOTHNESS

SWEETNESS

GREENS

LIQUIDS

GREENS

Arugula
Chard
Dandelion greens
Kale
Mustard greens
Radish greens
Romaine lettuce
Spinach
Swiss chard

MOJITO SMOOTHIE

PREP TIME: **5 minutes**   MAKES: **two 9-ounce (265-ml) servings**

EGG-FREE • NIGHTSHADE-FREE • VEGAN   OPTION: NUT-FREE

When I was vegan, my daily smoothie bowls were more like carb bowls. With so much fruit and so little fat, it's no wonder I was hungry an hour later. Not with this smoothie! There's loads of fat in each spoonful, meaning that you'll be satisfied for hours to come. If you love smoothie bowls as much as I do and want to make this a full meal, add collagen peptides or your favorite protein powder and top things off with a handful of berries, hulled hemp seeds, and perhaps more macadamia nuts.

1½ cups (350 ml) chilled brewed tea (green tea is my favorite for this recipe)

2 tablespoons plus 1 teaspoon fresh lime juice

2 tablespoons MCT oil

1 packed cup (70 g) fresh spinach

½ large Hass avocado, peeled and pitted (3 ounces/85 g flesh)

12 whole macadamia nuts, finely chopped if not using a high-powered blender

2 ice cubes

1 packed tablespoon fresh mint leaves

½ teaspoon vanilla extract or powder

4 to 6 drops liquid stevia (optional)

1. Place all the ingredients in a blender. Blend on high speed until the ice is crushed and the mixture is smooth, about 30 seconds if using a high-powered blender, or longer if using a regular blender.

2. Pour evenly into 2 glasses and enjoy!

> STORE IT: *Keep in an airtight container in the fridge for up to 1 day.*
>
> SERVE IT WITH: *To make this smoothie a complete meal, add collagen peptides or protein powder.*
>
> MAKE IT NUT-FREE: *Replace the macadamia nuts with 3 tablespoons of hulled hemp seeds.*

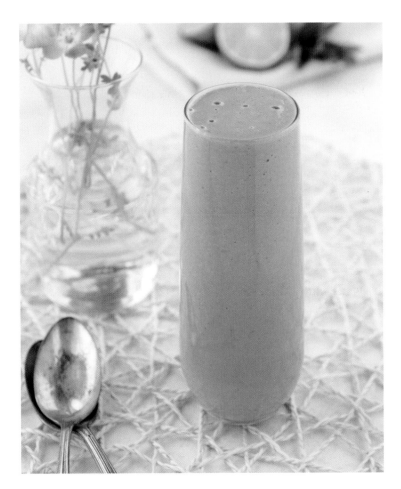

NUTRIENT INFORMATION (PER SERVING):

calories: 310 | calories from fat: 310 | total fat: 30.6g | saturated fat: 16.9g | cholesterol: 0mg

sodium: 25mg | carbs: 6.1g | dietary fiber: 4g | net carbs: 2.1g | sugars: 0.8g | protein: 2.6g

RATIOS:

fat:	carbs:	protein:
89%	**8%**	**3%**

ROCKET FUEL BONE BROTH

PREP TIME: **5 minutes**   MAKES: **two 9-ounce (270-ml) servings**

EGG-FREE • NUT-FREE   OPTIONS: **COCONUT-FREE • LOW-FODMAP • NIGHTSHADE-FREE**

When I prepare a batch of bone broth, I like to keep it rather "bland" so that I can spice it up as I wish, depending on the recipe I'm making. It's rare that I'll prepare an entire batch of bone broth only for sipping; instead, I usually freeze it in larger quantities for soups and the like and in 2-cup (475-ml) portions for this drink. To have everything ready to go in the morning, I thaw the frozen broth in the fridge overnight. This recipe is perfect for early-morning starts, extending your fast for another couple of hours.

2 cups (475 ml) hot bone broth (see page 152)

¼ cup (60 ml) MCT oil, melted coconut oil, or melted lard

1 small clove garlic, minced if not using a high-powered blender

½ teaspoon peeled and grated fresh ginger root

¼ teaspoon finely ground gray sea salt

Pinch of cayenne pepper

1. Place all the ingredients in a blender and blend on high speed for 10 to 30 seconds. The longer the mixture is blended, the stronger the garlic and ginger flavor will be.

2. Place a fine-mesh strainer over a large mug. Pour half of the blended mixture through the strainer, catching the garlic and ginger pulp. Strain the remaining mixture into a second mug. Enjoy!

STORE IT: *Let the strained broth cool completely and pour it into an airtight container. Store in the fridge for up to 3 days or in the freezer for up to 1 month. When cold, Rocket Fuel Bone Broth becomes gummy because of the gelatin in the broth. To restore it to a drinkable consistency, follow the reheating instructions below.*

REHEAT IT: *Scoop the Rocket Fuel Bone Broth into a saucepan and bring to a light simmer over medium heat, stirring often. Or you can use the microwave, heating until the desired temperature is reached.*

THAW IT: *Either defrost in the refrigerator until liquid or use while still frozen, then follow the reheating instructions above.*

PREP AHEAD: *Make the bone broth and keep it in the fridge for up to 3 days or in the freezer for up to 3 months. If using frozen broth, remember to defrost it in the fridge beforehand. When ready to prepare the drink, heat the broth on the stovetop or in the microwave, then follow the recipe instructions.*

MAKE IT COCONUT-FREE: *Use MCT oil or melted lard instead of coconut oil.*

MAKE IT LOW-FODMAP: *Replace the garlic with ½ teaspoon of peeled and grated fresh turmeric root.*

MAKE IT NIGHTSHADE-FREE: *Omit the cayenne pepper.*

NUTRIENT INFORMATION (PER SERVING):

calories: 273 | calories from fat: 231 | total fat: 25.7g | saturated fat: 10.1g | cholesterol: 24mg

sodium: 460mg | carbs: 1.5g | dietary fiber: 0g | net carbs: 1.5g | sugars: 0g | protein: 8.8g

RATIOS:

fat:	carbs:	protein:
85%	2%	13%

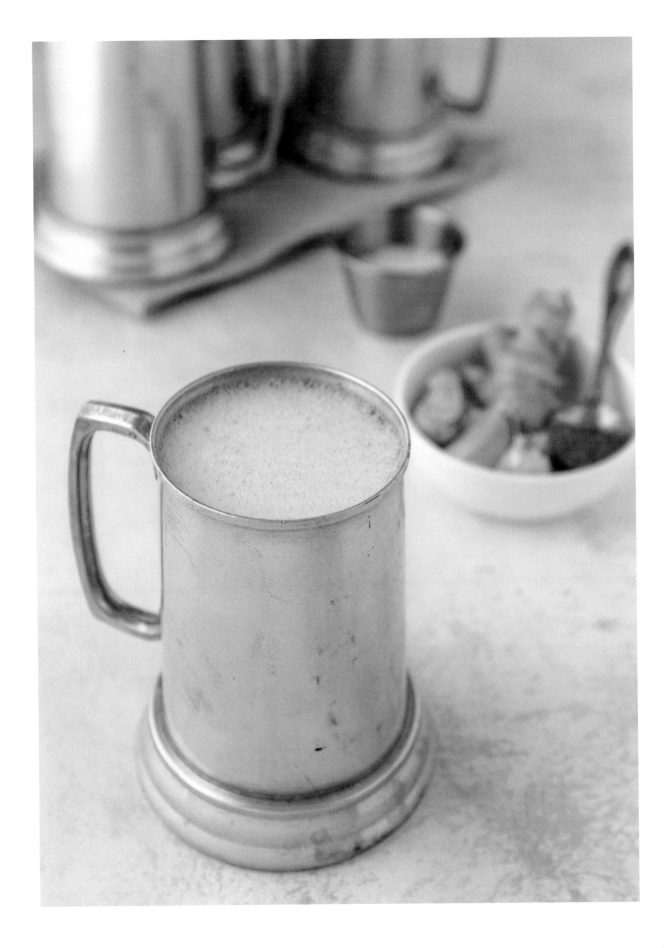

ROCKET FUEL LATTE

PREP TIME: **5 minutes**   MAKES: **one 16-ounce (475-ml) serving or two 8-ounce (240-ml) servings**

EGG-FREE • LOW-FODMAP • NIGHTSHADE-FREE • NUT-FREE OPTION: **VEGAN**

This creamy latte is an upgrade on the classic keto butter coffee, without the butter. And it has a hint of white chocolate flavor! I designed this beverage specifically to assist women with burning fat all morning long while regulating hormones and abolishing cravings. If you choose to enjoy your RFL in the morning, on its own, you'll continue your fast. If you enjoy eating breakfast, you could split your RFL into two servings, saving the other half for the next morning, and enjoy it alongside your favorite keto-friendly breakfast like bacon, eggs, and greens! If you don't have a high-powered blender to pulverize those hulled hemp seeds, substitute your favorite low-carb nut or seed butter.

1¾ cups (415 ml) hot brewed coffee (regular or decaf) or tea

1 tablespoon MCT oil or coconut oil

1 tablespoon cacao butter

1 tablespoon hulled hemp seeds

2 to 4 drops liquid stevia (optional)

¼ teaspoon vanilla extract or powder

Pinch of finely ground Himalayan rock salt (optional)

1 tablespoon collagen peptides or protein powder or 1½ teaspoons unflavored gelatin

Pinch of ground cinnamon, for garnish

1. Place the hot coffee, oil, cacao butter, hemp seeds, stevia (if using), vanilla, and salt in a high-powered blender (see note above). Blend on high speed for 1 minute, or until the hemp seeds are pulverized.

2. During the last 10 seconds, add the collagen and continue to blend.

3. Transfer to a mug, sprinkle with cinnamon, and enjoy.

VARIATION: HOT CACAO. *Combine 1¾ cups (415 ml) of hot brewed coffee or tea (peppermint tea is awesome in this version!), 1 tablespoon of cacao butter, 1 tablespoon of MCT oil or coconut oil, 1 tablespoon of chia seeds, 1 tablespoon of cacao powder, 2 to 4 drops of liquid stevia (optional), a pinch of finely ground Himalayan rock salt (optional), and 1 tablespoon of collagen peptides or protein powder or 1½ teaspoons of unflavored gelatin.*

VARIATION: COCONUT PARTY. *Combine 1¾ cups (415 ml) of hot brewed coffee or tea, 1 tablespoon of coconut oil, 1 tablespoon of MCT oil, 1 tablespoon of melted coconut butter, ¼ teaspoon of vanilla extract or powder, 2 to 4 drops of liquid stevia (optional), a pinch of finely ground Himalayan rock salt (optional), and 1 tablespoon of collagen peptides or protein powder or 1½ teaspoons of unflavored gelatin.*

VARIATION: GREEN TEA LATTE. *Combine 1¾ cups (415 ml) of hot water, 2 tablespoons of coconut oil, 2 tablespoons of full-fat coconut milk, 2 teaspoons of matcha powder, 2 to 4 drops of liquid stevia (optional), and 1 tablespoon of collagen peptides or protein powder or 1½ teaspoons of unflavored gelatin.*

VARIATION: EGGNOG. *Combine 1¾ cups (415 ml) of hot brewed coffee or tea, 2 tablespoons of full-fat coconut milk, 1 tablespoon of MCT oil, ½ teaspoon of ground cinnamon, ¼ teaspoon of ground nutmeg, 2 to 4 drops of liquid stevia (optional), and 1 tablespoon of collagen peptides or protein powder or 1½ teaspoons of unflavored gelatin.*

VARIATION: AYURVEDIC. *Combine 1¾ cups (415 ml) of hot brewed coffee or tea, 1 tablespoon of coconut oil, 1 tablespoon of MCT oil, 1 tablespoon of tahini, ½ teaspoon of turmeric powder, ¼ teaspoon of ground cardamom, ¼ teaspoon of ginger powder, 2 to 4 drops of liquid stevia (optional), a pinch of finely ground Himalayan rock salt (optional), and 1 tablespoon of collagen peptides or protein powder or 1½ teaspoons of unflavored gelatin.*

TIP. *Traveling with your Rocket Fuel Latte? Head on over to page 84.*

STORE IT: *Keep in an airtight container in the fridge for up to 3 days.*

REHEAT IT: *Pour the RFL into a saucepan and place over medium heat, stirring often, until it comes to a light simmer. Or you can use the microwave, heating until the desired temperature is reached.*

PREP AHEAD: *Brew the coffee or tea, let it cool, and store it in the fridge for up to 3 days. When ready to prepare the RFL, reheat the coffee or tea on the stovetop or in the microwave, then follow the instructions above.*

MAKE IT VEGAN: *Replace the collagen with an additional 2 tablespoons of hulled hemp seeds.*

NUTRIENT INFORMATION (PER 16-OZ/475-ML SERVING):

calories: 339 | calories from fat: 301 | total fat: 33.4g | saturated fat: 24.9g | cholesterol: 0mg

sodium: 192mg | carbs: 1g | dietary fiber: 1g | net carbs: 0g | sugars: 0g | protein: 8.5g

RATIOS:

fat:	carbs:	protein:
89%	1%	10%

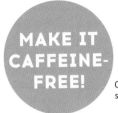
MAKE IT CAFFEINE-FREE!

Coffee
Caffeine per serving of RFL **164**

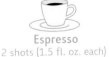
Yerba mate tea
Caffeine per serving of RFL **141**

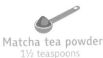
Espresso
2 shots (1.5 fl. oz. each)
Caffeine per serving of RFL **140**

Matcha tea powder
1½ teaspoons
Caffeine per serving of RFL **116**

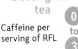 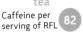
Black tea
Caffeine per serving of RFL **82**

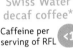
Four Sigma Foods mushroom coffee with cordyceps
2 packets
Caffeine per serving of RFL **79**

White tea
Caffeine per serving of RFL **46**

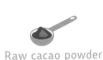 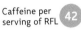
Green tea
Caffeine per serving of RFL **42**

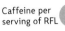 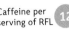 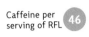
Raw cacao powder
1 tablespoon
Caffeine per serving of RFL **12**

Decaf black tea
Caffeine per serving of RFL **0** to **20**

Decaf green tea
Caffeine per serving of RFL **0** to **3**

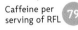
Swiss Water decaf coffee*
Caffeine per serving of RFL **<1**

Decaf espresso
2 shots (1.5 fl. oz. each)
Caffeine per serving of RFL **20**

Four Sigma Foods chaga mushroom elixir
2 packets
Caffeine per serving of RFL **0**

Herbal tea
Caffeine per serving of RFL **0**

Rooibos tea
Caffeine per serving of RFL **0**

Hot water
Caffeine per serving of RFL **0**

Swiss Water coffee is 100 percent chemical-free; water, coffee, time, and temperature are the only elements Swiss Water uses to remove caffeine.

For tea, caffeine amount is based on a 3-minute steep time. Steep time affects the caffeine content: a change from 1 minute to 5 minutes can increase the caffeine level by as much as 276 percent.

All caffeine levels are measured in mg.

SIGNS IT'S TIME TO LOWER YOUR CAFFEINE INTAKE: You can't go a day without it. You're slightly panicked, nervous, or anxious most days. Your sleep sucks. You experience rambling and random thoughts. You're thirstier than normal. You need that cuppa joe to get started in the morning or as a pick-me-up in the afternoon. If any of these sound familiar, transform your Rocket Fuel Latte into a less-stimulating version by replacing the coffee with lower-caffeine alternatives.

NOTE: *Caffeine levels in tea vary by brand. If you are concerned about your caffeine intake, it may be best to choose one of the 0 mg items.*

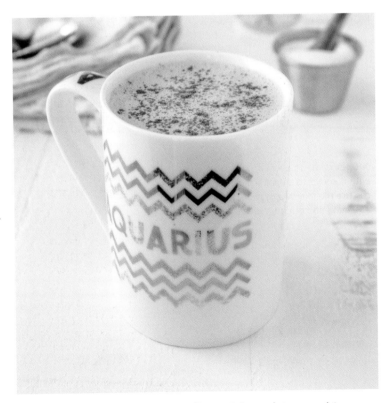

Get creative! Make your own flavor, take a picture, and tag it with #rocketfuellatte. A good amount of fat to start with is 2 tablespoons. I'd love to see what you create!

ROCKET FUEL ICED COFFEE

PREP TIME: **5 minutes**   MAKES: **one 16-ounce (475-ml) serving**

EGG-FREE · NIGHTSHADE-FREE · VEGAN   OPTIONS: LOW-FODMAP · NUT-FREE

This creamy, cooling iced coffee is a keto upgrade of the classic Rocket Fuel Latte (page 428), and since it's made without collagen, it's vegan! Like the RFL, I created this iced version to assist women in burning fat all morning long while regulating hormones and abolishing cravings. And if you're into fancy frosty coffee concoctions, I have you covered there with a frappé twist, whipped topping included!

If you don't have a high-powered blender to pulverize the hemp seeds, stick with the almond butter listed in the recipe.

1¾ cups (415 ml) chilled brewed coffee (regular or decaf)

1 tablespoon plus 1 teaspoon unsweetened smooth almond butter or 2 tablespoons hulled hemp seeds

1 tablespoon MCT oil

¼ teaspoon vanilla extract or powder

¼ teaspoon ground cinnamon

2 to 4 drops liquid stevia (optional)

Pinch of finely ground Himalayan rock salt (optional)

4 to 6 ice cubes

1. Put all the ingredients except the ice in a blender and blend until smooth.

2. Pour into a glass or mason jar, drop in the ice cubes, and enjoy!

STORE IT: *Keep in an airtight container in the fridge for up to 3 days. Give it a little shake before consuming.*

PREP AHEAD: *Brew the coffee up to 3 days in advance, let it cool, and store it in the fridge.*

VARIATION: ROCKET FUEL ICED TEA. *Replace the coffee with the brewed tea of your choice.*

VARIATION: ROCKET FUEL FRAPPÉ COFFEE. *After completing Step 1, add the ice cubes to the blender and blend until the ice is crushed and the drink is smooth, about 45 seconds. If you are not using a high-powered blender, crush the ice a bit before adding it to the blender. Otherwise, you'll need to run the motor quite a while, which will heat up your drink! Pour into a large glass or mason jar, top with ¼ cup (60 ml) of Coconut Whipped Cream (page 414) and 1 teaspoon of cacao nibs, and enjoy.*

MAKE IT LOW-FODMAP/NUT-FREE: *Use tahini in place of the almond butter.*

NUTRIENT INFORMATION FOR ICED COFFEE:

calories: 274 | calories from fat: 235 | total fat: 26.1g | saturated fat: 15.3g | cholesterol: 0mg

sodium: 242mg | carbs: 4.5g | dietary fiber: 3g | net carbs: 1.5g | sugars: 0.7g | protein: 5.2g

RATIOS:

fat:	carbs:	protein:
86%	6%	8%

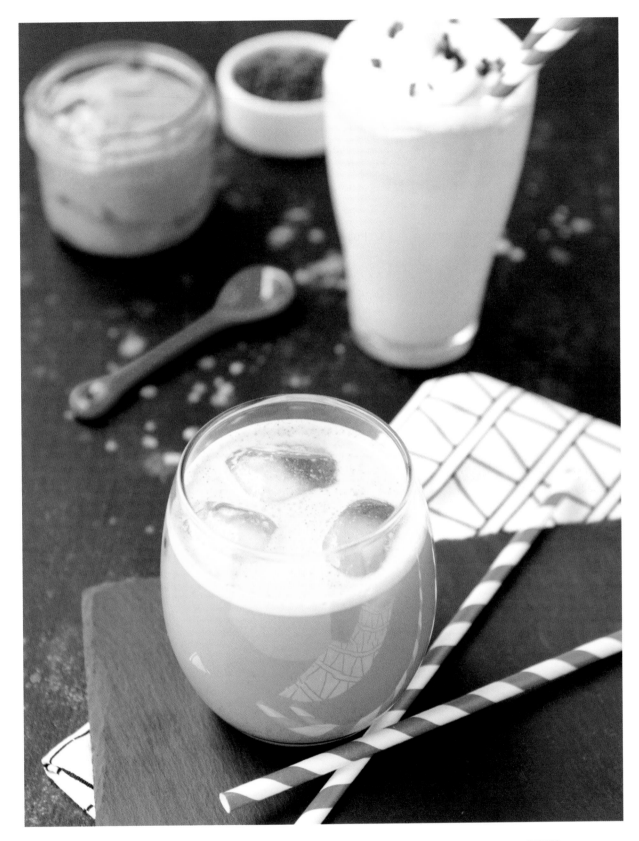

NUTRIENT INFORMATION FOR FRAPPÉ COFFEE WITH TOPPINGS:

calories: 357 | calories from fat: 331 | total fat: 36.8g | saturated fat: 24.9g | cholesterol: 0mg

sodium: 257mg | carbs: 8.7g | dietary fiber: 4.8g | net carbs: 3.9g | sugars: 0.7g | protein: 6.6g

RATIOS:

fat:	carbs:	protein:
84%	9%	7%

Recipe	PG	ck	pk	+	FAT	$	❄	📦	👥	⏱	COCONUT-FREE	EGG-FREE	LOW-FODMAP	NIGHTSHADE-FREE	NUT-FREE	VEGAN	VEGETARIAN
Cheese Sauce	218	•		•		•		•	•		O	•	O	•	•	O	O
Mayonnaise	220	•			•	•		•	•	•	•	O	•	•	•	O	•
Basil Avocado Spread	222	•			•	•		•	•	•	•	•	•	•	•	•	•
Kickin' Ketchup	223					•		•	•		•	•	O		•	•	•
Classic Caesar Dressing	224	•			•	•		•	•		O	O	O	•	•	O	O
Ranch Dressing	226	•			•	•		•	•	•	•	O	O	•	•	O	•
Red Wine Vinaigrette	227	•			•	•		•	•	•	•	•	O	•	•	•	•
Infused Oil	228	•			•	•		•			•	•	O	•	•	•	•
Greek Seasoning	232					•		•			•	•	O	•	•	•	•
Cajun Seasoning	232					•		•			•	•	O		•	•	•
Mediterranean Seasoning	233					•		•			•	•	O	•	•	•	•
Bahārāt Seasoning	233					•		•			•	•	O	•	•	•	•
Shichimi Seasoning	234					•		•			•	•	O		•	•	•
Italian Seasoning	234					•		•			•	•	O	•	•	•	•
Curry Powder	235					•		•			•	•	O	•	O	•	•
Seasoning Salt	235					•		•			•	•	O	•	O	•	•
Pancakes	236	•												•	O		
Allspice Muffins	238	•				•	•	•						•			
Flaxseed Cinnamon Bun Muffins	239	•				•	•	•			O			•	•		
Bacon Lovers' Quiche	240	•				•	•	•						•	•		O
Early-Day Jambalaya	242	•				•	•				•		•	O	•		
Sausage and Greens Hash Bowl	243	•					•				•	•	O	O	•		
Grain-Free Hemp Seed Porridge	244	•					•		•		O	•	O	•	O		
No-Nuts Granola with Clusters	246	•			•			•			O		•	•	•		
Chicken Crisps	248	•			•	•	•				•		O	O	•		
Italian Zucchini Rounds	250	•			•	•	•				•	•	O	O	•		
Zesty Nacho Cabbage Chips	252					•	•				•		O	O	•		
Bacon Crackers	254	•			•	•	•	•			•		O	•	•		
Bacon Spinach Dip	255					•	•				O		•	•	•	O	O
No-Beans Hummus	256	O		•	O	•	•		•		•		O	O	•	•	•
Pizza Pâté	258	•				•	•		•		O	•	O		O		
Kale Pâté	259	•				•	•		•		•		O	•	•		
MCT Guacamole	260					•	•		•		O	•	•	•	•		
Bahārāt Balls	261	•				•		•			O	•	O	O	•		
Bacon-Wrapped Asparagus	262	•			•	•	•		•		•	O	•	•	•		
Buffalo Chicken Tots	264	•	•			•	•				O	O	•	•	•		
Roasted Cajun Broccoli	266					•	•		•		O	•	O		•	O	
Nori Rolls with Almond Dipping Sauce	268			O		•	•		•		O	•	O	•		O	•
Salt and Pepper Chicken Wings	270					•	•		•		O	•	O	O	•		
Jerky Cookies	271	•	•			•	•				O	•	O	O	•		
Thanksgiving Balls	272	•			•	•	•				O	•	O	•	•		
The Only Way I'll Eat Liver	274		•			•	•				O	•	O	•	•		
Chicken Noodle Soup	276		•			•	•				O	•	O	•	•		
Shrimp Chowder	278	•				•	•				O	•	O	•	•		
Bacon Soup	280	•				•	•				O	•	O	•	•		
Vegan Cream of Broccoli Soup	282					•	•				O	•	O	•		•	•
Spinach Salad with Breaded Chicken Strips	284					•	•				O	O	O	O	•		
Cajun Pork Belly Chopped Salad	286					•	•	•			•	O	O	•	•		
Calamari Salad	288	•	•			•		•			•	O	O	•	•		
Verde Caesar Salad with Crispy Capers	289	•			•			•			O	O	•	•		O	O
Grilled Romaine and Scallop Salad	290	•		•				•	•		•	O	•	•	O		
Spinach Salad with Flank Steak	292					•	•				•	•	O	•	O		
Berry Avocado Salad	294					•			•		•	•	•	•		•	•

RECICE QUICK REFERENCE

RECIPE QUICK REFERENCE

• meets this criteria | O option | *(see page 173 for details)*

Recipe	PG	ck	pk	+	FAT*	$	❄	⊘	👤	⏱	COCONUT-FREE	EGG-FREE	LOW-FODMAP	NIGHTSHADE-FREE	NUT-FREE	VEGAN	VEGETARIAN
Marinated Bok Choy Salad	295				•		•		•	•	O	•		•	O	•	•
Curried Okra Salad	296	•			•	•	•		•	•	O	•		O	•	•	•
Shaved Cucumber and Smoked Salmon Salad	297		•					•	•	•	O	•	O	•	•	O	O
Bacon-Wrapped Mini Meatloaves	298		•			•	•	•	•	•	•	•	O	•	•		
Beef Stroganoff	300	•				•	•	•	•	•	O	•	O	•	•		
Bombay Sloppy Jolenes	302	•				•	•	•	•	•	O	•	O		O		
Chili-Stuffed Avocados	304	•				•	•	•	•	•	•	•			•		
Steak with Tallow Herb Butter	306	•		•			•	•	•	•	•	•	O	•	•		
Mind-Blowing Burgers	308	•				•	•	•	•	•	•	O	O	O	•		
One-Pot Hamburger Dinner	310		•	•		•	•	•	•	•	•	•		•	•		
Zucchini Rolls	311	•		•			•	•	•	•	•	•	O	O	•		
Michael's Pepperoni Meatzza	312	•				•	•	•	•	•	•	•	O		O		
Shredded Beef Tacos	314	•					•	•	•	•	•	•		•	•		
Coconut Lamb Curry	316	•				•	•	•	•	•		•			O		
Lamb Kebabs	318	•				•	•	•	•	•	O	•			O		
Bacon Mac 'n' Cheese	320		•			•	•	•	•	•	•	•			•		
Chipotle-Spiced Meatball Subs	322		•			•	•	•	•	•	•	•	•		O		
Cracked-Up Ham Salad Sandwiches	324	•					•		•	•	•	O		•	O		
Herb-Crusted Pork Chops	326		•	•		•	•	•	•	•	O	•	•	•	O		
Kung Pao Pork	328		•	•		•	•	•	•	•	O	•	O	O	O		
Salt and Pepper Ribs	330		•				•	•	•	•	•	•	O	O	•		
Shoulder Chops with Lemon-Thyme Gravy	332	•					•	•	•	•	•	•		•	•		
Stuffed Pork Roast with Herb Gravy	334		•				•	•	•	•	•	•		•	•		
Baked Olive Chicken	336		•	•			•	•	•	•	•	•	•	O	•		
Balsamic Turkey Thighs	338	•	•	•		•	•	•	•	•	•	•	•		•		
Butter Chicken	340		•	•		•	•	•	•	•	•	•	O		O		
Chicken Alfredo	342	•					•	•	•	•	O	•	O	•	•		
One-Pot Chicken Dinner	343	•		•			•	•	•	•	•	•		•	O		
Chicken Pot Pie Crumble	344	•				•		•	•	•	•	•			•		
Greek Chicken with Gravy and Asparagus	346		•	•			•	•	•	•	O	•	O	•	•		
Orange-Glazed Roasted Duck	348	•				•	•	•	•	•	•	•	O	•	•		
Sunflower Chicken Wings with Bok Choy	350	•				•	•	•	•	•	O	•	O	O	•		
Waldorf-Stuffed Tomatoes	351	•		•			•		•	•	•	O	O	O	O		
Lobster Pie	352						•	•	•	•	O	•	•		•		
Crab Tacos	354		•				•		•	•	•	•	O		•		
Stuffed Trout	355		•	•			•	•	•	•	•	•			•		
Crispy Salmon Steaks with Sweet Cabbage	356		•				•	•	•	•	•	•	O	•	O		
Prosciutto-Wrapped Fish Fillets	358		•	•			•	•	•	•	•	•	O	•	O		
Salmon Cakes with Dill Cream Sauce	360	•		•			•	•	•	•	O	•		•	O		
Sardine Fritter Wraps	362	•		•		•	•	•	•	•	•	•	O	O	O		
Cauliflower Rice	364			•		•	•	•	•	•	O	•		•	•	O	
Crusty Sandwich Bread	366			•		•	•	•	•	•	•	•			•		
Classic Butter Biscuits	368			•		•	•	•	•	•	•	•			•		
Bendy Tortillas	370		•	•		•	•	•	•	•	•	•		•	O		
Olive & Tomato Flaxseed Focaccia	372	•		•		•	•	•	•	•	O	O		•	•	O	•
Rosemary Garlic Croutons	374	•			O	•	•	•	•	•	•	O	O	•	•	O	•
Zoodles and Doodles	376		•			•	•	•	•	•	•	•		•	•	•	•
Avocado Fries with Dipping Sauce	378	•			•	•	•	•	•	•	•	O		O	•	O	•
Shichimi Collards	379		•				•	•	•	•	O	•			O	•	•
Creamy Baked Asparagus	380	•					•	•	•	•	•	O		•	•	O	O
Pesto Zoodles	381		•				•	•	•	•	•	•		•	•	•	•
Creamy Mashed Turnips	382		•				•	•	•	•	O	•	O	•	•	O	O
Herbed Radishes	384		•		•		•	•	•	•	•	•		•	•	O	O

RECICE QUICK REFERENCE

RECIPE QUICK REFERENCE

● meets this criteria | ○ option | *(see page 173 for details)*

Recipe	PAGE	ck	pk	+	FAT*	$	❄	🫙	👥	⏱	COCONUT-FREE	EGG-FREE	LOW-FODMAP	NIGHTSHADE-FREE	NUT-FREE	VEGAN	VEGETARIAN
Porky Cabbage	385					●		●	●		●	●	●	●	●		
Potato Salad...That Isn't	386			●		●		●	●		●	○		●	●	○	●
Roasted Brussels Sprouts with Walnut "Cheese"	388							●	●		○	●		●		○	○
Coconut Mounds	390				●	●	●		●			●			●	○	●	●
Almond Chai Truffles	392	●			●		●	●	●		●	●	●	●	○	●	●
Bacon Fudge	394	●			●		●		●		●	●	○	●	●		
Cardamom Orange Bark	395	●			●	●	●		●		○	●	○	●	○	●	●
Carrot Cake	396					●			●			●		●			
St. Louis Gooey "Butter" Cake	398	●				●		●	●			●		●			●
Rhubarb Microwave Cakes	400	●				●		●	●	●	●		●	○			
No-Bake N'Oatmeal Chocolate Chip Cookies	401	●				●			●		○	●		●	●	●	●
No-Nuts Brownies	402	●						●	●		○	●		●	●	●	●
Jelly Pie Jars	404					●			●		○		○	●			○
Iced Tea Lemonade Gummies	406		●					●	●		●	●	○	●	●	●	●
Lemon Drops	407	●			●		●	●			○	●	○	●	●	●	●
Chocolate-Covered Coffee Bites	408	●			●		●		●		●	●		●	●	●	●
Strawberry Butter Bites	409					●						●	○	●	●		●
Vanilla Ice Cream	410	●				●	●	●	●			●		●	○		●
Toasted Coconut Marshmallows	412				●	●	●	●	●		○	●		●	●		
Coconut Whipped Cream	414	●				●			●	●		●		●	●	●	●
Sweetened Condensed Coconut Milk	415					●						●		●	●	●	●
Fat-Burning Golden Milkshake	416	●				●			●		●	●	○	●	●		●
ACV Iced Tea	418					●			●		●	●	●	●	○	●	●
Fatty Green Tea	419	●				●			●		●	●		●	●		●
Iced Omega Tea	420					●			●	●	●	●	●	●	●	○	○
Keto Colada	421	●			●				●		●	●		●	●		●
Keto Lemonade	422					●			●		●	●	●	●	●		●
Keto Milkshake	423	●			●				●		●	○		●	●		
Mojito Smoothie	425	●			●		●		●		●	●		●	○	●	●
Rocket Fuel Bone Broth	426	●			●	●	●	●			●	○	●	○	○	●	
Rocket Fuel Latte	428	●			●				●		●		●		●	○	○
Rocket Fuel Iced Coffee	430				●				●		●		●	○		○	●

RECIPE INDEX

CHAPTER 13
SAUCY & SPICY

218 — Cheese Sauce

220 — Mayonnaise

222 — Basil Avocado Spread

223 — Kickin' Ketchup

224 — Classic Caesar Dressing

226 — Ranch Dressing

227 — Red Wine Vinaigrette

228 — Infused Oil

232 — Homemade Spice Mixtures

CHAPTER 14 — CLASSIC BREAKFAST

236
Pancakes

238
Allspice Muffins

239
Flaxseed Cinnamon
Bun Muffins

240
Bacon Lovers'
Quiche

242
Early-Day Jambalaya

243
Sausage and Greens
Hash Bowl

244
Grain-Free Hemp
Seed Porridge

246
No-Nuts Granola
with Clusters

CHAPTER 15 — SMALL BITES AND SNACKS

248
Chicken Crisps

250
Italian Zucchini
Rounds

252
Zesty Nacho
Cabbage Chips

254
Bacon Crackers

255
Bacon Spinach Dip

256
No-Beans Hummus

258
Pizza Pâté

259
Kale Pâté

260
MCT Guacamole

261
Bahārāt Balls

262
Bacon-Wrapped Asparagus
with Horseradish Sauce

264
Buffalo
Chicken Tots

266
Roasted Cajun
Broccoli

268
Nori Rolls with
Almond Dipping Sauce

270
Salt and Pepper
Chicken Wings

271
Jerky Cookies

272
Thanksgiving Balls

274
The Only Way
I'll Eat Liver

CHAPTER 16 — SOUPS AND SALADS

276
Chicken Noodle
Soup

278
Shrimp Chowder

280
Bacon Soup

282
Vegan Cream of
Broccoli Soup

284
Spinach Salad with
Breaded Chicken Strips

286
Cajun Pork Belly
Chopped Salad

288
Calamari Salad

289
Verde Caesar Salad
with Crispy Capers

290
Grilled Romaine and
Scallop Salad

292
Spinach Salad with
Flank Steak

294
Berry Avocado Salad

295
Marinated
Bok Choy Salad

296
Curried Okra Salad

297
Shaved Cucumber
and Smoked Salmon
Salad

CHAPTER 17
BEEF & LAMB

298
Bacon-Wrapped
Mini Meatloaves

300
Beef Stroganoff

302
Bombay Sloppy
Jolenes

304
Chili-Stuffed
Avocados

306
Steak with
Tallow Herb Butter

308
Mind-Blowing
Burgers

310
One-Pot
Hamburger Dinner

311
Zucchini Rolls

312
Michael's Pepperoni
Meatzza

314
Shredded Beef Tacos

316
Coconut Lamb Curry

318
Lamb Kebabs

CHAPTER 18
PORK

320
Bacon
Mac 'n' Cheese

322
Chipotle-Spiced
Meatball Subs

324
Cracked-Up Ham
Salad Sandwiches

326
Herb-Crusted
Pork Chops

328
Kung Pao Pork

330
Salt and Pepper Ribs

332
Shoulder Chops with
Lemon-Thyme Gravy

334
Stuffed Pork Roast
with Herb Gravy

CHAPTER 19
POULTRY

336
Baked Olive Chicken

338
Balsamic
Turkey Thighs

340
Butter Chicken

342
Chicken Alfredo

343
One-Pot
Chicken Dinner

344
Chicken Pot Pie
Crumble

346
Greek Chicken with
Gravy and Asparagus

348
Orange-Glazed
Roasted Duck

350
Sunflower Chicken
Wings with Bok Choy

351
Waldorf-Stuffed
Tomatoes

CHAPTER 20
SEAFOOD

352
Lobster Pie

354
Crab Tacos

355
Stuffed Trout

356
Crispy Salmon
Steaks with
Sweet Cabbage

358
Prosciutto-Wrapped
Fish Fillets with
Mediterranean
Vegetables

360
Salmon Cakes with
Dill Cream Sauce

362
Sardine Fritter
Wraps

CHAPTER 21 — SIDES AND ACCOMPANIMENTS

364 Cauliflower Rice

366 Crusty Sandwich Bread

368 Classic Butter Biscuits

370 Bendy Tortillas

372 Olive & Tomato Flaxseed Focaccia

374 Rosemary Garlic Croutons

376 Zoodles and Doodles

378 Avocado Fries with Dipping Sauce

379 Shichimi Collards

380 Creamy Baked Asparagus

381 Pesto Zoodles

382 Creamy Mashed Turnips

384 Herbed Radishes

385 Porky Cabbage

386 Potato Salad... That Isn't

388 Roasted Brussels Sprouts with Walnut "Cheese"

CHAPTER 22 — SWEET TOOTH SNACKS AND DESSERTS

390 Coconut Mounds

392 Almond Chai Truffles

394 Bacon Fudge

395 Cardamom Orange Bark

396 Carrot Cake

398 St. Louis Gooey "Butter" Cake

400 Rhubarb Microwave Cakes

401 No-Bake N'Oatmeal Chocolate Chip Cookies

402 No-Nuts Brownies

404 Jelly Pie Jars

406 Iced Tea Lemonade Gummies

407 Lemon Drops

408 Chocolate-Covered Coffee Bites

409 Strawberry Butter Bites

410 Vanilla Ice Cream

412 Toasted Coconut Marshmallows

414 Coconut Whipped Cream

415 Sweetened Condensed Coconut Milk

CHAPTER 23 — DRINKS

416 Fat-Burning Golden Milkshake

418 ACV Iced Tea

419 Fatty Green Tea

420 Iced Omega Tea

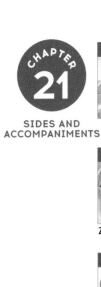
421 Keto Colada

422 Keto Lemonade

423 Keto Milkshake

425 Mojito Smoothie

426 Rocket Fuel Bone Broth

428 Rocket Fuel Latte

430 Rocket Fuel Iced Coffee

GENERAL INDEX

SOURCES

Abdel-Aal, El-Sayed M., Humayoun Akhtar, Khalid Zaheer, and Rashida Ali. "Dietary Sources of Lutein and Zeaxanthin Carotenoids and Their Role in Eye Health." *Nutrients* 5, no. 4 (2013): 1169–85. doi: 10.3390/nu5041169.

Afaghi, Ahmad, Helen O'Connor, and Chin Moi Chow. "High-Glycemic-Index Carbohydrate Meals Shorten Sleep Onset." *American Journal of Clinical Nutrition* 85, no. 2 (2007): 426–30. http://ajcn.nutrition.org/content/85/2/426.full.

Ainslie, Deborah A., Joseph Proietto, Barbara C. Fam, and Anne W. Thorburn. "Short-Term, High-Fat Diets Lower Circulating Leptin Concentrations in Rats." *American Journal of Clinical Nutrition* 71, no. 2 (2000): 438–42. http://ajcn.nutrition.org/content/71/2/438.full.

Alberts, Bruce, Alexander Johnson, Julian Lewis, Martin Raff, Keith Roberts, and Peter Walter. *Molecular Biology of the Cell.* 4th ed. New York: Garland Science, 2002.

Alirezaei, Mehrdad, Christopher C. Kemball, Claudia T. Flynn, Malcolm R. Wood, J. Lindsay Whitton, and William B. Kiosses. "Short-Term Fasting Induces Profound Neuronal Autophagy." *Autophagy* 6 no. 6 (2010): 702–10. doi: 10.4161/auto.6.6.12376.

Alsheikh-Ali, Alawi A., Prasad V. Maddukuri, Hui Han, and Richard H. Karas. "Effect of the Magnitude of Lipid Lowering on Risk of Elevated Liver Enzymes, Rhabdomyolysis, and Cancer." *Journal of the American College of Cardiology* 50, no. 5 (2007): 409–18. doi: 10.1016/j.jacc.2007.02.073.

Anson, Michael R., Zhihong Guo, Rafael de Cabo, Titilola Iyun, Michelle Rios, Adrienne Hagepanos, Donald K. Ingram, Mark A. Lane, and Mark P. Mattson. "Intermittent Fasting Dissociates Beneficial Effects of Dietary Restriction on Glucose Metabolism and Neuronal Resistance to Injury from Calorie Intake." *Proceedings of the National Academy of Sciences of the United States of America* 100, no. 10 (2003): 6216–20. doi: 10.1073/pnas.1035720100.

Bannai, Makoto, Nobuhiro Kawai, Kaori Ono, Keiko Nakahara, and Noboru Murakami. "The Effects of Glycine on Subjective Daytime Performance in Partially Sleep-Restricted Healthy Volunteers." *Frontiers in Neurology* 3 (2012): 61. doi: 10.3389/fneur.2012.00061.

Batterham, Rachel L., Helen Heffron, Saloni Kapoor, Joanna E. Chivers, Keval Chandarana, Herbert Herzog, Carel W. Le Roux, E. Louise Thomas, Jimmy D. Bell, and Dominic J. Withers. "Critical Role for Peptide YY in Protein-Mediated Satiation and Body-Weight Regulation." *Cell Metabolism* 4, no. 3 (2006): 223–33. doi: 10.1016/j.cmet.2006.08.001.

Béliveau, Richard, and Denis Gingras. "Role of Nutrition in Preventing Cancer." *Canadian Family Physician* 53, no. 11 (2007): 1905–11. www.ncbi.nlm.nih.gov/pmc/articles/PMC2231485/.

Berg, J. M., J. L. Tymoczko, L. Stryer. "Fuel Choice During Exercise Is Determined by Intensity and Duration of Activity." Section 30.4 in *Biochemistry*, 5th ed. New York: W. H. Freeman, 2002. www.ncbi.nlm.nih.gov/books/NBK22417/.

Bielohuby, Maximilian, Dominik Menhofer, Henriette Kirchner, Barbara J. M. Stoehr, Timo D. Müller, Peggy Stock, Madlen Hempel et al. "Induction of Ketosis in Rats Fed Low-Carbohydrate, High-Fat Diets Depends on the Relative Abundance of Dietary Fat and Protein." *Journal of Physiology—Endocrinology and Metabolism* 300, no. 1 (2010): E65–76. doi: 10.1152/ajpendo.00478.2010.

Bosse, John D., and Brian M. Dixon. "Dietary Protein to Maximize Resistance Training: A Review and Examination of Protein Spread and Change Theories." Journal of the International Society of Sports Nutrition 42, no. 9 (2012). doi: 10.1186/1550-2783-9-42.

Burdge, Graham C., and Philip C. Calder. "Conversion of Alpha-Linolenic Acid to Longer-Chain Polyunsaturated Fatty Acids in Human Adults." *Reproduction Nutrition Development* 45, no. 5 (2005): 581–97. doi: 10.1051/rnd:2005047.

Campbell-McBride, Natasha. "Cholesterol: Friend or Foe?" *Weston A. Price Foundation.* Posted on May 4, 2008. www.westonaprice.org/know-your-fats/cholesterol-friend-or-foe/.

Campos, Hannia, Jacques J. Genest, Jr., Erling Blijlevens, Judith R. McNamara, Jennifer L. Jenner, José M Ordovas, Peter W. F. Wilson, and Ernst J. Schaefer. "Low Density Lipoprotein Particle Size and Coronary Artery Disease." *Arteriosclerosis, Thrombosis, and Vascular Biology* 12, no. 2 (1992): 187–95.

Canadian Medical Association. "Intermittent Fasting: The Science of Going Without." *Canadian Medical Association Journal* 185, no. 9 (2013). doi: 10.1503/cmaj.109-4451.

Carr, Richard D., Marianne O. Larsen, Maria Sörhede Winzell, Katarina Jelic, Ola Lindgren, Carolyn F. Deacon, and Bo Ahrén. "Incretin and Islet Hormonal Responses to Fat and Protein Ingestion in Healthy Men." *American Journal of Physiology—Endocrinology and Metabolism* 295, no. 4 (1990): E779–84. doi: 10.1152/ajpendo.90233.2008.

Chalon, Sylvie, Sylvie Vancassel, Luc Zimmer, Denis Guilloteau, and Georges Durand. "Polyunsaturated Fatty Acids and Cerebral Function: Focus on Monoaminergic Neurotransmission." *Lipids* 36, no. 9 (2001): 937–44. doi: 10.1007/s11745-001-0804-7.

Chavarro, J. E., J. W. Rich-Edwards, B. Rosner, and Walter C. Willett. "A Prospective Study of Dairy Foods Intake and Anovulatory Infertility." *Human Reproduction* 22, no. 5 (2007): 1340–47. doi: 10.1093/humrep/dem019.

Conn, Jerome W. "The Advantage of a High Protein Diet in the Treatment of Spontaneous Hypoglycemia: Preliminary Report." *Journal of Clinical Investigation* 15, no. 6 (1936): 673–78. doi: 10.1172/JCI100819.

Conn, Jerome W., and L. H. Newburgh. "The Glycemic Response to Isoglucogenic Quantities of Protein and Carbohydrate." *Journal of Clinical Investigation* 15, no. 6 (1936): 665–71. doi: 10.1172/JCI100818.

Connor, William E., and Sonja L. Connor. "The Importance of Fish and Docosahexaenoic Acid in Alzheimer Disease." *American Journal of Clinical Nutrition* 85, no. 4 (2007): 929–30. http://ajcn.nutrition.org/content/85/4/929.full.

Dahl-Jorgensen, Knut, Geir Joner, and Kristian F. Hanssen. "Relationship Between Cows' Milk Consumption and Incidence of IDDM in Childhood." *Diabetes Care* 14, no. 11 (1991): 1081–83. doi: 10.2337/diacare.14.11.1081.

Daley, Cynthia A., Amber Abbott, Patrick S. Doyle, Glenn A. Nader, and Stephanie Larson. "A Review of Fatty Acid Profiles and Antioxidant Content in Grass-Fed and Grain-Fed Beef." *Nutrition Journal* 9, no. 10 (2010): doi: 10.1186/1475-2891-9-10.

Davis, P. G., and Stephen D. Phinney. "Differential Effects of Two Very Low Calorie Diets on Aerobic and Anaerobic Performance." *International Journal of Obesity* 14, no. 9 (1990): 779–87.

de Roos, Nicole M., Evert G. Schouten, and Martjin B. Katan. "Consumption of a Solid Fat Rich in Lauric Acid Results in a More Favorable Serum Lipid Profile in Healthy Men and Women than Consumption of a Solid Fat Rich in Trans-Fatty Acids." *Journal of Nutrition* 131, no. 2 (2001): 242–45.

de Souza, Russell J., Andrew Mente, Adriana Maroleanu, Adrian I. Cozma, Vanessa Ha, Teruko Kishibe, Elizabeth Uleryk et al. "Intake of Saturated and Trans Unsaturated Fatty Acids and Risk of All Cause Mortality, Cardiovascular Disease, and Type 2 Diabetes: Systematic Review and Meta-Analysis of Observational Studies." *British Medical Journal* 351 (2015): h3978. doi: 10.1136/bmj.h3978.

Dinan, T. G., and J. F. Cryan. "Melancholic Microbes: A Link Between Gut Microbiota and Depression?" *Neurogastroenterology and Motility* 25, no. 9 (2013): 713–19. doi: 10.1111/nmo.12198.

Dulloo, A. G., M. Fathi, N. Mensi, and L. Girardier. "Twenty-Four-Hour Energy Expenditure And Urinary Catecholamines Of Humans Consuming Low-To-Moderate Amounts Of Medium-Chain Triglycerides: A Dose-Response Study In A Human Respiratory Chamber." *European Journal of Clinical Nutrition* 50, no. 3 (1996): 152–58.

Eckel, Robert H., Alan S. Hanson, Arnold Y. Chen, Jeffrey N. Berman, Trudy J. Yost, and Eric P. Brass. "Dietary Substitution of Medium-Chain Triglycerides Improves Insulin-Mediated Glucose Metabolism in NIDDM Subjects." *Diabetes* 41, no. 5 (1992): 641–47. doi: 10.2337/diab.41.5.641.

Enig, Mary. "Saturated Fats and the Lungs." *Weston A. Price Foundation.* Posted on June 30, 2000. www.westonaprice.org/know-your-fats/saturated-fats-and-the-lungs/.

Enriori, Pablo J., Anne E. Evans, Puspha Sinnayah, and Michael A. Cowley. "Leptin Resistance and Obesity." *Obesity* 14, no. S8 (2006): 254S–58S. doi: 10.1038/oby.2006.319.

Faeh, David, Kaori Minehira, Jean-Marc Schwarz, Raj Periasamy, Seongsoo Park, and Luc Tappy. "Effect of Fructose Overfeeding and Fish Oil Administration on Hepatic De Novo Lipogenesis and Insulin Sensitivity in Healthy Men." *Diabetes* 54, no. 7 (2005): 1907–13. doi: 10.2337/diabetes.54.7.1907.

Faris, Mo'es Al-Islam E., Safia Kacimi, Ref'at A. Al-Kurd, Mohammad A. Fararjeh, Yasser K. Bustanji, Mohammad K. Mohammad, and Mohammad L. Salem. "Intermittent Fasting During Ramadan Attenuates Proinflammatory Cytokines and Immune Cells in Healthy Subjects." *Nutrition Research* 32, no. 12 (2012): 947–55. doi: 10.1016/j.nutres.2012.06.021.

Forsythe, Cassandra E., Stephen D. Phinney, Maria Luz Fernandez, Erin E. Quann, Richard J. Wood, Doug M. Bibus, William J. Kraemer, Richard D. Feinman, and Jeff S. Volek. "Comparison of Low Fat and Low Carbohydrate Diets on Circulating Fatty Acid Composition and Markers of Inflammation." *Lipids* 43, no. 1 (2008): 65–77. doi: 10.1007/s11745-007-3132-7.

Gao, Zhanguo, Jun Yin, Jin Zhang, Robert E. Ward, Roy J. Martin, Michael Lefevre, William T. Cefalu, and Jianping Ye.

"Butyrate Improves Insulin Sensitivity and Increases Energy Expenditure in Mice." *Diabetes* 58, no. 7 (2009): 1509–17. doi: 10.2337/db08-1637.

Gibson, A. A., R.V. Seimon, C. M. Lee, J. Ayre, J. Franklin, T. P. Markovic, I. D. Caterson, and A. Sainsbury. "Do Ketogenic Diets Really Suppress Appetite? A Systematic Review and Meta-Analysis." *Obesity Reviews* 16, no. 1 (2015): 64–76. doi: 10.1111/obr.12230.

Ginsberg, Henry, Jerrold M. Olefsky, George Kimmerling, Phyllis Crapo, and Gerald M. Reaven. "Induction of Hypertriglyceridemia by a Low-Fat Diet." *Journal of Clinical Endocrinology & Metabolism* 42, no. 4 (2016): 729–35. doi: 10.1210/jcem-42-4-729.

Hamazaki T., H. Okuyama, Y. Ogushi, and R. Hama. "Towards A Paradigm Shift in Cholesterol Treatment: A Re-Examination of the Cholesterol Issue in Japan." *Annals of Nutrition & Metabolism* 66, suppl. 4 (2015): 1–116. doi: 10.1159/000381654.

Hanif Palla, Amber, and Anwar-ul Hassan Gilani. "Dual Effectiveness of Flaxseed in Constipation and Diarrhea: Possible Mechanism." *Journal of Ethnopharmacology* 169 (2015): 60–8. doi: 10.1016/j.jep.2015.03.064.

Havemann, L., S. J. West, J. H. Goedecke, I. A. Macdonald, A. St. Clair Gibson, T. D. Noakes, and E. V. Lambert. "Fat Adaptation Followed by Carbohydrate Loading Compromises High-Intensity Sprint Performance." *Journal of Applied Physiology* 100, no. 1 (2006): 194–202. doi: 10.1152/japplphysiol.00813.2005.

Heilbronn, Leonie K., Steven R. Smith, Corby Martin, Stephen D. Anton, and Eric Ravussin. "Alternate-Day Fasting in Non-Obese Subjects: Effects on Body Weight, Body Composition, and Energy Metabolism." *American Journal of Clinical Nutrition* 81, no. 1 (2005): 69–73. http://ajcn.nutrition.org/content/81/1/69.long.

Henderson, Samuel T. "Ketone Bodies as a Therapeutic for Alzheimer's Disease." *Neurotherapeutics* 5, no. 3 (2008): 470–80. doi: 10.1016/j.nurt.2008.05.004.

Hibbeln, Joseph R., Levi R. G. Nieminen, Tanya L. Blasbalg, Jessica A. Riggs, and William E. M. Lands. "Healthy Intakes of N–3 and N–6 Fatty Acids: Estimations Considering Worldwide Diversity." *American Journal of Clinical Nutrition* 83, no. 6 (2006): S1483–1493S. http://ajcn.nutrition.org/content/83/6/S1483.full.

Higdon, Jane V., Barbara Delage, David E. Williams, and Roderick H. Dashwood. "Cruciferous Vegetables and Human Cancer Risk: Epidemiologic Evidence and Mechanistic Basis." *Pharmacological Research* 55, no. 3 (2007): 224–36.

Ho, K. Y., J. D. Veldhuis, M. L. Johnson, R. Furlanetto, W. S. Evans, K. G. Alberti, and M. O. Thorner. "Fasting Enhances Growth Hormone Secretion and Amplifies the Complex Rhythms of Growth Hormone Secretion in Man." *Journal of Clinical Investigation* 81, no. 4 (1988): 968–75. doi: 10.1172/JCI113450.

Hooper, Lee, Carolyn D. Summerbell, Julian P. T. Higgins, Rachel L. Thompson, Gillian Clements, Nigel Capps, George Davey Smith, Rudolph Riemersma, and Shah Ebrahim. "Reduced or Modified Dietary Fat for Preventing Cardiovascular Disease." *Cochrane Database of Systematic Reviews*, no. 2 (2000): CD002137. doi: 10.1002/14651858.CD002137.

Howard, Barbara V., Linda Van Horn, Judith Hsia, JoAnn E. Manson, Marcia L. Stefanick, Sylvia Wassertheil-Smoller, Lewis H. Kuller et al. "Low-Fat Dietary Pattern and Risk of Cardiovascular Disease the Women's Health Initiative Randomized Controlled Dietary Modification Trial." *Journal of the American Medical Association* 295, no. 6 (2006): 655–66. doi: 10.1001/jama.295.6.655.

Hu X, R.J. Jandacek, and W.S. White. "Intestinal Absorption of Beta-Carotene Ingested with a Meal Rich in Sunflower Oil or Beef Tallow: Postprandial Appearance in Triacylglycerolrich Lipoproteins in Women." *American Journal of Clinical Nutrition* 71, no. 5 (2000): 1170–80.

Jahoor, F., E. J. Peters, and R. R. Wolfe. "The Relationship Between Gluconeogenic Substrate Supply and Glucose Production in Humans." *American Journal of Physiology—Endocrinology and Metabolism* 258, no. 2 (1990): E288–96.

Johnson, James B., Warren Summer, Roy G. Cutler, Bronwen Martin, Dong-Hoon Hyun, Vishwa D. Dixit, M. Pearson et al. "Alternate Day Calorie Restriction Improves Clinical Findings and Reduces Markers of Oxidative Stress and Inflammation in Overweight Adults with Moderate Asthma." *Free Radical Biology and Medicine* 42, no. 5 (2005): 129–37. doi: 10.1016/j.freeradbiomed.2006.12.005.

Johnston, Carol S., Carol S. Day, and Pamela D. Swan. "Postprandial Thermogenesis Is Increased 100% on a High-Protein, Low-Fat Diet Versus a High-Carbohydrate, Low-Fat Diet in Healthy, Young Women." *Journal of the American College of Nutrition* 21, no. 1 (2002):55–61. doi: 10.1080/07315724.2002.10719194.

Johnstone, Alexandra M., Graham W. Horgan, Sandra D. Murison, David M. Bremner, and Gerald E. Lobley. "Effects of a High-Protein Ketogenic Diet on Hunger, Appetite, and Weight Loss in Obese Men

Feeding Ad Libitum." *American Journal of Clinical Nutrition* 87, no. 1 (2008): 44–55.

Kahlon, Talwinder S., Mei-Chen Chiu, and Mary H. Chapman. "Steam Cooking Significantly Improves In Vitro Bile Acid Binding of Collard Greens, Kale, Mustard Greens, Broccoli, Green Bell Pepper, and Cabbage." *Nutrition Research* 28, no. 6 (2008): 351–7. doi: 10.1016/j.nutres.2008.03.007.

Katayose, Yasuko, Mami Tasaki, Hitomi Ogata, Yoshio Nakata, Kumpei Tokuyama, and Makoto Satoh. "Metabolic Rate and Fuel Utilization During Sleep Assessed by Whole-Body Indirect Calorimetry." *Metabolism Clinical and Experimental* 58, no. 7 (2009): 920–26. doi: 10.1016/j.metabol.2009.02.025.

Koppes, Lando L. J., Jacqueline M. Dekker, Henk F. J. Hendriks, Lex M. Bouter, and Robert J. Heine. "Moderate Alcohol Consumption Lowers the Risk of Type 2 Diabetes." *Diabetes Care* 28, no. 3 (2005): 719–25. doi: 10.2337/diacare.28.3.719.

Krikorian, Robert, Marcelle D. Shidler, Krista Dangelo, Sarah C. Couch, Stephen C. Benoit, and Deborah J. Clegg. "Dietary Ketosis Enhances Memory in Mild Cognitive Impairment." *Neurobiology of Aging* 33, no. 2 (2012): 425e19–e27. doi: 10.1016/j.neurobiolaging.2010.10.006.

Kruger, Marlena C., and David F. Horrobin. "Calcium Metabolism, Osteoporosis and Essential Fatty Acids: A Review." *Progress in Lipid Research* 36, no. 2–3 (1997): 131–51.

Langfort, J., W. Pilis, R. Zarzeczny, K. Nazar, and H. Kaciuba-Uściłko. "Effect of Low-Carbohydrate-Ketogenic Diet on Metabolic and Hormonal Responses to Graded Exercise in Men." *Journal of Physiology Pharmacology* 47, no. 2 (1996): 361–71.

Lee, Changhan, Lizzia Raffaghello, Sebastian Brandhorst, Fernando M. Safdie, Giovanna Bianchi, Alejandro Martin-Montalvo, Vito Pistoia et al. "Fasting Cycles Retard Growth of Tumors and Sensitize a Range of Cancer Cell Types to Chemotherapy." *Science Translational Medicine* 4, no. 124 (2012): 124–27. doi: 10.1126/scitranslmed.3003293.

Linn, T., B. Santosa, D. Grönemeyer, S. Aygen, N. Scholz, M. Busch, and R. G. Bretzel. "Effect of Long-Term Dietary Protein Intake on Glucose Metabolism in Humans." *Diabetologia* 43, no. 10 (2000): 1257–65.

Malosse, D., H. Perron, A. Sasco, and J. M. Seigneurin. "Correlation Between Milk and Dairy Product Consumption and Multiple Sclerosis Prevalence: A Worldwide Study." *Neuroepidemiology* 11 (1992): 304–12. doi: 10.1159/000110946.

Martin, III., W. H., G. P. Dalsky, B. F. Hurley, D. E. Matthews, D. M. Bier, J. M. Hagberg, M. A. Rogers, D. S. King, and J. O. Holloszy. "Effect of Endurance Training on Plasma Free Fatty Acid Turnover and Oxidation During Exercise." *Journal of Physiology—Endocrinology and Metabolism* 265, no. 5 (1993): E708–14.

Mavropoulos, John C., William S. Yancy, Juanita Hepburn, and Eric C. Westman. "The Effects of a Low-Carbohydrate, Ketogenic Diet on the Polycystic Ovary Syndrome: A Pilot Study." *Nutrition & Metabolism* 2, no. 35 (2005). doi: 10.1186/1743-7075-2-35.

McBride, Patrick E. "Triglycerides and Risk for Coronary Heart Disease." *Journal of the American Medical Association* 298, no. 3 (2007): 336–38. doi: 10.1001/jama.298.3.336.

McClernon, F. Joseph, William S. Yancy, Jr., Jacqueline A. Eberstein, Robert C. Atkins, and Eric C. Westman. "The Effects of a Low-Carbohydrate Ketogenic Diet and a Low-Fat Diet on Mood, Hunger, and Other Self-Reported Symptoms." *Obesity* 15, no. 1 (2007): 182–87.

Nanji, Amin A., D. Zakim, Amir Rahemtulla, T. Daly, L. Miao, S. Zhao, S. Khwaja, S. R. Tahan, and Andrew J. Dannenberg. "Dietary Saturated Fatty Acids Down-Regulate Cyclooxygenase-2 and Tumor Necrosis Factor Alfa and Reverse Fibrosis in Alcohol-Induced Liver Disease in the Rat." *Hepatology* 26, no. 6 (1997): 1538–45. doi: 10.1002/hep.510260622.

Nanji, Amin A., Kalle Jokelainen, George L. Tipoe, Amir Rahemtulla, and Andrew J. Dannenberg. "Dietary Saturated Fatty Acids Reverse Inflammatory and Fibrotic Changes in Rat Liver Despite Continued Ethanol Administration." *Journal of Pharmacology and Experimental Therapeutics* 299, no. 2 (2001): 638–44.

Noakes, Manny, Jennifer B. Keogh, Paul R. Foster, and Peter M. Clifton. "Effect of an Energy-Restricted, High-Protein, Low-Fat Diet Relative to a Conventional High-Carbohydrate, Low-Fat Diet on Weight Loss, Body Composition, Nutritional Status, and Markers of Cardiovascular Health in Obese Women." *American Journal of Clinical Nutrition* 81, no. 6 (2005): 1298–306.

Odegaard, Andrew O., and Mark A. Pereira. "Trans Fatty Acids, Insulin Resistance, and Type 2 Diabetes." *Nutrition Reviews* 64, no. 8 (2006): 364–72. doi: 10.1111/j.17534887.2006.tb00221.x.

Phinney, S. D., B. R. Bistrian, W. J. Evans, E. Gervino, and G. L. Blackburn. "The Human Metabolic Response to Chronic Ketosis Without Caloric Restriction: Preservation of Submaximal Exercise Capability with Reduced Carbohydrate Oxidation." *Metabolism* 32, no. 8 (1983): 769–76.

Raatz, Susan K., Jeffrey T. Silverstein, Lisa Jahns, and Matthew J. Picklo, Sr. "Issues of Fish Consumption for Cardiovascular Disease Risk Reduction." *Nutrients* 5, no. 4 (2013): 1081–97. doi: 10.3390/nu5041081.

Redman, Leanne M., Leonie K. Heilbronn, Corby K. Martin, Lilian de Jonge, Donald A. Williamson, James P. Delany, and Eric Ravussin. "Metabolic and Behavioral Compensations in Response to Caloric Restriction: Implications for the Maintenance of Weight Loss." *PLoS ONE* (2009). doi: 10.1371/journal.pone.0004377.

Ridker, Paul M., Nader Rifai, Lynda Rose, Julie E. Buring, and Nancy R. Cook. "Comparison Of C-Reactive Protein and Low-Density Lipoprotein Cholesterol Levels in The Prediction of First Cardiovascular Events." *New England Journal of Medicine* 347 (2002): 1557–65. doi: 10.1056/NEJMoa021993.

Russo, Gian Luigi. "Dietary N-6 And N-3 Polyunsaturated Fatty Acids: From Biochemistry to Clinical Implications in Cardiovascular Prevention." *Biochemical Pharmacology* 77, no. 6 (2009): 937–46. doi: 10.1016/j.bcp.2008.10.020.

Santos, F. L., S. S. Esteves, A. da Costa Pereira, William S. Yancy, Jr., and J. P. L. Nunes. "Systematic Review and Meta-Analysis of Clinical Trials of the Effects of Low Carbohydrate Diets on Cardiovascular Risk Factors." *Obesity Reviews* 13, no. 1 (2012): 1048–66. doi: 10.1111/j.1467-789X.2012.01021.x.

Seale, J. L., and J. M. Conway. "Relationship Between Overnight Energy Expenditure and BMR Measured in a Room-Sized Calorimeter." *European Journal of Clinical Nutrition* 53, no. 2 (1999): 107–11.

Seely, Stephen, and David F. Horrobin. "Diet and Breast Cancer: The Possible Connection with Sugar Consumption." *Medical Hypotheses* 11, no. 3 (1983): 319–27. doi: 10.1016/0306-9877(83)90095-6.

Seyfried, Thomas N., and Laura M. Shelton. "Cancer as a Metabolic Disease." *Nutrition & Metabolism* 7, no. 7 (2010). doi: 10.1186/1743-7075-7-7.

Shimomura, Iichiro, Robert E. Hammer, Shinji Ikemoto, Michael S. Brown, and Joseph L. Goldstein. "Letters to Nature." *Nature* 401 (1999): 73–76. doi: 10.1038/43448.

Siri-Tarino, Patty W., Qi Sun, Frank B. Hu, and Ronald M. Krauss. "Saturated Fat, Carbohydrate, and Cardiovascular Disease." *American Journal of Clinical Nutrition* 91, no. 3 (2010): 502–9. doi: 10.3945/ajcn.2008.26285.

Slavin, Joanne. "Fiber and Prebiotics: Mechanisms and Health Benefits." *Nutrients* 5, no. 4 (2013): 1417–35. doi: 10.3390/nu5041417.

Sofer, Sigal, Abraham Eliraz, Sara Kaplan, Hillary Voet, Gershon Fink, Tzadok Kima, and Zecharia Mada. "Greater Weight Loss and Hormonal Changes After 6 Months Diet with Carbohydrates Eaten Mostly at Dinner." *Obesity* 19, no. 10 (2011): 2006–14. doi: 10.1038/oby.2011.48.

St-Onge, Marie-Pierre, and Aubrey Bosarge. "Weight-Loss Diet That Includes Consumption of Medium-Chain Triacylglycerol Oil Leads to a Greater Rate of Weight and Fat Mass Loss Than Does Olive Oil." *American Journal of Clinical Nutrition* 87, no. 3 (2008): 621–26. http://ajcn.nutrition.org/content/87/3/621.long.

St-Pierre, Annie C., Bernard Cantin, Gilles R. Dagenais, Pascale Mauriège, Paul-Marie Bernard, Jean-Pierre Després, and Benoît Lamarche. "Low-Density Lipoprotein Subfractions And the Long-Term Risk of Ischemic Heart Disease in Men: 13-Year Follow-Up Data from the Québec Cardiovascular Study." *Arteriosclerosis, Thrombosis, and Vascular Biology* 25, no. 3 (2005): 553–59, doi: 10.1161/01.ATV.0000154144.73236.f4.

Stubbs, R. J., and C. G. Harbron. "Covert Manipulation of the Ratio of Medium- to Long-Chain Triglycerides in Isoenergetically Dense Diets: Effect on Food Intake in Ad Libitum Feeding Men." *International Journal of Obesity and Related Metabolic Disorders* 20, no. 5 (1996): 435–44.

Sumithran, P., L. A. Prendergast, E. Delbridge, K. Purcell, A. Shulkes, A. Kriketos, and J. Proietto. "Ketosis and Appetite-Mediating Nutrients and Hormones After Weight Loss." *European Journal of Clinical Nutrition* 67, no. 7 (2013): 759–64. doi: 10.1038/ejcn.2013.90.

Swallow, Dallas M. "Genetics of Lactase Persistence and Lactose Intolerance." *Annual Review of Genetics* 37 (2003): 197–219. doi: 10.1146/annurev.genet.37.110801.143820.

Swanson, Danielle, Robert Block, and Shaker A. Mousa. "Omega-3 Fatty Acids EPA and DHA: Health Benefits Throughout Life." *Advances in Nutrition* 3 (2012): 1–7. doi: 10.3945/an.111.000893.

Tarpila, S., A. Aro, I. Salminen, A. Tarpila, P. Kleemola, J. Akkila, and H. Adlercreutz. "The Effect of Flaxseed Supplementation in Processed Foods on Serum Fatty Acids and Enterolactone." *European Journal of Clinical Nutrition* 56, no. 2 (2002): 157–65. doi: 10.1038/sj.ejcn.1601298.

Taubes, Gary. "The Soft Science of Dietary Fat." *Science* 291 (2001): 2536–45. doi: 10.1126/science.291.5513.2536.

Thomas, Jaya Mary, Joyamma Varkey, and Bibin Baby Augustine. "Association Between Serum Cholesterol, Brain Serotonin, and Anxiety: A Study in Simvastatin Administered Experimental Animals." *International Journal of Nutrition, Pharmacology, Neurological Diseases* 4, no. 1 (2014): 69–73. doi: 10.4103/2231-0738.124617.

Toth, Peter P. "The 'Good Cholesterol': High-Density Lipoprotein." *Circulation* 111 (2005): e89–91. doi: 10.1161/01.CIR.0000154555.07002.CA.

Van Wymelbeke, V., A. Himaya, J. Louis-Sylvestre, and M. Fantino. "Influence of Medium-Chain and Long-Chain Triacylglycerols on the Control of Food Intake in Men." *American Journal of Clinical Nutrition* 68, no. 2 (1998): 226–34.

Veldhorst, Margriet A. B., Margriet S. Westerterp-Plantenga, and Klaas R. Westerterp. "Gluconeogenesis and Energy Expenditure After a High-Protein, Carbohydrate-Free Diet." *American Journal of Clinical Nutrition* 90, no. 3 (2009): 519–26. doi: 10.3945/ajcn.2009.27834.

Verhoeven, D. T. H., R. A. Goldbohm, G. van Poppel, H. Verhagen, and P. A. van den Brandt. "Epidemiological Studies on Brassica Vegetables and Cancer Risk." *Cancer Epidemiology, Biomarkers & Prevention* 5, no. 9 (1996): 733–48.

Volek, Jeff S., Maria Luz Fernandez, Richard D. Feinman, and Stephen D. Phinney. "Dietary Carbohydrate Restriction Induces a Unique Metabolic State Positively Affecting Atherogenic Dyslipidemia, Fatty Acid Partitioning, and Metabolic Syndrome." *Progress in Lipid Research* 47 (2008): 307–18. doi: 10.1016/j.plipres.2008.02.003.

Volkow, N. D., G. J. Wang, J. S. Fowler, D. Tomasi, and R. Baler. "Food and Drug Reward: Overlapping Circuits in Human Obesity and Addiction." In *Brain Imaging in Behavioral Neuroscience*, edited by Cameron S. Carter and Jeffrey W. Dailey, 1–24. Heidelberg: Springer Berlin Heidelberg, 2012. doi: 10.1007/7854_2011_169.

Wake Forest University Baptist Medical Center. "Trans Fat Leads to Weight Gain Even on Same Total Calories, Animal Study Shows." Published June 19, 2006. www.wakehealth.edu/News-Releases/2006/Trans_Fat_Leads_To_Weight_Gain_Even_on_Same_Total_Calories,_Animal_Study_Shows.htm.

Watras, Abigail C., A. C. Buchholz, R. N. Close, Z. Zhang, and D. A. Schoeller. "The Role of Conjugated Linoleic Acid in Reducing Body Fat and Preventing Holiday Weight Gain." *International Journal of Obesity* 31, no. 3 (2007): 481–87. doi: 10.1038/sj.ijo.0803437.

Weigle, David S., Patricia A. Breen, Colleen C. Matthys, Holly S. Callahan, Kaatje E. Meeuws, Verna R. Burden, and Jonathan Q. Purnell. "A High-Protein Diet Induces Sustained Reductions in Appetite, Ad Libitum Caloric Intake, and Body Weight Despite Compensatory Changes in Diurnal Plasma Leptin and Ghrelin Concentrations." *American Journal of Clinical Nutrition* 82, no. 1 (2005): 41–48. http://ajcn.nutrition.org/content/82/1/41.long.

Westman, Eric C., and Mary C. Vernon. "Has Carbohydrate-Restriction Been Forgotten as a Treatment for Diabetes Mellitus? A Perspective on the ACCORD Study Design." *Nutrition & Metabolism* 5 (2008): 10. doi: 10.1186/1743-7075-5-10.

Wolk, Alicja, Reinhold Bergström, David Hunter, Walter C. Willett, Håkan Ljung, Lars Holmberg, Leif Bergkvist, Åke Bruce, and Hans-Olov Adami. "A Prospective Study of Association of Monounsaturated Fat and Other Types of Fat with Risk of Breast Cancer." *Archives of Internal Medicine* 158, no. 1 (1998): 41–45. doi: 10.1001/archinte.158.1.41.

Wu, Felicia, Shaina L. Stacy, and Thomas W. Kensler. "Global Risk Assessment of Aflatoxins in Maize and Peanuts: Are Regulatory Standards Adequately Protective?" *Toxicological Sciences* 135, no. 1 (2013): 251–59. doi: 10.1093/toxsci/kft132.

Yancy Jr., William S., Marjorie Foy, Allison M. Chalecki, Mary C. Vernon, and Eric C. Westman. "A Low-Carbohydrate, Ketogenic Diet to Treat Type 2 Diabetes." *Nutrition & Metabolism* 2, no. 34 (2005). doi: 10.1186/1743-7075-2-34.

Zhong, Zhi, Michael D. Wheeler, Xiangli Li, Matthias Froh, Peter Schemmer, Ming Yin, Hartwig Bunzendaul, Blair Bradford, and John J. Lemasters. "L-Glycine: A Novel Antiinflammatory, Immunomodulatory, and Cytoprotective Agent." *Current Opinion in Clinical Nutrition & Metabolic Care* 6, no. 2 (2003): 229–40.

For a more complete list of sources used in the writing of this book, visit healthfulpursuit.com/ketodietsources.